Fetal Alcohol Spectrum Disorders

Omar A. Abdul-Rahman • Christie L. M. Petrenko
Editors

Fetal Alcohol Spectrum Disorders

A Multidisciplinary Approach

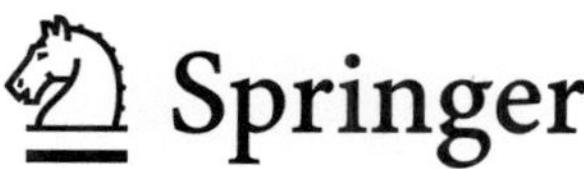 Springer

Editors
Omar A. Abdul-Rahman
Division of Medical Genetics, Department
of Pediatrics
Weill Cornell Medicine
New York, NY, USA

Christie L. M. Petrenko
Mt. Hope Family Center, Department of
Psychology
University of Rochester
Rochester, NY, USA

ISBN 978-3-031-32388-1   ISBN 978-3-031-32386-7   (eBook)
https://doi.org/10.1007/978-3-031-32386-7

This Springer imprint is published by the registered company Springer Nature Switzerland AG
The registered company address is: Gewerbestrasse 11, 6330 Cham, Switzerland

Foreword

When I first started investigating the effects of prenatal alcohol exposure (PAE) in the mid-1970s, I naively thought that it would be a short-term research project. Over 45 years have passed and the issues that I felt would be resolved rather quickly, were more complex than I and most others had imagined. In the ensuing years, I have participated in several expert panels, attended numerous town hall meetings across the globe, written hundreds of papers, and edited a few books of my own. I am still absorbed with fetal alcohol spectrum disorders (FASD), remain active in the field, and look forward to new research and insights into this major public health issue with tentacles reaching far and wide into many medical, educational, and social institutions.

Drs. Petrenko and Abdul-Rahman have assembled a book that superbly presents a variety of these issues and the complexities of FASD. This is not surprising in that Christie and Omar both follow the scientist/practitioner model, where previous research findings guide their clinical practices while they allow their clinical experiences to help formulate their own research questions. I met Dr. Petrenko when she started as my graduate student (one of the best) nearly 20 years ago, and I have known Dr. Abdul-Rahman for about the same length of time, as we did trainings together for the World Health Organization (WHO). Christie is a remarkable neuropsychologist with an interest in capacity building and interventions. Omar is recognized in the field of teratology not only for his clinical skills but also for research in medical genetics. Both have a real commitment to including stakeholders in their work.

Even though fetal alcohol syndrome (FAS) was met with much skepticism when it was initially reported in 1973, over the next decade or so, alcohol was recognized as a teratogen and then as a behavioral teratogen. Although there were differences in diagnostic criteria and complex terminologies used to refer to FASD by various groups (e.g., alcohol embryopathy, fetal alcohol syndrome, fetal alcohol effects, alcohol-related neurodevelopment disorder, static encephalopathy—alcohol exposed), the clinical and basic research studies coalesced about alcohol's teratogenic effects based upon the dose, timing, and duration of exposure. Nutritional and genetic factors also played a role, and it was clear that PAE could cause a range of outcomes.

At the time of these early studies on the teratogenicity of alcohol, alcohol was different than most other known teratogens. Alcohol was a legal substance, widely used throughout most of the world, and generally considered safe during pregnancy; it was even used to suppress preterm labor in the late 60s and early 70s. With its low molecular weight, alcohol freely passed into the embryo/fetus and had direct effects on developing cells, organs, and organ systems; it also impacted the pregnant person, thus having effects on the parent/fetal unit. The brain of the fetus, given its protracted period of development, was seen as especially vulnerable to PAE, and autopsy studies and structural brain imaging soon provided evidence that many of the behavioral issues described in FASD had biological underpinnings. Looking back on the early years in the field of FASD, animal models developed soon after FAS was recognized gave credence to the field, by providing data at least partially unconfounded by the numerous factors present in early case reports and clinical studies. These animal models provided important data on critical periods of exposure, dysmorphia, behavioral effects, putative mechanisms, and risk/resiliency factors. Importantly, and much to the field's credit, there was solid collegiality among the clinicians, epidemiologists, basic science researchers, and stakeholders, which is still true today.

This book presents an outstanding compendium on many of the issues facing the field of FASD. As with any disorder or disease, among the first questions asked is "What is it?" which in the case of FASD turns out to be a complex question. Thus, several chapters address this question taking us through preconceptional to prenatal periods, through the various issues surrounding the diagnostic methods to the behavioral, brain, and whole-body effects caused by prenatal alcohol. The next question usually asked is "How common is it?" and there are excellent chapters on epidemiology and risk/resiliency factors. "Why it happens and what can we do about it?" is addressed in chapters relying on those animal models I discussed above and on the intervention process. Then the chapters delve into the complexities of living life faced by individuals with an FASD. As I stated, FASD is a complex issue requiring interaction with a variety of institutions and these last chapters clearly demonstrate the lifelong challenges faced by the incredible people with this disorder. In testimonies provided at town hall meetings, camps, and other interactions with stakeholders through my years in the field, I've learned about the mindboggling multitude of medical, educational, legal, and socioeconomic barriers affected individuals, their families and caretakers face to try and obtain desperately needed services. A parent once shared a chart showing the spiderweb of systems of care that her child had been routed through, and no one should have to navigate this type of quagmire, not to mention while experiencing the social and institutional stigma that can accompany this disorder.

I'd like to share just a few other points. In 2015, I coauthored a paper "What Happens When Children with Fetal Alcohol Spectrum Disorders Become Adults?" At that time, in a PubMed search of over 3000 publications with "fetal alcohol" as a keyword and restricted to human studies, only a handful dealt with anyone older than a young adult. Also, I've always been an advocate of FASD being primarily a brain disorder. This book puts these two ideas in a new context. FASD is a lifelong condition, many of the facets we are only beginning to discover, and while the cognitive/behavioral issues are indeed important, FASD is a disorder impacting several major organ systems besides the brain. What happens to us perinatally can have long-term effects as we age. We need to identify individuals at risk for having an impacted child and recognize that in FASD we have at minimum two clients, the impacted person and that person's parent. We need to destigmatize the cloud around FASD and screen for alcohol use beginning in the teen years so it becomes as routine as asking about smoking. We need to deal with factors that might exacerbate the impact of PAE such as other drugs and adverse childhood experiences. Finally, we need to be very cognizant of the fact that the capacity for screening, diagnosis, and intervention for FASD is far less than the numbers impacted, especially in areas where alcohol consumption is increasing among pregnant people. We need to think outside the normal channels, outside of the box, and utilize technological advances to improve access to services.

Drs. Abdul-Rahman and Petrenko have provided a valuable resource for those who may come into contact with someone impacted by FASD. Healthcare professionals from all disciplines and teachers and/or staff within school districts need to be able to, at a minimum, screen for FASD and make referrals to experts when a case may be suspected. For example, clinical psychologists and occupational therapists interact with individuals with FASD regularly, yet only a relatively small percent feels confident in recognizing the disorder. This book, with chapters by leading experts in the field, can help to change that and open the door for a continuum of care, services, and support.

Center for Behavioral Teratology   Edward P. Riley
San Diego State University, San Diego, CA, USA

Preface

Fetal alcohol spectrum disorders (FASD) represent a range of physical, mental, and behavioral disabilities associated with prenatal alcohol exposure (PAE). FASDs are among the most common causes of developmental disability, with an estimated 2–5% of children being born with FASD each year in the world. Despite its high prevalence, FASD is often missed or misdiagnosed, making prevention and intervention more challenging. A multidisciplinary team of providers who understand the diagnostic requirements is crucial for an accurate FASD diagnosis.

As we approach the 50th anniversary of the description of fetal alcohol syndrome by Jones and Smith in 1973, significant progress has been made on multiple fronts in understanding FASD. Advancements in screening and diagnostic criteria are allowing for improved identification of individuals across the spectrum, with novel tools being developed to facilitate early diagnosis and treatment. Numerous studies on the epidemiology, embryology, and neuropsychological impacts of PAE on development have provided the foundation for prevention and intervention programs aimed at reducing its effects. Finally, systems-level barriers have been identified and efforts are underway to test innovative strategies to increase access to care and improve quality of life.

In developing the outline for this text, we sought to take a lifespan approach and provide the reader with a broad perspective of FASD. This textbook will provide a comprehensive, state-of-the art review of this field, and will serve as a valuable resource for clinicians, patients, families, advocates, and researchers with an interest in FASD. The book will provide a detailed overview for clinicians of various backgrounds on the diagnostic process, extensive mechanistic and embryologic data, neuropsychologic aspects of the condition, prevention and treatment approaches, foundational knowledge to navigate the educational, legal and child welfare systems, and policy perspectives that impact patients and families. The textbook will be organized parallel to the journey of individuals who experience alcohol-related conditions, beginning with the prenatal period addressing epidemiology of alcohol exposure, prevention and interventions, continuing through the fetal experience with a focus on embryology. Experiences of people with FASD and their families are considered next including the diagnostic process and health effects. Finally, issues related to systems of care for individuals with FASD and the broader community will be addressed. The global context of FASD will be presented throughout the textbook.

This textbook is intended to serve as a very useful resource for healthcare providers and researchers dealing with, and interested in, FASD. Primary care providers, obstetricians, pediatricians, neurologists, psychiatrists, psychologists, educators, behavioral health professionals, counselors, lawyers, and child advocates who care for or support individuals with FASD will benefit from the material presented. The book will provide a concise yet comprehensive summary of the current status of the field that will help guide prevention efforts, the diagnostic process, school and community interventions, and global policy efforts. By ensuring content is accessible to diverse audiences, the textbook will also provide a foundation that will facilitate translational research across basic and clinical science researchers in the field. All chapters will be written by experts in their fields and will include the most up-to-date scientific and clinical information.

New York, NY, USA   Omar A. Abdul-Rahman
Rochester, NY, USA   Christie L. M. Petrenko

Contents

Contributors

Omar A. Abdul-Rahman Division of Medical Genetics, Department of Pediatrics, Weill Cornell Medicine, New York, USA

Lisa K. Akison The Child Health Research Centre, The University of Queensland, Brisbane, QLD, Australia

School of Biomedical Sciences, The University of Queensland, Brisbane, QLD, Australia

Dorothy Badry Faculty of Social Work, University of Calgary, Calgary, AB, Canada

Kerryn Bagley Department of Community and Allied Health, La Trobe University, Melbourne, VIC, Australia

Gretchen Bandoli Department of Pediatrics, University of California San Diego, La Jolla, CA, USA

Herbert Wertheim School of Public Health, University of California San Diego, La Jolla, CA, USA

Nora Byington Masonic Institute for the Developing Brain, University of Minnesota, Minneapolis, MN, USA

Christina D. Chambers Department of Pediatrics, University of California San Diego, La Jolla, CA, USA

Herbert Wertheim School of Public Health, University of California San Diego, La Jolla, CA, USA

Peter Choate Department of Child Studies and Social Work, Mount Royal University, Calgary, AB, Canada

Child Studies and Social Work, Mount Royal University, Calgary, AB, Canada

Dae Chung Department of Neuroscience and Experimental Therapeutics, Texas A & M School of Medicine, Bryan, TX, USA

Lynn L. Cole Division of Developmental and Behavioral Pediatrics, University of Rochester Medical Center, Rochester, NY, USA

Natalie Collins Department of Neuroscience and Experimental Therapeutics, Texas A&M College of Medicine, Bryan, TX, USA

Natasia S. Courchesne-Krak Center for Behavioral Teratology and Department of Psychology, San Diego State University, San Diego, CA, USA

Ana Hanlon Dearman Max Rady College of Medicine, Pediatrics and Child Health, University of Manitoba, Winnipeg, MB, Canada

Katherine N. DeJong Department of Obstetrics and Gynecology, Addiction Medicine, Swedish Medical Center, Seattle, WA, USA

Kirsten A. Donald Division of Developmental Paediatrics, Department of Paediatrics and Child Health, Red Cross War Memorial Children's Hospital, Cape Town, South Africa
Neuroscience Institute, University of Cape Town, Cape Town, South Africa

Danijela Dozet Institute for Mental Health Policy Research, Centre for Addiction and Mental Health, Toronto, ON, Canada

Johann K. Eberhart Department of Molecular Biosciences, Waggoner Center for Alcohol and Addiction Research, Institute for Neuroscience, University of Texas at Austin, Austin, TX, USA

Diego A. Gomez Mayo Clinic Alix School of Medicine, Scottsdale, AZ, USA

Jessica Hanson Department of Applied Human Sciences, University of Minnesota Duluth, Duluth, MN, USA

Nicole Hayes The Child Health Research Centre, The University of Queensland, Brisbane, QLD, Australia

H. Eugene Hoyme Department of Pediatrics, University of South Dakota Sanford School of Medicine, Sioux Falls, SD, USA
Sanford Children's Genomic Medicine Consortium, Sanford Health, Sioux Falls, SD, USA

Matthew T. Hyland Center for Behavioral Teratology and Department of Psychology, San Diego State University, San Diego, CA, USA

Tracy Jirikowic Department of Rehabilitation Medicine, University of Washington School of Medicine, Seattle, WA, USA

Jessica J. Joseph 6-131 Education North, University of Alberta, Edmonton, AB, Canada

Carson Kautz-Turnbull Mt. Hope Family Center, University of Rochester, Rochester, NY, USA

Jordan Kuhlman Department of Neuroscience and Experimental Therapeutics, Texas A & M School of Medicine, Bryan, TX, USA

Jamie O. Lo Department of Obstetrics and Gynecology, Oregon Health & Science University, Portland, OR, USA

Lenora Marcellus School of Nursing, University of Victoria, Victoria, BC, Canada

Sarah N. Mattson Center for Behavioral Teratology and Department of Psychology, San Diego State University, San Diego, CA, USA

Kaitlyn McLachlan Department of Psychology, University of Guelph, Guelph, ON, Canada

Mansfield Mela Department of Psychiatry, College of Medicine, University of Saskatchewan, Saskatoon, Canada

Molly N. Millians Department of Child Psychiatry and Behavioral Sciences, Emory University School of Medicine, Atlanta, GA, USA

Rajesh Miranda Department of Neuroscience and Experimental Therapeutics, Texas A & M School of Medicine, Bryan, TX, USA

Karen M. Moritz The Child Health Research Centre, The University of Queensland, Brisbane, QLD, Australia

School of Biomedical Sciences, The University of Queensland, Brisbane, QLD, Australia

Heather Carmichael Olson Department of Psychiatry and Behavioral Sciences, University of Washington School of Medicine, Seattle, WA, USA

Center on Child Health, Development and Behavior, Seattle Children's Research Institute, Seattle, WA, USA

Scott E. Parnell Department of Cell Biology and Physiology, Bowles Center for Alcohol Studies, Carolina Institute for Developmental Disabilities, University of North Carolina at Chapel Hill, Chapel Hill, NC, USA

Jacqueline Pei Department of Educational Psychology, University of Alberta, Edmonton, AB, Canada

Department of Pediatrics, University of Alberta, Edmonton, AB, Canada

Canada FASD Research Network, Vancouver, BC, Canada

6-131 Education North, University of Alberta, Edmonton, AB, Canada

Christie L. M. Petrenko Mt. Hope Family Center, University of Rochester, Rochester, NY, USA

Marisa Pinson Department of Neuroscience and Experimental Therapeutics, Texas A & M School of Medicine, Bryan, TX, USA

Svetlana Popova Institute for Mental Health Policy Research, Centre for Addiction and Mental Health, Toronto, ON, Canada

Misty Pruner Center on Child Health, Development and Behavior, Seattle Children's Research Institute, Seattle, WA, USA

Natasha Reid The Child Health Research Centre, The University of Queensland, Brisbane, QLD, Australia

Madeline N. Rockhold Mt. Hope Family Center, University of Rochester, Rochester, NY, USA

Siara Kate Rouzer Department of Neuroscience and Experimental Therapeutics, Texas A & M School of Medicine, Bryan, TX, USA

Vincent C. Smith Division of Newborn Medicine, Department of Pediatrics, Boston Medical Center, Boston University Medical School, Boston, MA, USA

Chloe M. Sobolewski Center for Behavioral Teratology and Department of Psychology, San Diego State University, San Diego, CA, USA

Christina Tortorelli Department of Child Studies and Social Work, Mount Royal University, Calgary, AB, Canada

Robyn Williams Curtin Medical School, Faculty of Health Sciences, Perth, WA, Australia

Carissa Zambrano Center for Behavioral Teratology and Department of Psychology, San Diego State University, San Diego, CA, USA

Chapter 1
Epidemiology of Prenatal Alcohol Exposure

Svetlana Popova and Danijela Dozet

Abbreviations

AD	Alcohol dependence
APC	Alcohol per capita
AUD	Alcohol use disorder
DALYs	Disability-adjusted life years
FAS	Fetal alcohol syndrome
FASD	Fetal alcohol spectrum disorder
HED	Heavy episodic drinking
PAE	Prenatal alcohol exposure
US	United States
WHO	World Health Organization

Introduction

The World Health Organization (WHO) has indicated that women of childbearing age (15–49 years of age) and pregnant women are at particular risk of harm from alcohol and special attention needs to be given to these populations [1]. The prevention of prenatal alcohol exposure (PAE) is aligned with the *WHO Global Action Plan for the Prevention and Control of Non-communicable Diseases* [2], which calls for health care systems to respond more effectively to the health care needs of individuals with NCDs and to target risk factors. This endeavor has the capacity to

S. Popova (✉) · D. Dozet
Institute for Mental Health Policy Research, Centre for Addiction and Mental Health, Toronto, ON, Canada
e-mail: lana.popova@camh.ca; danijela.dozet@camh.ca

improve maternal and child health outcomes and prevent PAE, and therefore, new cases of fetal alcohol spectrum disorder (FASD), and therefore save service systems substantial costs. Understanding the epidemiology of alcohol use among women of childbearing age, alcohol use during pregnancy and FASD globally, is a critical first step to implementing effective prevention and intervention strategies to serve the needs of these populations.

Alcohol Use Among Women of Childbearing Age

The most accurate measure of alcohol use at the population level is adult per capita consumption of alcohol (APC), which is based on taxation and production statistics as well as population survey data [3]. Globally, women consumed an average of 2.3 L per capita in 2016 [4]. This ranged significantly across WHO regions, with 0.1 L in the Eastern Mediterranean Region and 3.1 L adult per capita in the Americas. Globally, an estimated 32.1% of women are "current" drinkers; this ranges from a 1.3% prevalence in the Eastern Mediterranean Region (lowest) and 53.9% prevalence in the European Region (highest) [5]. An estimated 56.7% women globally are categorized as "former" drinkers; this ranges from a 25.0% prevalence in the American Region (lowest) and 97.8% prevalence in the Eastern Mediterranean Region (highest) [5]. An estimated 11.3% of women of childbearing age globally are lifetime abstainers from alcohol; with the European (15.9%) and American (32.0%) Regions showing the highest rates of lifetime abstention among all WHO regions [5].

According to the WHO, there is a steady increase in the number of women of childbearing age in WHO regions who consume alcohol [6]. Relative to men, women are less likely to regularly consume alcohol and are more likely to abstain from alcohol, or be "former" drinkers. When women do drink alcohol regularly, they typically consume alcohol at lower levels than men do, which means a lower risk of alcohol-related harms for women. With the exception of the Western Pacific and South-East Asian Regions, the prevalence of currently drinking women has decreased in the last couple decades; however, due to a growing population size, the absolute number of currently drinking women is increasing [6]. This is especially of concern in highly populated countries such as China or India, where the risk of alcohol-related harms is markedly increasing for women in the general population.

An estimated 46 million women of childbearing age globally (1.7% of all women) have alcohol use disorders (AUDs), which pose the most significant disease burden [6]. AUDs among women are generally more prevalent in high-income countries, with the highest prevalence being in the European Region (3.5%) and the Region of the Americas (5.1%) [6]. Worldwide, approximately 8.7% of women of childbearing age engage in heavy episodic drinking (HED), defined as consuming at least 60 g of pure alcohol on at least one occasion in the past 30 days [5]. The definition of what constitutes a "standard drink" ranges across countries: one standard drink in the United States (U.S.) contains 14 g of pure alcohol and one European standard drink contains approximately 10 g of pure alcohol. The prevalence of HED among women of childbearing age was lowest in the Eastern Mediterranean region (0.1%) and highest in the European region (18.7%) [5]. Indeed, high-income countries display the highest liters per capita consumption among women of childbearing age (4.5 L), which is over three times higher than that seen in low-income countries (1.2 L) [5]. Stratified by income, countries with very high-income economies reported the highest prevalence of AUDs and AD (5.0% AUDs and 2.4% AD), while the prevalence of AUDs was lowest in lower-middle-income economies (0.6% AUDs), and the prevalence of AD was lowest in low-income economies (0.3%) [5] (using DSM-IV criteria). In most countries, predictors of high-risk drinking among women include higher levels of job/occupational status and higher levels of education obtained, as well as being in an affluent, non-Muslim majority society [6].

Alcohol use among women of childbearing age is increasing overall due to various factors, including the convergence of gender roles in some countries, regional economic development, increased availability and accessibility of alcohol, and increased exposure to alcohol advertising [7]. In some countries, the alcohol industry is an additional factor, wherein alcohol advertising is targeted specifically toward women (i.e., the "pinking" of the alcohol industry), which often promotes consumption by appealing to women's preferences or advertising cultural events [7]. These societal trends are important to observe, as alcohol use has important consequences on individual and systemic levels. Among both men and women, mortality resulting for alcohol consumption is higher compared to deaths caused by HIV/AIDS, tuberculosis, or diabetes [6]. In 2016 alone, there were 700,000 deaths resulting from alcohol and 26.1 disability-adjusted life years (DALYs) attributed to alcohol use, among women in WHO regions [6]. The leading contributors to alcohol-related deaths among women in the same year included unintentional injuries (15.5% of all alcohol-attributable deaths), digestive disorders (22.0% of all alcohol-attributable deaths), and cardiovascular diseases (41.6% of all alcohol-attributable deaths) [6]. The leading causes of DALYs attributed to alcohol use among women included unintentional injuries (28.1% of all alcohol-attributable DALYs), digestive diseases (19.5% of all alcohol-attributable DALYs), and cardiovascular diseases (19.0% of all alcohol-attributable DALYs) [6].

As alcohol consumption increases in general among women and men globally, so does the disease burden, as alcohol consumption is associated with over 200 diseases and conditions [8]. The reported morbidity and mortality related to women's alcohol use, or alcohol-attributable harms, often do not include secondary effects of alcohol such as assaults and domestic violence and therefore do not capture the full spectrum of the adverse effects of alcohol use globally [6]. As well, women may be at risk of motor vehicle injuries from drivers under the influence of alcohol, which is more commonly perpetrated by drivers who are men. Lastly, morbidity and mortality related to women's alcohol use may not capture secondary harms such as the fetal harms that can occur if alcohol is consumed during pregnancy, which can result in FASD.

Alcohol Use During Pregnancy

It is well-established that alcohol use during pregnancy can pose significant risks to the health of the mother and child. Understanding women's alcohol use patterns is critical to predicting PAE, which occurs in an estimated 10% of all pregnancies globally [9]. Since the absolute number of drinkers among women of childbearing age is increasing, and an estimated 44% of pregnancies globally are unintended [10], this means millions of pregnancies globally are at risk of PAE. This is especially the case as the use of alcohol and other substances can delay pregnancy recognition [6]. For example, in Canada, women who consumed alcohol during pregnancy were less likely to receive an early prenatal ultrasound and adequate prenatal care [11]. As with prevalence rates of alcohol among women of childbearing age, the prevalence of alcohol use during pregnancy also varies according to WHO region: alcohol use during pregnancy is the lowest in the Eastern Mediterranean Region (0.2%) and the highest in the European Region (25.2%) [12]. A systematic review and meta-analyses show that alcohol use during pregnancy is the highest among countries including Ireland (60%), Belarus (47%), Denmark (46%), the United Kingdom (41%), and Russia (37%) [9]. Alcohol use during pregnancy is lowest in countries including Oman, United Arab Emirates, Saudi Arabia, Qatar, and Kuwait; all of which belong to the Eastern Mediterranean WHO Region and are Muslim-majority countries.

Binge drinking (consumption of four or more drinks on a single occasion) during pregnancy is the most detrimental pattern of alcohol consumption, posing the highest risk of fetal harm in particular. Binge drinking tends to comprise a very small portion of alcohol-exposed pregnancies. For example, in Canada, an estimated 10% of women consume alcohol during pregnancy, and among those women, only 3% engage in binge drinking [12]. At the country level, the prevalence of binge drinking during pregnancy among alcohol-exposed pregnancies ranges from 0.2% in Brunei Darussalam to 13.9% in Paraguay [13]. Among countries included in a systematic review and meta-analysis, binge drinking during pregnancy is the highest in Paraguay (13.9%), Moldova (10.6%), Ireland (10.5%), Lithuania (10.5%), and Czech Republic (9.4%) [13]. Countries with the lowest prevalence of binge drinking during pregnancy include Brunei Darussalam (0.2%), Singapore (0.2%), Luxembourg (0.3%), Italy (0.7%), and the Republic of Korea (0.8%) [13]. In 40 of the countries with available data, over 25% of women who consumed any alcohol during pregnancy engaged in binge drinking [13].

Many countries such as Australia, Denmark, Canada, France, and the United States, have obstetric and/or low-risk drinking guidelines that specify that abstention from alcohol is the safest choice during pregnancy. The WHO also published guidelines for the management of substance use during pregnancy, where alcohol use screening is outlined [14]. Despite these guidelines, screening for alcohol use during pregnancy and education about the effects of PAE is under-utilized in healthcare settings. Alcohol use during pregnancy also occurs due to a variety of additional individual and systemic factors. For example, predictors of alcohol use during pregnancy include exposure to intimate partner violence, attitudes toward the current pregnancy and pre-pregnancy alcohol use patterns [15]. Women are more likely to have an alcohol-exposed pregnancy if they have limited access to education and/or prenatal care, have a substance use disorder, have a history of mental health issues, have FASD themselves, or have previously given birth to a child with FASD [16, 17]. As well, certain sub-populations of women within countries may be more likely to consume alcohol use during pregnancy, including women in marginalized cultural groups [16]. In one systematic review, one of the most commonly provided reasons for alcohol consumption during pregnancy included women's belief that alcohol consumption was only harmful if consumed in excessive quantities or in certain forms (i.e., beer or wine instead of hard liquor) [18]. As well, women often stated being pressured to drink alcohol while pregnant or while hiding a pregnancy, or related their consumption of alcohol due to a lack of awareness of the harmful effects of alcohol to the fetus [18]. Indeed, there is a great deal of misinformation related to alcohol use in general and during pregnancy, globally. Many countries lack specific guidance related to alcohol in pregnancy in their published obstetric guidelines, and there is also a lack of consensus in what is published [19]. Furthermore, only 19 countries have low-risk drinking guidelines for the general population published in some form wherein it is specified that alcohol should be avoided while pregnant or breastfeeding [20]. Globally, there is a lack of training among prenatal care providers with respect to alcohol use screening for pregnant women and the adverse effects of PAE. Unfortunately, some women receive incorrect or misleading information from their prenatal care providers related to alcohol use, which they attribute as being related to their alcohol use during pregnancy [18].

Prenatal care providers have the opportunity to screen pregnant women for alcohol use using one or more of the following: (1) clinician-directed questions at antenatal care encounters; (2) structured, validated alcohol use screening instruments; and/or (3) laboratory-based tools and biomarkers [21]. Screening pregnant women for alcohol use varies across provider types (e.g., midwife or obstetrician) and countries. For example, only 38% of medical doctors in the U.S. reported consistently screening pregnant women for alcohol use [22], whereas midwives in Sweden reported routinely asking pregnant women about alcohol use from 81% to 85% of the time [23]. Globally, however, it is estimated that only 1–3% of women drinking during pregnancy are identified by health care providers as doing so [24]. Alcohol use during pregnancy is underestimated based on underutilization of screening as well as the inherent social desirability bias that is present in prenatal care encounters. Studies have found, however, that simply engaging pregnant women in conversation about their alcohol use has significant potential to change their alcohol use behavior [25, 26]. As well, building rapport, providing non-judgmental support and increasing trust within the patient–provider relationship, is key to engaging women in honest conversations about their alcohol use during pregnancy. This also facilitates referrals and provision of brief interventions to women consuming alcohol during pregnancy, which are generally very effective in helping women abstain from alcohol for the remainder of their pregnancy, or minimize alcohol use if abstention is not possible.

The use of structured, validated screening questionnaires offers a high degree of clinical utility, and this can be valuable in screening pregnant women for any level of alcohol use, as well as AUDs. For example, studies show that the T-ACE ("Tolerance, Annoyance, Cut Down, Eye-opener") instrument has been validated for use in pregnant women and offers between 69–100% sensitivity and 19–89% specificity [21]. Other validated instruments include the TWEAK ("Tolerance, Worried, Eye-opener, Amnesia, K/Cut Down") (59–100% sensitivity; 36–83% specificity); the AUDIT-C (Alcohol Use Disorders Identification Test) (18–100% sensitivity; 71–100% specificity); the AUDIT (7–87% sensitivity; 86–100% specificity); the CAGE (38–59% sensitivity; 82–93% specificity); the SMAST (Short Michigan Alcohol Screening Test; 7.5–15% sensitivity; 96–98% specificity); and the NET ("Normal Drinker, Eye Opener, Tolerance"; 24–71% sensitivity; 86–99% specificity) [21]. Furthermore, a recently developed 1-Question Screen has been utilized in sub-Saharan countries and offers 97% sensitivity and 98% specificity; this is very resource-effective and can be useful in increasing alcohol abstention among pregnant women [21]. Further information about screening tools for alcohol use in pregnancy is available in Chap. 4.

Due to stigma associated with alcohol use during pregnancy and FASD, maternal self-report generally underestimates PAE [21]. For this reason, it may also be useful to screen for alcohol use using laboratory-based screening tools, such as ethanol biomarkers (e.g., fatty acid ethyl esters) found in blood, maternal and neonatal hair, placenta, cord blood, and meconium [21]. The testing of meconium, or an infant's first few bowel movements, is considered the gold standard for assessing PAE. Meconium testing produces estimates that are four times higher as compared to self-report [27], however, meconium testing only captures PAE which occurred during second and third trimesters and likely detects continuous drinking through pregnancy; therefore, meconium testing may miss many cases of alcohol-exposed pregnancies [21]. Screening for maternal alcohol use using any of these biomarkers may be a second step, following an indication of alcohol use risk behavior using other measures, including maternal self-report. These biomarkers, however, are significantly more resource-intensive as compared to routine screening based on self-report. Other laboratory tests that are inexpensive, such as ethanol detection in blood, urine, and saliva, only capture recent alcohol use relative to the time of the sample and therefore are not a comprehensive screen for alcohol use during pregnancy [21].

Fetal Alcohol Spectrum Disorder

Alcohol is a teratogen that can readily cross the placenta, resulting in central nervous system and physical damage to the developing embryo and fetus. PAE is linked with numerous adverse fetal health outcomes, including stillbirth, spontaneous abortion, intrauterine growth restriction, preterm birth, low birthweight, and FASD [28–32]. FASD is an umbrella term describing a wide range of effects, including central nervous system damage, prenatal or postnatal growth restrictions, congenital anomalies, characteristic dysmorphic facial features, and deficits in cognitive, behavioral, emotional, and adaptive functioning (See Chap. 9).

Globally, there are 130 million live births each year. Based on global estimates, about 10% of pregnancies are alcohol-exposed and one in every 13 alcohol-exposed pregnancies will result in FASD in the child [9, 33]. This means there are 1 million pregnancies per year will comprised new cases of FASD each year. Additionally, an estimated one in every 67 alcohol-exposed pregnancies will result in Fetal Alcohol Syndrome (FAS) in the child [9]. Binge drinking is the most detrimental drinking pattern during pregnancy and is a significant predictor of FASD in the child. Unfortunately, binge drinking most often occurs before pregnancy recognition, which can cause significant fetal harm. The risk of developing FASD is related to the patterns of alcohol consumption during pregnancy (i.e., the quantity, frequency, duration); however, both animal and human studies consistently show that larger quantities of PAE and continued drinking throughout all trimesters result in greater physical and cognitive deficits, and the appearance of facial features in FAS [34, 35]. While binge drinking is associated with the highest risk of fetal damage, it is important to note that that low and moderate levels of drinking during pregnancy are also associated with fetal damage. Other risk and moderating factors for the development of FASD following PAE include a smaller body profile of mother (height, weight, and body mass index [BMI]), higher maternal age, low socioeconomic status and smoking, poor nutrition, and paternal alcohol consumption (see Chap. 2).

FASD affects an estimated 0.7% of the general population globally, or 77.3 per 10,000 individuals [12]. This ranges from 1.3 per 10,000 individuals in the Eastern Mediterranean Region to 198 per 10,000 individuals in the European Region [12]. FAS affects considerably fewer individuals who are prenatally alcohol-exposed, seen in the estimate of 9.4 per 10,000 individuals with FAS in the global general population [12]. The prevalence range of FAS corresponds with that of FASD: the lowest is seen in the Eastern Mediterranean Region (0.2 per 10,000) and the highest is seen in the European Region (24.7 per 10,000) [12]. However, FASD is significantly underdiagnosed or misdiagnosed globally, and this is due to the lack of training among doctors, the lack of a consensus on diagnostic guidelines and the lack of an ICD code that captures the full spectrum of FASD [36]. For example, less than 1% of individuals with FASD are diagnosed each year and 99.9% of individuals with FASD in prison are undiagnosed or misdiagnosed [24]. As well, the diagnostic capacity using the current FAS phenotype is approximately 2% for individuals with FASD [24]. Currently, FASD is not widely recognized by healthcare practitioners and in many countries, there are little to no FASD cases being diagnosed [36]. Mandatory training on FASD screening, diagnosis, and treatment to common service providers of individuals with FASD (e.g., doctors, mental health professionals, individuals working within the justice system) would significantly increase the referral rate and improve the available regional and global data on the incidence and prevalence of FASD.

Studies using active case ascertainment (ACA), which is the gold standard for estimating the prevalence of FASD, have generated much higher prevalence estimates of FASD regionally as compared to what is available in administrative health databases or studies relying on passive surveillance. In Canada, an estimated 2–3% of the general population has FASD [37], and recent multi-site ACA studies in the USA have obtained estimates as high as 5% in the general population [38]. Remarkably, within these studies, nearly all of the students who participated in the diagnostic study had not been previously diagnosed with FASD. Depending on the prevalence estimates for the general population, this means there are between 3562 and 17,810 new FASD cases per day globally (assuming 1% and 5% prevalence rates, respectively) [24].

The prevalence of FASD is considerably higher among certain sub-populations. A recent systematic review and meta-analysis have shown that FASD is more prevalent among children in care, special education populations, correctional populations, and specialized clinical populations [39]. Compared to a recent global prevalence estimate of 7.7 FASD cases per 1000 people in the general population [16], prevalence in the selected sub-populations was 10–40 times higher. For example, compared to the general population, the prevalence of FASD among children in care was 32 times higher in the U.S. and 40 times higher in Chile, the prevalence of FASD among adults in the Canadian correctional system was 19 times higher, and the prevalence of FASD among special education populations in Chile was over 10 times higher [20]. The pooled prevalence of FASD among children in out-of-home care/foster care was estimated to be 31.2% in Chile and 25.2% in the U.S [40]. The pooled prevalence of FAS was estimated to be 9.6% among children in care in Russia [40]. The pooled FASD prevalence among adults in the Canadian correctional system was estimated to be 14.7% [40]. Additionally, some individual studies not included in the meta-analysis yielded alarmingly high prevalence rates. For example, the prevalence of FASD was 62% among children with intellectual disabilities in care in Chile [41], over 52% among adoptees from Eastern Europe [42], and approximately 40% among children residing in orphanages in Lithuania [43]. Among Russian orphanages for children with developmental abnormalities, the prevalence of FAS ranged from 46% to 68% [44]. Furthermore, the prevalence of FASD for youth in correctional services in Canada was over 23% [45] and among U.S. populations in psychiatric care, it was over 14% [46].

FASD has a broad phenotype, and its common misdiagnosis or lack of diagnosis is related to its high rates of comorbidity. FASD is highly comorbid, as a recent systematic review found that over 400 disease conditions have been reported to co-occur in people diagnosed with FASD [47]. Of these conditions, the most prevalent conditions are found within the categories of congenital malformations, deformities, and chromosomal abnormalities (43%) and mental and behavioral disorders (18%) [47]. Some comorbid conditions that are highly prevalent among people with FASD include language, auditory, visual, developmental, cognitive, mental, and behavioral issues, with prevalence estimates of these conditions ranging from 50% to 91% [47]. The number of comorbid disorders found to co-occur in individuals with FASD may overshadow the underlying condition of FASD, as clinicians often seek to diagnose the immediate health concern and its impact on daily life as opposed to the underlying adverse consequences of PAE.

The comorbidity of FASD and its related adverse health and social impacts affect the individual with FASD, their family and the utilized service systems. Individuals with FASD may require long-term support services such as health care, social assistance, and remedial or special education. Individuals with FASD often struggle with substance use, employment, independent living, and interpersonal relationships. One estimate suggests that, on any given day in a specific year, children and adolescents with FASD are 19 times more likely to be incarcerated compared to children and adolescents without FASD [48]. Individuals with FASD are also more likely to be victimized. For these reasons, there is often a continued reliance on support services, and repeated presence in various service systems. FASD presents an enormous cost burden, with an estimated $2.3 billion in related costs seen in Canada, assuming only 1% FASD prevalence [49]. FASD has a substantial impact on any society, and it has been estimated that the lifetime cost for a complex case of FASD to be more than $1 million CAD [50]. Globally, the annual costs of care per child and adult with FASD are $22,810 and $24,308, respectively [51]. Alternatively, it has been estimated that preventing one case of FASD incurs only 3% of the costs required to provide support services to individuals with FASD [52]. Based on these estimates, prevention of PAE demonstrates immense potential to prevent new cases of FASD and therefore reduce cost and service burdens on related service systems globally. Prevention of PAE through the provision of support services for pregnant women, including screening and access to brief interventions, is a worthy endeavor to support healthy pregnancies and improve the quality of life for families and communities.

Understanding the life course of individuals with FASD and the context of PAE also helps to shed light on the higher prevalence rates of FASD in specific subpopulations globally. For example, children are often placed in the child welfare system (i.e., foster care, orphanages, or adoption) due to unfavorable circumstances, such as parental alcohol and/or drug use, child maltreatment, abandonment, and young maternal age. These circumstances suggest a higher likelihood of PAE among children in care. As well, the high prevalence rates of FASD among special education and specialized clinical populations are not surprising given that individuals with FASD are at an increased risk of having learning difficulties and mental health problems, and of experiencing developmental delays [47].

Reducing stigma associated with PAE and FASD is another essential priority in order to improve data collection and to provide adequate diagnostic and treatment services. Birth mothers of children with FASD are more likely to experience stigma and discrimination compared to women with mental illness, previous involvement with the legal system, or women with substance use disorders [53]. In order to reduce this stigma that can negatively impact the patient, birth mother, and family members, one idea is to use an alternative term that does not specify fetal alcohol exposure, to minimize barriers to maternal self-report of alcohol consumption and its facilitation of earlier diagnoses for individuals living with FASD. While this may be effective in reducing stigma related to PAE (particularly stigma against birth mothers of children with FASD), the elimination of the exposure from the name may create confusion in terms of how FASD can be prevented. While there are many moderating factors for FASD when there is PAE (e.g., poor nutrition, other substances, etc.) [16], indeed PAE is the only cause of this disorder.

Across the lifespan, individuals with FASD are faced with numerous challenges. Less is known about individuals with FASD over the age of 65 years because the elderly population is largely undiagnosed, and also because individuals with FASD are at high risk of premature mortality. The majority of people who may have met the diagnostic criteria for FASD spend their entire lives without receiving a diagnosed, and die before they are included in any statistics. For example, infants with FASD may have passed from stillbirth, infectious diseases, or Sudden Infant Death Syndrome (SIDS) [54]. Individuals with FASD are five times more likely to suffer from premature death as compared to individuals without FASD [54]. Premature mortality is also more common for mothers of children with FASD, who are at a 44.82-fold increased risk in mortality compared to mothers of the same age who have children without FASD [54]. Siblings of individuals with FASD are also at increased risk of premature mortality, even if they themselves do not have the condition. Unfortunately, individuals living with FASD are at greater risk of premature mortality and the estimated life expectancy is far shorter than that of the general population. For example, a study in Alberta, Canada, estimated a life expectancy of 34 years for individuals with FAS [55], however, this study is based on administrative health data, which greatly underestimates the prevalence of FAS in the population as it relies on recorded diagnoses (i.e., life expectancy may be longer for the entire population of individuals with FAS, who are largely undiagnosed).

COVID-19 Pandemic

While it is clear that the COVID-19 pandemic has had various effects on different regions, the data show that mental health outcomes and substance use patterns have been altered during this time period [56]. It is clear that the pandemic has made a disproportionately more negative impact on women's mental health as compared to men [57]. Women have reported higher rates of anxiety, frustrations, household burden, and more disturbances in productivity, mood, and sleep [57]. There are mixed findings for changes in alcohol use patterns globally during the pandemic, and this is moderated by restrictions related to alcohol sales during regional lockdowns. For example, some countries deemed alcohol sales as an essential commodity during lockdown, which could explain the 262% past-year increase in online sales of alcohol in 2020 in the US [58]. Among women in the U.S. specifically, there were significant past-year increases in drinking frequency (14%), number of heavy drinking occasions (41%), and alcohol-related problems (39%) among women in 2020 [58]. Early indications from Australia (April–May 2020), for example, noted increases in AUDIT scores among women aged 36–50 years who indicated higher levels of stress [59]. Similarly, a study from the U.S. found that exposure to high levels of stress from COVID-19 pandemic was associated with changes in women's drinking behavior, wherein women more closely approximated alcohol use patterns of men based on several indices [60]. This pattern of gender convergence in alcohol use patterns is especially harmful as similar quantities of alcohol have greater adverse health effects for women [61]. A study in Switzerland shows that on average, a person would have 0.105 Years of Life Lost (YLL) due to alcohol use disorder as a psychological consequence of isolation during the COVID-19 pandemic [62]. In high-income countries, advertising alcohol as a way for women to cope with daily stress [63] may also be an influencing factor on increased alcohol use during the pandemic.

The COVID-19 pandemic may also influence alcohol use during pregnancy, which may be mediated by mental health status. One U.S. study found that pregnant women's psychological distress was predictive of the number of substances they used during the first and second COVID waves [64], whereas a Canadian study found no associations between COVID-19 concerns or mental health outcomes with alcohol use during pregnancy [65]. Generally, depressive symptoms and financial difficulties have been found to be linked with increased tobacco, cannabis, and polysubstance use during pregnancy [65]. Prenatal polysubstance exposure can further increase the risk of FASD if there is already some exposure to alcohol as well [16]. This is further complicated by the fact that global maternal and fetal outcomes have worsened during the pandemic, with an increase in maternal depression, maternal death, ruptured ectopic pregnancies, and stillbirth [66].

A global event such as a pandemic must be examined through the lens of trauma and how this affects the context of PAE. Any event that impacts mental health outcomes, family dynamics, and/or substance use patterns also impacts alcohol use that occurs during pregnancy, and therefore PAE. Firstly, women with adverse childhood experiences (ACEs) are more likely to have anxiety or depression and more likely to consume alcohol during pregnancy [16, 17], making their pregnancies extremely vulnerable to PAE during the COVID-19 pandemic. As well, individuals with FASD are more likely to have ACEs as compared to individuals without FASD [67], and the added stress of the pandemic and perhaps lack of availability or access to support services, may worsen mental health outcomes and contribute to the development of added comorbid disorders [67, 68]. Understanding the role of trauma and ACEs in women who consume alcohol during pregnancy and among individuals living with FASD can facilitate referrals to appropriate prevention and intervention services and prevent FASD familial recurrence during the COVID-19 pandemic.

Conclusions

Alcohol use and binge drinking levels are increasing among women of childbearing age in the majority of countries globally, especially the most populous countries such as India and China. Increased alcohol consumption among childbearing age women, combined with the fact that 44% of pregnancies globally are unplanned, indicates that millions of pregnancies are at risk of alcohol exposure. Therefore, countries can expect an increase in the incidence and prevalence of FASD, which will continue to incur high-cost burden to healthcare and other service systems and impact affected individuals and their families.

Alcohol use screening stands to greatly benefit all childbearing age and pregnant women, and it is one of the most important public health initiatives to minimize the disease burden of alcohol and prevent FASD and other teratogenic effects. Alcohol use should be assessed at during every visit of primary health care settings, especially for visits related to conditions known to be comorbid with alcohol use among women of childbearing age (e.g., cardiovascular disease). For women of childbearing age who screen positive for an AUD, referrals to substance use programs and access to contraceptive counseling are critical to prevent alcohol-exposed pregnancies.

Prenatal alcohol screening should be universal, mandatory, and implemented consistently among all prenatal care providers, including physicians, obstetricians, midwives, and nurses. All prenatal care providers must be trained in FASD prevention and must have the capacity to educate childbearing age and pregnant women about the risks of PAE while empowering them to make the healthiest choice using a trusting, non-judgmental rapport. The level of alcohol screening must be carefully selected, based on individualized needs, such as the cultural context, pre-pregnancy alcohol use patterns, health status history, and the resources required to implement the screening measure. If simply asking about alcohol use in pregnancy has the potential to change alcohol use behavior [25, 26], it is imperative that prenatal care providers take this opportunity. Furthermore, consistent PAE screening will result in more complete, high-quality data in population-based birth registries, which will allow researchers to measure the true prevalence of PAE and to design, implement, and evaluate PAE interventions over time.

Several evidence-based alcohol use screening instruments have been validated as a means to screen for PAE: the AUDIT-C, 1-Question screen, the TWEAK, T-ACE, and CAGE. Further research must be conducted to validate other existing screening instruments in pregnant women, in various cultural groups and settings. Prenatal care providers can choose from the recommended instruments based on their respective practitioner guidelines, while keeping in mind that there is no safe level of alcohol consumption during pregnancy and it is imperative to detect even low levels so as to ensure the healthiest outcomes for the mother and child. Providers should encourage all women to avoid consuming any alcohol throughout their pregnancy and while trying to become pregnant, emphasizing the benefits of doing so to the health and well-being of the mother and child. These providers must dispel common myths about alcohol use during pregnancy (e.g., "only high levels of drinking are harmful") and provide guidance in accordance with their regional obstetric guidelines. Prenatal care providers must also be knowledgeable about the existing interventions in their communities that can support maternal and child health during pregnancy and in the postpartum period.

Screening for PAE could lead to close monitoring of a child's development, facilitate early diagnosis, and the implementation of timely interventions, if necessary. It would also prevent the occurrence of adverse health and social outcomes later in life and the occurrence and/or recurrence of prenatal and postnatal alcohol exposure within families at risk for FASD. Improved access to FASD diagnosis also is an opportunity to identify mothers who not only have maternal risk factors for FASD but also have children with FASD. This is a priority population for the prevention of alcohol exposure in future pregnancies. Among people diagnosed with FASD, specific efforts must be made to make support services readily available and to improve the quality of life for individuals with FASD, their families and communities. Support services can help individuals with FASD achieve their goals in terms of academic success, obtaining/maintaining employment, being safe and staying healthy (e.g., preventing victimization of substance use disorders). From an epidemiological standpoint, increased screening of PAE and FASD can help establish regional surveillance systems which can monitor the prevalence of PAE/FASD over time and measure incidence rates as well. This data collection effort can help identify vulnerable populations, develop resources, and evaluate the effectiveness of prevention and research strategies. Regional surveillance systems can eventually be synchronized in order to initiate a global effort to prevent PAE and FASD, and to diagnose individuals living with FASD.

FASD is present in all populations globally and is not restricted to disadvantaged groups or any particular socioeconomic status, education, or ethnicity. Large-scale efforts to achieve public health awareness of the harmful effects of PAE and the life course of individuals with FASD can dispel common myths surrounding PAE. Increased public awareness can also assist women's partners and families in helping pregnant women have alcohol-free pregnancies. Lastly, these prevention efforts must be combined with the provision of diagnostic and support services for individuals with FASD in order to reduce stigma and improve their overall quality of life.

References

1. World Health Organization. Global strategy to reduce the harmful use of alcohol. Geneva: World Health Organization; 2010.
2. World Health Organization. Global action plan for the prevention and control of NCDs 2013–2020. Geneva: World Health Organization; 2013.
3. Rehm J, et al. What is the best indicator of the harmful use of alcohol? A narrative review. Drug Alcohol Rev. 2020;39(6):624–31.
4. World Health Organization. Global information system on alcohol and health. Geneva: World Health Organization; 2018.
5. Popova S, Rehm J, Shield K. Global alcohol epidemiology: focus on women of childbearing age. In: The Routledge handbook of social work and addictive behaviors. Routledge; 2020.
6. World Health Organization. Global status report on alcohol and health, 2018. Geneva: World Health Organization; 2018.
7. Popova S, et al. Alcohol industry–funded websites contribute to ambiguity regarding the harmful effects of alcohol consumption during pregnancy: a commentary on Lim et al. (2019). J Stud Alcohol Drugs. 2019;80(5):534–6.

8. Rehm J, et al. The relation between different dimensions of alcohol consumption and burden of disease: an overview. Addiction (Abingdon, England). 2010;105(5):817–43.
9. Popova S, et al. Estimation of national, regional, and global prevalence of alcohol use during pregnancy and fetal alcohol syndrome: a systematic review and meta-analysis. Lancet Glob Health. 2017;5(3):e290–9.
10. Bearak J, et al. Global, regional, and subregional trends in unintended pregnancy and its outcomes from 1990 to 2014: estimates from a Bayesian hierarchical model. Lancet Glob Health. 2018;6(4):e380–9.
11. Abdullah P, et al. Factors associated with the timing of the first prenatal ultrasound in Canada. BMC Pregnancy Childbirth. 2019;19(1):164–14.
12. Popova S, et al. Global prevalence of alcohol use and binge drinking during pregnancy, and fetal alcohol spectrum disorder. Biochem Cell Biol. 2018;96(2):237–40.
13. Lange S, et al. Prevalence of binge drinking during pregnancy by country and World Health Organization region: systematic review and meta-analysis. Reprod Toxicol. 2017;73:214–21.
14. World Health Organization. Guidelines for the identification and management of substance use and substance use disorders in pregnancy. Geneva: World Health Organization; 2014.
15. Skagerstróm J, Chang G, Nilsen P. Predictors of drinking during pregnancy: a systematic review. J Women's Health (Larchmont, N.Y. 2002). 2011;20(6):91–913.
16. McQuire C, et al. The causal web of foetal alcohol spectrum disorders: a review and causal diagram. Eur Child Adolesc Psychiatry. 2020;29(5):575–94.
17. Popova S, et al. Maternal alcohol use, adverse neonatal outcomes and pregnancy complications in British Columbia, Canada: a population-based study. BMC Pregnancy Childbirth. 2021;21(1):74–13.
18. Popova S, et al. Why do women consume alcohol during pregnancy or while breastfeeding? Drug Alcohol Rev. 2021;41:759.
19. Furtwængler NAFF, de Visser RO. Lack of international consensus in low-risk drinking guidelines. Drug Alcohol Rev. 2013;32(1):11–8.
20. International Alliance for Responsible Drinking. Drinking guidelines: general population. IARD; 2019.
21. Dozet D, Burd L, Popova S. Screening for alcohol use in pregnancy: a review of current practices and perspectives. Int J Ment Heal Addict. 2021;21:1220.
22. Arnold K, et al. Fetal alcohol spectrum disorders: knowledge and screening practices of university hospital medical students and residents. J Popul Ther Clin Pharmacol. 2013;20(1):e18–25.
23. Lemola S, et al. Midwives' engagement in smoking- and alcohol-prevention in prenatal care before and after the introduction of practice guidelines in Switzerland: comparison of survey findings from 2008 and 2018. BMC Pregnancy Childbirth. 2020;20(1):31.
24. Burd L, Popova S. Fetal alcohol spectrum disorders: fixing our aim to aim for the fix. Int J Environ Res Public Health. 2019;16(20):3978.
25. Tzilos GK, Sokol RJ, Ondersma SJ. A randomized phase I trial of a brief computer-delivered intervention for alcohol use during pregnancy. J Womens Health (Larchmt). 2011;20(10):1517–24.
26. Floyd RL, et al. Preventing alcohol-exposed pregnancies: a randomized controlled trial. Am J Prev Med. 2007;32(1):1–10.
27. Lange S, et al. A comparison of the prevalence of prenatal alcohol exposure obtained via maternal self-reports versus meconium testing: a systematic literature review and meta-analysis. BMC Pregnancy Childbirth. 2014;14(1):127.
28. O'Connor MJ, Kogan N, Findlay R. Prenatal alcohol exposure and attachment behavior in children. Alcohol Clin Exp Res. 2002;26(10):1592–602.
29. Kesmodel U, Olsen SF, Secher NJ. Does alcohol increase the risk of preterm delivery? Epidemiology (Cambridge, Mass.). 2000;11(5):512–8.
30. Kesmodel U, et al. Moderate alcohol intake during pregnancy and the risk of stillbirth and death in the first year of life. Am J Epidemiol. 2002;155(4):305–12.

31. Patra J, et al. Dose–response relationship between alcohol consumption before and during pregnancy and the risks of low birthweight, preterm birth and small for gestational age (SGA)—a systematic review and meta-analyses. BJOG. 2011;118(12):1411–21.
32. Yang Q, et al. A case-control study of maternal alcohol consumption and intrauterine growth retardation. Ann Epidemiol. 2001;11(7):497–503.
33. Lange S, et al. Global prevalence of fetal alcohol spectrum disorder among children and youth: a systematic review and meta-analysis. JAMA Pediatr. 2017;171(10):948–56.
34. Chambers CD, et al. Fetal alcohol spectrum disorders in a Pacific Southwest City: maternal and child characteristics. Alcohol Clin Exp Res. 2019;43(12):2578–90.
35. Caputo C, Wood E, Jabbour L. Impact of fetal alcohol exposure on body systems: a systematic review: impact of fetal alcohol exposure on body systems. Birth Defects Res. 2016;108(2):174–80.
36. Popova S, Dozet D, Burd L. Fetal alcohol Spectrum disorder: can we change the future? Alcohol Clin Exp Res. 2020;44(4):815–9.
37. Popova S, et al. Population-based prevalence of fetal alcohol spectrum disorder in Canada. BMC Public Health. 2019;19(1):845.
38. May PA, et al. Prevalence of fetal alcohol spectrum disorders in 4 US communities. JAMA. 2018;319(5):474–82.
39. Popova S, et al. Prevalence of fetal alcohol spectrum disorder among special subpopulations: a systematic review and meta-analysis. Addiction (Abingdon, England). 2019;114(7):1150–72.
40. Popova S, et al. Prevalence of fetal alcohol spectrum disorder among special subpopulations: a systematic review and meta-analysis. Addiction. 2019;114(7):1150–72.
41. Mena M, et al. Alcohol drinking in parents and its relation with intellectual score of their children. Rev Med Chile. 1993;121(1):98–105.
42. Landgren M, et al. Prenatal alcohol exposure and neurodevelopmental disorders in children adopted from eastern Europe. Pediatrics. 2010;125(5):e1178–85.
43. Kuzmenkovienė E, Prasauskienė A, Endzinienė M. The prevalence of fetal alcohol spectrum disorders and concomitant disorders among orphanage children in Lithuania. J Popul Ther Clin Pharmacol. 2012;19(3):e423.
44. Legonkova SV. Kliniko-funktcionalnaia kharakteristika fetalnogo alkogolnogo sindroma u detei rannego vozrasta [Clinical and functional characteristics of Fetal Alcohol Syndrome in early childhood]. St. Petersburg: St. Peterburg's State Paediatric Medical Academy; 2011.
45. Fast DK, Conry J, Loock CA. Identifying fetal alcohol syndrome among youth in the criminal justice system. J Dev Behav Pediatr. 1999;20(5):370–2.
46. Bell CC, Chimata R. Prevalence of neurodevelopmental disorders among low-income African Americans at a clinic on Chicago's south side. Psychiatr Serv. 2015;66(5):539–42.
47. Popova S, et al. Comorbidity of fetal alcohol spectrum disorder: a systematic review and meta-analysis. Lancet (Br Ed). 2016;387(10022):978–87.
48. Popova S, et al. Fetal alcohol spectrum disorder prevalence estimates in correctional systems: a systematic literature review. Can J Public Health. 2011;102(5):336–40.
49. Popova S, Shannon L, Burd L, Rehm J. The economic burden of fetal alcohol Spectrum disorder in Canada in 2013. Alcohol Alcohol. 2016;51(3):367–75.
50. Popova S, et al. What do we know about the economic impact of fetal alcohol spectrum disorder? A systematic literature review. Alcohol Alcohol. 2011;46(4):490–7.
51. Greenmyer JR, et al. A multicountry updated assessment of the economic impact of fetal alcohol spectrum disorder: costs for children and adults. J Addict Med. 2018;12(6):466–73.
52. Greenmyer JR, et al. Fetal alcohol spectrum disorder: a systematic review of the cost of and savings from prevention in the United States and Canada. Addiction (Abingdon, England). 2020;115(3):409–17.
53. Corrigan PW, et al. The public stigma of birth mothers of children with fetal alcohol Spectrum disorders. Alcohol Clin Exp Res. 2017;41(6):1166–73.
54. Popova S, et al. Alcohol's impact on the fetus. Nutrients. 2021;13(10):3452.

55. Thanh NX, Jonsson E. Life expectancy of people with fetal alcohol syndrome. J Popul Ther Clin Pharmacol. 2016;23(1):e53–9.
56. Murthy P, Narasimha VL. Effects of the COVID-19 pandemic and lockdown on alcohol use disorders and complications. Curr Opin Psychiatry. 2021;34(4):376–85.
57. Palsson OS, Ballou S, Gray S, The US. National Pandemic Emotional Impact report. University of North Carolina, Harvard Medical School; 2020.
58. Pollard MS, Tucker JS, Green JHD. Changes in adult alcohol use and consequences during the COVID-19 pandemic in the US. JAMA Netw Open. 2020;3(9):e2022942.
59. Callinan S, et al. Shifts in alcohol consumption during the COVID-19 pandemic: early indications from Australia. Addiction (Abingdon, England). 2021;116(6):1381–8.
60. Rodriguez LM, Litt DM, Stewart SH. Drinking to cope with the pandemic: the unique associations of COVID-19-related perceived threat and psychological distress to drinking behaviors in American men and women. Addict Behav. 2020;110:106532.
61. Stewart SH, Gavric D, Collins P. Women, girls, and alcohol. In: Women and addiction: a comprehensive handbook. New York: The Guilford Press; 2009. p. 341–59.
62. Moser DA, et al. Years of life lost due to the psychosocial consequences of COVID-19 mitigation strategies based on Swiss data. Eur Psychiatry. 2020;63(1):e58.
63. Esser MB, Jernigan DH. Policy approaches for regulating alcohol marketing in a global context: a public health perspective. Annu Rev Public Health. 2018;39(1):385–401.
64. Smith CL, et al. Substance use and mental health in pregnant women during the COVID-19 pandemic. J Reprod Infant Psychol. 2022;40:465–78.
65. Kar P, et al. Alcohol and substance use in pregnancy during the COVID-19 pandemic. Drug Alcohol Depend. 2021;225:108760.
66. Chmielewska B, et al. Effects of the COVID-19 pandemic on maternal and perinatal outcomes: a systematic review and meta-analysis. Lancet Glob Health. 2021;9(6):e759–72.
67. Kambeitz C, et al. Association of adverse childhood experiences and neurodevelopmental disorders in people with fetal alcohol spectrum disorders (FASD) and non-FASD controls. BMC Pediatr. 2019;19(1):498.
68. Weyrauch D, et al. Comorbid mental disorders in fetal alcohol Spectrum disorders: a systematic review. J Dev Behav Pediatr. 2017;38(4):283–91.

Chapter 2
Protective and Risk Factors

Gretchen Bandoli and Christina D. Chambers

Risk and Protective Factors for Alcohol Use Among Women of Childbearing Ages

Historical Trends in Alcohol Use

Alcohol Use Among Women of Childbearing Age

The Centers for Disease Control and Prevention (CDC) analyzed 2011–2013 Behavioral Risk Factor Surveillance System (BRFSS) data among pregnant and non-pregnant women ages 18–44 in the United States. Among non-pregnant women, the prevalence of any alcohol use in the past 30 days was 53.6%, while the prevalence of heavy episodic or "binge" drinking (defined in this survey as ≥4 drinks on at least one occasion) was 18.2% [1]. From more recent data in the National Surveys on Drug Use and Health, prevalence of past 30-day alcohol use among non-pregnant women ages 18–44 was estimated at 58.2% in 2017 [2]. These estimates could have substantial public health impact, as up to 50% of pregnancies are unplanned, and the gestational timing of pregnancy recognition can vary widely from pregnancy to pregnancy. Thus, even pregnancies with intended cessation of alcohol use upon

---

Statement on inclusivity—The authors would like to acknowledge that alcohol and fetal spectrum disorder research must be inclusive of all individuals, including gender non-conforming people. We use the term "women" to refer to all pregnancy capable individuals and those with female reproductive organs regardless of gender identity.

G. Bandoli (✉) · C. D. Chambers
Department of Pediatrics, University of California San Diego, La Jolla, CA, USA

Herbert Wertheim School of Public Health, University of California San Diego,
La Jolla, CA, USA
e-mail: gbandoli@health.ucsd.edu; chchambers@health.ucsd.edu

recognition have the potential for a few to several weeks of alcohol exposure to the developing fetus. With the estimated amount of alcohol use and binge alcohol use among women of childbearing ages, a non-trivial number of pregnancies is very likely exposed to alcohol during the crucial developmental window of organogenesis and structural development. Several studies have concluded that the most important predictor of alcohol consumption during pregnancy is frequent consumption outside of pregnancy [3]. Ideally, education and intervention targets should be aimed at reducing alcohol consumption among individuals during their reproductive years, before conception occurs, impacting both the health of the pregnant person and optimizing outcomes for future pregnancies.

Alcohol Use Among Pregnant People

The weighted prevalence of any past 30-day drinking reported by pregnant individuals in the BRFSS increased from 9.2% in 2011 to 11.3% in 2018 [4]. Similar trends were reported for binge drinking in pregnancy, which increased from 2.5% to 4.0% over the same time frame. Further, between those same two time periods, the average number of drinks consumed on drinking days increased from 2.1 to 2.2 drinks, and the average number of days having at least one alcoholic beverage increased from 5.8 to 7.0 days [4].

In a separate data source, the National Survey on Drug Use and Health (NSDUH), approximately 8–12% of pregnant people surveyed between 2015 and 2018 reported alcohol use in the past month (Fig. 2.1) [5]. When examined by trimester of pregnancy, 19.6% of respondents in their first trimester endorsed any past 30-day alcohol use, while 4.7% of respondents in their second or third trimester of pregnancy endorsed past 30-day alcohol use [6]. Binge drinking was reported by 10.5% of first trimester respondents, and 1.4% of second or third trimester respondents [6]. From the full NSDUH survey, 11–15% of pregnant people reported past month tobacco use, and 3–7% reported past month marijuana use (Fig. 2.1) [5]. When examined by

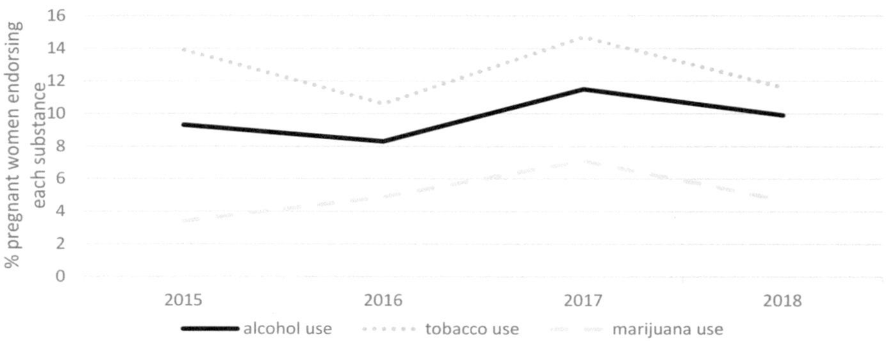

Fig. 2.1 Past month substance use among pregnant women in the National Survey on Drug use and Health, 2018. (Data taken from Center for Behavioral Health Statistics and Quality [5])

alcohol use status, 38.2% of respondents who reported current drinking also reported one or more other substances, most often tobacco (28.1%) or marijuana (20.6%) [6].

Global Prevalence Estimates for Alcohol Use During Pregnancy

Globally, the prevalence of alcohol consumption during pregnancy, both as any use and as binge drinking, varies widely. Popova and colleagues estimated the global prevalence of any alcohol use during pregnancy to be 9.8% (95% CI 8.9, 11.1) [7, 8] of the 2012 population. Estimates ranged from very low prevalence in the Eastern Mediterranean Region (0.2%, 95% CI 0.1, 0.9) and the South East Asia Region (1.8%, 95% CI 0.5, 9.1), to very high prevalence in the European Region (25.2, 95% CI 21.6, 29.6) (Fig. 2.2). The African Region, Region of the Americas, and Western Pacific Region all had estimated prevalence rates of 9–11%. When examined by individual countries, Russia, United Kingdom, Belarus, Denmark, and Iceland had the highest prevalence of alcohol use during pregnancy, while Oman, United Arab Emirates, Saudi Arabia, Qatar, and Kuwait had the lowest prevalence estimates. Binge drinking behaviors varied by region, at times dissimilar to overall alcohol use prevalence estimates. The European Region, which had the highest prevalence of any alcohol use, had a lower proportion of binge drinking (defined as $\geq$4 drinks on at least one occasion) during pregnancy (10.7%) compared with the African Region (31.0%), Region of the Americas (25.0%), or Western Pacific Region (20.9%). It should be noted, however, that the lower proportion in the European Region is from

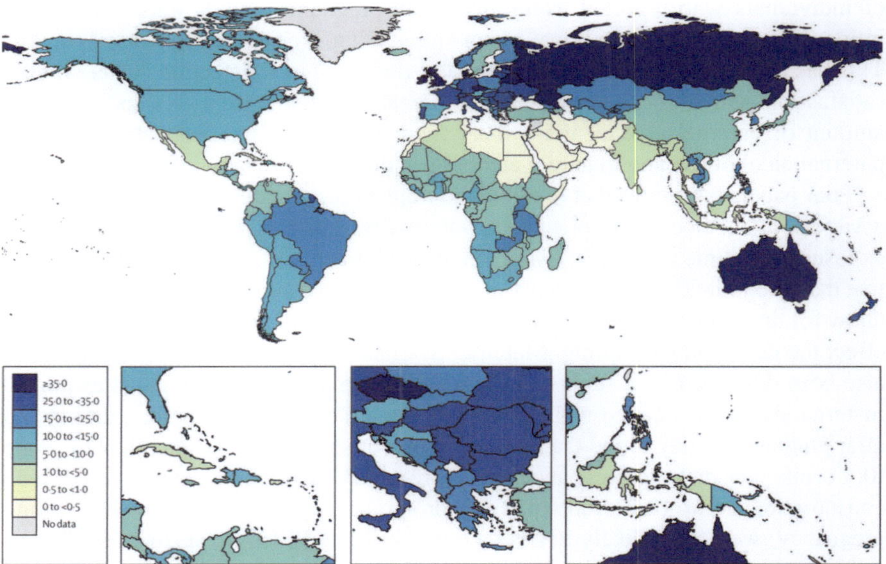

Fig. 2.2 Global prevalence (%) of alcohol use (any amount) during pregnancy among the general population in 2012. (Reproduced with permission [7])

a much higher base prevalence of any alcohol use in pregnancy, which corresponds to the evidence that, as a region, it has the highest prevalence of fetal alcohol syndrome (FAS) and fetal alcohol spectrum disorders (FASD) in the world [8].

Risk Factors for Alcohol Use

In the 2011–2013 BRFSS survey [1], the prevalence of any alcohol use among non-pregnant women ages 18–44 was highest among those in their twenties, who identified as non-Hispanic White or non-Hispanic Black, those who had a college degree, and who were employed. Alcohol consumption did not differ by marital status. The picture was slightly different among women who reported binge drinking. There, the highest prevalence was still among women in their twenties, and women who identified as non-Hispanic White, followed by those who identified as "other" race. The prevalence was also higher among women with some college or a college degree, those who were employed, and those who were not married.

Interestingly, the profile of pregnant people in the BRFSS survey who consumed alcohol was different [1]. The prevalence of any reported alcohol use in pregnancy was highest among individuals ages 35–44, those who identified as non-Hispanic Black or other races, those with a college degree, who were employed, and those not married. These patterns were generally observed among pregnant people who reported binge drinking as well, although estimates became increasingly small and unstable. The 2015–2017 BRFSS report found essentially the same characteristics of individuals who reported using alcohol in pregnancy [9]. In addition, partner influence has been reported as a factor influencing prenatal alcohol use [10, 11]. This has been observed both with respect to relationship satisfaction (where higher satisfaction was associated with lower prenatal alcohol use [11]) and with the amount of paternal alcohol use (where there was a positive correlation between paternal alcohol use and maternal alcohol use during pregnancy [10]).

Four papers have looked at longitudinal trajectories of alcohol use, which through a variety of methods attempt to incorporate the timing, quantity, and duration of exposure over time (Fig. 2.3). Using longitudinal trajectories may be more informative than the individual constituents of exposure when estimating risk for FASD and allow for the estimation of how highly variable patterns of prenatal alcohol exposure effect the developing offspring. Maternal risk factors by pattern of alcohol use have also been described. In a study of over 6000 women in Australia, authors examined maternal factors associated with patterns of alcohol consumption before, during and after pregnancy. They found that compared to women within the light alcohol group (0.4 drinks per day pre-pregnancy, early pregnancy cessation), women in the high consumption group (2.5 drinks per day pre-pregnancy, 0.6 drinks per day during pregnancy) were more likely to have a lower income, be single or divorced, be primiparous, not attend church, to report depression or anxiety, to have high maternal adversity, and to have select negative health-related lifestyle behaviors (smoking, little exercise, poor sleep) [12]. In the Safe Passage study, authors assessed maternal

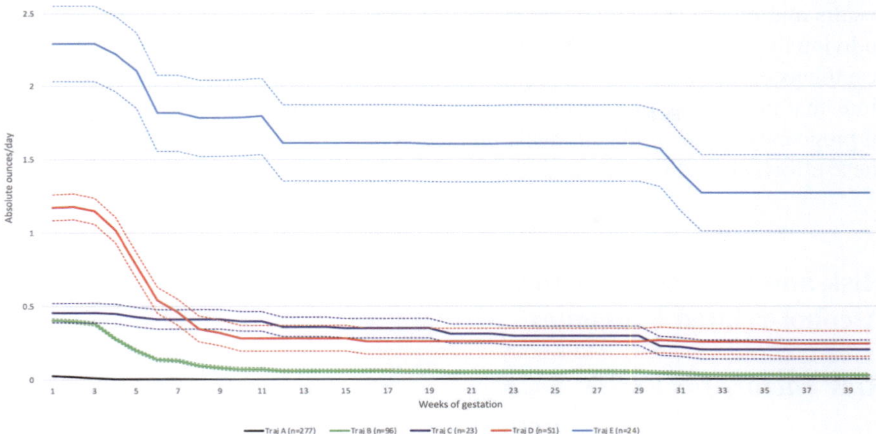

Fig. 2.3 Trajectory groups of mean absolute ounces of alcohol per day (solid lines) and 95% confidence intervals (hashed lines) from a pregnancy cohort in Ukraine. (Reproduced with permission [26])

demographics by patterns of prenatal alcohol use in high-risk samples from the United States and South Africa. There, compared to women who had moderate consumption with early cessation, women who either had high or low consumption with continued alcohol use during pregnancy were much more likely to report mixed-race ancestry, were less likely to have at least a high-school education, were more likely to have symptoms of depression, were slightly more likely to receive government assistance, and were more likely to smoke during pregnancy [13]. In the third study of patterns of prenatal alcohol use (Fig. 2.3), women in Ukraine who continued alcohol use longer into pregnancy were more likely to be older, have less educational achievement, be single or divorced, and not use prenatal vitamins [14]. In the latter two studies, maternal characteristics and sociodemographic profiles were more similar by duration of alcohol use in pregnancy than by initial quantity of use, highlighting that pre-pregnancy level of alcohol consumption is not necessarily indicative of who will abstain from alcohol after recognition of pregnancy. Finally, using data from 2002 to 2009 Pregnancy Risk Assessment Monitoring System, authors looked at predictors of drinking behaviors in pregnancy (reduction vs. no reduction of prenatal alcohol use in the last 3 months of pregnancy compared to the preconceptual period) [15]. Compared to women who reduced alcohol use in pregnancy, women who did not were more likely to be young, identify as non-Hispanic Black or other race, to report Hispanic ethnicity, to have fewer years of education, be married, be overweight or obese, have higher parity, and report having difficulty paying the bills. Interestingly, they were less likely to have smoked in the previous trimester, and were less likely to report someone close to them having a drinking or substance use problem [15].

The results from these four studies demonstrate that there is not a single profile for individuals who are likely to consume large quantities of alcohol in pregnancy, or those that continue consumption later in pregnancy. However, based on these results and others, it may be beneficial to target cessation efforts toward pregnant individuals with lower educational achievement, who are divorced or single, who use tobacco, and who have depression, anxiety, or adversity. In addition, interventions that include the partner may be more effective. Finally, as alcohol use outside of pregnancy is one of the strongest predictors of alcohol use during pregnancy [3], these efforts should be extended to all women during their reproductive years.

Risk and Protective Factors for Fetus and Child Alcohol-related Outcomes

Risk Factors for FASD

Although alcohol is a necessary exposure and the cause of FASD, there are other risk and protective factors that contribute to the outcome. Popov and colleagues estimated that one in every 67 individuals who consumed alcohol in pregnancy had a child with FAS [7], highlighting the role that other factors play in addition to prenatal alcohol exposure.

Prenatal Alcohol Exposure: Quantity, Timing, and Frequency

FASD and other neurodevelopmental deficits not rising to the level to meet diagnostic criteria for FASD have been consistently associated with prenatal exposure to heavy or binge drinking [16–19]. Findings regarding low to moderate levels of prenatal alcohol exposure (PAE) have been less consistent, with some systematic reviews and meta-analyses reporting no deficits in functional domains [16, 19–21], while other studies have suggested that there are effects even at lower levels of consumption [16, 22, 23].

In recognition of the importance of the quantity, timing, and frequency of PAE on the risk of FASD, many studies have focused on these three parameters in an attempt to produce more precise risk estimates. In studies of first-grade children in South Africa, the quantity and frequency of PAE were consistently higher among children with FAS, followed by partial FAS (pFAS) and alcohol-related neurodevelopmental disorder (ARND) compared to control children [17, 24]. These findings were observed in all each of the three trimesters of pregnancy. Although sample sizes were smaller, these findings were replicated in a low-risk, community-based sample of first-grade children in the Southwest region of the United States [25].

As previously discussed, a few authors have summarized all three parameters into PAE trajectories, which allows for the incorporation of quantity, timing, and frequency of PAE into a single measure. Although several methodologies exist, the underlying premise of longitudinal exposure modeling is to create groups with similar longitudinal exposure patterns in order to minimize heterogeneity within the assigned trajectory group and maximize heterogeneity between trajectories. One finding that has emerged from the longitudinal trajectory studies is that the duration of PAE, often described as "sustained" exposure, is a very important factor when assessing outcomes. In the study of PAE trajectories in Ukraine, sustained alcohol ("Traj C" in blue in Fig. 2.3), even at relatively low levels, was associated with modest reductions in neurodevelopmental performance at 6 and 12 months of age compared with trajectories of higher PAE with earlier pregnancy reduction/cessation ("Traj D" in red in Fig. 2.3) [14]. Similar results were observed when the trajectories were examined with select alcohol-related malformations and the total dysmorphology score [26]. In the Safe Passage Study, the sustaining trajectory (modeled as maximum drinks per drinking day) was associated with sudden infant death syndrome (SIDS), while the trajectories with similar consumption early in pregnancy but earlier cessation were not [27]. It is unlikely that researchers will identify a "threshold" of PAE that results in FASD; rather, the use of longitudinal trajectory analysis will continue efforts toward understanding how the timing, quantity, and frequency of PAE interact, and the individuals that are most susceptible to different exposure patterns.

Maternal Characteristics and the Intrauterine Environment

Multiple risk factors are associated with FASD, although it is unclear the extent to which these are causal or they are simply associated with PAE. Prenatal tobacco exposure is higher among children with FASD and is independently associated with growth restriction and neurocognitive deficits [28, 29]. Animal models have suggested synergistic effects between prenatal alcohol and tobacco on FASD-related outcomes [28], and human studies have noted the synergistic effects between prenatal alcohol and tobacco on the risk of SIDS [27]. There is also an increased prevalence of other licit and illicit substance use associated with PAE, including marijuana, opioids, and other substances [25, 28]. Marijuana is of particular concern given the increasing prevalence of use (Fig. 2.1), including co-use with alcohol among youth [30]. Animal models [31, 32] have also demonstrated synergistic effects between prenatal alcohol and marijuana exposure and will be an increasingly urgent area of study in the coming years.

Although higher levels of drinking are often associated with younger ages, having a child with FASD is associated with increased maternal age [25, 28, 29, 33]. Reasons for this are unclear, though may involve decreased liver functioning of women as they age due to longer exposure to alcohol, as well as altered nutrition transport due to chronic alcohol exposure. Maternal age may also confound other factors that are associated with age, such as parity, which has previously been noted as a risk factor for FASD. In animal studies, when maternal age is held constant, birth defects in alcohol-exposed rats are similar. In contrast, when parity was held constant and age was varied, there were more alcohol-related defects in litters born to older dams [28].

Finally, in a systematic review, in addition to the aforementioned characteristics, authors reported the following maternal risk factors for having an offspring with

FAS: lower education, less religiosity, rural residence, psychiatric morbidity, maternal history of physical or sexual abuse, and having a partner/spouse with disordered alcohol use [34].

Biologic Factors

In addition to the maternal and environmental factors, biologic factors of both the pregnant person and the child also contribute to the risk of FASD. There are several reviews on the genetic contributors to FASD [35, 36] which provide more detail on previous findings and directions of future research. Briefly, there is strong human evidence for the role of genetics in conferring susceptibility to FASD: monozygotic twins have been found to be 100% concordant on FASD diagnosis, while concordance fell to 54% in dizygotic twins pairs, 41% in full siblings and 22% in half-sibling pairs [35, 37]. In one examined discordant pair, an 18q12.3-q21.1 microdeletion was detected in the affected twin, which resides in a region associated with growth restriction, developmental delay, and abnormal facial features [38].

Candidate genes have also been examined, primarily polymorphisms of one of the genes for the alcohol dehydrogenase enzyme family, the ADH1B, which is involved in alcohol metabolism. The functioning and examination of these alleles are thoroughly described in the review by Warren and Li [36]. Briefly, in one study examining maternal and child phenotypes and alcohol-related outcomes, there was little to no association between PAE and adverse outcomes among offspring born to mothers with the ADH1B*3 allele, which is associated with faster alcohol metabolism. In contrast, there were no consistent findings by absence or presence of the ADH1B*3 allele in the offspring [39]. Several other studies have found similar protective effects from the ADH1B*2 variant as compared to ADH1B*1 [36]. However, it remains unclear to what extent the protective effects noted in the ADH1B polymorphisms are actually due to reducing consumption of alcohol, leading to lower levels of PAE [35].

More recently, researchers have begun to focus on the epigenetic modifications associated with PAE, including alterations to DNA methylation, histone modification, and microRNAs. Most studies have focused on specific loci, such as insulin-like growth factor [35], although others have examined methylation through epigenome-wide association studies (EWAS). The latter have reported many differentially methylated CpG sites, although to date, studies have not replicated well. The studies have been small, used different cell types, and had great variability in age, timing and amount of exposure, and sociodemographic backgrounds and criteria for diagnosis of FASD for participants [35]. Future work in the field has already begun to address these limitations, as well as expanding into novel areas including paternal preconception alcohol consumption, and maternal and paternal transgenerational transmission of PAE-induced epigenetic alterations [35].

Biologic sex may also factor into FASD. In a study of over 1500 children from community studies, males and females had mostly similar physical and neurocognitive development associated with PAE [40]. However, sex ratios indicated lower viability and survival of males by first grade, and females had more dysmorphology and neurocognitive impairment than males. This pronouncement of FASD features may lead to earlier diagnosis for females and better outcomes in the long run [41].

Postnatal Factors

Although the intrauterine environment is where PAE occurs, the postnatal environment should also be considered as a crucial period during which factors may modify, in either direction, the effects of intrauterine exposure to alcohol. Some factors, such as maternal socioeconomic status, are discussed in the context of pregnancy but endure, likely with little change, through the child's postnatal life. Other exposures, such as maternal use of nicotine or other substances in pregnancy, may endure, but would have different mechanisms by which they shape the offspring's development. With this acknowledgment, here we focus specifically on postnatal factors that exclusively occur in that period.

Children with physical malformations or neurodevelopmental impairment are at a higher risk for maltreatment. Maltreatment alone has the potential to impact brain development, leading to deficits in cognitive, social, and behavioral domains. Many of these domains are already affected in children with FASD. A recent review found tremendous comorbidity between trauma and PAE; in a sample of fostered children with PAE 58% were neglected by birth parents, 36% witnessed violence, 16% were physically abused, and 5% were sexually abused. In a second sample of kids with FASD, 85% experienced some level of trauma. Similarly, in a sample of children with trauma, 40% had PAE. The authors concluded from reviewing the evidence that deficits in speech, language, attention intelligence, memory, and emotional and behavioral issues occurred to a greater extent when both exposures were present, highlighting the negative and likely synergistic effects of trauma in children with FASD [42].

In addition to abuse, other postnatal risk factors for outcomes of FASD include time in residential care, a lower dysmorphology score (likely leading to later detection and intervention) [43, 44], frequent changes in living arrangements [44], poor sleep in childhood [45], and continued alcohol exposure through breastmilk [46].

The postnatal period also presents opportunity to mitigate PAE. In a study in rats, researchers found increased positive environmental stimuli during adolescence (tested in the form of environmental enrichment) ameliorated or mitigated select prenatal alcohol-related cognitive deficits [47]. In human studies, specialized educational intervention for math learning disabilities associated with FASD proved beneficial, although interventions with a task-oriented framework for gross motor skills were less consistent [48]. Early detection and intervention through evidence-based measures are key to optimizing development of children affected by PAE.

Protective Factors

In addition to the protective factors previously mentioned, there are other factors that appear to, at least partially, mitigate the effects of PAE. In recent years, many have investigated the role of nutrition for its potential in preventing or alleviating symptomatology due to FASD [49]. Maternal nutritional status is compromised by alcohol and may mediate some of the effects of alcohol observed in children with FASD. Thus, suggestions that supplementation of select nutrients in pregnancy may alleviate the severity of FASD warrant our full attention.

There are few nutrients in FASD studies that have received greater interest than the essential B vitamin, choline. In a study of dietary choline levels and PAE in rats, the most severe alcohol-related effects were observed in offspring where the dam received 40% of recommended choline in the diet, suggesting suboptimal intake of a single nutrient can exacerbate some of prenatal alcohol's teratogenic effects [50]. Human studies have reported similar, although inconsistent, benefit of choline as reviewed by Wozniak and colleagues, which included studies of choline supplementation to the mother in pregnancy as well postnatal administration to children with FASD [51].

In addition to choline, many other nutrients have been hypothesized to mitigate PAE, which include vitamin A, docosahexaenoic acid (DHA), folic acid, zinc, vitamin E, and selenium [52]. Further research into individual and multiple-nutrient supplementation is necessary.

Finally, the relationship between socioeconomic factors and FASD is nuanced. Although higher socioeconomic status (SES) and full-time employment are associated with alcohol use in pregnancy, binge use is more common among women of low SES [28]. Further, prenatal alcohol exposure and *being affected* by prenatal alcohol are not synonymous. Studies have demonstrated that children born to women of higher economic means are less likely to be affected by PAE [28, 29], potentially due to different patterns of PAE, as well as the protective effects afforded by being raised in a high-resource environment. From this understanding, it is hypothesized that studies that report a protective effect (or reduced risk) of low amounts of alcohol on childhood neurodevelopmental outcomes are confounded by SES. The confounding would arise when women of higher SES are more likely to consume low to moderate amounts of alcohol in pregnancy with relatively early cessation, and also are more likely to have children with good neurodevelopmental outcomes afforded by their environment. Thus, in summary, high SES is considered to be a protective factor for FASD, although it is likely due to many factors, including pattern of exposure, intrauterine, and postnatal environment.

Risk and Protective Factor Summary

In summary, previous studies have revealed that quantity, frequency, and timing of PAE all contribute to the risk of FASD, as do co-exposures such as tobacco and other substances. Maternal factors such as advanced age and low socioeconomic status likely increase the risk, while nutritional factors or being born into a high-resource environment decrease developmental sequelae of FASD. Many of these findings were from retrospective studies that compared the factors in children with FAS, pFAS, ARND, and control children, which makes it hard to decouple high amounts of alcohol exposure from other correlated factors such as poverty, low maternal education, co-exposures, etc. In order to expand our collective understanding of protective and risk factors, more cohort studies are necessary that begin by following individuals exposed to different levels of PAE and psychosocial factors to more fully determine the risk and protective factors associated with development. This includes studying children affected by relatively low levels of alcohol, and children seemingly unaffected by relatively high levels of alcohol, to expand on risk and protective factors. In addition, it involves understanding the health and development of exposed children whose neurobehavioral and cognitive outcomes do not rise to the level of FASD. Through that work, a more inclusive framework of the risk and protective factors associated with PAE and health outcomes can emerge.

Future Projections

As previously noted, the prevalence of alcohol use in pregnancy increased from 2011 to 2018 [4]. This was despite public health efforts to reduce alcohol consumption, including the recommendation by the CDC in 2016 that women of reproductive ages who are sexually active and not using birth control abstain from alcohol. There may be additional reasons to be wary of near-term projections of the impact of alcohol exposure in pregnancy in the population. At the end of 2019, a novel coronavirus, SARS-CoV-2, began circulating around the world, resulting in the enforcement of stay-at-home orders and social distancing measures. There was tremendous global disruption and stress during the pandemic, including financial burden, emotional struggles, impact to healthcare, including family planning and prenatal care, and food and housing insecurity. During this time, there has been a documented increase in alcohol consumption, including among women in the United States [53]. From 2019 to 2020, women ages 18 or older reported more days that they consumed alcohol in the past 30 (a change of 0.78 days), no change in the number of drinks consumed in the past 30 days, an 41% increase in the number of heavy drinking in the past 30 days (0.18 additional days), and a 39% increase in the average score on the Short Inventory of Problems scale, which is indicative of alcohol related problems [53]. In contrast, a small study of pregnancies in Denmark during the COVID-19 pandemic found no reported change in alcohol consumption compared to a historical cohort 1 year prior, and a slight decrease in the among of binge episodes [54]. Suffice to say, it is reasonable to expect that alcohol consumption during pregnancy was higher in the pandemic period than otherwise would have been expected, at least in some populations. The near-term effects of this have yet to be fully realized.

Despite these setbacks, there may be cause for future optimism. Among youth, alcohol consumption trends are changing. Between 1999 and 2015, there were decreasing trends in weekly alcohol use and monthly heavy episodic drinking among adolescent females in Europe [55]. During a similar period in the United States, the single use of alcohol, and the dual use of alcohol and tobacco declined among high-school students. However, these public health gains were slightly reduced by an increase in the dual use of alcohol and marijuana [30]. Although these trends highlight the urgency behind further study of marijuana in pregnancy, they also should be seen as an opportunity to continue to promote alcohol reduction among our youth in the hopes of a reduction of alcohol-exposed pregnancies in the future.

References

1. Tan CH, Denny CH, Cheal NE, Sniezek JE, Kanny D. Alcohol use and binge drinking among women of childbearing age —United States, 2011–2013. MMWR Morb Mortal Wkly Rep. 2015;64:1042–6.
2. Hasin DS, Shmulewitz D, Keyes K. Alcohol use and binge drinking among U.S. men, pregnant and non-pregnant women ages 18–44: 2002–2017. Drug Alcohol Depend. 2019;205:107590.
3. Corrales-Gutierrez I, Mendoza R, Gomez-Baya D, Leon-Larios F. Understanding the relationship between predictors of alcohol consumption in pregnancy: towards effective prevention of FASD. Int J Environ Res Public Health. 2020;17:1–15.
4. Denny CH, Acero CS, Terplan M, Kim SY. Trends in alcohol use among pregnant women in the U.S., 2011–2018. Am J Prev Med. 2020;59:768–9.
5. Center for Behavioral Health Statistics and Quality. The National Survey on Drug Use and Health: 2018. Results from 2018 National Survey of Drug Use and Health detail tables. 2020. p. 1–58.
6. England LJ, Bennett C, Denny CH, Honein MA, Gilboa SM. Alcohol use and co-use of other substances among pregnant females aged 12–44 years—United States, 2015–2018. MMWR Morb Mortal Wkly Rep. 2020;69:1009.
7. Popova S, Lange S, Probst C, Gmel G, Rehm J. Estimation of national, regional, and global prevalence of alcohol use during pregnancy and fetal alcohol syndrome: a systematic review and meta-analysis. Lancet Glob Health. 2017;5:e290–9.
8. Popova S, Lange S, Probst C, Gmel G, Rehm J. Global prevalence of alcohol use and binge drinking during pregnancy, and fetal alcohol spectrum disorder. Biochem Cell Biol. 2018;96:237–40.
9. Denny CH, Acero CS, Naimi TS, Kim SY. Consumption of alcohol beverages and binge drinking among pregnant women aged 18–44 years — United States, 2015–2017. MMWR Morb Mortal Wkly Rep. 2019;68:2015–7.
10. Bakhireva LN, Wilsnack SC, Kristjanson A, Yevtushok L, Onishenko S, Wertelecki W, Chambers CD. Paternal drinking, intimate relationship quality, and alcohol consumption in pregnant Ukrainian women. J Stud Alcohol Drugs. 2011;72:536–44.
11. Kautz-Turnbull C, Petrenko CLM, Handley ED, Coles CD, Kable JA, Wertelecki W, Yevtushok L, Zymak-Zakutnya N, Chambers CD. Partner influence as a factor in maternal alcohol consumption and depressive symptoms, and maternal effects on infant neurodevelopmental outcomes. Alcohol Clin Exp Res. 2021;45:1265–75.

12. Tran NT, Najman JM, Hayatbakhsh R. Predictors of maternal drinking trajectories before and after pregnancy: evidence from a longitudinal study. Aust N Z J Obstet Gynaecol. 2015;55:123–30.
13. Dukes K, Tripp T, Willinger M, et al. Drinking and smoking patterns during pregnancy: development of group-based trajectories in the safe passage study. Alcohol. 2017;62:49–60.
14. Bandoli G, Coles CD, Kable JA, Wertelecki W, Yevtushok L, Zymak-Zakutnya N, Wells A, Granovska IV, Pashtepa AO, Chambers CD. Patterns of prenatal alcohol use that predict infant growth and development. Pediatrics. 2019;143:e20182399.
15. Kitsantas P, Gaffney KF, Wu H, Kastello JC. Determinants of alcohol cessation, reduction and no reduction during pregnancy. Arch Gynecol Obstet. 2014;289:771–9.
16. Flak AL, Su S, Bertrand J, Denny CH, Kesmodel US, Cogswell ME. The association of mild, moderate, and binge prenatal alcohol exposure and child neuropsychological outcomes. Alcohol Clin Exp Res. 2014;38:214–26.
17. May PA, Blankenship J, Marais A-SS, et al. Maternal alcohol consumption producing fetal alcohol spectrum disorders (FASD): quantity, frequency, and timing of drinking. Drug Alcohol Depend. 2013;133:502–12.
18. Conover EA, Jones KL. Safety concerns regarding binge drinking in pregnancy: a review. Birth Defects Res A Clin Mol Teratol. 2012;94:570–5.
19. Bay B, Kesmodel US. Prenatal alcohol exposure—a systematic review of the effects on child motor function. Acta Obstet Gynecol Scand. 2011;90:210–26.
20. Henderson J, Gray R, Brocklehurst P. Systematic review of effects of low-moderate prenatal alcohol exposure on pregnancy outcome. BJOG. 2007;114:243–52.
21. Kesmodel US, Bertrand J, Støvring H, Skarpness B, Denny C, Mortensen EL. The effect of different alcohol drinking patterns in early to mid pregnancy on the child's intelligence, attention, and executive function. BJOG. 2012;119:1180–90.
22. Sood B, Delaney-Black V, Covington C, Nordstrom-Klee B, Ager J, Templin T, Janisse J, Martier S, Sokol RJ. Prenatal alcohol exposure and childhood behavior at age 6 to 7 years: I. Dose-response effect. Pediatrics. 2001;108:e34.
23. Willford JA, Richardson GA, Leech SL, Day NL. Verbal and visuospatial learning and memory function in children with moderate prenatal alcohol exposure. Alcohol Clin Exp Res. 2004;28:497–507.
24. May PA, Marais AS, De Vries MM, et al. The prevalence, child characteristics, and maternal risk factors for the continuum of fetal alcohol spectrum disorders: a sixth population-based study in the same South African community. Drug Alcohol Depend. 2021;218:108408.
25. Chambers CD, Coles C, Kable J, Akshoomoff N, Xu R, Zellner JA, Honerkamp-Smith G, Manning MA, Adam MP, Jones KL. Fetal alcohol spectrum disorders in a Pacific Southwest City: maternal and child characteristics. Alcohol Clin Exp Res. 2019;43:2578–90.
26. Bandoli G, Jones K, Wertelecki W, Yevtushok L, Zymak-Zakutnya N, Granovska I, Plotka L, Chambers C. Patterns of prenatal alcohol exposure and alcohol-related dysmorphic features. Alcohol Clin Exp Res. 2020;44:2045–52.
27. Elliott AJ, Kinney HC, Haynes RL, et al. Concurrent prenatal drinking and smoking increases risk for SIDS: safe passage study report. EClinicalMedicine. 2020;19:100247.
28. McQuire C, Daniel R, Hurt L, Kemp A, Paranjothy S. The causal web of foetal alcohol spectrum disorders: a review and causal diagram. Eur Child Adolesc Psychiatry. 2020;29:575–94.
29. May PA, Gossage JP. Maternal risk factors for fetal alcohol spectrum disorders: not as simple as it might seem. Alcohol Res Heal. 2011;34:15–26.
30. Young-Wolff KC, Sarovar V, Tucker LY, Conway A, Alexeeff S, Weisner C, Armstrong MA, Goler N. Self-reported daily, weekly, and monthly cannabis use among women before and during pregnancy. JAMA Netw Open. 2019;2:1–10.
31. Fish EW, Murdaugh LB, Zhang C, et al. Cannabinoids exacerbate alcohol teratogenesis by a CB1-hedgehog interaction. Sci Rep. 2019;9:1–16.
32. Breit KR, Zamudio B, Thomas JD. The effects of alcohol and cannabinoid exposure during the brain growth spurt on behavioral development in rats. Birth Defects Res. 2019;111:760–74.

33. May PA, Gossage JP, Marais A-S, Hendricks LS, Snell CL, Tabachnick BG, Stellavato C, Buckley DG, Brooke LE, Viljoen DL. Maternal risk factors for fetal alcohol syndrome and partial fetal alcohol syndrome in South Africa: a third study. Alcohol Clin Exp Res. 2008;32:738–53.
34. Esper LH, Furtado EF. Identifying maternal risk factors associated with fetal alcohol spectrum disorders: a systematic review. Eur Child Adolesc Psychiatry. 2014;23:877–89.
35. Kaminen-Ahola N. Fetal alcohol spectrum disorders: genetic and epigenetic mechanisms. Prenat Diagn. 2020;40:1185–92.
36. Warren KR, Li T-K. Genetic polymorphisms: impact on the risk of fetal alcohol spectrum disorders. Birth Defects Res Part A Clin Mol Teratol. 2005;73:195–203.
37. Astley Hemingway SJ, Bledsoe JM, Brooks A, Davies JK, Jirikowic T, Olson EM, Thorne JC. Twin study confirms virtually identical prenatal alcohol exposures can lead to markedly different fetal alcohol spectrum disorder outcomes-fetal genetics influences fetal vulnerability. Adv Pediatr Res. 2018;5:23.
38. Kahila H, Marjonen H, Auvinen P, Avela K, Riikonen R, Kaminen-Ahola N. 18q12.3-q21.1 microdeletion detected in the prenatally alcohol-exposed dizygotic twin with discordant fetal alcohol syndrome phenotype. Mol Genet Genomic Med. 2020;8:e1192.
39. Jacobson SW, Carr LG, Croxford J, Sokol RJ, Li T-K, Jacobson JL. Protective effects of the alcohol dehydrogenase-ADH1B allele in children exposed to alcohol during pregnancy. J Pediatr. 2006;148:30–7.
40. May PA, Tabachnick B, Hasken JM, et al. Who is most affected by prenatal alcohol exposure: boys or girls? Drug Alcohol Depend. 2017;177:258–67.
41. Inkelis SM, Moore EM, Bischoff-Grethe A, Riley EP. Neurodevelopment in adolescents and adults with fetal alcohol spectrum disorders (FASD): a magnetic resonance region of interest analysis. Brain Res. 2020;1732:146654.
42. Price A, Cook PA, Norgate S, Mukherjee R. Prenatal alcohol exposure and traumatic childhood experiences: a systematic review. Neurosci Biobehav Rev. 2017;80:89–98.
43. Fagerlund Å, Autti-Rämö I, Hoyme HE, Mattson SN, Korkman M. Risk factors for behavioural problems in foetal alcohol spectrum disorders. Acta Paediatr. 2011;100:1481–8.
44. Rasmussen C, Andrew G, Zwaigenbaum L, Tough S. Neurobehavioural outcomes of children with fetal alcohol spectrum disorders: a Canadian perspective. Paediatr Child Health. 2008;13:185–91.
45. McDonald SW, Kehler HL, Tough SC. Protective factors for child development at age 2 in the presence of poor maternal mental health: results from the All Our Babies (AOB) pregnancy cohort. BMJ Open. 2016;6:e012096.
46. May PA, Hasken JM, Blankenship J, et al. Breastfeeding and maternal alcohol use: prevalence and effects on child outcomes and fetal alcohol spectrum disorders. Reprod Toxicol. 2016;63:13–21.
47. Brancato A, Castelli V, Lavanco G, Cannizzaro C. Environmental enrichment during adolescence mitigates cognitive deficits and alcohol vulnerability due to continuous and intermittent perinatal alcohol exposure in adult rats. Front Behav Neurosci. 2020;14:583122.
48. Wozniak JR, Riley EP, Charness ME. Clinical presentation, diagnosis, and management of fetal alcohol spectrum disorder. Lancet Neurol. 2019;18:760–70.
49. Bastons-Compta A, Astals M, Andreu-Fernandez V, Navarro-Tapia E, Garcia-Algar O. Postnatal nutritional treatment of neurocognitive deficits in fetal alcohol spectrum disorder. Biochem Cell Biol. 2018;96:213–21.
50. Idrus NM, Breit KR, Thomas JD. Dietary choline levels modify the effects of prenatal alcohol exposure in rats. Neurotoxicol Teratol. 2017;59:43–52.
51. Wozniak JR, Fink BA, Fuglestad AJ, et al. Four-year follow-up of a randomized controlled trial of choline for neurodevelopment in fetal alcohol spectrum disorder. J Neurodev Disord. 2020;12:9.
52. Young JK, Giesbrecht HE, Eskin MN, Aliani M, Suh M. Nutrition implications for fetal alcohol spectrum disorder. Adv Nutr. 2014;5:675–92.

53. Pollard MS, Tucker JS, Green HD Jr. Changes in adult alcohol use and consequences during the COVID-19 pandemic in the US. JAMA Netw Open. 2020;3:e2022942.
54. Hegaard HK, Rom AL, Christensen KB, Broberg L, Høgh S, Christiansen CH, Nathan NO, de Wolff MG, Damm P. Lifestyle habits among pregnant women in Denmark during the first COVID-19 lockdown compared with a historical period-a hospital-based cross-sectional study. Int J Environ Res Public Health. 2021;18:7128.
55. Kraus L, Seitz N-N, Piontek D, et al. 'Are The Times A-Changin'? Trends in adolescent substance use in Europe. Addiction. 2018;113:1317–32.

Chapter 3
Prevention of Exposure During the Preconception Period

Jessica Hanson

Introduction

Alcohol consumption during pregnancy, especially binge drinking, has the potential to cause lifelong physical and cognitive effects, as highlighted in other chapters of this book [1–3]. Fetal alcohol spectrum disorders (FASD) is the continuum of outcomes in those prenatally exposed to alcohol and includes diagnoses of fetal alcohol syndrome (FAS), partial-FAS, alcohol-related neurodevelopmental disorders (ARND), or alcohol-related birth defects (ARBD) [1]. Although most professional health boards advise against any drinking during pregnancy, the Centers for Disease Control and Prevention (CDC) found between 2% and 5% of people report binge drinking during pregnancy and 9–13% of those who are pregnant consume any amounts of alcohol [4].

Many types of interventions have been implemented to prevent alcohol-exposed pregnancies, most of which have promoted alcohol cessation among pregnant people, including behavioral interventions to encourage complete alcohol abstention during pregnancy [5–10]. A 2020 review of literature found 34 peer-reviewed interventions for those who are pregnant or postpartum, with nearly half of these utilizing screening and brief intervention techniques [11]. Additionally, examples of more general prevention efforts with all individuals who are pregnant to encourage alcohol abstinence include the use of mass media campaigns [12, 13], as well as policies to regulate drinking during pregnancy, which have limited evidence of any impact on drinking during pregnancy [14–17].

J. Hanson (✉)
Department of Applied Human Sciences, University of Minnesota Duluth, Duluth, MN, USA
e-mail: jdhanson@d.umn.edu

Preconceptual Approach to Prevention

Recent research concludes that prevention of FASD must begin preconceptually, or before a person even becomes pregnant [18]. According to experts on preconceptual approaches to alcohol-exposed pregnancy (AEP) prevention, focusing alcohol reduction efforts *only* on individuals who are already pregnant or who are planning to get pregnant ignores a large segment of those at risk for AEP: those not wanting or planning a pregnancy [19]. Nearly 20 years ago, the National Task Force on Fetal Alcohol Syndrome and Fetal Alcohol Effect in the United States stated that screening and providing interventions for those at risk for an AEP are essential, specifically by preventing unintended pregnancies or by discouraging alcohol consumption in people who are at risk for pregnancy [20]. Two of the task force's recommendations focused on universal prevention of FASD through reducing alcohol-related problems in people of child-bearing age who might become pregnant. There are several key areas in understanding prevention of FASD and AEP among non-pregnant individuals, including the relationship between alcohol consumption and sexual activity, particularly risky drinking in people at risk for an unintended pregnancy.

More specifically, there are three factors that influence risk for an AEP: alcohol use, sexual activity, and birth control use [18, 21]. In terms of alcohol use, behaviors around risky drinking are most concerning. Risky drinking can be conceptualized in one of two ways: binge drinking or heavy drinking. According to the CDC (2019), *binge drinking* is defined as a pattern of drinking that brings a person's blood alcohol concentration (BAC) to 0.08 g/dL or above. This typically happens when an individual consumes 4 or more drinks in about 2 h [22]. *Heavy drinking* is defined by the National Institute on Alcohol Abuse and Alcoholism (NIAAA) as consuming more than 3 drinks on any day or more than 7 drinks per week [23]. Risky drinking is increasing, with an estimated 5.3 million people in the United States currently drink in a way that "threatens their health, safety, and general well-being" [24]. Young people in their 20s and early 30s are more likely to drink than older individuals, and a previous history of physical or sexual abuse may make it more likely that an individual has a drinking problem [24].

Many people are vulnerable for an AEP because of continued risky drinking while being at risk for an unintended pregnancy, defined as being sexually active and able to get pregnant but using ineffective, inconsistent, or no birth control methods [25, 26]. Worldwide, 40% of pregnancies are unplanned [27], which ranges from 16% in the United Kingdom [28] to nearly one-half of in the United States [29], largely due to lack of effective or any type of contraception [19]. Although there has been a large increase in the use of birth control services among the general population [30], 38% of people who were sexually active and able to get pregnant in one study reported having missed at least one active pill in the prior 3 months, and 61% of condom users had not used a condom at every sexual encounter [26]. People who are able to get pregnant but who are less likely to use birth control during sex include those who have less than a college education; are of younger reproductive age; and believe that health care providers did not respond adequately to method-related questions [26, 28, 31–33]. In addition, individuals over 30 years old and those who are nonwhite tend to express more ambivalence about their intentions to become pregnant, a factor that has been associated with using less effective birth control methods [26, 31, 34].

As noted in a recent review article on causes and risk factors for FASD, unplanned pregnancy is a risk factor for FASD [35], as unplanned pregnancy appears to be more common among those who drink regularly or exhibit risky drinking patterns [28, 32, 33, 36]. In fact, in a sample of individuals in the U.S. who gave birth to a child later diagnosed with FAS, 73% of their pregnancies were unplanned [37]. Unintended pregnancies are problematic when those at risk for an unplanned pregnancy are drinking at risky levels, as these individuals may not realize they are pregnant for several weeks and are thus exposing the fetus to alcohol during an especially vulnerable developmental period [38]. Often, the level of drinking during the first trimester and before confirmation of pregnancy may have already been detrimental to the developing fetus [18, 36, 38]. According to the previous research, alcohol can cause "severe and permanent brain damage as early as the third week of pregnancy" [19]. In addition, central nervous system (CNS), heart, and eye and limb development can be impacted by prenatal alcohol exposure in the first trimester [39]. Though many significantly reduce their alcohol use once they know they are pregnant [40], alcohol use before pregnancy is a strong predictor of alcohol use during pregnancy, especially during the first trimester [36, 41–45]. In a sample of individuals with pregnancies that ended in a live birth, preconception binge drinkers were more likely to engage in other risky behaviors, including drinking during pregnancy [32]. Likewise, as synthesized in a recent review article, people who gave birth to a child with an FASD have been found to be more likely to drink at risky levels prior to pregnancy and had a history of alcohol abuse when compared to those without a child with an FASD [35, 46–48].

Alcohol consumption can also have an impact on the prevention of pregnancy, specifically method and consistency of birth control utilization [49], especially with "casual" partners [50]. Unplanned sexual intercourse under the influence of alcohol or other drugs has been found to be an "independent risk factor for multiple sexual partners and inconsistent condom use" [51]. In particular, binge drinking is associated with not using contraception during sex consistently or at all [52]. A study with both White/European Americans and Black/African Americans in the U.S. found that binge drinking in the preconception period was associated with unintended pregnancies; specifically, individuals with the highest reported binge drinking episodes also had the highest rate of unplanned pregnancies [32]. Several studies with adolescents and young adults have also found relationships between alcohol and other substance use and risky sexual behaviors, such as multiple sexual partners and sexual intercourse without use of a condom [53–57]. While other studies contradict these findings somewhat [58, 59], this research highlights the ongoing relationship between alcohol use and sexual behaviors. In fact, a national U.S. study of young adults aged 18–20 found that those who were at risk for an AEP were more likely to use alcohol to enhance sexual activity, such as feeling closer to a partner, being less nervous during sex, and enjoying sex [60].

Therefore, the dyadic relationship of alcohol and sexual behavior influences birth control use and causes an increased risk for an AEP among the offspring of those of reproductive age. In fact, among individuals who are susceptible to an unintended pregnancy, approximately 55% consume some amount of alcohol, with 12.4–13.1% either binge drinking or drinking frequently [61]. A separate study from the CDC estimated that the weighted prevalence of AEP risk in the U.S. among those who are aged 15–44 years was 7.3%, which means that during a 1-month period, approximately 3.3 million in the U.S. were at risk for an AEP [62]. Another study from a team of CDC researchers found that 3.4%, or 1 in 30, of all non-pregnant people were at risk of an AEP, and that pregnancy intention was strongly associated with AEP risk [63]. A study from South Africa found that over 20% of those who were sexually active were at risk for an AEP [64], and a study from Russia showed that between 32% and 54% would be classified as at risk for an AEP [65], showing the disparity between geographic regions.

A separate study attempted to provide a more definitive number of those at risk of AEP and alcohol-exposed births in the United States using data from preconceptual individuals aged 15–44 years from the 2011–2013 National Survey of Family Growth. This project used three criteria: (1) included data only on people "likely to have drunk alcohol after pregnancy was established" and that included binge drinking regardless of frequency; (2) included individuals likely to have become pregnant during a month when both drinking and unprotected sex occurred; and (3) accounted for three pregnancy outcomes: miscarriage, abortion, and birth. Using these assumptions, there were an estimated 2.5 million fewer expected cases of AEPs in the United States compared to the 2016 CDC estimate. More specifically, the research found that the estimated prevalence of AEPs was 1.2% (95% confidence interval, 0.9–1.7), which means an estimated 731,000 (range 104,000–1,242,000) of individuals from this study were at risk for an AEP during a 1-month time period [66]. Additional studies to more clearly understand risk for AEP are outlined in the last section of this chapter.

Levels of Prevention

Prevention of AEP during the preconceptual time period is challenging because many people do not believe that AEP prevention applies to them. The drinking threshold above which AEPs can occur, particularly risky or heavy drinking as defined earlier, may not be considered problematic by many [19]. Those who are younger, single, or in college, may drink above risky levels but think their drinking is normal or even less when compared to their peers [67, 68]. In addition, traditional FASD messages that focus on pregnant people and/or on stopping drinking completely may generate reasons that FASD and AEP prevention doesn't apply to them

[19]. Fortunately, there is a continuum of interventions to prevent FASD at the preconceptual level, including universal, selective, and indicated interventions [69]. First, universal prevention provides AEP and FASD prevention messages for all, without regard to differential risk factors. In FASD prevention, this has been seen with regard to public education on FASD, such as public service announcements, posters, and social media posts, as well as labels that warn against drinking during pregnancy and other laws and regulations [69]. These types of universal interventions have appeared to increase knowledge about the harms of drinking during pregnancy, although there is little evidence that these broad prevention efforts change actual behaviors around FASD and AEP risk [69].

Second, selective prevention targets groups that are thought to be at risk for alcohol-exposed pregnancies but does not focus on specific individuals. These efforts are targeted to a population subgroup of people at high risk of delivering a child with FASD simply by virtue of belonging to that subgroup. With FASD, this would include groups with higher rates of drinking during pregnancy, such as those individuals who are older [36, 38, 70]. In addition, those who gave birth to children who have a diagnosis of FASD tended to have increased depression, later recognition that they were pregnant, lower educational attainment, and other drug use during pregnancy [71], which may be subgroups included in a selective prevention effort. Selective prevention for AEP with the preconceptual population is challenging because it technically includes any person of reproductive age who drinks alcohol at a risky level who may be sexually active, is able to get pregnant, and not using effective or any type of contraception [69]. As highlighted in the next section, these selective AEP prevention efforts at the preconceptual level might occur on college campuses where risky drinking often occurs.

Finally, indicated prevention interventions are targeted to high-risk individuals who meet specific criteria for being at risk. Often, indicated prevention is focused on individuals with genetic or other biological markers indicating a predisposition to a certain disease. For FASD and AEP, much is unknown about a genetic predisposition to having a child born with FASD, although it is well-known that genetic factors play a role in risk for certain alcohol-related harms [72], and more is being discovered on the role of genetics on the impact of prenatal alcohol exposure [73–76]. Research does show that individuals who have previously given birth to a child with an FASD are at higher risk of having another child with FASD [37], and the Institute of Medicine (1996) specifically recommends that a pregnant person who currently or previously drank alcohol or who has already given birth to a child with an FASD be provided with an indicated intervention [69]. For those who are preconceptual, the risk for AEP is less clear, as what "high risk" is for AEP is convoluted. In those with a diagnosed alcohol dependence, a referral for a formal treatment and specific counsel on prenatal alcohol exposure is important, but addiction is not a prerequisite for AEP risk [69]. Regardless, there is a plethora of indicated AEP prevention efforts when compared to universal or selective efforts. As with selective prevention, indicated prevention of AEP with preconceptual individuals is complicated but distinctly possible.

Universal Prevention of AEP

Screening for AEP Risk

Universal prevention efforts with preconceptual individuals typically focus on general screening for risk and health education on AEP in general. While most information in published literature is focused on those who are pregnant, there are relatively new recommendations to utilize with preconceptual people. The first step when providing general screening for AEP risk is to identify risky (e.g., heavy and binge) drinking, defined earlier. For example, the U.S. Preventive Services Task Force recommends that all people aged 18 years and older be screened for heavy and binge drinking when seeking primary care [77]. Risky drinking patterns can be cross-tabulated with risk for an unintended pregnancy, and a brief intervention focused on AEP risk may be appropriate. Likewise, asking a single question of all preconceptual individuals seen at a healthcare facility can help facilitate discussions on risky drinking. This idea of *One Key Question*, where healthcare providers screen for pregnancy intent, has shown success in one state in the U.S. and is gaining traction nationally. Those who do not desire a pregnancy in the next year can be referred to counseling and contraceptive care [78]. Additional details on the *One Key Question* program are located later in this chapter with other research recommendations.

To implement screening for AEP risk generally, training health care providers on ethical and appropriate ways to screen for alcohol, pregnancy intent, and AEP risk is often necessary [79–81]. Researchers supported by the CDC have suggested a multi-disciplinary training program in order to reach a wide variety of health care providers [82]. Training health care providers on evidence-based communication styles such as motivational interviewing (MI) or other brief intervention techniques can aid in the response to any positive screens, while also boosting confidence in health care providers in addressing this sensitive issue with preconceptual individuals [81, 83]. Examples of collaborations between academic, research-based training units, and health care providers can be found in recent literature, as well as lessons learned in implementing these multi-level screening programs [82, 84]. These interventions should occur at multiple levels to include policy and health system change strategies to promote required alcohol and AEP screening practices [82].

Health Education Campaigns

In addition to screening for AEP risk in health care settings, health education campaigns are often used as a way to prevent AEP on a universal level. While many efforts have been focused on reducing drinking during pregnancy, there are some campaigns that have been developed and implemented with preconceptual populations and that utilize multiple mediums to disseminate messages. Researchers in the Netherlands developed a campaign to promote healthy behaviors in preconceptual couples who were planning pregnancy. Included in the posters, flyers, a website, and social media feeds were messages about alcohol cessation when planning a pregnancy. It appeared the health campaign was successful, with 62.4% of preconceptual participants who were exposed to the intervention reducing or completing quitting alcohol consumption, which was higher than the 48.7% in the comparison group who were not exposed to the intervention [85]. An FASD and AEP prevention campaign developed in South Africa used similar mediums and also include community health workers who led community and facility/hospital-level "health talks" to address drinking prior to and during pregnancy. Similar to the Netherlands campaign, the health education campaign in South Africa saw increases in knowledge in those with multiple exposures to the different messages, and most who had been exposed to FASD educational media believed they would modify their drinking behaviors during future pregnancies [86].

Within these examples are questions of what specific elements of persuasion contribute to an impactful health education campaign (e.g., *why* does a message work in reducing risk for AEP). A study in Australia tested different messages, specifically those that included either threat messages, self-efficacy messages, or both. This study found that the two experimental threat concepts were significantly more effective than the positive appeal (self-efficacy alone) with respect to intention and confidence to not drink in future pregnancies [87]. In addition to carefully considering the types of messaging of health education campaigns when preventing AEP is *how* these messages are created. In developing prevention efforts on the sensitive topics of risky drinking and unintended pregnancy, community input and involvement from the inception of such campaigns is recommended [88, 89]. For example, a broad health education campaign on AEP prevention with three American Indian tribal communities in the Great Plains of the U.S. was developed by conducting focus groups in each of the communities to better understand media preferences, wording, and use of traditional language and images. Additional input involved having community members provide input into the final versions of each of the messages and dissemination practices [90].

Selective Prevention of AEP

Selective AEP prevention occurs in places or with groups where high AEP risk occurs, not specifically with individuals screening positive for AEP risk, as is seen with indicated prevention. There are fewer examples of selective AEP interventions for preconceptual individuals, and often these interventions include screening for AEP risk in specific settings or providing education those groups who may be at higher risk, such as those seeking out emergency contraception to prevent a pregnancy [91]. For example, a multi-site AEP prevention intervention was implemented at sexually transmitted disease (STD) clinics that served patients with a high prevalence of heavy alcohol consumption coupled with ineffective contraceptive use [92]. Such interventions are also often targeted on college campuses where high bingeing and risky sexual behaviors often occur, although knowledge of FASD is relatively high in college-aged individuals [93]. General education in combination with MI-based interventions (e.g., Project CHOICES, described in the next section) is often successful with college-aged individuals [94, 95] and has been shown to be also feasible and acceptable with those who are younger than college-aged [96].

Finally, a web-based intervention with people seeking Women Infant and Children (WIC) services focused on both alcohol and contraception in attempts to lower AEP risk [97], as lower levels of education and income have been identified as risk factors for FASD [98, 99] (although it should be noted that research has found individuals within higher socioeconomic classes are more likely to drink during pregnancy [35]). A similar example of a selective intervention occurred with American Indian and Alaska Natives in Southern California (U.S.). It utilized Screening, Brief Intervention, and Referral to Treatment (SBIRT) concepts to reduce AEP risk for individuals of childbearing age, but enrolled anyone who completed a survey regarding alcohol and contraceptive use, even those who were pregnant; about one-third were at risk for an AEP. Participants were randomized into either a "treatment as usual" or intervention group, where the intervention group received an online, web-based intervention. Both the intervention and control group significantly decreased their drinking and therefore AEP risk, and there were no differences between the treatment groups, indicating that just participating in the screening assessment may have been sufficient to change behaviors [100].

Indicated Prevention of AEP

The majority of preconceptual approaches to AEP prevention in peer-reviewed, published literature are focused on indicated interventions with individuals who screen positive for AEP risk. The reason that there are a great number of indicated intervention efforts is likely because of the cost–benefit relationship with these interventions: although these interventions may not reach as many people as more universal interventions (e.g., health campaigns), they are more likely to impact behaviors and therefore reduce risk for AEP in higher risk individuals. Indicated prevention of AEP focuses on two behaviors: reducing risky drinking (e.g., heavy or binge drinking) in individuals who can become pregnant, are sexually active, and are not using effective or any contraception during sex, meaning they are at risk for an unintended pregnancy.

Project CHOICES

One of the major efforts to decrease risk for AEPs among non-pregnant individuals was Project CHOICES (Changing High-risk alcOhol use and Increasing Birth control Effectiveness Study). This intervention focused on reducing risk for AEPs through alcohol reduction and pregnancy prevention for those at risk for AEP. The original CHOICES research utilized four motivational interviewing (MI) sessions, a counseling style that "guides the individual to explore and resolve ambivalence about changing [behavior], highlighting and increasing perceived discrepancy between current behaviors and overall goals and values" [101]. Elements of the brief motivational intervention utilized for this intervention included personalized feedback about drinking and utilization of birth control compared to population norms and goal setting regarding birth control and drinking [101]. The intervention also included a separate session to discuss birth control methods.

Participants in the original Project CHOICES were non-pregnant individuals from various settings in three Southern states who were at high risk for an AEP. They were randomized to receive information plus the brief intervention sessions or information only. Overall, the Project CHOICES intervention significantly decreased the risk of an AEP in the intervention group. Of the participants who completed all the intervention sessions, 68.5% were no longer at risk for an AEP through either increasing birth control or decreasing binge drinking rates; a large proportion of those who reduced risk changed both behaviors. There was a statistically significant difference in risky drinking and birth control utilization between the two groups, with the intervention group having significantly lower drinking rates and increased birth control use 9 months after completing the four intervention sessions [21, 40, 101, 102].

There have been several ancillary studies from the original Project CHOICES. Project BALANCE (Birth control and ALcohol Awareness: Negotiating Choices Effectively) was an intervention with non-pregnant, college-aged individuals that adapted the Project CHOICES curriculum to include a single session of personalized feedback with a MI-based intervention. People from one university who binge drank and were using birth control ineffectively were recruited and assigned to either the intervention or control group (education only). While both groups reduce AEP risk, the intervention condition was more likely to change both contraception use and risky drinking and fewer of the individuals in this group changed neither [95, 103]. Also, when compared to the original CHOICES study, the college-aged participants of Project BALANCE were proportionately less likely to reduce risky drinking but more likely to achieve effective contraception [95].

Project EARLY (no acronym definition given), another spin-off of Project CHOICES, was a randomized control trial to test the efficacy of a one-session MI intervention (compared to the original four-sessions) to reduce the risk for AEPs in a general population of women from one U.S. state. This ancillary study was particularly focused on the impact of the one-session intervention on the Transtheoretical Model Stages of Change (precontemplation, contemplation, preparation, action, and maintenance) regarding alcohol use and consistent use of birth control. The results indicated that there were differences in drinking behavior and birth control use depending on where a person fell in the Stages of Change continuum. Specifically, there were significant differences found in the total number of drinks consumed in the past 90 days for participants in the respective five stages of change, with individuals in the preparation stage reporting drinking a significantly higher amount of alcohol. In addition, significant differences in birth control ineffectiveness were found for participants at different stages of change, with individuals in precontemplation reporting higher levels of birth control ineffectiveness [104]. These findings indicate that an intervention, like Project CHOICES, that focuses on moving people along the Stages of Change continuum can have a significant impact on reducing risk for AEP. Project EARLY has been additionally tested for feasibility using remote-delivery methods, which showed short-term success in reducing AEP risk [105].

Like remote Project EARLY, additional ancillary studies from Project CHOICES have utilized remote ways of interacting to prevent AEP. The Healthy Choices intervention compared the results of a telephone versus in-person application of CHOICES, in this case with two sessions versus the original four. A project with three tribes in the Great Plains of the United States also utilized a telephone-based intervention that included the CHOICES curriculum [106]. Both telephone interventions of CHOICES—Healthy CHOICES and the tribal project—were successful in showing decreases in AEP risk, particularly in regard to increasing utilization of contraception [106, 107]. A similarly named Project Healthy CHOICES focused on implementing a self-administered, mail-based version of Project CHOICES [94]; data specifically with the Hispanic participants of this study found outcomes similar to the original Project CHOICES intervention, although this sample reduced AEP risk primarily by practicing effective birth control [108]. Finally, the CHOICES intervention has been adapted into a scalable Internet intervention called the Contraception and Alcohol Risk Reduction Internet Intervention (CARRII). A feasibility study of the CARRII intervention showed that it was acceptable and feasible to the study population, and the promising impact it had on AEP risk needs additional testing [109]. Another web-based AEP intervention with preconceptual individuals used self-guided change materials that were similar to CHOICES and found similar preliminary successes in reducing AEP risk [110].

The CHOICES intervention has also addressed additional behaviors in addition to AEP. In particular, CHOICES Plus was created to address both AEP prevention and also smoking-exposed pregnancies (SEP). Research from the original CHOICES study found that over 17% of the participants were also at risk for a SEP, in addition to being at risk for an AEP. In fact, the co-occurrence of AEP and SEP was more prevalent (16.4%) than AEP risk (5.5%) or SEP risk (14.0%) alone [111]. Several factors differentiated individuals at dual risk for SEP/AEP versus just AEP alone, such as lower socioeconomic level, higher frequency of sexual intercourse without use of contraception, and higher frequency of alcohol use and mental disorders [112]. Therefore, CHOICES Plus was designed using the CHOICES curriculum with additional activities for smoking cessation and was subsequently tested in a randomized controlled trial. CHOICES Plus subsequently reduced both AEP and SEP risk both [113]. Of interest is that those at risk for SEP were more likely to reduce their risk by utilizing effective contraception when compared to reducing their risk through smoking cessation [113].

Finally, the CHOICES intervention has been implemented in several diverse subpopulations. Tribal communities in the Great Plains of the United States led efforts to adapt and pilot the two-session, in-person CHOICES intervention with American

Indian individuals at risk for AEP [114]. A feasibility study of the adapted in-person CHOICES with American Indians found significant reductions in AEP risk [115], and a subsequent randomized controlled trial is underway to more thoroughly test the intervention effectiveness with tribal communities [116]. The feasibility study did show that individuals who reduced risk were more likely to do so by improving their use of effective contraception when compared to reducing risky drinking [106]. The in-person CHOICES intervention was also modified for use in a group MI session and pilot tested with American Indians; while success of CHOICES in a group setting is pending, this was an important expansion of CHOICES that could be utilized in future studies [117]. In addition to CHOICES with American Indian communities, the intervention has been used with adolescent and adult Latinx individuals in the Southwest of the United States, including within Project Healthy CHOICES as described above, which reduced AEP primarily by improving birth control use [108]. Another implementation of Project CHOICES with Hispanics who were currently seeking alcohol treatment showed preliminary success in reducing risk for AEP in this population by improving both alcohol abstinence and contraception use [118]. Finally, an intervention similar to Project CHOICES that included multiple in-person MI sessions adapted the curriculum for use in South Africa and found that AEP risk was reduced mainly by a significant uptake in contraception.

Parent-Child Assistance Program (PCAP)

Another indicated effort to prevent AEP is the Parent-Child Assistance Program (PCAP). While PCAP was primarily focused on providing home visitation services to pregnant people who were drinking alcohol and using other drugs, it also provided the intervention in the postpartum period in order to prevent future alcohol- and drug-exposed births among those who already delivered at least one exposed child. Participants were therefore enrolled for approximately 3 years, and PCAP case managers assisted them in obtaining alcohol and drug treatment and linked them with comprehensive community resources. PCAP participants worked with the case managers during regular home visitations to identify personal goals and steps necessary to achieve them. An analysis of PCAP participants found reduced risk for AEP via improved abstinence from alcohol and other drugs and increased use of regular and reliable contraception [119]. An economic analysis of PCAP estimated that the number of FASD cases prevented by the PCAP programs varied from 20 to 43, and the net monetary benefit from $13 to $31 million [120].

Like CHOICES, PCAP has several ancillary studies to test the impact of the intervention with various groups. For example, the Washington State (U.S.) legislature funded PCAP sites in nine counties and on the Spokane Reservation, creating a capacity to serve nearly 700 families state-wide. As well, the Alberta First Steps intervention is modeled after PCAP and aims to prevent alcohol- and drug-exposed births among individuals who have already had an exposed child. These PCAP replications appeared successful in reducing AEP risk. The Alberta First Steps intervention, for example, had a significant increase in birth control use and at program exit, many participants were abstinent from alcohol and/or drugs and the majority did not experience a subsequent pregnancy [9]. A comparison between rural-urban differences in PCAP outcomes revealed that people living in rural areas reported higher use of alcohol at the end of PCAP, were less likely to complete outpatient substance abuse treatment compared to urban participants, and used fewer services during the last year of PCAP [121]. However, a qualitative evaluation of PCAP services found the relational and trauma-informed nature of PCAP was "perceived to have positive impacts and be well suited for use with Indigenous communities" [122].

Prevention of AEP in Special Populations

Adolescents

There is a need to focus on AEP prevention with adolescents as few of the prevention efforts detailed in this chapter was specifically with this population besides those in college. One of the few studies on teen substance use during pregnancy found that pregnant teens reported elevated levels of substance use prior to becoming pregnant, with varying substance use by subgroups of pregnant adolescents [123, 124]. A recent study found 24.9% of pregnant teenagers reported using one or more substances in the past 30 days, although the majority quit using substances when they found out they were pregnant [123]. In regard to preconceptual adolescents, unplanned sexual intercourse under the influence of alcohol or other drugs has been found to be an independent risk factor for multiple sexual partners and inconsistent condom use among adolescents [51]. In addition, certain demographic characteristics are more prevalent in younger, non-pregnant individuals who consume alcohol and are at risk for an unintended pregnancy. For example, older adolescence (i.e., those between 18 and 24), a single marital status, and a higher income are each associated with high rates of alcohol consumption [125, 126], and one study of college-aged individuals found that 49% reported binge drinking and using withdrawal as their birth control, a method that has a 22% failure rate [103].

Health campaigns and multimedia programs have also been targeted to younger populations as a way to provide general education on FASD and the preconceptual prevention of AEP [127, 128]. While these health campaigns show preliminary changes in knowledge, none show any changes in behaviors related to AEP prevention. To further reach this population, recent indicated interventions have been developed to target both unintended pregnancy and risky drinking, as seen in a randomized controlled trial with indigenous youth in the U.S. [129]. Also, as noted earlier, the CHOICES intervention has been shown to be successful with those who are college-aged (e.g., Project BALANCE), and CHOICES has been shown to be feasible and acceptable with younger individuals, aged 14–17. This study, called

CHOICES-TEEN, showed preliminary success in reducing AEP risk in teens in the juvenile justice system [96]. There have also been efforts to evaluate the feasibility and acceptability of an eHealth intervention, modeled after Project CHOICES, with American Indian/Alaska Native teens in the U.S. [130, 131]. Both CHOICES-TEEN and the eHealth intervention need further testing to determine its impact on drinking and contraception behaviors in adolescents but highlight both the feasibility and acceptability of AEP prevention in younger individuals potentially at risk for AEP.

Diverse Populations

As noted throughout this chapter, many AEP prevention efforts have focused on diverse populations. The original Project CHOICES research study screened 2672 participants aged 18–44 for AEP risk at six settings: an urban jail, a drug/alcohol treatment facility, a gynecology clinic, two primary care clinics, and respondents to a media solicitation. The samples who were screened for AEP were of lower socio-economic status (e.g., 70% reported a household income of <$20,000 and 68% had a high school or equivalent education), and 62% were African American [101]. Of those who screened *positive* for AEP risk (e.g., 12.5% of those screened), nearly half were Black/non-Hispanic and single. As well, many of the ancillary CHOICES studies have focused on diverse subpopulations. For example, much of the expansion of CHOICES, PCAP, and other preconceptual AEP prevention work has been focused with indigenous communities in the United States and Canada, as well as with Hispanic communities in the U.S. and in the Western Cape in South Africa [9, 90, 96, 100, 106–108, 115–118, 122, 129, 130, 132].

While prevention and intervention efforts have been focused on diverse populations, issues surrounding AEP is not a health issue that only impacts communities of color. More specifically, the concern in this is not that half of all Black/non-Hispanic people in the original Project CHOICES study received the intervention, or that there are several examples of AEP prevention in indigenous communities. Indeed, these are important efforts that are often instigated and guided by community leaders, as shown in much of the research around adaptations to Project CHOICES and other AEP prevention efforts with indigenous communities [89, 100, 114, 116, 129]. Instead, the question is why other, more general populations are underrepresented in AEP prevention research and that additional implementation or dissemination research has not yet focused on more general populations of individuals who have certain risk factors based on previous research studies [32, 36, 44, 46, 47, 133–135]. The lack of dissemination to more general populations may be because of some of the controversies around AEP prevention detailed later in this chapter, but it may also be because this is seen as a health problem in certain, more diverse communities when in fact that is not necessarily the case, at least not based on what is known in the published literature. In addition to future efforts of more universal or selective AEP interventions, more research is needed on the surveillance of AEP risk. Additional recommendations for research surrounding this issue are in the last section of this chapter.

Historical Trends and Future Predictions

Historical Trends

While these efforts to move preconceptual prevention of AEP continue to move forward, this field is historically not without its controversies, particularly with universal prevention efforts. In 2016, the CDC published and disseminated new data on preconceptual risk for AEP in the U.S. Noted earlier, the CDC analyzed data from the 2011–2013 National Survey of Family Growth and included information from 4303 non-pregnant people aged 15–44 years. An individual was considered at risk for an AEP during the past month if they were having vaginal intercourse, drank any alcohol, did not (and the sexual partner did not) use contraception during sex in the past month, and were able to get pregnant (e.g., neither partner was sterile) [62]. The authors of the study estimated that approximately 7.3%, or 3.3 million people in the U.S., aged 15–44 were at risk for an AEP during a 1-month period. Along with the publication, the CDC developed infographics and talking points for health care providers to talk to individuals about risky drinking if they were at risk for an unintended pregnancy. These handouts had descriptors such as *Alcohol and Pregnancy: Why take the risk?* and *Drinking too much can have many risks for women.* They emphasized the brief nature of many alcohol screening tools, and that "this clinical service is effective, inexpensive, and can be accomplished in 6–15 min, although follow-up sessions might be needed. Health care providers should advise women not to drink at all if they are pregnant or might be pregnant." The updated versions of these materials are still available on the CDC website as of 2021 [136].

When the publication and health education materials were released, there were some key recommendations that were viewed as controversial. There was information in one of the infographics that focused on the potential increased risks for any person (who identifies as a woman) who is drinking at risky levels, including increased risk for injuries/violence, heart disease, cancer, sexually transmitted infections, and unintended pregnancy. This information and recommendations were viewed as victim blaming for people who were sexually or otherwise assaulted. It also appeared to miss a clear explanation of the complicated link between alcohol and sexual activity, which includes issues of inhibitions, coercion, and consent; this is very different to the cause-and-effect relationship between alcohol and birth defects. In response to the controversy, there were opinion pieces and editorials in major newspapers and other media outlets, such as the Washington Post, Los Angeles Times, the BBC, and National Public Radio. The titles of these op-eds included *The CDC's Alcohol Warning Shames and Discriminates against Women* and *The CDC Can Rip the Wine Glass Out of My Childbearing-Aged Hand.* Within these editorials were quotes such as, "The CDC's rec nails the trifecta of impractical, sexist, and alarmist," and "If having a drink was really unsafe for sexually active women, that danger would be manifest in an incredibly high number of births with FASD not only in this country, but around the world."

As the original data and subsequent infographics and recommendations came from a subgroup at the CDC that aims to decrease FASD and other preventable disabilities, it was apparent that the message of reducing risk for AEP was being lost in the controversy. The health education materials were subsequently updated with a focus on individual issues: alcohol has health risks for everyone; alcohol is a teratogen; many people drink when they don't realize they are pregnant; and many are at risk for an unplanned pregnancy. The health education materials were also edited to include more information on FASD specifically. However, this controversy repeated itself in 2021 with recommendations from the World Health Organization's (WHO) *Global Alcohol Action Plan 2022–2030*, which included statements on reducing or abstaining from alcohol to prevent the effects of drinking while pregnant or of childbearing ages [137]. Editorials speaking against these recommendations were titled things such as *The WHO Alcohol-Pregnancy Warning for Childbearing Women Overlooks Men, As Usual.* One editorial stated, "It is extremely disturbing to see the World Health Organization risk hard-won women's rights by attempting to control their bodies and choices in this way" and another news story included this quote: "As well as being sexist and paternalistic, and potentially restricting the freedoms of most women, it goes well beyond their remit and is not rooted in science." The response from the scientific community has attempted to redirect the issue back to AEP and FASD prevention in both the CDC and WHO examples, and future research is needed to better discuss AEP and FASD as public health issues.

Future Goals

The future of research in AEP risk and prevention must consider several questions, starting with sifting through the convoluted nature of AEP risk. First, *what is the impact of AEP?* In other words, what is the health outcome related to AEP and what is the best way to communicate this risk? As noted, the CDC estimated that the weighted prevalence of AEP risk among in the U.S. among those aged 15–44 years was 7.3%, or approximately 3.3 million individuals per month [62]. A separate study accounted for different pregnancy outcomes, actual likelihood of a pregnancy in any given month, and assumptions about continuing to drink while pregnant; this study found a much more conservative estimated prevalence of 1.2%, or about 731,000 individuals per month, and an additional 0.8%, or 481,000 people, at risk for an alcohol-exposed birth [66]. Within the range of 1.2–7.3% of *potential* risk for AEP, which may vary based on geographically and among different subpopulations of a community, most people who do become pregnant will stop drinking when they find out they are pregnant [138]. As there have been no studies linking risk for AEP with later having a child diagnosed with FAS or another FASD, the health outcomes of AEP are unclear, one of the main critiques of the CDC and WHO recommendations.

With the CDC/WHO controversy and not knowing the short- or long-term health impact of AEP, discussing AEP risk is something that many health professionals do not tackle. One potential way to overcome the sensitivity of AEP risk is to focus more on birth control rather than alcohol. Unintended pregnancies (either due to contraceptive failure or sex without contraceptives) account for 80% (75–87%) of pregnancies unknowingly exposed to alcohol [139]. An effort called "One Key Question" is attracting national interest for its easy way of addressing pregnancy risk and a person's health status prior to becoming pregnant. The one key question—"would you like to become pregnant in the next year?"—could potentially be asked as a general screen for all individuals of childbearing age, who are able to become pregnant, coming in for well visits. For individuals who choose not to become pregnant or are not definitive in their pregnancy intent, there provides an opportunity to focus on birth control and pregnancy prevention, as well as education on behaviors (e.g., nutrition, substance use) that could impact a pregnancy, should one occur [78]. While the adoption of One Key Question may take a paradigm shift in many medical practices, contraception is an extremely promising and effective way of reducing one's risk to AEP as highlighted in much of the Project CHOICES ancillary studies.

Secondly, future research must better understand *who is at risk?* As noted earlier, prevention of AEP with diverse populations has been the main focus of AEP intervention development, particularly with indicated interventions. However, researchers continue to make assumptions about AEP risk based on certain demographic features that are currently unsupported by surveillance data. For example, several of the CHOICES ancillary studies in the U.S. have been focused in indigenous communities. While many of these are community driven, American Indian/Alaska Natives have been found to be less likely to report pre-pregnancy alcohol use in the years preceding pregnancy when compared to White/European Americans (56% vs. 76%) [133]. Among this same sample, similar percentages of American Indian/Alaska Native and Caucasian American participants reported not drinking alcohol during pregnancy (89% and 87%, respectively) [133]. Parallel to this, recent FAS surveillance data from an active case ascertainment study in the Great Plains area of the United States, which oversampled for indigenous children, found no difference in FAS when comparing indigenous children to other races [140]. Note there were also no socioeconomic differences when comparing those with FAS in this sample. As well, a study with one tribal community in California had similar rates of FAS when compared to U.S. national rates (e.g., no difference between tribe and national, more general rates) [141].

Ultimately, prevention of FASD with preconceptual individuals has great potential, and there are several examples of universal, selective, and indicated prevention that can be expanded upon. Before beginning such implementation and dissemination efforts on AEP interventions, additional surveillance is vital to have a clear picture of who is actually at risk, as well as the short- and long-term outcomes of

AEP. More universal AEP screening efforts are likely to impact what we know in terms of prevalence of AEP risk and outcomes and can better inform selective and indicated prevention of AEP in particular. There is also opportunity for more inclusive prevention efforts, such as reaching more rural communities through e- and mHealth interventions as well as changing the language around AEP prevention to include people who are non-binary and gender non-conforming. The issue of FASD is a spectrum, as are the intervention efforts needed to prevent the health outcomes related to prenatal alcohol consumption.

References

1. Hoyme HE, Kalberg WO, Elliott AJ, et al. Updated clinical guidelines for diagnosing fetal alcohol spectrum disorders. Pediatrics. 2016;138 https://doi.org/10.1542/peds.2015-4256.
2. May PA, Blankenship J, Marais AS, et al. Maternal alcohol consumption producing fetal alcohol spectrum disorders (FASD): quantity, frequency, and timing of drinking. Drug Alcohol Depend. 2013;133:502–12. https://doi.org/10.1016/j.drugalcdep.2013.07.013.
3. May PA, Chambers CD, Kalberg WO, et al. Prevalence of fetal alcohol spectrum disorders in 4 US communities. JAMA. 2018;319:474–82. https://doi.org/10.1001/jama.2017.21896.
4. Denny CH, Acero CS, Terplan M, et al. Trends in alcohol use among pregnant women in the U.S., 2011-2018. Am J Prev Med. 2020;59:768–9. https://doi.org/10.1016/j.amepre.2020.05.017.
5. May PA, Miller JH, Goodhart KA, et al. Enhanced case management to prevent fetal alcohol spectrum disorders in Northern Plains communities. Matern Child Health J. 2008;12:747–59. https://doi.org/10.1007/s10995-007-0304-2.
6. Chang G, McNamara TK, Orav EJ, et al. Brief intervention for prenatal alcohol use: the role of drinking goal selection. J Subst Abus Treat. 2006;31:419–24. https://doi.org/10.1016/j.jsat.2006.05.016.
7. Handmaker NS, Miller WR, Manicke M. Findings of a pilot study of motivational interviewing with pregnant drinkers. J Stud Alcohol. 1999;60:285–7. https://doi.org/10.15288/jsa.1999.60.285.
8. Armstrong MA, Kaskutas LA, Witbrodt J, et al. Using drink size to talk about drinking during pregnancy: a randomized clinical trial of Early Start Plus. Soc Work Health Care. 2009;48:90–103. https://doi.org/10.1080/00981380802451210.
9. Rasmussen C, Kully-Martens K, Denys K, et al. The effectiveness of a community-based intervention program for women at-risk for giving birth to a child with Fetal Alcohol spectrum Disorder (FASD). Community Ment Health J. 2012;48:12–21. https://doi.org/10.1007/s10597-010-9342-0.
10. Deshpande S, Basil M, Basford L, et al. Promoting alcohol abstinence among pregnant women: potential social change strategies. Health Mark Q. 2005;23:45–67. https://doi.org/10.1300/J026v23n02_04.
11. Erng MN, Smirnov A, Reid N. Prevention of alcohol-exposed pregnancies and fetal alcohol spectrum disorder among pregnant and postpartum women: a systematic review. Alcohol Clin Exp Res. 2020;44:2431–48. https://doi.org/10.1111/acer.14489.
12. Lowe JB, Baxter L, Hirokawa R, et al. Description of a media campaign about alcohol use during pregnancy. J Stud Alcohol Drugs. 2010;71:739–41. https://doi.org/10.15288/jsad.2010.71.739.
13. Glik D, Prelip M, Myerson A, et al. Fetal alcohol syndrome prevention using community-based narrowcasting campaigns. Health Promot Pract. 2008;9:93–103. https://doi.org/10.1177/1524839907309044.

14. Roberts SCM, Mericle AA, Subbaraman MS, et al. Variations by education status in relationships between alcohol/pregnancy policies and birth outcomes and prenatal care utilization: a legal epidemiology study. J Public Health Manag Pract. 2020;26(Suppl 2):S71–83. https://doi.org/10.1097/phh.0000000000001069.

15. Roberts SCM, Berglas NF, Subbaraman MS, et al. Racial differences in the relationship between alcohol/pregnancy policies and birth outcomes and prenatal care utilization: a legal epidemiology study. Drug Alcohol Depend. 2019;201:244–52. https://doi.org/10.1016/j.drugalcdep.2019.04.020.

16. Subbaraman MS, Roberts SCM. Costs associated with policies regarding alcohol use during pregnancy: results from 1972-2015 vital statistics. PLoS One. 2019;14:e0215670. https://doi.org/10.1371/journal.pone.0215670.

17. Roberts SCM, Mericle AA, Subbaraman MS, et al. State policies targeting alcohol use during pregnancy and alcohol use among pregnant women 1985-2016: evidence from the behavioral risk factor surveillance system. Womens Health Issues. 2019;29:213–21. https://doi.org/10.1016/j.whi.2019.02.001.

18. Floyd RL, Jack BW, Cefalo R, et al. The clinical content of preconception care: alcohol, tobacco, and illicit drug exposures. Am J Obstet Gynecol. 2008;199:S333–9. https://doi.org/10.1016/j.ajog.2008.09.018.

19. Velasquez MM, Ingersoll KS, Sobell MB, et al. Women and drinking: preventing alcohol-exposed pregnancies. Hogrefe Publishing; 2016.

20. Weber MK, Floyd RL, Riley EP, et al. National Task Force on Fetal Alcohol Syndrome and Fetal Alcohol Effect: defining the national agenda for fetal alcohol syndrome and other prenatal alcohol-related effects. MMWR Recomm Rep. 2002;51:9–12.

21. Floyd RL, Sobell M, Velasquez MM, et al. Preventing alcohol-exposed pregnancies: a randomized controlled trial. Am J Prev Med. 2007;32:1–10. https://doi.org/10.1016/j.amepre.2006.08.028.

22. Centers for Disease Control and Prevention. Binge drinking. 2019. https://www.cdc.gov/alcohol/fact-sheets/binge-drinking.htm. Accessed 19 Jul 2021.

23. National Institute on Alcohol Abuse and Alcoholism. Drinking levels defined. https://www.niaaa.nih.gov/alcohol-health/overview-alcohol-consumption/moderate-binge-drinking. Accessed 19 Jul 2021.

24. National Institute on Alcohol Abuse and Alcoholism. Alcohol: a women's health issue. 2008. https://www.una.edu/manesafety/Alcohol%20Brochures/WomanHealthIssue.pdf. Accessed 19 Jul 2021.

25. Fabbri S, Farrell LV, Penberthy JK, et al. Toward prevention of alcohol exposed pregnancies: characteristics that relate to ineffective contraception and risky drinking. J Behav Med. 2009;32:443–52. https://doi.org/10.1007/s10865-009-9215-6.

26. Frost JJ, Darroch JE. Factors associated with contraceptive choice and inconsistent method use, United States, 2004. Perspect Sex Reprod Health. 2008;40:94–104. https://doi.org/10.1363/4009408.

27. Sedgh G, Singh S, Hussain R. Intended and unintended pregnancies worldwide in 2012 and recent trends. Stud Fam Plan. 2014;45:301–14. https://doi.org/10.1111/j.1728-4465.2014.00393.x.

28. Wellings K, Jones KG, Mercer CH, et al. The prevalence of unplanned pregnancy and associated factors in Britain: findings from the third National Survey of Sexual Attitudes and Lifestyles (Natsal-3). Lancet. 2013;382:1807–16. https://doi.org/10.1016/s0140-6736(13)62071-1.

29. Finer LB, Zolna MR. Declines in unintended pregnancy in the United States, 2008-2011. N Engl J Med. 2016;374:843–52. https://doi.org/10.1056/NEJMsa1506575.

30. Frost JJ. Trends in US women's use of sexual and reproductive health care services, 1995-2002. Am J Public Health. 2008;98:1814–7. https://doi.org/10.2105/ajph.2007.124719.

31. Frost JJ, Singh S, Finer LB. Factors associated with contraceptive use and nonuse, United States, 2004. Perspect Sex Reprod Health. 2007;39:90–9. https://doi.org/10.1363/3909007.

32. Naimi TS, Lipscomb LE, Brewer RD, et al. Binge drinking in the preconception period and the risk of unintended pregnancy: implications for women and their children. Pediatrics. 2003;111:1136–41.
33. Oulman E, Kim TH, Yunis K, et al. Prevalence and predictors of unintended pregnancy among women: an analysis of the Canadian Maternity Experiences Survey. BMC Pregnancy Childbirth. 2015;15:260. https://doi.org/10.1186/s12884-015-0663-4.
34. Schwarz EB, Lohr PA, Gold MA, et al. Prevalence and correlates of ambivalence towards pregnancy among nonpregnant women. Contraception. 2007;75:305–10. https://doi.org/10.1016/j.contraception.2006.12.002.
35. McQuire C, Daniel R, Hurt L, et al. The causal web of foetal alcohol spectrum disorders: a review and causal diagram. Eur Child Adolesc Psychiatry. 2020;29:575–94. https://doi.org/10.1007/s00787-018-1264-3.
36. Ethen MK, Ramadhani TA, Scheuerle AE, et al. Alcohol consumption by women before and during pregnancy. Matern Child Health J. 2009;13:274–85. https://doi.org/10.1007/s10995-008-0328-2.
37. Astley SJ, Bailey D, Talbot C, et al. Fetal alcohol syndrome (FAS) primary prevention through FAS diagnosis: II. A comprehensive profile of 80 birth mothers of children with FAS. Alcohol Alcohol. 2000;35:509–19. https://doi.org/10.1093/alcalc/35.5.509.
38. Centers for Disease Control and Prevention. Alcohol use among pregnant and nonpregnant women of childbearing age—United States, 1991-2005. MMWR Morb Mortal Wkly Rep. 2009;58:529–32.
39. Sulik KK. Genesis of alcohol-induced craniofacial dysmorphism. Exp Biol Med (Maywood). 2005;230:366–75. https://doi.org/10.1177/15353702-0323006-04.
40. Velasquez MM, Ingersoll KS, Sobell MB, et al. A dual-focus motivational intervention to reduce the risk of alcohol-exposed pregnancy. Cogn Behav Pract. 2010;17:203–12. https://doi.org/10.1016/j.cbpra.2009.02.004.
41. Parackal SM, Parackal MK, Harraway JA. Prevalence and correlates of drinking in early pregnancy among women who stopped drinking on pregnancy recognition. Matern Child Health J. 2013;17:520–9. https://doi.org/10.1007/s10995-012-1026-7.
42. Mullally A, Cleary BJ, Barry J, et al. Prevalence, predictors and perinatal outcomes of peri-conceptional alcohol exposure—retrospective cohort study in an urban obstetric population in Ireland. BMC Pregnancy Childbirth. 2011;11:27. https://doi.org/10.1186/1471-2393-11-27.
43. Parackal S, Parackal M, Harraway J. Associated factors of drinking prior to recognising pregnancy and risky drinking among New Zealand women aged 18 to 35 years. Int J Environ Res Public Health. 2019;16:16. https://doi.org/10.3390/ijerph16101822.
44. Strandberg-Larsen K, Rod Nielsen N, Nybo Andersen AM, et al. Characteristics of women who binge drink before and after they become aware of their pregnancy. Eur J Epidemiol. 2008;23:565–72. https://doi.org/10.1007/s10654-008-9265-z.
45. McDonald SW, Hicks M, Rasmussen C, et al. Characteristics of women who consume alcohol before and after pregnancy recognition in a Canadian sample: a prospective cohort study. Alcohol Clin Exp Res. 2014;38:3008–16. https://doi.org/10.1111/acer.12579.
46. Cannon MJ, Dominique Y, O'Leary LA, et al. Characteristics and behaviors of mothers who have a child with fetal alcohol syndrome. Neurotoxicol Teratol. 2012;34:90–5. https://doi.org/10.1016/j.ntt.2011.09.010.
47. Kvigne VL, Leonardson GR, Borzelleca J, et al. Characteristics of mothers who have children with fetal alcohol syndrome or some characteristics of fetal alcohol syndrome. J Am Board Fam Pract. 2003;16:296–303. https://doi.org/10.3122/jabfm.16.4.296.
48. May PA, Gossage JP, Marais AS, et al. Maternal risk factors for fetal alcohol syndrome and partial fetal alcohol syndrome in South Africa: a third study. Alcohol Clin Exp Res. 2008;32:738–53. https://doi.org/10.1111/j.1530-0277.2008.00634.x.
49. Campo S, Askelson NM, Spies EL, et al. Preventing unintended pregnancies and improving contraceptive use among young adult women in a rural, Midwestern state: health

promotion implications. Women Health. 2010;50:279–96. https://doi.org/10.1080/0363024 2.2010.480909.

50. Kiene SM, Barta WD, Tennen H, et al. Alcohol, helping young adults to have unprotected sex with casual partners: findings from a daily diary study of alcohol use and sexual behavior. J Adolesc Health. 2009;44:73–80. https://doi.org/10.1016/j.jadohealth.2008.05.008.

51. Poulin C, Graham L. The association between substance use, unplanned sexual intercourse and other sexual behaviours among adolescent students. Addiction. 2001;96:607–21. https://doi.org/10.1046/j.1360-0443.2001.9646079.x.

52. Ingersoll KS, Ceperich SD, Nettleman MD, et al. Risk drinking and contraception effectiveness among college women. Psychol Health. 2008;23:965–81. https://doi.org/10.1080/08870440701596569.

53. Hingson RW, Strunin L, Berlin BM, et al. Beliefs about AIDS, use of alcohol and drugs, and unprotected sex among Massachusetts adolescents. Am J Public Health. 1990;80:295–9. https://doi.org/10.2105/ajph.80.3.295.

54. McEwan RT, McCallum A, Bhopal RS, et al. Sex and the risk of HIV infection: the role of alcohol. Br J Addict. 1992;87:577–84. https://doi.org/10.1111/j.1360-0443.1992.tb01959.x.

55. Logie CH, Lys C, Okumu M, et al. Pathways between depression, substance use and multiple sex partners among northern and indigenous young women in the Northwest Territories, Canada: results from a cross-sectional survey. Sex Transm Infect. 2018;94:604–6. https://doi.org/10.1136/sextrans-2017-053265.

56. Green KM, Musci RJ, Matson PA, et al. Developmental patterns of adolescent marijuana and alcohol use and their joint association with sexual risk behavior and outcomes in young adulthood. J Urban Health. 2017;94:115–24. https://doi.org/10.1007/s11524-016-0108-z.

57. Moylett S, Hughes BM. The associations among personality, alcohol-related protective behavioural strategies (PBS), alcohol consumption and sexual intercourse in Irish, female college students. Addict Behav Rep. 2017;6:56–64. https://doi.org/10.1016/j.abrep.2017.08.001.

58. Tucker JS, Shih RA, Pedersen ER, et al. Associations of alcohol and Marijuana use with condom use among young adults: the moderating role of partner type. J Sex Res. 2019;56:957–64. https://doi.org/10.1080/00224499.2018.1493571.

59. Marcantonio TL, Jozkowski KN, Angelone DJ, et al. Students' alcohol use, sexual behaviors, and contraceptive use while studying abroad. J Community Health. 2019;44:68–73. https://doi.org/10.1007/s10900-018-0554-5.

60. Thompson EL, Litt DM, Griner SB, et al. Cognitions and behaviors related to risk for alcohol-exposed pregnancies among young adult women. J Behav Med. 2021;44:123–30. https://doi.org/10.1007/s10865-020-00183-w.

61. Centers for Disease Control and Prevention. Alcohol consumption among women who are pregnant or who might become pregnant—United States, 2002. MMWR Morb Mortal Wkly Rep. 2004;53:1178–81.

62. Green PP, McKnight-Eily LR, Tan CH, et al. Vital signs: alcohol-exposed pregnancies—United States, 2011–2013. MMWR Morb Mortal Wkly Rep. 2016;65:91–7. https://doi.org/10.15585/mmwr.mm6504a6.

63. Cannon MJ, Guo J, Denny CH, et al. Prevalence and characteristics of women at risk for an alcohol-exposed pregnancy (AEP) in the United States: estimates from the National Survey of Family Growth. Matern Child Health J. 2015;19:776–82. https://doi.org/10.1007/s10995-014-1563-3.

64. Watt MH, Knettel BA, Choi KW, et al. Risk for alcohol-exposed pregnancies among women at drinking venues in Cape Town, South Africa. J Stud Alcohol Drugs. 2017;78:795–800. https://doi.org/10.15288/jsad.2017.78.795.

65. Balachova T, Bonner B, Chaffin M, et al. Women's alcohol consumption and risk for alcohol-exposed pregnancies in Russia. Addiction. 2012;107:109–17. https://doi.org/10.1111/j.1360-0443.2011.03569.x.

66. Roberts SCM, Thompson KM. Estimating the prevalence of United States women with alcohol-exposed pregnancies and births. Womens Health Issues. 2019;29:188–93. https://doi.org/10.1016/j.whi.2018.11.001.
67. Neighbors C, Larimer ME, Lewis MA. Targeting misperceptions of descriptive drinking norms: efficacy of a computer-delivered personalized normative feedback intervention. J Consult Clin Psychol. 2004;72:434–47. https://doi.org/10.1037/0022-006x.72.3.434.
68. Winograd RP, Steinley D, Sher K, Searching for Mr. Hyde: a five-factor approach to characterizing "types of drunks". Addict Res Theory. 2016;24:1–8. https://doi.org/10.3109/16066359.2015.1029920.
69. Institute of Medicine. Fetal alcohol syndrome: diagnosis, epidemiology, prevention, and treatment. Washington, DC: National Academy Press; 1996.
70. Wilsnack SC, Wilsnack RW, Kantor LW. Focus on: women and the costs of alcohol use. Alcohol Res. 2013;35:219–28.
71. May PA, Keaster C, Bozeman R, et al. Prevalence and characteristics of fetal alcohol syndrome and partial fetal alcohol syndrome in a Rocky Mountain Region City. Drug Alcohol Depend. 2015;155:118–27. https://doi.org/10.1016/j.drugalcdep.2015.08.006.
72. Edenberg HJ, Foroud T. The genetics of alcoholism: identifying specific genes through family studies. Addict Biol. 2006;11:386–96. https://doi.org/10.1111/j.1369-1600.2006.00035.x.
73. Liyanage VR, Curtis K, Zachariah RM, et al. Overview of the genetic basis and epigenetic mechanisms that contribute to FASD pathobiology. Curr Top Med Chem. 2017;17:808–28. https://doi.org/10.2174/1568026616666160414124816.
74. Green RF, Stoler JM. Alcohol dehydrogenase 1B genotype and fetal alcohol syndrome: a HuGE minireview. Am J Obstet Gynecol. 2007;197:12–25. https://doi.org/10.1016/j.ajog.2007.02.028.
75. Gemma S, Vichi S, Testai E. Metabolic and genetic factors contributing to alcohol induced effects and fetal alcohol syndrome. Neurosci Biobehav Rev. 2007;31:221–9. https://doi.org/10.1016/j.neubiorev.2006.06.018.
76. Eberhart JK, Parnell SE. The genetics of fetal alcohol spectrum disorders. Alcohol Clin Exp Res. 2016;40:1154–65. https://doi.org/10.1111/acer.13066.
77. U.S. Preventive Services Task Force. Unhealthy alcohol use in adolescents and adults: screening and behavioral counseling interventions. 2018. https://www.uspreventiveservices-taskforce.org/uspstf/recommendation/unhealthy-alcohol-use-in-adolescents-and-adults-screening-and-behavioral-counseling-interventions. Accessed 19 Jul 2021.
78. Allen D, Hunter MS, Wood S, et al. One key question(®): first things first in reproductive health. Matern Child Health J. 2017;21:387–92. https://doi.org/10.1007/s10995-017-2283-2.
79. Edwards A, Kelsey B, Pierce-Bulger M, et al. Applying ethical principles when discussing alcohol use during pregnancy. J Midwifery Womens Health. 2020;65:795–801. https://doi.org/10.1111/jmwh.13159.
80. Rhoads S, Mengel M. Make your office alcohol-exposed pregnancy prevention friendly. J Ark Med Soc. 2011;108:62–4.
81. Mwansa-Kambafwile J, Rendall-Mkosi K, Jacobs R, et al. Evaluation of a service provider short course for prevention of fetal alcohol syndrome. J Stud Alcohol Drugs. 2011;72:530–5. https://doi.org/10.15288/jsad.2011.72.530.
82. Tenkku Lepper L, King D, Doll J, et al. Partnering with the health professions to promote prevention of an alcohol-exposed pregnancy: lessons learned from an academic-organizational collaborative. Int J Environ Res Public Health. 2019;16 https://doi.org/10.3390/ijerph16101702.
83. Manwell LB, Fleming MF, Mundt MP, et al. Treatment of problem alcohol use in women of childbearing age: results of a brief intervention trial. Alcohol Clin Exp Res. 2000;24:1517–24.
84. Payne J, France K, Henley N, et al. Changes in health professionals' knowledge, attitudes and practice following provision of educational resources about prevention of prenatal alcohol exposure and fetal alcohol spectrum disorder. Paediatr Perinat Epidemiol. 2011;25:316–27. https://doi.org/10.1111/j.1365-3016.2011.01197.x.

85. Poels M, van Stel HF, Franx A, et al. The effect of a local promotional campaign on preconceptional lifestyle changes and the use of preconception care. Eur J Contracept Reprod Health Care. 2018;23:38–44. https://doi.org/10.1080/13625187.2018.1426744.

86. Chersich MF, Urban M, Olivier L, et al. Universal prevention is associated with lower prevalence of fetal alcohol spectrum disorders in Northern Cape, South Africa: a multicentre before-after study. Alcohol Alcohol. 2012;47:67–74. https://doi.org/10.1093/alcalc/agr145.

87. France KE, Donovan RJ, Bower C, et al. Messages that increase women's intentions to abstain from alcohol during pregnancy: results from quantitative testing of advertising concepts. BMC Public Health. 2014;14:30. https://doi.org/10.1186/1471-2458-14-30.

88. Hanson J, Mohawk C, Shrestha U, et al. The importance of understanding social context in the reduction of AEP risk among native women. Alcohol Clin Exp Res. 2020;44:2154–7. https://doi.org/10.1111/acer.14470.

89. Hanson JD, Weber TL. Commentary on Montag et al. (2017): The importance of CBPR in FASD prevention with American Indian communities. Alcohol Clin Exp Res. 2018;42:6–8. https://doi.org/10.1111/acer.13524.

90. Hanson JD, Winberg A, Elliott A. Development of a media campaign on fetal alcohol spectrum disorders for Northern Plains American Indian communities. Health Promot Pract. 2012;13:842–7. https://doi.org/10.1177/1524839911404232.

91. Walker DS, Fisher CS, Sherman A, et al. Fetal alcohol spectrum disorders prevention: an exploratory study of women's use of, attitudes toward, and knowledge about alcohol. J Am Acad Nurse Pract. 2005;17:187–93. https://doi.org/10.1111/j.1745-7599.2005.0031.x.

92. Hutton HE, Chander G, Green PP, et al. A novel integration effort to reduce the risk for alcohol-exposed pregnancy among women attending urban STD clinics. Public Health Rep. 2014;129(Suppl 1):56–62. https://doi.org/10.1177/00333549141291s109.

93. Brems C, Johnson ME, Metzger JS, et al. College students' knowledge about fetal alcohol spectrum disorder. J Popul Ther Clin Pharmacol. 2014;21:e159–66.

94. Sobell LC, Sobell MB, Johnson K, et al. Preventing alcohol-exposed pregnancies: a randomized controlled trial of a self-administered version of project CHOICES with college students and nonstudents. Alcohol Clin Exp Res. 2017;41:1182–90. https://doi.org/10.1111/acer.13385.

95. Ceperich SD, Ingersoll KS. Motivational interviewing + feedback intervention to reduce alcohol-exposed pregnancy risk among college binge drinkers: determinants and patterns of response. J Behav Med. 2011;34:381–95. https://doi.org/10.1007/s10865-010-9308-2.

96. Parrish DE, von Sternberg K, Benjamins LJ, et al. CHOICES-TEEN: reducing substance-exposed pregnancy and HIV among juvenile justice adolescent females. Res Soc Work Pract. 2019;29:618–27. https://doi.org/10.1177/1049731518779717.

97. Delrahim-Howlett K, Chambers CD, Clapp JD, et al. Web-based assessment and brief intervention for alcohol use in women of childbearing potential: a report of the primary findings. Alcohol Clin Exp Res. 2011;35:1331–8. https://doi.org/10.1111/j.1530-0277.2011.01469.x.

98. Esper LH, Furtado EF. Identifying maternal risk factors associated with fetal alcohol spectrum disorders: a systematic review. Eur Child Adolesc Psychiatry. 2014;23:877–89. https://doi.org/10.1007/s00787-014-0603-2.

99. May PA, de Vries MM, Marais AS, et al. The continuum of fetal alcohol spectrum disorders in four rural communities in South Africa: prevalence and characteristics. Drug Alcohol Depend. 2016;159:207–18. https://doi.org/10.1016/j.drugalcdep.2015.12.023.

100. Montag AC, Brodine SK, Alcaraz JE, et al. Preventing alcohol-exposed pregnancy among an American Indian/Alaska Native population: effect of a screening, brief intervention, and referral to treatment intervention. Alcohol Clin Exp Res. 2015;39:126–35. https://doi.org/10.1111/acer.12607.

101. Project CHOICES Intervention Research Group. Reducing the risk of alcohol-exposed pregnancies: a study of a motivational intervention in community settings. Pediatrics. 2003;111:1131–5.

102. Centers for Disease Control and Prevention. Motivational intervention to reduce alcohol-exposed pregnancies—Florida, Texas, and Virginia, 1997–2001. MMWR Morb Mortal Wkly Rep. 2003;52:441–4.
103. Ingersoll KS, Ceperich SD, Nettleman MD, et al. Reducing alcohol-exposed pregnancy risk in college women: initial outcomes of a clinical trial of a motivational intervention. J Subst Abus Treat. 2005;29:173–80. https://doi.org/10.1016/j.jsat.2005.06.003.
104. Ingersoll KS, Ceperich SD, Hettema JE, et al. Preconceptional motivational interviewing interventions to reduce alcohol-exposed pregnancy risk. J Subst Abus Treat. 2013;44:407–16. https://doi.org/10.1016/j.jsat.2012.10.001.
105. Farrell-Carnahan L, Hettema J, Jackson J, et al. Feasibility and promise of a remote-delivered preconception motivational interviewing intervention to reduce risk for alcohol-exposed pregnancy. Telemed J E Health. 2013;19:597–604. https://doi.org/10.1089/tmj.2012.0247.
106. Hanson JD, Miller AL, Winberg A, et al. Prevention of alcohol-exposed pregnancies among nonpregnant American Indian women. Am J Health Promot. 2013;27:S66–73. https://doi.org/10.4278/ajhp.120113-QUAN-25.
107. Wilton G, Moberg DP, Van Stelle KR, et al. A randomized trial comparing telephone versus in-person brief intervention to reduce the risk of an alcohol-exposed pregnancy. J Subst Abus Treat. 2013;45:389–94. https://doi.org/10.1016/j.jsat.2013.06.006.
108. Letourneau B, Sobell LC, Sobell MB, et al. Preventing alcohol-exposed pregnancies among Hispanic women. J Ethn Subst Abus. 2017;16:109–21. https://doi.org/10.1080/15332640.2015.1093991.
109. Ingersoll K, Frederick C, MacDonnell K, et al. A pilot RCT of an internet intervention to reduce the risk of alcohol-exposed pregnancy. Alcohol Clin Exp Res. 2018;42:1132–44. https://doi.org/10.1111/acer.13635.
110. Tenkku LE, Mengel MB, Nicholson RA, et al. A web-based intervention to reduce alcohol-exposed pregnancies in the community. Health Educ Behav. 2011;38:563–73. https://doi.org/10.1177/1090198110385773.
111. Parrish DE, von Sternberg K, Velasquez MM, et al. Characteristics and factors associated with the risk of a nicotine exposed pregnancy: expanding the CHOICES preconception counseling model to tobacco. Matern Child Health J. 2012;16:1224–31. https://doi.org/10.1007/s10995-011-0848-z.
112. Ingersoll KS, Hettema JE, Cropsey KL, et al. Preconception markers of dual risk for alcohol and smoking exposed pregnancy: tools for primary prevention. J Womens Health (Larchmt). 2011;20:1627–33. https://doi.org/10.1089/jwh.2010.2633.
113. Velasquez MM, von Sternberg KL, Floyd RL, et al. Preventing alcohol and tobacco exposed pregnancies: CHOICES plus in primary care. Am J Prev Med. 2017;53:85–95. https://doi.org/10.1016/j.amepre.2017.02.012.
114. Hanson JD, Pourier S. The Oglala Sioux Tribe CHOICES program: modifying an existing alcohol-exposed pregnancy intervention for use in an American Indian community. Int J Environ Res Public Health. 2015;13:ijerph13010001. https://doi.org/10.3390/ijerph13010001.
115. Hanson JD, Nelson ME, Jensen JL, et al. Impact of the CHOICES intervention in preventing alcohol-exposed pregnancies in American Indian women. Alcohol Clin Exp Res. 2017;41:828–35. https://doi.org/10.1111/acer.13348.
116. Hanson JD, Oziel K, Sarche M, et al. A culturally tailored intervention to reduce risk of alcohol-exposed pregnancies in American Indian communities: rationale, design, and methods. Contemp Clin Trials. 2021;104:106351. https://doi.org/10.1016/j.cct.2021.106351.
117. Hanson JD, Ingersoll K, Pourier S. Development and implementation of CHOICES group to reduce drinking, improve contraception, and prevent alcohol-exposed pregnancies in American Indian women. J Subst Abus Treat. 2015;59:45–51. https://doi.org/10.1016/j.jsat.2015.07.006.

118. Russell T, Craddock C, Kodatt S, et al. Preventing fetal alcohol spectrum disorders: an evidence-based prevention program for adolescent and adult Hispanic females in the South Texas border region. 2017.
119. Grant TM, Ernst CC, Streissguth A, et al. Preventing alcohol and drug exposed births in Washington state: intervention findings from three parent-child assistance program sites. Am J Drug Alcohol Abuse. 2005;31:471–90. https://doi.org/10.1081/ada-200056813.
120. Thanh NX, Jonsson E, Moffatt J, et al. An economic evaluation of the parent-child assistance program for preventing fetal alcohol spectrum disorder in Alberta, Canada. Adm Policy Ment Health. 2015;42:10–8. https://doi.org/10.1007/s10488-014-0537-5.
121. Shaw MR, Grant T, Barbosa-Leiker C, et al. Intervention with substance-abusing mothers: are there rural-urban differences? Am J Addict. 2015;24:144–52. https://doi.org/10.1111/ajad.12155.
122. Pei J, Carlson E, Tremblay M, et al. Exploring the contributions and suitability of relational and community-centered fetal alcohol spectrum disorder (FASD) prevention work in First Nation communities. Birth Defects Res. 2019;111:835–47. https://doi.org/10.1002/bdr2.1480.
123. Salas-Wright CP, Vaughn MG, Ugalde J, et al. Substance use and teen pregnancy in the United States: evidence from the NSDUH 2002-2012. Addict Behav. 2015;45:218–25. https://doi.org/10.1016/j.addbeh.2015.01.039.
124. Salas-Wright CP, Vaughn MG, Ugalde J. A typology of substance use among pregnant teens in the United States. Matern Child Health J. 2016;20:646–54. https://doi.org/10.1007/s10995-015-1864-1.
125. Caetano R, Ramisetty-Mikler S, Floyd LR, et al. The epidemiology of drinking among women of child-bearing age. Alcohol Clin Exp Res. 2006;30:1023–30. https://doi.org/10.1111/j.1530-0277.2006.00116.x.
126. Zammit SL, Skouteris H, Wertheim EH, et al. Pregnant women's alcohol consumption: the predictive utility of intention to drink and prepregnancy drinking behavior. J Womens Health (Larchmt). 2008;17:1513–22. https://doi.org/10.1089/jwh.2007.0595.
127. Lachausse RG. The effectiveness of a multimedia program to prevent fetal alcohol syndrome. Health Promot Pract. 2008;9:289–93. https://doi.org/10.1177/1524839906289046.
128. Boulter LT. The effectiveness of peer-led FAS/FAE prevention presentations in middle and high schools. J Alcohol Drug Educ. 2007;51:7–26.
129. Chambers RA, Begay J, Patel H, et al. Rigorous evaluation of a substance use and teen pregnancy prevention program for American Indian girls and their female caregivers: a study protocol for a randomized controlled trial. BMC Public Health. 2021;21:1179. https://doi.org/10.1186/s12889-021-11131-x.
130. Hanson JD, Weber TL, Shrestha U, et al. Acceptability of an eHealth intervention to prevent alcohol-exposed pregnancy among American Indian/Alaska Native teens. Alcohol Clin Exp Res. 2020;44:196–202. https://doi.org/10.1111/acer.14229.
131. Shrestha U, Hanson J, Weber T, et al. Community perceptions of alcohol exposed pregnancy prevention program for American Indian and Alaska Native teens. Int J Environ Res Public Health. 2019;16:16. https://doi.org/10.3390/ijerph16101795.
132. Rendall-Mkosi K, Morojele N, London L, et al. A randomized controlled trial of motivational interviewing to prevent risk for an alcohol-exposed pregnancy in the Western Cape, South Africa. Addiction. 2013;108:725–32. https://doi.org/10.1111/add.12081.
133. Hebert LE, Sarche MC. Pre-pregnancy and prenatal alcohol use among American Indian and Alaska Native and non-Hispanic white women: findings from PRAMS in five states. Matern Child Health J. 2021;25:1392. https://doi.org/10.1007/s10995-021-03159-7.
134. Smith IE, Lancaster JS, Moss-Wells S, et al. Identifying high-risk pregnant drinkers: biological and behavioral correlates of continuous heavy drinking during pregnancy. J Stud Alcohol. 1987;48:304–9. https://doi.org/10.15288/jsa.1987.48.304.

135. Testa M, Reifman A. Individual differences in perceived riskiness of drinking in pregnancy: antecedents and consequences. J Stud Alcohol. 1996;57:360–7. https://doi.org/10.15288/jsa.1996.57.360.
136. Centers for Disease Control and Prevention. Alcohol and pregnancy. 2016. https://www.cdc.gov/vitalsigns/fasd/index.html. Accessed 20 Jul 2021.
137. World Health Organization. Global alcohol action plan 2022–2030 to strengthen implementation of the global strategy to reduce the harmful use of alcohol. 2021. https://cdn.who.int/media/docs/default-source/alcohol/action-plan-on-alcohol_first-draft-final_formatted.pdf?sfvrsn=b690edb0_1&download=true. Accessed 27 Jul 2021.
138. Pryor J, Patrick SW, Sundermann AC, et al. Pregnancy intention and maternal alcohol consumption. Obstet Gynecol. 2017;129:727–33. https://doi.org/10.1097/aog.0000000000001933.
139. Yaesoubi R, Mahin M, Martin G, et al. Reducing the prevalence of alcohol-exposed pregnancies in the United States: a simulation modeling study. Med Decis Mak. 2021;42:272989x211023203. https://doi.org/10.1177/0272989x211023203.
140. May PA, Hasken JM, Baete A, et al. Fetal alcohol spectrum disorders in a Midwestern City: child characteristics, maternal risk traits, and prevalence. Alcohol Clin Exp Res. 2020;44:919–38. https://doi.org/10.1111/acer.14314.
141. Montag AC, Romero R, Jensen T, et al. The prevalence of fetal alcohol spectrum disorders in an American Indian Community. Int J Environ Res Public Health. 2019;16 https://doi.org/10.3390/ijerph16122179.

Chapter 4
Care During the Prenatal Period

Katherine N. DeJong and Jamie O. Lo

Introduction

Alcohol consumption in pregnancy is associated with an increased risk of miscarriage, stillbirth, premature birth, impaired fetal growth, congenital anomalies, and fetal alcohol spectrum disorders (FASD), the leading environmental cause of developmental disabilities worldwide [1, 2]. In a cross-sectional study of first-grade children in four regions of the United States, the estimated prevalence for FASD was 1.1–5% [3]. Fetal alcohol spectrum disorder can lead to long-term difficulties with school and employment because it includes birth defects that can impair the central nervous system, affect intellectual development, and result in behavioral disorders [3]. It also carries a significant economic impact in part due to substantial costs to support individuals with FASD. Children with FASD enrolled in Medicaid have annual mean medical expenses that are nine times higher than children without. This equates to a median annual expenditure of $6670 per child with FASD versus $518 in children without FASD [4, 5]. The evidence also suggests that costs per-person for FASD exceed those for other common conditions, estimated costs for children with FASD are $23,000 versus $17,000 for children with autism [6].

A primary contributor to the high prevalence of FASD and other adverse perinatal outcomes is prenatal alcohol exposure prior to pregnancy awareness. This is

K. N. DeJong
Department of Obstetrics and Gynecology, Addiction Medicine, Swedish Medical Center, Seattle, WA, USA
e-mail: Katherine.Dejong@swedish.org

J. O. Lo (✉)
Department of Obstetrics and Gynecology, Oregon Health & Science University, Portland, OR, USA
e-mail: Loj@ohsu.edu

because half of all pregnancies in the United States are unintended and unrecognized until at least 4–6 weeks in gestation, during a period of increased teratogen susceptibility [7–9]. As treatments for FASD are currently limited, there is no known safe level of alcohol intake in pregnancy, and consumption at any point in the pregnancy can be associated with an increased risk of adverse perinatal outcomes, the Surgeon General, Center for Disease Control (CDC), American College of Obstetricians and Gynecologists (ACOG), and other medical societies including the Society of Obstetricians and Gynaecologists of Canada all recommend complete abstinence during pregnancy [10–13].

Despite these recommendations and public health initiatives, more than half of reproductive age women in the United States report current alcohol use [14] and the prevalence of prenatal alcohol consumption is on the rise. A recent study of pregnant individuals in the United States from 2011 to 2018, using data from the Behavioral Risk Factor Surveillance System (BRFSS), noted that current drinking, consumption of at least one alcohol beverage in the past 30 days, had increased from 9.2% to 11.3%, respectively [15] (Table 4.1). This study also noted that binge drinking, consuming four or more alcohol beverages in one occasion during the past 30 days, also increased from 2.5% to 4% in the same time period [15]. This is concerning because prior animal studies have found that binge-like drinking patterns are particularly dangerous, especially to fetal neurodevelopment, even if the total amount of alcohol consumed is less [16]. An earlier study using 2015 to 2017 BRFSS data found that of women who engaged in binge drinking, the average frequency was 4.5 episodes in the past 30 days and the average intensity of binge drinking (the average largest number of drinks reported consumed on any occasion) was six drinks [17].

Pregnancy is a window to future health. It is a critical time of significant fetal development that is highly sensitive and vulnerable to environmental exposures, such as prenatal alcohol exposure, with potential long-term implications on adult disease. Within this chapter, we will review the existing literature and explore the potential harmful effects of prenatal alcohol exposure on perinatal and fetal outcomes as well as strategies to screen for maternal alcohol use and intervene.

Table 4.1 Definition of 1 drink [10]

Beverage	Quantity (ounces)
Beer or wine cooler	12
Table wine	5
Malt liquor	8–9
80-Proof spirits	1.5

Prevalence of Alcohol Use in Pregnancy

A recent CDC study using 2015–2018 data from the National Survey on Drug Use and Health (NSDUH) focused on estimating the overall and trimester-specific prevalence of self-reported alcohol consumption in the past 12 months, current drinking and binge drinking [18]. Women studied were aged 12–44 years old and among pregnant respondents, the estimated prevalence of past drinking (12 months), current drinking (at least one drink in the past 30 days), and binge drinking (four or more drinks on at least one occasion in the past 30 days) were 64.7%, 9.8%, and 4.5%, respectively [18]. Responses by trimester of current drinking were notable for 19.6% in the first trimester, and 4.7% in their second or third trimester [18]. Binge drinking by trimester was noted by 10.5% of individuals in the first trimester and 1.4% in the second or third trimester. Past 12 months drinking by trimester was reported by 76.1% of individuals in the first trimester of pregnancy and 59.8% of those in the second or third trimester [18]. Other studies of individuals drinking in late pregnancy have shown that the highest prevalence was among individuals who were white non-Hispanic, college graduates, 35 years or older, and undergoing social stressors [19, 20]. There is also an increased risk of FASD in those who are of older maternal age, high parity, and African-American or Native American ethnicities [21, 22].

Screening for Alcohol Use in Pregnancy

Screening, Brief Intervention, Referral to Treatment (SBIRT)

Several national organizations, including the National Institute on Alcohol Abuse and Alcoholism [23], the American College of Obstetricians and Gynecologists (ACOG) [24], and the United States Preventive Services Task Force (USPSTF) [25], recommend the use of SBIRT (Screening, Brief Intervention, and Referral to Treatment) for all pregnant individuals as a routine part of prenatal care. The initial screening identifies individuals who continue to drink during pregnancy. The brief intervention is aimed to prevent ongoing drinking. If problematic alcohol use in pregnancy continues or if an alcohol use disorder is diagnosed using DSM-5 criteria [26, 27], timely referral for substance use disorder treatment becomes the next step in providing services and minimizing risk [28]. Although utilizing SBIRT remains part of national practice guidelines, barriers do exist for routine adherence to these guidelines and include lack of time, lack of knowledge, misconceptions about alcohol use in pregnancy, discomfort with the subject matter, inability to obtain reimbursement, and concern for treatment usefulness or availability [29–31].

Structured Questionnaires

Screening for alcohol use in pregnancy should be performed using validated screening tools. ACOG and USPSTF both recommend routine screening of pregnant individuals via the TWEAK (tolerance, worries, eye-opener, amnesia, cut-down) and T-ACE (tolerance, annoyed-, cut-down, eye-opener) questionnaires [25, 30]. The T-ACE questionnaire was the first validated sensitive screen for risky drinking developed for use in obstetric-gynecologic practices (Table 4.2). The TWEAK questionnaire is a five-item screening tool that includes questions from the Michigan Alcohol Screening Test (MAST), CAGE (cut-down, annoyed, guilty, eye-opener), and T-ACE questionnaires and additionally has been validated for use in the pregnant population as well (Table 4.3) [34, 35]. Of the two, the T-ACE has the highest at-risk drinking sensitivity (69–88%) [32, 36]. One limitation of both screening questionnaires is that they were originally developed to screen the general population for moderate or heavy alcohol use, instead of any current alcohol use, which should be the overall goal of any screening tool.

Other commonly used screening tests for alcohol use have not been validated or found to be effective in the pregnant population and therefore should not be used include CAGE, the Michigan Alcoholism Screening Test (MAST), and the

Table 4.2 T-ACE screening tool [32]

T	**Tolerance**: How many drinks does it take to make you feel high?
A	Have people **Annoyed** you by criticizing your drinking?
C	Have you ever felt you ought to **Cut down** on your drinking?
E	**Eye-opener**: Have you ever had a drink first thing in the morning to steady your nerves or get rid of a hangover?

The T-ACE is used to screen for pregnancy risk drinking, defined as the consumption of 1 ounce or more of alcohol per day while pregnant. Scores are calculated as follows: a reply of "more than two drinks" to question T is considered a positive response and scores 2 points, and an affirmative answer to question A, C, or E scores 1 point, respectively. A total score of 2 or more points on the T-ACE indicates a positive outcome for pregnancy risk drinking

Table 4.3 TWEAK screening tool [33]

T	**Tolerance**: How many drinks can you hold?
W	Have close friends or relatives **Worried** or complained about your drinking in the past year?
E	**Eye opener**: Do you sometimes take a drink in the morning when you get up?
A	**Amnesia**: Has a friend or family member ever told you about things you said or did while you were drinking that you could not remember?
K (C)	Do you sometimes feel the need to **Cut down** on your drinking?

The TWEAK is used to screen for pregnancy risk drinking, defined here as the consumption of 1 ounce or more of alcohol per day while pregnant. Scores are calculated as follows: A positive response to question T on Tolerance (i.e., consumption of more than five drinks) or question W on Worry yields 2 points each; an affirmative reply to question E, A, or K scores 1 point each. A total score of 2 or more points on the TWEAK indicates a positive outcome for pregnancy risk drinking

Table 4.4 The 5 P's screening tool [39]

Parents	Did any of your *parents* have a problem with alcohol or drugs?	Yes	No	No answer
Peers	Do any of your friends (*peers*) have problems with alcohol or drug use?	Yes	No	No answer
Partner	Does your *partner* have a problem with alcohol or drug use?	Yes	No	No answer
Past	Before you knew you were pregnant (*past*), how often did you drink beer, wine, wine coolers or liquor?	Not at all Sometimes	Rarely Frequently	
Present	In the past month, did you drink beer, wine or liquor, or use other drugs? (*Pregnancy*)	Not at all Sometimes	Rarely Frequently	

ShortMAST [28]. These screening tools were developed and tested primarily in male populations.

Two other screening tools remain appropriate as preliminary screening instruments for pregnant individuals: the validated "4 Ps Plus" and the "5 P's" Behavior Risk Screening Tool. These are both designed to elicit information about multiple risk factors, including any current use of alcohol, without solely focusing on alcohol consumption [28]. The original 4 P's (Parents, Partner, Past, Pregnancy) screening tool was developed by Dr. Hope Ewing. The "4 P's Plus" was another iteration by Dr. Ira Chasnoff and is a copyrighted instrument that requires a licensing fee [37, 38]. The 5 P's screening tool was developed by the Institute for Health and Recovery through funding by the Maternal and Child Health Bureau for the *Alcohol Screening Assessment in Pregnancy Project* and remains in the public domain (Table 4.4) [39]. There are now multiple slight iterations of these screening tools available.

The AUDIT-C (alcohol use disorders identification test-consumption subset) captures alcohol use frequency and quantity, but does not distinguish timepoints of alcohol use with respect to pre-pregnancy, pregnancy recognition, and during pregnancy time periods. Although it has been validated for use in pregnant women, it has been found to be unreliable in certain countries for assessing alcohol use during pregnancy.

Despite the utility of validated screening tools and their ability to be used as the first step in SBIRT, they are subject to underreporting bias of prenatal alcohol use due to inaccurate patient recall, embarrassment, or denial regarding actual consumption [34, 40–42]. Additionally, some individuals may have already modified their alcohol use upon learning they were pregnant and may not accurately report on prior use, even if it occurred earlier in the pregnancy.

Laboratory-Based Screening

Despite the utility of laboratory testing to definitively detect and quantify alcohol use during the prenatal period, there is no such available test at this time [43]. Several limitations include the short half-life of alcohol in the blood stream, inability to rule out alcohol use with a single negative result of a test and the lack of information gathered regarding pattern of use from a single positive result. While maternal and neonatal urine and blood samples have been used to determine prenatal alcohol use [44, 45], the biomarkers measured most accurately reflect alcohol exposure within 2–3 days prior to delivery and therefore provide limited information.

Other bodily fluids and tissue samples, including meconium, have been considered as a means for laboratory-based screening. Meconium, often used to detect prenatal exposure to drugs, has been studied to measure fatty acid ethyl esters (FAEE) as a biomarker for prenatal alcohol use that may reflect exposure since the 13th week of pregnancy when meconium first begins to form [43, 46–48]. However, the correlation between FAEE in meconium and prenatal alcohol use has limitations [43, 47]. FAEE may accumulate unevenly in meconium over time, there are genetic variations in alcohol metabolism that may influence the synthesis of FAEE, and illness, medications, or food additives can also affect FAEE concentrations.

Risk Factors for Alcohol Use in Pregnancy

Prior studies have demonstrated that the main risk factors for alcohol use in pregnancy include low socioeconomic status, homelessness, preconception substance use, substance use by one's partner, comorbid psychiatric illness, and a personal history of physical or sexual abuse [49–52]. A recent study by Shmulewitz et al. noted a higher risk of prenatal alcohol use in adolescents (aOR = 1.5) and those with higher education (aOR = 1.4) while a decreased risk was observed in individuals with lower incomes (aORs = 0.7) [53]. An older study by Bayatpour et al. also found a higher incidence of alcohol use in teen pregnancies, especially those with other psychiatric illnesses and a history of child abuse [54]. Similarly, a systematic review of 14 international studies, including 4 from the United States and 4 from Europe, between 2002 and 2009 noted that predictors of prenatal alcohol use most consistently identified were pre-pregnancy alcohol consumption, both quantity and frequency of typical drinking, and a history of abuse or violence [55]. Other predictors of prenatal drinking that were less consistently reported included high income/ social class and a positive dependence screen [55]. Factors less consistently predictive, but also examined were unemployment, marital status, and education level. See Chap. 2 for a more in-depth review of risk factors associated with alcohol use in pregnancy.

The CDC conducted a study of United States individuals from 2011 to 2013 and noted slightly different findings than above. In their study, characteristics associated with the highest prevalence of prenatal alcohol use were maternal age between 35 and 44 (18.6%), non-Hispanic black (13.9%), college degree (13%), and employment (12%) [56].

Risk Factors for Binge Drinking in Pregnancy

A pattern of binge drinking in pregnancy is associated with a higher risk for FASD as well as other prenatal complications such as miscarriage, stillbirth, and prematurity [57]. Data from the Pregnancy Risk Assessment Monitoring System (PRAMS) suggest that individuals who binge drink prior to pregnancy are more likely to drink and binge drink prenatally than those who did not engage in binge drinking before pregnancy [58]. In another CDC study using BRFSS data, pregnant individuals that were binge drinking in the past 30 days reported an average frequency of 4.5 (CI 3.1–5.9) episodes and an average largest intensity of 6 (CI 5.0–7.0) drinks [17].

A prior NSDUH study surveyed over 13,000 pregnant individuals from 2002 to 2017 regarding either any alcohol use or binge drinking the past 2 months. Shmulewitz et al. found that risk factors for any or binge drinking in pregnancy were in individuals that engaged in other substance use (aORs 2.9–25.9), had alcohol use disorder (aORs 4.5–7.5), depression (aORs = 1.6), and were unmarried (aORs 1.6–3.2) [53]. Similar findings were reported in a former CDC study, which noted that the most significant demographic factor for prenatal binge drinking was non-married status, likely secondary to a multitude of socioeconomic factors, with a prevalence of 4.6 times greater than married pregnant individuals [56]. Of those who binge drank while pregnant, there was a significantly higher frequency of binge drinking (4.6 vs. 3.1 episodes) and greater alcohol consumption per episode (7.5 vs. 6 drinks) compared with non-pregnant binge drinkers [56].

Alcohol Use in Pregnant Individuals with Substance Use Disorder

Polysubstance use is common among individuals who consume alcohol in pregnancy. Bakhrieva et al. studied self-reported prevalence of alcohol use in patients enrolled in a prenatal care program for individuals with substance use disorder [59]. A total of 295 individuals were studied, of which 95% were treated for opioid use disorder, and found that 28.8% and 24.1% reported at least 1 binge drinking episode in the periconceptional period and in early pregnancy respectively. Of those who reported drinking in early pregnancy, the median number of binge drinking episodes was higher among patients at the substance use disorder clinic versus the general obstetrics group (median = 3 versus 1, $p < 0.001$). This study demonstrated a high prevalence of prenatal alcohol use in early pregnancy and highlights the need for targeted screening and intervention for maternal alcohol use in all pregnancies, but especially those with substance use disorders such as opioid use disorder.

Protective Factors Against Prenatal Alcohol Consumption

A prior study examined social determinants of tobacco and alcohol use during pregnancy in a rural tribal nation located in the Central United States that have unique challenges to preventing prenatal substance use because it is influenced by isolation, cultural barriers, and historical trauma [60]. Data collected as part of the Safe Passages Study from 421 pregnancies were used, and substance use rates were found to be higher than the national averages. This study found that five factors that were protective against prenatal substance use were as follows: (1) living with someone (92% less likely to smoke and drink), (2) having at least 12 years of education (126% less likely to smoke and drink), (3) having over 12 years of education (206% less likely to smoke and drink), (4) being employed (111% less likely to smoke and drink), and (5) not being depressed (229% less likely to smoke and drink) [60]. See Chap. 2 for a more in-depth review of protective factors associated with alcohol use in pregnancy.

Reducing Risk and Interventions

Brief Interventions (Please See Chap. 3 for Further Details)

The next step in the performance of SBIRT after the previously discussed use of validated screening tools is for providers to engage with patients in brief interventions. Brief interventions are a collection of time-limited counseling strategies geared toward facilitating reduction or elimination of at-risk alcohol use in patients. There is strong evidence that brief counseling interventions effectively reduce the incidence of alcohol-exposed pregnancies when performed in the preconception, prenatal or postpartum periods [61–63] and that individuals who receive brief interventions are more than five times as likely than individuals who do not receive the same intervention to abstain from subsequent alcohol consumption [62]. Components of successful brief intervention include (1) awareness raising and assessment for readiness to change, (2) advice and discussion of strategies for reducing or eliminating problematic alcohol use, and (3) assistance in the form of eliciting ideas about change strategies, goal setting, positive reinforcement, and referrals to supportive services [64, 65]. This approach is often referred to as the "3 A's: Assess, Advise, Assist." Motivational interviewing remains a crucial component of brief intervention, with the goal to motivate individuals to change behaviors through exploring and resolving discrepancy and ambivalence. Motivational interviewing has consistently been shown to be more effective at supporting change than traditional advice-giving and studies have not shown it to be any more time-consuming [66]. In the preconception period, there is strong evidence for the use of brief interventions that have a dual focus of reducing alcohol use and increasing use of effective contraception, such as the CHOICES approach [67]. See Chap. 3 for a more in-depth review of interventions to reduce alcohol use in pregnancy.

One reason health care providers may abstain from screening for alcohol use and providing brief interventions is their lack of knowledge about where to refer individuals with at-risk alcohol consumption or alcohol use disorders. Knowledge of community-based outreach programs, as well as substance use treatment facilities that serve women and/or pregnant patients, in one's area of practice may inspire more providers to engage in SBIRT.

Behavior Modification Treatments

Individuals with at-risk drinking or a diagnosis of alcohol use disorder in pregnancy benefit from participation in treatment, regardless of the kind of treatment program they engage in. However, there is a paucity of data regarding the effectiveness of specific psychosocial interventions in this population [68]. Ideally, these treatment programs will include multi-disciplinary care teams, with members such as physicians, chemical dependency counselors/substance use disorder professionals, and mental health professionals. Low-level alcohol use in pregnancy is often amenable to treatment that involves brief intervention, motivational interviewing, and cognitive behavioral therapy [65]. However, more intensive care is required by many individuals, including management of withdrawal, pharmacologic treatment, and relapse prevention. Involvement in peer support groups (such as Alcoholics Anonymous) and residential rehabilitation programs or substance-free housing remain part of the holistic approach to treating and supporting individuals with alcohol use disorder in pregnancy.

Harm reduction is another approach that has been found to be helpful in assisting individuals with establishing realistic and attainable goals aimed at decreasing their alcohol consumption or minimizing the risks associated with prenatal alcohol exposure [69]. This method strives to shift away from stigma, guilt, confrontation, and shame, which are often associated with maternal use of substances in pregnancy. Instead, the goal of harm reduction is to meet individuals where they are and empower them through patient-centered, compassionate, and non-judgmental care. One example of employing a harm reduction approach is working with individuals who are ambivalent about quitting on cutting back their alcohol consumption.

Pharmacotherapy for Treatment of Alcohol Use Disorder

The goal of treatment can either be complete abstinence or reduced alcohol consumption. The reduction or complete cessation of alcohol use often causes withdrawal symptoms, which are commonly treated by short courses of benzodiazepines and a variety of other medications aimed at easing the associated withdrawal symptoms. Detoxification for pregnant individuals who are alcohol dependent is generally done in a specialized setting that allows for regular dosing of benzodiazepines, close monitoring in order to decrease risk of withdrawal-related seizures and administration of adjunctive medications [52, 65].

In order to support ongoing abstinence following withdrawal, there are several first-line evidence-based pharmacologic treatments available for individuals with alcohol use disorder in the general population. A review of their safety in pregnancy can be found in Graves et al. [65] and Kelty et al. [70] and will be summarized. Despite the extensive data on the harms of alcohol use in pregnancy, there is little data on the safety of medications for the treatment of alcohol use disorder in pregnancy. First-line pharmacologic options for the treatment of alcohol use disorder in the non-pregnant population (naltrexone, acamprosate, disulfiram) are not approved for use in pregnancy. When making decisions about initiation of a medication in pregnancy, a core principal remains that potential benefits to mother and fetus should outweigh any potential harms.

Naltrexone is a non-selective opioid antagonist with high affinity for mu opioid receptors. It is used as one of the first-line treatments for alcohol use disorder in individuals not on opioid therapy in the general population and functions to reduce alcohol cravings and positive reinforcing effects of alcohol use. It has also been shown to be effective in decreasing the incidence of relapse to heavy drinking [71]. Only limited data is available for its use in pregnancy, with most of the available data extrapolated from animal studies or for its use in opioid use disorder in pregnancy [71].

The exact mechanism of acamprosate is unknown, but it is thought to stabilize glutamatergic neurotransmission that is altered in a withdrawal state and reduce abstinence cravings. While there is some animal data about acamprosate in pregnancy [70], there is a paucity of human data and acamprosate is generally thought to be contraindicated in pregnancy.

Disulfiram inhibits aldehyde dehydrogenase and therefore prevents metabolism of alcohol's primary metabolite, acetaldehyde, which causes an acute reaction that often involves sweating, headache, nausea, and emesis if alcohol is taken alongside the drug. It is not recommended in pregnancy given concern for potential teratogenicity and has been found to predispose to maternal hypertension and autonomic instability in all trimesters [65].

Gabapentin is an antiepileptic drug used to treat a variety of medical conditions. It is a γ-aminobutyric acid analog that functions in part by inhibition of dopamine release in parts of the central nervous system. In the general population, there is data that gabapentin is effective in decreasing the incidence and severity of protracted alcohol withdrawal symptoms, cravings, and heavy drinking days [72]. In regard to safety data in pregnancy, there has not been shown to be any increase in risk of malformations [68, 73].

Nutrition and Supplementation with Folic Acid

Regular alcohol consumption can impair quality nutrition and energy intake during the preconception and prenatal period. Heavy alcohol consumption not only impairs consumption of a balanced diet but can also interfere with the nutritional status of the individual. In addition to the adverse effects of decreased consumption of daily recommended amounts of carbohydrates, proteins, fats, calcium, and iron, alcohol can interfere with absorption and utilization of essential amino acids and vitamins, including B_1 (thiamine), B_2 (riboflavin), B_6 (pyridoxine), vitamin A, vitamin C, choline, and folic acid [74, 75]. The lack of micronutrients and subsequent reduction in antioxidants, in addition to the toxic metabolites of alcohol, likely play a role in potential for altered neurodevelopment, as well as other potential adverse effects in the offspring.

Chronic alcohol use can also lead to thiamine deficiency. Thiamine plays an essential role in the body's energy metabolism, and thiamine deficiency is a factor in the development of Wernicke-Korsakoff syndrome. Supplementation with at least 100 mg thiamine should be initiated in anyone undergoing alcohol withdrawal, especially before a glucose load is given [76]. Therefore, pregnant individuals in alcohol withdrawal should receive 100–200 mg IV or IM thiamine daily (depending on nutritional status) for 3–5 days in order to correct any nutritional deficiencies caused by excessive alcohol use and prevent Wernicke-Korsakoff syndrome. Additionally, pregnant individuals, regardless of drinking status, have an increased need for dietary thiamine and should receive at least 1.4 mg/day in their diet or in the form of supplementation. There are no known adverse effects of high thiamine levels in pregnancy.

Individuals who have folic acid deficiency during pregnancy are more likely to give birth to premature and low birth weight infants, in addition to infants with neural tube defects [76]. Folic acid is converted to tetrahydrofolate (folate), which is important in the production of methyl groups. This ability to move methyl groups has implicated folate as a key coenzyme in multiple metabolic pathways and in methylation of DNA [77]. Alcohol impairs many processes where folate plays a key role and therefore folic acid supplementation, especially in the first trimester, may be risk reducing. The current USPSTF and ACOG recommendations for folic acid supplementation in pregnancy in order to reduce risk of neural tube defects are 0.4 mg daily, ideally initiated at least 1 months before conception and continued for the first trimester of pregnancy. It is recommended that individuals at high risk of neural tube defects (e.g., history of previous affected pregnancy, individuals affected with neural tube defect themselves, partner who is affected, partner with a previously affected child, and ingestion of certain antiseizure medications) supplement with 4 mg of folic acid daily, ideally initiating 3 months before pregnancy and continuing for the first trimester of pregnancy [78]. In the United States, the recommended upper limit for folic acid intake in the general adult population is

1 mg daily. The 4 mg high dose supplementation is generally believed to be nontoxic in the short term, but the dose should be decreased after the first trimester of pregnancy when no longer beneficial for prevention of neural tube defects. Unclear guidance remains in regard to dose of supplemental folic acid in pregnancies where alcohol is consumed. According to the Society of Obstetricians and Gynaecologists in Canada, 1 mg folic acid supplementation initiated 3 months prior to conception and continued for the first trimester of pregnancy should be recommended for pregnant individuals consuming alcohol in order to decrease risk of neural tube defects [79]. This is often recommended by expert opinion in the United States as well.

Perinatal Outcomes of Maternal Alcohol Use

Risk of Stillbirth and Miscarriage with Maternal Alcohol Use

Alcohol is a teratogen and adverse developmental effects in the fetus can occur, especially depending on whether the drinking occurred during critical stages of organ formation [80]. The most significant consequences of prenatal alcohol exposure are stillbirth and FASD. Kesmodel et al. prospectively studied pregnant individuals using self-administered questionnaires and hospital files found that maternal consumption of greater than or equal to five drinks per week was associated with a risk ratio for stillbirth of 2.96 (CI 1.37–6.41) compared to individuals who consumed less than one drink per week [81]. The rate of stillbirth secondary to fetal-placental function also increased across alcohol categories from 1.37 per 1000 births in individuals consuming less than one drink per week to 8.83 per 1000 births in individuals consuming greater than or equal to five drinks per week [81]. However, the study was unable to associate the risk for stillbirth directly to prenatal alcohol exposure [81].

Sundermann et al. studied the association between week-by-week alcohol consumption in the first trimester and spontaneous abortion in 5353 individuals of which 49.7% reported alcohol consumption during early pregnancy and 12% miscarried [82]. Alcohol use in weeks 5–10 from last menstrual period were associated with increased miscarriage risk with the highest risk peaking for alcohol consumption in week 9 [83]. Each successive week of alcohol consumption was associated with an 8% increase in miscarriage relative to individuals who did not consume alcohol in pregnancy (aHR 1.08, CI 1.04–1.12) that was not related to the number of drinks consumed per week, the type of drink or binge drinking [82].

Adverse Perinatal and Offspring Outcomes Associated with Prenatal Alcohol Exposure

A prior systematic review and meta-analysis of 36 studies on the effect of prenatal alcohol exposure on the risk of low birthweight, preterm birth, and small for gestational age (SGA) noted that compared with abstainers, the overall dose–response relationships for low birthweight and SGA showed no effect up to 10 g pure alcohol/day (an average of about 1 drink/day) and preterm birth showed no effect up to 18 g pure alcohol/day (an average of 1.5 drinks/day) [83]. However, the risk of impaired fetal growth or preterm birth increased with consumption of an average of two or more drinks per day in each of the trimesters. The study concluded that a dose–response relationship indicates that heavy alcohol consumption during pregnancy increases the risks of all three outcomes whereas light to moderate alcohol consumption shows no effect [83].

Muggli et al. performed a prospective study from 2011 to 2014 examining the association between dose, frequency, and timing of prenatal alcohol exposure and craniofacial phenotype in children at 12 months of age [2]. A total of 415 children were studied, and a consistent association between craniofacial shape and prenatal alcohol exposure was observed even at low levels of prenatal alcohol consumption and regardless of timing of exposure. Craniofacial areas of difference were concentrated around the midface, nose, lips, and eyes [2].

In a recent large retrospective study of 9719 youth ages 9–10.9 years old, 2518 (25.9%) were exposed to alcohol in utero based on parental report and any alcohol use during pregnancy was found to be associated with subtle yet significant psychopathology, attention deficits, and impulsiveness in offspring [84]. Some of these effects even demonstrated a dose-dependent response. Several studies from Denmark studied the effects of maternal low to moderate alcohol consumption (less than nine drinks a week) in early to mid-pregnancy on developmental outcomes in offspring at the age of 5 years old and no significant effects to intelligence quotient (IQ), attention, executive function, motor function, or behavior were found [85–90].

Pregnancy Management

As comprehensive prenatal care can mitigate some of the perinatal, fetal, and offspring complications secondary to prenatal alcohol exposure, it is recommended that healthcare providers should screen all pregnant individuals for substance use, including alcohol use, counsel and educate pregnant individuals regarding the risks of alcohol consumption, and intervene as necessary. As prenatal alcohol exposure can be associated with craniofacial anomalies, decreased fetal growth and preterm birth, an early dating ultrasound, detailed fetal anatomic survey, serial fetal growth ultrasounds throughout gestation, and antenatal surveillance should be considered [10].

Guidance for Delivery and Postnatal Planning

Accessing prenatal care and disclosing substance use is often the first step an individual takes toward improving their health and investing in the health of their child and families. It often takes immense courage and becomes not only an opportunity to receive interventions and treatment, but also to support preparation for parenting. Birth becomes a time where ongoing support and services of parenting mothers and families become essential to short- and long-term health and stability, while bonding and attachment with stable caregivers remain crucial for infant health, safety, and development. During pregnancy and the postpartum period, availability of and access to culturally responsive, trauma-informed and evidence-based services for pregnant and parenting women with substance use disorders remains a barrier to quality compassionate care.

No specific guidance exists around planning for the delivery of an infant exposed to alcohol in utero. Labor management for individuals with alcohol use disorder often does not differ greatly from routine care. However, many of the principles for caring for substance-exposed infants and their mothers likely apply to the peripartum period. Multi-disciplinary teams, including obstetric care providers, pediatricians, social workers, case managers, and chemical dependency providers well-versed in the care of individuals with substance use disorders are often beneficial. Social workers, chemical dependency providers, proactive legal counsel, and peer support workers can assist and support individuals in navigating state-based child welfare programs. Obstetric care providers can support or initiate referrals for treatment for birthing parents if indicated. Pediatricians can identify potentially substance-exposed infants and initiate a comprehensive care plan regarding developmental assessment and support.

Safe housing, ongoing social support, relapse prevention, and postpartum contraception remain crucial aspects of postnatal planning. Stable housing and safe home environments enhance protective measures and reduce social risk factors that can negatively impact infants, children, and women. Individual and family stressors are often compounded in the postpartum period, contributing to an increased risk of relapse. Therefore, ongoing involvement in peer support programs, access to psychosocial interventions and initiation of pharmacotherapy when indicated become crucial components of relapse prevention. Close postpartum follow-up can also be beneficial, as can proactive referral for mental health services when necessary. Postpartum contraceptive plans should be addressed in the prenatal period and individuals should have immediate, easily access to contraception of their choice. Long-acting reversible contraception remains an excellent choice for a variety of reasons, including its ability to empower individuals to choose if and when she feels ready for any future pregnancy.

Alcohol Use While Breastfeeding

The prevalence of alcohol consumption throughout the lactation period has been reported to be 35–80% [91]. Of great concern is the lack of counseling and education surrounding drinking while breastfeeding. Pepino et al. found that only 13% of lactating mothers reported receiving advice from their healthcare provider about the detrimental effects of drinking while breastfeeding [92]. The lack of communication by healthcare providers is likely in part because of the limited data on alcohol consumption while breastfeeding [93]. Currently, the consensus is that avoiding alcohol is the safest option for breastfeeding mothers, but for those who choose to still consume during lactation, binge drinking should be avoided. The World Health Organization (WHO) recommends avoiding any alcohol during lactation [94] whereas the American Academy of Pediatrics and the Academy of Breastfeeding Medicine state that consuming 8 oz of wine or two cans of beer daily is acceptable and waiting 2 h after the last drink to breastfeed is sufficient [95–97]. Alternatively, ACOG recommends waiting at least 2 h, but preferably 3–4 h, after a single drink before breastfeeding [10, 98]. Similarly, the CDC also echoes that moderate alcohol consumption (up to one drink per day) while breastfeeding is not known to be harmful to the infant, especially if nursing occurs at least 2 h after a single drink [99]. It is not necessary to pump and dump milk after alcohol consumption, but if nursing is delayed then expressing milk can help maintain supply and avoid complications of breast engorgement.

Bioavailability of Alcohol in Breastmilk

Breastmilk alcohol levels are similar to blood alcohol levels with the highest alcohol levels in breastmilk occurring 30–60 min after consumption of an alcoholic beverage, but this can be delayed if food is also being ingested [93, 100]. The overall bioavailability of alcohol in lactating individuals is approximately 25% lower than non-lactating individuals, which results in lower peak alcohol blood levels, but the duration of time to achieve peak blood alcohol levels is the same [101]. The rate of alcohol elimination from breastmilk depends on the amount consumed and maternal weight. In an average 60 kg person, alcohol is detected in breastmilk for approximately 2.5 h after consuming a standard single drink, about 5 h after a second drink is consumed, and more than 9 h if binge drinking occurs [101]. If breastfeeding occurs during peak maternal blood alcohol levels, the amount of alcohol the infant consumes is approximately 5–6% of the weight-adjusted maternal intake [92]. The infant metabolizes alcohol at half the rate of an adult due to immature metabolism [102].

Risk to Offspring When Drinking During Lactation

Long-term offspring effects of daily drinking while breastfeeding are unknown. The existing data suggesting an adverse effect on infant growth and motor function from one drink or more daily is inconsistent. It is likely that a 2–2.5 h delay in nursing per drink and limiting consumption to casual drinking only (no more than 1 glass of wine or beer daily) will minimize the risk of any adverse short-term or long-term offspring effects [94]. However, heavy daily drinking (two or more drinks daily) is associated with decreased breastfeeding duration and excessive sedation, fluid retention, and hormone imbalances in breastfed infants [93, 103].

Little et al. found that although maternal alcohol use during lactation did not affect cognitive outcomes in infants at 12 months of age, a measurable decrease in motor function development was observed at 12 months that was no longer detectable at 18 months of age [104, 105]. In a different study, first-grade students that were exposed to alcohol during breastfeeding were noted to have worse grammatical comprehension than children that were not exposed [106]. Gibson et al. noted that infants exposed to alcohol through breastmilk may have dose-dependent reductions in their cognitive abilities observed at age 6–7 years old that was not present at age 10–11 years old [107, 108]. Preliminary studies have not demonstrated an increased risk of autism spectrum disorder or attention deficit hyperactivity disorder in offspring of mothers who consumed alcohol during lactation [93, 109].

Effect of Alcohol Consumption on Milk Production

Alcohol consumption can also impact the neuroendocrine axis and as a result, a decreased ability to breastfeed. Two major hormones play a vital role in breastfeeding: oxytocin, which is essential for contraction of mammary glands, and prolactin, which stimulates the production of breast milk [100]. Alcohol consumption can inhibit oxytocin and decrease milk production. Even after one or two drinks, including beer, an infant's milk intake can be decreased by 20–23% and result in infant irritability and poor sleep patterns [93]. This decrease in infant milk intake is mostly because of a lack of milk production rather than palatability or decreased feeding time [100]. Decreased feeding volumes are often compensated by increased breastfeeding frequency in the 8–16 h following maternal drinking [100]. Milk let down can also be delayed by about 30 s after consuming lower doses of alcohol or as high as 330 s after consuming higher doses of alcohol [110]. Consumption of five drinks or more can decrease milk let down and disrupt nursing until maternal alcohol levels decrease [93]. If nursing or pumping occurs within an hour prior to alcohol consumption, this may slightly reduce the subsequent amount of alcohol in breastmilk.

Conclusion

The current research is sufficient to demonstrate that prenatal alcohol use is a serious public health problem associated with tremendous adverse health outcomes and economic burden. Healthcare professionals caring for reproductive age individuals, especially those that are pregnant, have a unique opportunity to screen for alcohol use, educate, and intervene. A recent study suggests that interventions and education regarding the harms of prenatal alcohol use for frequent users prior to conception may reduce maternal drinking in pregnancy [111]. Pregnant individuals are also typically highly motivated to modify their behavior if it may potentially benefit their child [112]. As binge drinking behavior is associated with a higher risk of FASD, to prevent severe prenatal harm, healthcare providers should pay attention to individuals that are at risk for binge drinking including those with polysubstance use, depression, unmarried, Black or of lower socioeconomic class [53]. Ultimately, to reduce the prevalence of alcohol-exposed pregnancies, a combination of evidence-based community-level interventions, prevention programs aimed at reducing risk behaviors, substance use screening, counseling, and more research to identify groups of individuals at risk is needed.

Acknowledgment None.

References

1. Henderson J, Gray R, Brocklehurst P. Systematic review of effects of low-moderate prenatal alcohol exposure on pregnancy outcome. BJOG. 2007;1114(3):243–52.
2. Muggli E, Matthews H, Penington A, Claes P, O'Leary C, Forster D, et al. Association between prenatal alcohol exposure and craniofacial shape of children at 12 months of age. JAMA Pediatr. 2017;171(8):771–80.
3. May PA, Chambers CD, Kalberg WO, et al. Prevalence of fetal alcohol spectrum disorders in 4 US communities. JAMA. 2018;319:474–82.
4. Denny L, Coles S, Blitz R. Fetal alcohol syndrome and fetal alcohol spectrum disorders. Am Fam Physician. 2017;96(8):515–22.
5. Amendah DD, Grosse SD, Bertrand J. Medical expenditures of children in the United States with fetal alcohol syndrome. Neurotoxicol Teratol. 2011;33(2):322.
6. Greenmeyer JR, Klug MG, Kambeitz C, Popova S, Burd L. A multicountry updated assessment of the economic impact of fetal alcohol spectrum disorder: costs for children and adults. J Addict Med. 2018;12(6):466–73.
7. Edwards EM, Werler MM. Alcohol consumption and time to recognition of pregnancy. Matern Child Health J. 2006;10(6):467–72.
8. Floyd RL, Decoufle P, Hungerford DW. Alcohol use prior to pregnancy recognition. Am J Prev Med. 1999;17(2):101–7.
9. Finer LB, Zolna MR. Unintended pregnancy in the United States: incidence and disparities, 2006. Contraception. 2011;84(5):478–85.

10. American College of Obstetricians and Gynecologists. Committee on Health Care for Underserved Women. Committee opinion no. 496: At-risk drinking and alcohol dependence obstetric and gynecologic implications. Obstet Gynecol. 2011;118(2 Pt 1):383–8.

11. Carson G, Cox LV, Crane J, Croteau P, Graves L, Kluka S, Koren G, et al. No. 245—Alcohol use and pregnancy consensus clinical guidelines. J Obset Gynaecol Can. 2017;39(9):e220–54.

12. Williams JF, Smith VC. Committee on substance abuse. Fetal alcohol spectrum disorders. Pediatrics. 2015;136(5):e1395–406.

13. Centers for Disease Control and Prevention. Fetal alcohol spectrum disorders (FASDs). http://www.cdc.gov/ncbddd/fasd/alcohol-use.html. Accessed on 14 Aug 2021.

14. McHugh RK, Wigderson S, Greenfield SF. Epidemiology of substance use in reproductive-age women. Obstet Gynecol Clin N Am. 2014;41(2):177–89.

15. Denny CH, Acero CS, Terplan M, Kim SY. Trends in alcohol use among pregnant women in the U.S., 2011-2018. Am J Prev Med. 2020;59(5):768–9.

16. Maier SE, West JR. Drinking patterns and alcohol-related birth defects. Alcohol Res Health. 2001;25:168–74.

17. Denny CH, Acero CS, Naimi TS, Kim SY. Consumption of alcohol beverages and binge drinking among pregnant women aged 18-44 years—United States, 2015-2017. MMWR Morb Mortal Wkly Rep. 2019;68:365–8.

18. England LJ, Bennett C, Denny CH, Honein MA, Gilboa SM, Kim SY, Guy GP, Tran EL, Rose CE, Bohm MK, Boyle CA. Alcohol use and co-use of other substances among pregnant females aged 12–44 years—United States, 2015–2018. MMWR Morb Mortal Wkly Rep. 2020;69(31):1009–14.

19. Cheng D, Kettinger L, Uduhiri K, Hurt L. Alcohol consumption during pregnancy: prevalence and provider assessment. Obstet Gynecol. 2011;117(2 Pt 1):212–7.

20. Kitsantas P, Gaffney K, Wu H, Kastello J. Determinants of alcohol cessation, reduction and no reduction during pregnancy. Arch Gynecol Obstet. 2014;289(4):771–9.

21. Floyd RL, O'Connor MJ, Sokol RJ, Bertrand J, Cordero JF. Recognition and prevention of fetal alcohol syndrome. Obstet Gynecol. 2005;106(5 Pt 1):1059–64.

22. CDC. Fetal alcohol syndrome-Alaska, Arizona, Colorado, and New York, 1995-1997. MMWR Morb Mortal Wkly Rep. 2002;51(20):433–5.

23. United States Department of Health & Human Services. National Institutes of Health. National Institute on Alcohol Abuse and Alcoholism. Helping patients who drink too much: a clinician's guide. Bethesda, MD: National Institute on Alcohol Abuse and Alcoholism; 2007. NIH publication no. 07-3769. http://pubs.niaaa.nih.gov/publications/Practitioner/CliniciansGuide2005/guide.pdf. Accessed 20 Aug 2021.

24. Committee opinion no. 496: At-risk drinking and alcohol dependence: obstetric and gynecologic implications. Obstet Gynecol. 2011;118(2 Pt 1):383–8.

25. Screening and behavioral counseling interventions in primary care to reduce alcohol misuse: recommendation statement. U.S. Preventive Services Task Force. Ann Intern Med. 2004;140(7):554–6.

26. American Psychiatric Association. Diagnostic and statistical manual of mental disorders. 5th ed (DSM-5). Washington, DC: American Psychiatric Publishing; 2013.

27. National Institute on Alcohol Abuse and Alcoholism (NIAAA). Alcohol use disorder: a comparison between DSM-IV and DSM-5. NIH Publication No. 13-7999. 2016. Available at: https://pubs.niaaa.nih.gov/publications/dsmfactsheet/dsmfact.pdf. Last accessed 21 Aug 2021.

28. O'Brien PL. Performance measurement: a proposal to increase use of SBIRT and decrease alcohol consumption during pregnancy. Matern Child Health J. 2014;18(1):1–9.

29. Taylor P, Zaichkin J, Pilkey D, Leconte J, Johnson BK, Peterson AC. Prenatal screening for substance use and violence: findings from physician focus groups. Matern Child Health J. 2007;11(3):241–7.

30. ACOG committee opinion no. 422: At-risk drinking and illicit drug use: ethical issues in obstetric and gynecologic practice. Obstet Gynecol. 2008;112(6):1449–60.

31. Clarren SK, Salmon A. Prevention of fetal alcohol spectrum disorder: proposal for a comprehensive approach. Expert Rev Obstet Gynecol. 2010;5(1):23–30.
32. Sokol RJ, Martier SS, Ager JW. The T-ACE questions: practical prenatal detection of risk-drinking. Am J Obstet Gynecol. 1989;160(4):863–8; discussion 868–70.
33. Chan AK, Pristach EA, Welte JW, Russell M. The TWEAK test in screening for alcoholism/heavy drinking in three populations. Alcohol Clin Exp Res. 1993;17(6):1188–92.
34. Chang G. Alcohol-screening instruments for pregnant women. Alcohol Res Health. 2001;25(3):204–9.
35. Russell M. New assessment tools for risk drinking during pregnancy. Alcohol Health Res World. 1994;18(1):55–61.
36. Burns E, Gray R, Smith LA. Brief screening questionnaires to identify problem drinking during pregnancy: a systematic review. Addiction. 2010;105(4):601–14.
37. Chasnoff IJ, McGourty RF, Bailey GW, Hutchins E, Lightfoot SO, Pawson LL, et al. The 4P's Plus screen for substance use in pregnancy: clinical application and outcomes. J Perinatol. 2005;25(6):368–74.
38. Chasnoff IJ, Wells AM, McGourty RF, Bailey LK. Validation of the 4P's Plus screen for substance use in pregnancy. J Perinatol. 2007;27(12):744–8.
39. Kennedy C, Finkelstein N, Hutchins E, Mahoney J. Improving screening for alcohol use during pregnancy: the Massachusetts ASAP program. Matern Child Health J. 2004;8(3):137–47.
40. Morrow-Tlucak M, Ernhart CB, Sokol RJ, Martier S, Ager J. Underreporting of alcohol use in pregnancy: relationship to alcohol. Alcohol Clin Exp Res. 1989;13(3):399–401.
41. Verkerk PH. The impact of alcohol misclassification on the relationship between alcohol and pregnancy outcome. Int J Epidemiol. 1992;21(Suppl 1):S33–7.
42. Jacobson SW, Jacobson JL, Sokol RJ, Martier SS, Ager JW, Kaplan MG. Maternal recall of alcohol, cocaine, and marijuana use during pregnancy. Neurotoxicol Teratol. 1991;13(5):535–40.
43. Bearer CF, Jacobson JL, Jacobson SW, Barr D, Croxford J, Molteno CD, et al. Validation of a new biomarker of fetal exposure to alcohol. J Pediatr. 2003;143(4):463–9.
44. Wisniewski KE, Pullarkat RK, Harin A, Vartolo M. Increased urinary dolichol in newborns whose mothers were heavy alcohol users. Ann Neurol. 1983;14:382A.
45. Halmesmaki E, Roine R, Salaspuro M. Gamma-glutamyltransferase, aspartate and alanine aminotransferases and their ratio, mean cell volume and urinary dolichol in pregnant alcohol abusers. Br J Obstet Gynaecol. 1992;99(4):287–91.
46. Bearer CF, Lee S, Salvator AE, Minnes S, Swick A, Yamashita T, et al. Ethyl linoleate in meconium: a biomarker for prenatal ethanol exposure. Alcohol Clin Exp Res. 1999;23(3):487–93.
47. Chan D, Bar-oz B, Pellerin B, Paciorek C, Klein J, Kapur B, et al. Population baseline of meconium fatty acid ethyl esters among infants of nondrinking women in Jerusalem and Toronto. Ther Drug Monit. 2003;25(3):271–8.
48. Niemela O, Halmesmaki E, Ylikorkala O. Hemoglobin-acetaldehyde adducts are elevated in women carrying alcohol-damaged fetuses. Alcohol Clin Exp Res. 1991;15(6):1007–10.
49. Regier DA, Farmer ME, Rae DS, et al. Comorbidity of mental disorders with alcohol and other drug abuse: results from the Epidemiological Catchment Area (ECA) study. JAMA. 1990;264:2511–8.
50. Kissin WB, Svikis DS, Moylan P, et al. Identifying pregnant women at risk for early attrition from substance abuse treatment. J Subst Abus Treat. 2004;27:31–8.
51. Velez M, Montoya I, Jansson L, et al. Exposure to violence among substance-dependent pregnant women and their children. J Subst Abus Treat. 2006;30:31–8.
52. Bhuvaneswar CG, Chang G, Epstein LA, Stern TA. Alcohol use during pregnancy: prevalence and impact. Prim Care Companion J Clin Psychiatry. 2007;9(6):455–60.
53. Shmulewitz D, Hasin DS. Risk factors for alcohol use amongst pregnant women ages 15-44, in the United States, 2002 to 2017. Prev Med. 2019;124:75–83.
54. Bayatpour M, Wells RD, Holford S. Physical and sexual abuse as predictors of substance use and suicide among pregnant teenagers. J Adolesc Health. 1992;13:128–32.

55. Skagerstrom J, Chang G, Nilsen P. Predictors of drinking during pregnancy: a systematic review. J Womens Health (Larchmt). 2011;20(6):901–13.
56. Tan CH, Denny CH, Cheal NE, Sniezek JE, Kanny D. Alcohol use and binge drinking among women of childbearing age—United States, 2011-2013. MMWR Morb Mortal Wkly Rep. 2015;64(37):1042–6.
57. May PA, Gossage JP. Maternal risk factors for fetal alcohol spectrum disorders. Alcohol Res Health. 2011;34(1):15–26.
58. Naimi TS, Lipscomb LE, Brewer RD, Gilbert BC. Binge drinking in the preconception period and the risk of unintended pregnancy: implications for women and their children. Pediatrics. 2003;111(5 Pt 2):1136–41.
59. Bakhrieva LN, Shrestha S, Garrison L, Leeman L, Rayburn WF, Stephen JM. Prevalence of alcohol use in pregnant women with substance use disorder. Drug Alcohol Depend. 2018;187:305–10.
60. Jorda M, Conant BJ, Sandstrom A, Klug MG, Jyoti A, Burd L. Protective factors against tobacco and alcohol use among pregnant women from a tribal nation in the Central United States. PLoS One. 2021;16(2):e0243924.
61. O'Connor MJ, Whaley SE. Brief intervention for alcohol use by pregnant women. Am J Public Health. 2007;97(2):252–8.
62. Carson G, Cox LV, Crane J, Croteau P, Graves L, Kluka S, et al. Alcohol use and pregnancy consensus clinical guidelines. Society of Obstetricians and Gynecologists of Canada. J Obstet Gynaecol Can. 2010;32(8 Suppl 3):S1–31.
63. Carson G, Cox LV, Crane J, Croteau P, Graves L, Kluka S, Koren G, et al. No. 245—Alcohol use and pregnancy consensus clinical guidelines. J Obstet Gynaecol Can. 2017;39(9):e220–54.
64. Wilk A, Jensen NM, Havighurstt TC. Meta-analysis of randomized control trials addressing brief interventions in heavy alcohol drinkers. J Gen Intern Med. 1997;12(5):274–83.
65. Graves L, Carson G, Poole N, Patel T, Bigalky J, Green CR, Cook JL. Guideline No. 405: Screening and counselling for alcohol consumption during pregnancy. J Obstet Gynaecol Can. 2020;42(9):1158–1173.e1.
66. Rubak S, Sandbaek A, Lauritzen T, Christensen B. Motivational interviewing: a systematic review and meta-analysis. Br J Gen Pract. 2005;55(513):305–12.
67. Centers for Disease Control and Prevention C. CHOICES as a program to prevent alcohol-exposed pregnancies. Available at: www.cdc.gov/ncbddd/fasd/choices-program-prevent-alcohol-exposed-pregnancies.html. Accessed 20 Aug 2021.
68. Furieri FA, Nakamura-Palacios EM. Gabapentin reduces alcohol consumption and craving: a randomized, double-blind, placebo-controlled trial. J Clin Psychiatry. 2007;68(11):1691–700.
69. Dejong K, Olyaei A, Lo JO. Alcohol use in pregnancy. Clin Obstet Gynecol. 2019;62(1):142–55.
70. Kelty E, Terplan M, Greenland M, Preen D. Pharmacotherapies for the treatment of alcohol use disorders during pregnancy: time to reconsider? Drugs. 2021;81(7):739–48.
71. Rosner S, Hackl-Herrwerth A, Leucht S, Vecchi S, Srisurapanont M, Soyka M. Opioid antagonists for alcohol dependence. Cochrane Database Syst Rev. 2010;12:CD001867.
72. Mason BJ, Quello S, Goodell V, Shadan F, Kyle M, Begovic A. Gabapentin treatment for alcohol dependence: a randomized clinical trial. JAMA Intern Med. 2014;174(1):70–7.
73. Fujii H, Goel A, Bernard N, Pistelli A, Yates LM, Stephens S, et al. Pregnancy outcomes following gabapentin use: results of a prospective comparative cohort study. Neurology. 2013;80(17):1565–70.
74. Sebastiani G, Borrás-Novell C, Casanova MA, Pascual M, Ferrero S, Gómez-Roig MD, García-Algar O. The effects of alcohol and drugs of abuse on maternal nutritional profile during pregnancy. Nutrients. 2018;10(8):1008.
75. Lieber CS. Relationships between nutrition, alcohol use, and liver disease. Alcohol Res Health. 2003;27(3):220–31.

76. Molloy AM, Brody LC, Mills JL, Scott JM, Kirke PN. The search for genetic polymorphisms in the homocysteine/folate pathway that contribute to the etiology of human neural tube defects. Birth Defects Res A Clin Mol Teratol. 2009;85(4):285–94.
77. Ballard MS, Sun M, Ko J. Vitamin A, folate, and choline as a possible preventive intervention to fetal alcohol syndrome. Med Hypotheses. 2012r;78(4):489–93.
78. Cheschier N, ACOG Committee on Practice Bulletins-Obstetrics. ACOG practice bulletin. Neural tube defects. Number 44, July 2003. Int J Gynaecol Obstet. 2003;83(1):123–33.
79. Wilson RD, Genetics Committee, Wilson RD, Audibert F, Brock JA, Carroll J, Cartier L, Gagnon A, Johnson JA, Langlois S, Murphy-Kaulbeck L, Okun N, Pastuck M, Contributors S, Deb-Rinker P, Dodds L, Leon JA, Lowel HL, Luo W, MacFarlane A, McMillan R, Moore A, Mundle W, O'Connor D, Ray J, Van den Hof M. Pre-conception folic acid and multivitamin supplementation for the primary and secondary prevention of neural tube defects and other folic acid-sensitive congenital anomalies. J Obstet Gynaecol Can. 2015;37(6):534–52.
80. Alledeck P, Olsen J. Alcohol and fetal damage. Alcohol Clin Exp Res. 1998;22(7 Suppl):329S–32S.
81. Kesmodel U, Wisborg K, Olsen SF, Henriksen TB, Secher NJ. Moderate alcohol intake during pregnancy and the risk of stillbirth and death in the first year of life. Am J Epidemiol. 2002;155(4):305–12.
82. Sundermann AC, Velez Edwards DR, Slaughter JC, et al. Week-by-week alcohol consumption in early pregnancy and spontaneous abortion risk: a prospective cohort study. Am J Obstet Gynecol. 2021;223:97.e1.
83. Patra J, Bakker R, Irving H, Jaddoe VWV, Malini S, Rehm J. Dose-response relationship between alcohol consumption before and during pregnancy and the risks of low birthweight, preterm birth and small for gestational age (SGA)—a systematic review and meta-analyses. BJOG. 2011;118(12):1411–21.
84. Lees B, Mewton L, Jacobus J, Valadez EA, Stapinski LA, Teesson M, Tapert SF, Squeglia LM. Association of prenatal alcohol exposure with psychological, behavioral, and neurodevelopmental outcomes in children from the adolescent brain cognitive development study. Am J Psychiatry. 2020;177(11):1060–72.
85. Falgreen Eriksen HL, Mortensen EL, Kilburn T, et al. The effects of low to moderate prenatal alcohol exposure in early pregnancy on IQ in 5-year-old children. BJOG. 2012;119:1191.
86. Underbjerg M, Kesmodel US, Landro NI, et al. The effects of low to moderate alcohol consumption and binge drinking in early pregnancy on selective and sustained attention in 5 year-old children. BJOG. 2012;119:1211.
87. Skogerbo A, Kesmodel US, Wimberley T, et al. The effects of low to moderate alcohol consumption and binge drinking in early pregnancy on executive function in 5-year-old children. BJOG. 2012;119:1201.
88. Kesmodel US, Bertrand J, Stovring H, et al. The effect of different alcohol drinking patterns in early to mid pregnancy on the child's intelligence, attention, and executive function. BJOG. 2012;119:1180.
89. Bay B, Stovring H, Wimberley T, et al. Low to moderate alcohol intake during pregnancy and risk of psychomotor deficits. Alcohol Clin Exp Res. 2012;36:807.
90. Skogerbo A, Kesmodel US, Denny CH, et al. The effects of low to moderate alcohol consumption and binge drinking in early pregnancy on behavior in 5-year-old children: a prospective cohort study on 1628 children. BJOG. 2013;120:1042.
91. Davidson S, Alden L, Davidson P. Changes in alcohol consumption after childbirth. J Adv Nurs. 1981;6(3):195–8.
92. Pepino MY, Mennella JA. Advice given to women in Argentina about breast-feeding and the use of alcohol. Rev Panam Salud Publica. 2004;16(6):408–14.
93. Drugs and lactation database (LactMed). Bethesda, MD: National Library of Medicine (US); 2006. Alcohol [Updated 2021 May 17]. Available from: https://www.ncbi.nlm.nih.gov/books/NBK501469/.

94. Guidelines for the identification and management of substance use and substance use disorders in pregnancy. World Health Organization; 19 Nov 2014. https://www.who.int/publications/i/item/9789241548731. Accessed 11 Jun 2021.
95. Section on Breastfeeding. Breastfeeding and the use of human milk. Pediatrics. 2012;129(3):e827–41. https://doi.org/10.1542/peds.2011-3552.
96. Sachs HC, Committee on Drugs. The transfer of drugs and therapeutics into human breast milk: an update on selected topics. Pediatrics. 2013;132(3):e796–809. https://doi.org/10.1542/peds.2013-1985.
97. Reece-Stremtan S, Marinelli KA. ABM clinical protocol #21: guidelines for breastfeeding and substance use or substance use disorder, revised 2015. Breastfeed Med. 2015;10(3):135–41.
98. American College of Obstetricians and Gynecologists. Breastfeeding your baby. Updated May 2021. https://www.acog.org/womens-health/faqs/breastfeeding-your-baby. Last accessed 11 Jun 2021.
99. Alcohol. CDC. Updated 9 Feb 2021. Accessed 14 Aug 2021. https://www.cdc.gov/breastfeeding/breastfeeding-special-circumstances/vaccinations-medications-drugs/alcohol.html.
100. Mennella JA. Regulation of milk intake after exposure to alcohol in mothers' milk. Alcohol Clin Exp Res. 2001;25(4):590–3.
101. Anderson PO. Alcohol use during breastfeeding. Breastfeed Med. 2018;13(5):315–7. https://doi.org/10.1089/bfm.2018.0053.
102. Horst PG, Madjunkov M, Chaudry S. Alcohol: a pharmaceutical and pharmacological point of view during lactation. J Popul Ther Clin Pharmacol. 2016;23(2):e145–50.
103. Haastrup MB, Pottegard A, Damkier P. Alcohol and breastfeeding. Basic Clin Pharmacol Toxicol. 2014;114:168–73.
104. Little RE, Anderson KW, Ervin CH, Worthington-Roberts B, Clarren SK. Maternal alcohol use during breast-feeding and infant mental and motor development at one year. N Engl J Med. 1989;321(7):425–30.
105. Little RE, Northstone K, Golding J, ALSPAC Study Team. Alcohol, breastfeeding, and development at 18 months. Pediatrics. 2002;109(5):E72.
106. May PA, Hasken JM, Blankenship J, et al. Breastfeeding and maternal alcohol use: prevalence and effects on child outcomes and fetal alcohol spectrum disorders. Reprod Toxicol. 2016;63:13–21.
107. Gibson L, Porter M. Drinking or smoking while breastfeeding and later cognition in children. Pediatrics. 2018;142(2):e20174266.
108. Gibson L, Porter M. Drinking or smoking while breastfeeding and later academic outcomes in children. Nutrients. 2020;12(3):829.
109. Gibson L, Porder M. Alcohol and tobacco use while breastfeeding and risk of autism spectrum disorder or attention deficit/hyperactivity disorder. J Autism Dev Disord. 2022;52:1223.
110. Cobo E. Effect of different doses of ethanol on the milk-ejecting reflex in lactating women. Am J Obstet Gynecol. 1973;115(6):817–21.
111. Young-Wolff KC, Sarovar V, Alexeeff SE, Adams SR, Tucker LY, Conway A, Ansley D, Goler N, Armstrong MA, Weisner C. Trends and correlates of self-reported alcohol and nicotine use among women before and during pregnancy, 2009-2017. Drug Alcohol Depend. 2020;214:108168.
112. Lindqvist M, Lindkvist M, Eurenius E, Persson M, Mogren I. Change of lifestyle habits—motivation and ability reported by pregnant women in northern Sweden. Sex Reprod Health. 2017;13:83–90.

Chapter 5
Mechanisms of Teratogenesis

Siara Kate Rouzer, Dae Chung, Marisa Pinson, Natalie Collins, Jordan Kuhlman, and Rajesh Miranda

Historical Recognition of Deficits Associated with Prenatal Alcohol Exposure

The diagnosis of "Fetal Alcohol Syndrome" (FAS) was first clinically defined in a British medical journal, *The Lancet*, in 1973 [1]. However, observational links between ethanol exposure during pregnancy and adverse health outcomes have been documented for centuries. Published historical reports have cited the Old Testament[1] and lectures by ancient Greek and Roman philosophers,[2] including Aristotle, as the first written acknowledgments of alcohol's teratogenic effects on a developing fetus

---

[1] *Judges 13:3–4*, The angel of the Lord appeared to her and said, "You are barren and childless, but you are going to become pregnant and give birth to a son. Now see to it that you drink no wine or other fermented drink and that you do not eat anything unclean."

[2] In *Anatomy of Melancholia* (1621), Robert Burton quotes Roman author Aulus Gellius (130–180 AD): "If a drunken man get a child, it will never likely have a good brain" and Greek philosophers Plutarch (~120 AD): "one drunkard begets another" and Aristotle (322 BC): "foolish, drunken or hare-brain women, most part bring forth children like unto themselves." Plutarch further describes lawgiver Lycurgus' advice for child-rearing in ancient Sparta in *Life of Lycurgus* (reproduced in 1914): "In order to the good education of their youth (which, as I said before, he thought the most important and noblest work of a lawgiver), he [Lycurgus] went so far back as to take into consideration their very conception and birth, by regulating their marriages… he had tried all ways to reduce the women to more modesty and sobriety…" This thinking may have influenced ancient laws in the cities of Carthage and Sparta, which prohibited the use of alcohol by newly married couples to prevent conception during intoxication, according to Warner & Rosett, *The Effects of Drinking on Offspring* (1975).

S. K. Rouzer (✉) · D. Chung · M. Pinson · N. Collins · J. Kuhlman · R. Miranda
Department of Neuroscience and Experimental Therapeutics, Texas A & M School of Medicine, Bryan, TX, USA
e-mail: srouzer@tamu.edu; daehyukchung@tamu.edu; marisa_pinson@tamu.edu; ncollins19@tamu.edu; kuhlman.jordan@tamu.edu; rmiranda@tamu.edu

© The Author(s), under exclusive license to Springer Nature Switzerland AG 2023
O. A. Abdul-Rahman, C. L. M. Petrenko (eds.), *Fetal Alcohol Spectrum Disorders*,
https://doi.org/10.1007/978-3-031-32386-7_5

[2, 3]. Artist William Hogarth painted "Gin Lane" in 1751 in response to England's Gin Epidemic, possibly one of the earliest artistic renderings of harm to children following prenatal alcohol exposure. The painting centers on a mother engaging in "exuberant drinking" while dropping a baby with notable facial malformations, which are now recognized as a symptom of FAS. Within the next century, recognition of alcohol as a teratogen would appear in academic works, including Charles Darwin's "On the Origin of Species," as well as in popular literature, including Charles Dickens' novel *The Posthumous Papers of the Pickwick Club*.[3] Indeed, by the time Aldous Huxley references a child who is "stunted" by prenatal alcohol exposure in his 1932 novel *Brave New World*, there appears to be a societal consensus that alcohol exposure during pregnancy can produce negative developmental outcomes.

At the turn of the twentieth century, clinical researchers associated intrauterine alcohol exposure with distinct health risks during pregnancy and birthing, including spontaneous abortion, premature labor, and higher mortality rates in newborns [3]. Furthermore, the ability of alcohol to cross the placental barrier, and to be transmitted through breast milk, was discovered in 1900. A boom of research incorporating animal models, leading up through 1922, reported that offspring exhibited physical malformations after birth and throughout the lifespan. However, with the onset of Prohibition in the 1920s, research into the harmful effects of alcohol exposure declined suddenly and considerably, viewed unnecessary following the ban of alcohol consumption in the United States. This mindset carried through to the 1950s, well after the repeal of the 21st Amendment, when alcohol consumption among the general population was once again socially accepted. It was recognition of physical malformations in developing children exposed to radiation—specifically, explosions in Hiroshima and Nagasaki [4]—as well as widespread prescription of *thalidomide* to pregnant women in the 1950s–60s [5], that caused the resurgence of research into teratogenic exposures during pregnancy. Still, research investigating prenatal alcohol exposure remained minimal until Jones and Smith defined FAS in 1973, supplementing their diagnostic criteria with supporting evidence of prenatal alcohol exposure-induced deficits in humans. Follow-up investigations by Jones' research group incorporated animal models and accounted for confounding environmental and socioeconomic variables, providing compelling evidence that prenatal alcohol exposure directly produced not only physical impairments in exposed offspring, but behavioral deficits as well.

---

[3] Dickens writes, "Betsy Martin, widow, one child, and one eye. Goes out charring and washing, by the day; never had more than one eye, but knows her mother drank bottled stout, and shouldn't wonder if that caused it… Thinks it not impossible that if she had always abstained from spirits she might have had two eyes by this time."

Investigating the Toxic and Teratogenic Effects of Prenatal Alcohol Exposure: Factors of Consideration in Research

Research Models and Subjects

Just as our societal views on alcohol consumption during pregnancy have changed, so has the strict classification of alcohol as a poisonous agent. It is tempting to assume, based on observable deficits in children with a history of prenatal alcohol exposure, that alcohol behaves exclusively as a toxin. However, the field of fetal alcohol spectrum disorder (FASD) research has advanced to recognize that not all of alcohol's effects are toxic—rather, prenatal alcohol can also contribute to the adaptive reprogramming of cells and tissues, without directly inhibiting cell survival (a.k.a., *teratology*), which we will describe in this chapter.

It is important to acknowledge that the history of research investigating prenatal alcohol exposure began with clinical observation—recognizing an association between fetal alcohol exposure and distinct morphological and behavioral phenotypes in these same children after birth [1, 6]. These observations have led to numerous associative studies in humans—from reduced arousal and reflex scores on the Brazelton Newborn Behavioral Assessment Scale, to abnormal development of frontal lobe gray and white matter in magnetic resonance and diffusion tension imaging [7]—which have informed our ability to recognize and diagnose FASD in clinical settings. However, there are also a vast number of studies that incorporate non-human subjects, including simple systems (cells, organoids, and tissues) and living animals, to investigate prenatal alcohol teratology. These investigations have been crucial for identifying and manipulating biological mechanisms impaired by intrauterine alcohol exposure. There are several benefits and practical reasons for performing these types of non-human research.

First, no single medical assessment can definitively diagnose an individual with FASD; often, diagnoses rely on self-reports of prenatal alcohol exposure by pregnant individuals. Unfortunately, such behaviors are largely unreported, in part due to social stigmatization and shame. In a 2017 survey of adults, mothers of children with FASD were perceived with more disdain than women with mental illnesses, substance use disorders, and histories of incarceration [8]. In experiments incorporating animal subjects, exposures to alcohol are tightly regulated, allowing researchers to obfuscate the ethical and social concerns with prenatal alcohol exposure in humans. Another notable consideration of data collected from human subjects is that relationships between prenatal alcohol exposure and reported symptoms are associative, but not necessarily causal. In real-world cases of FASD, child outcomes often reflect comorbidities (i.e., high maternal stress, neglect, poly-drug exposures) which confound our ability to distinguish which observed outcomes are attributable to a history of alcohol exposure. Preclinical research allows for highly controlled exposure paradigms, which may examine these co-exposures and environmental factors in combination with prenatal alcohol exposure while incorporating appropriate control groups/conditions. Finally, from the breadth of existing research, we have observed common features of prenatal alcohol exposure across animal models—including non-human primates, rodents, sheep, and zebrafish—which correspond with features observed in humans (see review [9]). With the added benefit of shorter gestational periods, as well as the potential for using invasive techniques to identify mechanistic contributions to offspring outcomes (i.e., physiology, histology, and genetics), animals provide unique benefits and insights for researchers, informing future therapeutic and clinical treatments of FASD symptoms.

In addition to animal models, cells derived from humans and animals can serve as the simplest model for investigating alcohol's effects on cellular processes, including differentiation, proliferation, and programmed cell death (apoptosis). In these models, alcohol can be applied acutely to cell cultures derived from the neuroepithelium, whole brain extracts, or neuronal/glial cell lines. Human-induced pluripotent stem cells (iPSCs), for instance, can be differentiated into every cell type of the human body, and allow for in vitro investigations of alcohol's toxicity to different subcellular populations. Prior research of iPSC-derived neurospheres—three-dimensional systems of clustered neural precursor cells—has demonstrated that alcohol exposure causes premature apoptosis [10]. Furthermore, human iPSCs can be grown to generate cerebral organoids ("mini brains"), which allow cells to differentiate into layers which structurally mimic real, developing brains. Although these cell lines are the least translational models to humans, in terms of the complexity of the FASD phenotype, cell culture investigations have been pivotal to scientists' understanding of alcohol-induced changes to epigenetic profiles, cell cycle function, and transcriptional regulation during development [11].

Dose/Levels of Alcohol Exposure During Pregnancy

One challenge faced by researchers investigating prenatal alcohol exposure is factoring in the amount of alcohol consumed at a particular time point during pregnancy. People often underestimate their levels of consumption [12], in part due to the variety of cup/glass sizes (i.e., pint, bottle, wine glass), variation in how much beverage is poured into a glass, and a lack of knowledge about the alcohol by volume (ABV) associated with a particular beverage (for instance, beer has a substantially lower ABV than wine, which in turn has a much lower ABV than spirits). To properly assess one's alcohol consumption, an individual would have to multiply their beverage's ABV by the total volume of liquid, and sum all beverages into alcohol "units." Not only is this uncommon by everyday drinkers, but when we consider the sedative effects of alcohol that lead to memory impairments, which are also dose dependent [13], its unsurprising that drinkers often struggle to accurately self-report how much alcohol they have consumed.

Despite the difficulties with reliably assessing alcohol consumption, existing literature has demonstrated that the amount of alcohol fetuses are exposed to dictates the extent of their impairments, across a multitude of measures. Newborns exposed to >1 drink per day during the first trimester of pregnancy were more likely to express FASD symptoms, including lower birth weight, shorter body length, and increased facial dysmorphology, compared to newborns exposed to <1 drink per day [14]; importantly, infants exposed to these lower alcohol levels still exhibited FASD symptoms compared to non-exposed infants. To more accurately determine the effects of alcohol dose on offspring survival, Clarren and colleagues [15] performed a controlled series of experiments in pregnant macaques investigating the effects of a range of alcohol doses, delivered once a week throughout gestation. Alcohol exposures that produced blood alcohol levels of at least 205 mg/dL significantly increased the risk for spontaneous abortion. (For reference, 205 mg/dL can be achieved by a 150 lb woman after 7 drinks, with drinks defined as 1.25 oz of liquor, 12 oz of beer, or 5 oz of wine [16].) Furthermore, as blood alcohol levels continued to increase, pregnant individuals experienced even greater risk of pregnancy loss, with 83% of pregnancies ending early when alcohol levels exceeded 250 mg/dL. In the United States, a blood alcohol level above 80 mg/dL is legally qualified as intoxication; however, humans are capable of drinking considerably more (exceeding levels of 400 mg/dL [17]), depending upon the individual and the amount of alcohol consumed.

Importantly, 80 mg/dL is not a cutoff for "safe" alcohol exposure during pregnancy. In a series of experiments performed in rodents, pregnant females received liquid diets of 2%, 3%, and 5% ethanol throughout gestation, leading to average blood alcohol levels of 7, 30, and 83 mg/dL, respectively. Importantly, when their exposed offspring grew into adulthood, they demonstrated dose-dependent deficits in hippocampal synaptic activity and spatial learning tasks, with deficits increasing incrementally with dose [18]. These data are further supported by research in humans, with pregnant individuals who report low, moderate, or high levels of alcohol use: meta-analyses have demonstrated that even low-moderate exposures impact child development, cognitive performance, and mental health [19, 20]. Although considerably more research is necessary to investigate the consequences of sub-intoxicating prenatal exposures, many scientists today challenge the notion of a "safe" level of alcohol exposure during pregnancy.

Timing and Frequency of Alcohol Exposure During Pregnancy

Another factor to consider in understanding alcohol's impact on a developing fetus is the time during gestation in which alcohol exposure occurs. During the first few weeks after fertilization, alcohol exposure can impede the proper implantation of a developing blastocyst in a woman's uterus, resulting in early termination of a pregnancy even prior to detection [21]. Within 4–6 weeks after fertilization, differentiation of cardiac myocytes occurs, and alcohol exposure can inhibit proper growth, migration, and specification of cardiac progenitor cells. Furthermore, during this period of time, alcohol exposure can damage neural progenitor cells, which has been tied to the facial dysmorphology associated with FAS [21]. This window of development for facial features may carry into the second half of the first trimester, as alcohol exposure within this time period corresponds with incidence of a smooth philtrum and thin vermillion border in exposed children [14]. Fetal exposure to alcohol is most common during the first month of pregnancy [22], likely because the pregnancy has not been detected, and alcohol exposure during this month of life has been associated with low infant birth weight, reduced body length, and smaller head circumference [14]. Importantly, there are numerous critical periods of development for embryonic tissues and structures within each gestational trimester. Preclinical and clinical research have cohesively informed the theory that fetal organs and tissues forming at the time of alcohol exposure are particularly vulnerable to long-term damage [23–25].

Related to the timing of alcohol exposure, the frequency of alcohol exposure during pregnancy also corresponds with the degree of impairment observed in exposed children. In a series of experiments by Clarren and colleagues, pregnant female macaques were exposed to alcohol once a week during the first 3 or 6 weeks of pregnancy or for the entire 24 weeks of gestation [26]. Offspring exposed to either 6 or 24 weeks of alcohol exposure experienced significant delays in memory and learning tasks, which were most pronounced in the offspring exposed for 24-weeks, as well as greater difficulty walking and climbing compared to both 3-week-alcohol-exposed and non-exposed offspring [26]. Importantly, these experiments demonstrated that early-gestation alcohol exposure (6 weeks) followed by abstinence failed to recover deficits in offspring, producing cognitive and behavioral outcomes comparable to exposure throughout pregnancy. However, these data should be interpreted with caution, as research in humans has found that in several measures of FAS—including infant growth and neurodevelopmental outcomes—avoiding alcohol exposure early in pregnancy can reduce the severity of symptoms expressed by children [27]. This conclusion was supported regardless of whether developing fetuses were exposed to low-moderate or high alcohol levels during pregnancy. Indeed, when alcohol exposure was significantly reduced or eliminated within the first ~6 weeks of pregnancy, children exhibited less severe FAS symptoms than those who were exposed to alcohol throughout pregnancy.

Taken together, there does not appear to be a point during embryonic development in which prenatal alcohol exposure lacks consequences. Rather, specific deficits expressed by children may correspond with the timing of exposure, as well as the amount and frequency of alcohol exposure during pregnancy.

The Toxicology of Prenatal Alcohol Exposure

Across diverse exposure paradigms and subject models, a substantial body of literature has demonstrated that alcohol can be toxic to an exposed organism, contributing to the physical, mental, and behavioral abnormalities that we associate with FASD [28]. Here, we will briefly discuss mechanisms commonly associated with the toxicity of ethanol, including increased oxidative stress, mitochondrial damage, and apoptosis/cell death (Fig. 5.1).

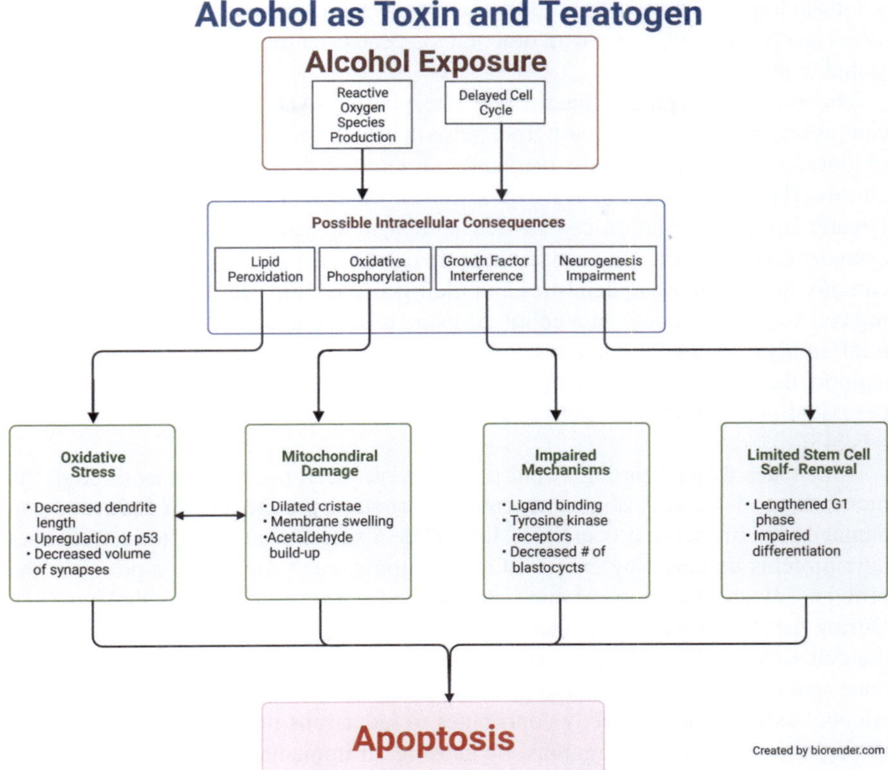

Fig. 5.1 Alcohol as a toxin and teratogen. This figure summarizes alcohol's direct effects as a poisonous toxin, as well as indirect effects as a teratogen, which contribute to increased rates of apoptosis following prenatal alcohol exposure

Oxidative Stress

Oxygen is required for molecular electron transfer and energy (or ATP) production in aerobic species. However, excess amounts of oxygen can produce harmful side effects, such as oxidative stress. Oxidative stress is the imbalance of reactive oxygen species (ROS) and antioxidant defenses [29] and serves as a driving mechanism to change mitochondrial structure/function, and damage lipids, proteins, and DNA [30–34]. Such imbalance caused by oxidative stress can lead to free radicals damaging DNA, proteins, and fatty tissue in an individual, with prolonged damage leading to a variety of diseases over time [35]. Prenatal alcohol exposure has a direct relationship with the aggregation of free radicals, with alcohol causing an increase in free radicals, ROS, and, consequently, oxidative stress [36, 37]. When free radicals attack other biological molecules—for example, lipids—they can damage cell membranes and induce lipid peroxidation [30, 33, 35]. Lipid peroxidation is often used as an indicator of oxidative stress, as this chain reaction of lipid degeneration results in high volumes of ROS [38]. The increase in ROS and subsequent oxidative stress can potentially, along with other factors, cause neuronal deficits that are associated with FASD [39].

Nicotinamide adenine dinucleotide phosphate (NADPH) is another ROS that can initiate reactions to increase lipid peroxidation by generating high quantities of oxidoreductases during early pregnancy, including the enzyme family of cytochrome P450, which are directly involved in the metabolism of alcohol [35, 40]. Greater lipid peroxidation can be detrimental to structures required for *in utero* synapse formation during early development as well [41]. An *in vitro* rat hippocampus study looking at dendrites and their synapses showed that, without affecting cell survival, six days of alcohol exposure resulted in an overall decrease in the total number, length, and synapse of dendrites [42]. Taken together, these further support the negative effects, through higher levels of oxidative stress and lipid peroxidation, that alcohol can have on a fetus during the early gestational periods [43].

Aldehydes formed through lipid peroxidation reactions, as well as through the metabolism of alcohol, also contribute to increased productions of ROS and can damage proteins in the process [31, 36]. While research attempting to identify specific proteins damaged by excess ROS is ongoing, such damage compromises the proteins' overall structures, which can prevent normal cellular metabolism [31]. During the metabolism of alcohol, acetaldehyde is oxidized to acetate along one of the cell's metabolic pathways, which increases respiratory chain activity and can once again lead to greater oxidative stress through the overproduction of ROS [36]. Alcohol exposure also directly contributes to reductions in the number of neurons throughout multiple brain regions, by causing an immediate increase in ROS and oxidative stress, leading to mitochondria-mediated apoptotic cell death of neurons [44, 45].

In conclusion, alcohol-induced oxidative stress negatively alters the role that oxygen plays within the cell, leading to the hindrance of other intracellular mechanisms that contribute to the expression of FASD symptoms [46]. Further research is necessary to explore these respiratory reactions, and specifically how they can be stimulated to self-repair following alcohol exposure. This research would inform therapeutic interventions to potentially minimize the damage of oxidative stress during fetal development.

Mitochondrial Damage

Mitochondria are organelles essential for the production of ATP, for maintaining reduction potential and ionic balance, and for normally-occurring apoptosis. They are also crucial in supporting multiple cellular signaling pathways, cell-cell communication, and overall healthy cellular function [47]. When mitochondria are damaged, such as following alcohol exposure, the cell's primary energy source is compromised, increasing the probability of ROS developments (and possibly the overproduction of ROS), disturbing ionic balances, and inducing inappropriate apoptosis [47]. Alcohol exposure has toxic effects on both the structure and function of the mitochondria [48, 49], producing elongation, cristae (the folds of the inner mitochondrial membrane), disorientation, and overcrowding of material within the mitochondrial matrix [50]. Cumulatively, this means that alcohol exposure can disrupt mitochondrial functions of generating ATP and cell-cell communication [51, 52].

Additionally, alcohol exposure inhibits the function of the electron transport chain (ETC) located in the inner mitochondrial membrane [51, 52], which can lead to the overproduction of ROS [53, 54]. Subsequently, stray electrons escape the ETC and react with oxygen outside the ETC to form superoxide or hydrogen peroxide; this is why the mitochondria is the primary source of ROS [53, 54]. This increase in ROS removes electrons ("oxidizes") from the ETC complex subunits, which results in oxidative phosphorylation and decreased ATP levels, leading to insufficient mitochondrial energy production [51, 52]. In response to the impaired production of ATP, the internal integrity of the mitochondria is compromised, and the cristae become dilated [55, 56]. Because the proper formation and folding of cristae are crucial for its function and capacity to synthesize ATP, dilated cristae are associated with oxidative stress through either elevated ROS production or reductions in ROS protective mechanisms, i.e., antioxidants [43, 57]. Importantly, this connection between dilated cristae and ROS overproduction caused by alcohol exposure illustrates how alcohol can directly induce oxidative stress and lead to mitochondrial damage. Furthermore, there is evidence that the introduction of foreign substances (such as alcohol) leads to a mitochondrial response which incites an independent increase in ROS production and oxidative stress [55, 58]. Together, these findings imply that ethanol exacerbates the relationship between oxidative stress and mitochondrial damage.

Furthermore, alcohol exposure reduces mitochondrial glutathione, an antioxidant, and may lead to more oxidative damage, including lipid peroxidation, that changes how much ATP the mitochondria synthesizes [51, 57]. There is additional evidence that alcohol alters various signaling pathways to the mitochondria, including Complex I, Complex IV, succinate dehydrogenase, and ADP translocase activities. These changes produce a rapid onset of oxidative stress that precedes cellular apoptosis [44, 48]. Lipid peroxidation also affects the permeability of mitochondrial membranes, which produces mitochondrial swelling. This swelling is a result of increased cytochrome c release, caspase activation, and DNA fragmentation that also can lead to increased rates of cellular death [51, 59, 60].

In summary, the mitochondria play an integral role in balancing out ROS production and limiting oxidative stress. When function of this organelle is impeded by alcohol, the cell becomes more susceptible to destructive reactions [61]. Research investigating therapeutic treatments that are specific to maintaining the functional and structural integrity of the mitochondria would yield valuable information for combatting the toxicity of alcohol exposure and ensuring the maintenance of healthy levels of ROS [51].

Apoptosis

Optimal brain development requires a homeostatic degree of programmed cell death (PCD), with apoptosis serving as the controlled process of cell death via specific cellular pathways. During apoptosis, various membrane receptors, such as Fas, TNFR, and cytochrome c, trigger signal transduction steps that activate cysteine proteases, i.e., caspases [30, 62–64]. The initiation of apoptosis involves the loss of cell division controls, interference with growth factors, changes to cell attachment to tissue surface, and the activation of specific proteins that trigger cell death [30, 65–67]. Cells undergoing apoptosis show membrane blebbing, chromatin condensation, and DNA fragmentation until the cells eventually break down into smaller membrane-bound fragments, apoptotic bodies, and are no longer viable [68–70]. PCD is essential in fetal development and organ formation, occurring throughout embryonic development in normally-developing children. However, excessive embryonic cell death can disrupt the formation of organs or tissues and cause structural or functional abnormalities [68, 71].

Alcohol, as a toxic substance, can affect specific tissues and cell types more than others, depending on a multitude of factors including the amount and timing of exposure during gestation [30, 72]. These critical developmental windows are an essential consideration when investigating the tissues or cell types that are most susceptible to harm following alcohol exposure. Importantly, because cells are already biologically primed for apoptosis, exposure to alcohol may cause a dramatic increase in cell death, especially during embryonic development [73]. Cellular impairment in response to alcohol exposure has been attributed to several deficiencies, including vitamin A compound levels, antioxidant compounds levels (high oxidative stress), and an interference with normal internal cellular communication pathways [30]. Retinoic acid (RA) is an active form of vitamin A and a key regulator of morphogenesis. Importantly, RA deficiencies are linked to increased apoptosis in neural crest cell populations [30, 74]. These deficiencies can be compounding factors to the negative effects of alcohol, including increased apoptosis, during development.

As stated previously, alcohol increases the abundance of free radicals that are associated with elevated levels of oxidative stress. These free radicals can further damage embryonic cells by inciting unnecessary apoptosis [30, 33]. In addition, cell membrane-associated proteins act as communication signals from the outside of the cell to the inside. Alcohol interferes with this process by inhibiting this central communication pathway of the cell (inhibiting intracellular signaling kinases or increasing intracellular calcium), augmenting further cell death [30, 75, 76]. There may also be a direct neurotoxic effect of alcohol on the nervous system, both inciting apoptosis and reducing the density of synapses [30]. Several studies have found higher rates of apoptosis and neural crest populations resulting from alcohol exposure [30, 33, 77], once again highlighting the vulnerability of specific brain regions and tissues in the central nervous system at different timepoints and gestational periods. It is important to note that this is not an exhaustive explanation of alcohol-induced apoptosis, as research is currently underway to further understand the mechanisms through which alcohol increases rates of cell death. The goal of this research is to identify cellular targets with the potential to be therapeutically regulated, and to ultimately reduce the frequency and magnitude of physical, behavioral, and mental abnormalities in developing fetuses.

The Teratology of Prenatal Alcohol Exposure

Aside from its toxic effects, alcohol is also a prominent teratogen—a substance that disrupts normal fetal developmental pathways and programs. Prenatal alcohol exposure is the most prevalent cause of neurobehavioral deficits in Western countries [30], creating long-term cellular damage that contributes to the development of FASD. These lasting effects of alcohol exposure *in utero* can occur during the cell cycle or during stem cell self-renewal/growth (Fig. 5.2) and can interfere with

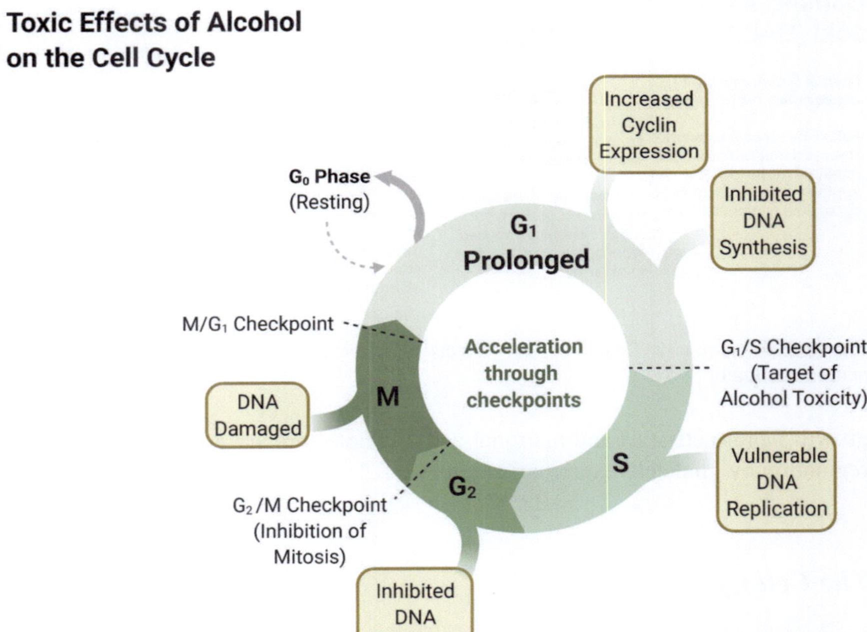

Fig. 5.2 The toxic effects of alcohol on the cell cycle. Alcohol toxicity impacts cellular function within each stage of the cell cycle, altering cell cycle progression and subsequent proliferation in exposed cells. These effects may furthermore be cell-type specific and dependent on the stage of development at which alcohol exposure occurs. G_0 phase: a class of cells that have the potential to divide but have not yet entered the cell cycle; interphase stages of the cell cycle—G_1: cell growth, S: DNA synthesis, G_2: preparation for mitosis, and M: mitotic

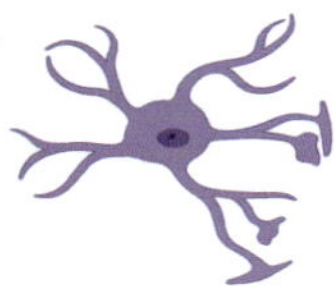
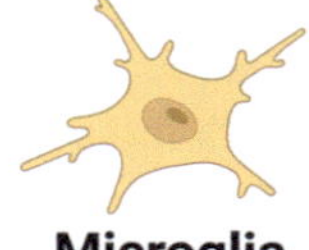
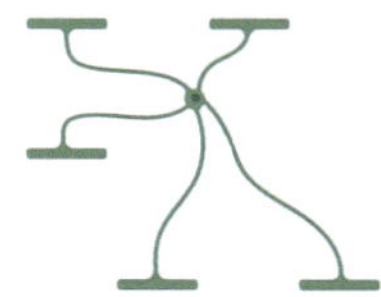
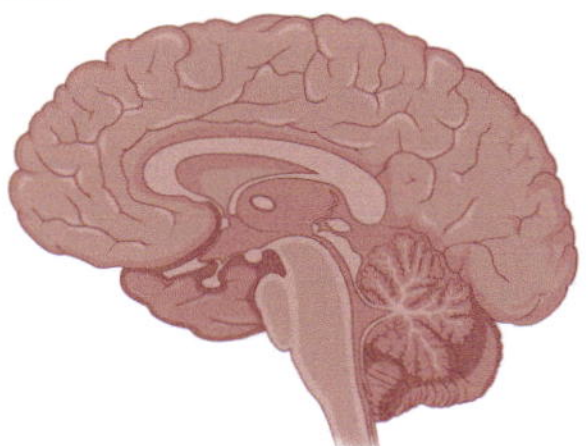
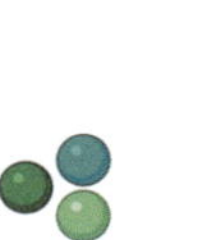
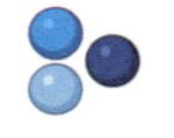
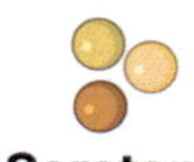

Fig. 5.3 A summary figure of the effects of prenatal alcohol exposure on glia and neurotransmitters

growth factor activities and neuronal activity, both directly and indirectly through regulation by glial cells (summarized in Fig. 5.3).

The Cell Cycle

The cell cycle is the multifaceted process in which cells grow (interphase) and divide (mitosis). The interphase stages of the cell cycle include G_1 (cell growth), S (DNA synthesis), G_2 (preparation for mitosis), and M (mitotic) phases (Fig. 5.2). The M phase, consisting of four sub-phases, prophase, metaphase, anaphase, and telophase, results in the division of a parent cell into two daughter cells. An additional G_0 phase encompasses a class of cells that have the potential to divide but have not yet entered the cell cycle [78]. Cell cycle is very important in early embryonic development because the growth and duplication of DNA are crucial in transmitting generational information [79, 80]. It is vital for each cell to follow the proper order of the cell cycle to ensure each daughter cell has equally distributed DNA [79, 81], and there are certain embedded biological controls to verify that this process is undisturbed. However, when these controls are compromised, such as following alcohol exposure, cells will stall in certain cyclic phases depending on the duration, volume, and timing of alcohol exposure, resulting in apoptosis, premature maturation, or inappropriate differentiation [79].

Chronic alcohol exposure can have a lasting effect on cell cycle proteins and on cell proliferation. For instance, alcohol exposure induces an increase in G_1 cyclins and E2F Transcription Factor 1, which can alter cell cycle progression [82]. However, it has also been found that, depending on the cell type (such as neural progenitor cells), alcohol does not induce apoptosis but instead stimulates progression through the cell cycle [83]. An *in vitro* study of fetal cerebral cortical neuroepithelial cells found that alcohol exposure of 120 and 620 mg/dL, compared to alcohol-free controls, resulted in a significantly higher percentage of these cells in S-phase and G_2/M phase, without causing apoptosis [83]. The same study observed that these alcohol-exposed cells exhibited decreased proliferation capacity and asymmetric cell division of the stem cells, possibly depleting the fetal stem cell population. Contrastingly, in a study using neuronal-like cells, alcohol increased the amount of cells in the G_1 phase, but the proliferation capacity varied depending on the volume and length of alcohol exposure [72]. This implies that alcohol exposure prolongs time within the G_1 phase, possibly caused by a reduction in proliferation, the increase of apoptosis, and DNA damage, making the G_1/S checkpoint a prime target for alcohol toxicity [82, 84]. Additionally, there is evidence of slowed S-phase progression that is dose-dependent following exposure to alcohol [82], as well as inhibition of DNA synthesis and subsequently, mitosis [85]. Vulnerable tissue cells may also exhibit a prolonged G_2 phase, due to the diminished ability to repair DNA damage, and may eventually die from stalling at the G_2/M and G_0/G_1 checkpoints once exposed to alcohol [85]. Another study reports that alcohol exposure prolonged the G_2/M checkpoint due to the inactivation of the cyclin-dependent kinase protein, which functionally allows cells to progress through mitosis [86]. In summary, such diverse and seemingly contrasting alcohol effects on the cell cycle exemplify how various factors, including cell types and developmental periods, play a role in the immediate toxic effects of prenatal alcohol exposure on development, as well as long-lasting teratogenic effects on an individual with FASD.

DNA methylation is also compromised from exposure to alcohol [84]. The methylation of DNA is crucial to early fetal development because it facilitates embryonic cell differentiation while simultaneously protecting cells from regressing into an altered state [87, 88]. When cells experience a delay in any phase of the cell cycle, the potential for DNA damage and genetic mutations increases. However, the specific mechanisms responsible for delays in G_1 and S phases are still unknown and require further study.

Mechanisms for Stem Cell Self-Renewal and Growth

Stem cells may divide into daughter cells that either retain or loose the parent cell's potential to self-renew. Self-renewal is necessary to ensure that sufficient quantities of stem cells are retained throughout development and into adulthood [89]. Specific cellular mechanisms are responsible for promoting or limiting self-renewal, and maintaining the genomic integrity of stem cells. Disrupting these mechanisms may lead to inappropriate aging of stem cells, limiting their ability to grow, self-renew, and repair injury [89, 90]. Embryonic stem cells have the capacity to divide nearly endlessly, while preserving their self-renewal and differentiation potential [79]. Embryonic stem cells, like other self-renewing stem cells, possess a unique ability to maintain a state of proliferation [79], with rapid self-renewal of embryonic stem cells being associated with a shortened G_1 phase [91]. Because a shortened G_1 phase alters how fast and effectively embryonic stem cells grow, alcohol introduction may limit the stem cells' ability to fully and efficiently self-renew [91]. There are multiple immediate detrimental effects to embryonic stem cells, along with long-lasting effects that persist into adulthood in individuals who are exposed to alcohol during early development.

Immediate effects of prenatal alcohol exposure on fetal neural stem cells include the inhibition of microRNAs (miRNAs), DNA methylation, overproduction of ROS, and decreased neurogenesis. Exposure to alcohol may also have the potential to alter the migration, neuronal formation, and growth processes of neural stem cells' (NSCs) ability to self-renew or differentiate. It also prevents the cell from being able to repair itself when alcohol inhibits its primary function of self-renewing. Prenatal alcohol exposure has been found to hinder the expression of specific miR-NAs (such as miR-9, miR-21, miR-153, and miR-335) that may help stem cells maintain their ability to self-renew [92–94]. These miRNAs are especially sensitive to alcohol and can cause premature differentiation in neural stem cells and negatively affect NSC populations [92]. Increased DNA methylation (or hypermethylation) also occurs when exposed to alcohol, which may further contribute to the reduction of NSCs that provide proteins to stimulate cell cycle phases (G_1 and G_2 especially) [95]. Oxidative stress and the overproduction of ROS also disrupt certain mechanisms for stem cell self-renewal and growth. This imbalance of ROS may suggest a decline in the function of stem cells that play a role in self-renewal, which is therefore altered due to alcohol exposure [96, 97]. Additionally, low levels of nicotinamide adenine dinucleotide (NAD+) may indicate the reduction of stem cell self-renewal and the differentiation of NSCs [96, 97]. Alcohol can also be detrimental to embryonic neurogenesis (the development of new neurons in specific brain regions) during early development. The regulation of neurogenesis is associated with intrinsic properties of NSCs, including cell surface receptors and intracellular signaling, that are negatively affected by alcohol [98]. Exposure to alcohol decreases NSC populations and causes them to become vulnerable as they mature. This can contribute to persistent neural abnormalities, leading to symptoms such as memory deficits, which have been observed in cells with a history of intrauterine exposure to alcohol [99–101].

Alcohol effects on embryonic neurogenesis can potentially persevere and affect other developmental stages up to adulthood [98, 102]. An *in vitro* study using adult mice exposed to alcohol prenatally reported a decrease in neurospheres, neuronal differentiation, and overall neurogenesis in the adult hippocampus [98]. The decrease in hippocampal neurogenesis was not mediated by enriched environments, and was associated with impaired memory and learning functionality [102]. Furthermore, early postnatal alcohol exposure can result in lasting deficits of adult hippocampal neurogenesis that correspond with neuronal and behavioral deficits associated with FASD [103]. In addition, individuals with FASD may be predisposed to early onset cancer, higher chance of congenital heart disease, and impaired immunity as an adult, which may all contribute to a higher mortality rate due to the teratogenic effects of alcohol [93, 104–107]. Stem cells play a key role in preventing early aging by proliferating throughout each developmental stage. Alcohol disrupts this proliferative ability, acutely and persistently affecting stem cell function and in turn fetal development, eventually contributing to the behavioral and physical abnormalities linked to FASD.

Interference with the Activity of Growth Factors

Growth factors are secreted proteins that are released to influence the behavior of recipient cells, to facilitate cell division and differentiation, stimulate the development of tissues and organs, and protect against apoptosis and other mechanisms of cell death [108]. Prenatal alcohol exposure can disrupt growth factor expression and signaling [109–112] and consequently may prevent crucial cellular functions from occurring, including differentiation and cell division, or protecting against apoptosis [113–115].

The uterus is a source of a number of growth factors that have important mitogenic and differentiation effects on embryo and fetal maturation [114]. During embryonic development, blastocysts (small orbs of rapidly developing cells) divide into an inner group (or morula) and outer group (trophoblast) [116]. The inner group of cells eventually transform into embryonic cells [117]. Epidermal growth factor (EGF) increases blastocyst cell numbers, which reflects mitogenic and differentiating effects on fetal development [114]. Normal blastocyst and embryonic cell development are boosted by the production of growth factors throughout pregnancy, and when these growth factors are inhibited, it may alter the amount of blastocysts that contribute to fetal development [114]. Apoptosis in embryos negatively affects embryonic neurogenesis and consequently leads to an increase in oxidative stress in the placenta [109]. Alcohol exposure increases the amount of EGF-like growth factors, especially during increased levels of oxidative stress [109], perhaps as a compensatory mechanism to protect against apoptosis and oxidative stress [109]. Altered expression of growth factors negatively influences fetal growth and development, which can eventually lead to FASD [118]. Brain-derived neurotrophic factor (BDNF), for example, a neurotrophic factor which plays a key role in maintaining the survival of neurons by promoting cell growth, differentiation, and maintenance to prevent apoptosis, was reported to be increased in amniotic fluid of small-for-gestational age fetuses [113], a common outcome following prenatal alcohol exposure. Such a response may constitute a maladaptation to an unhealthy environment and reflect an aberrant speeding up of cell maturation.

Lastly, Insulin-like growth factor (IGF)-I and II are associated with mediating neuronal growth and survival, metabolizing energy, and facilitating synapse formation [41]. Prenatal alcohol exposure has been shown to interfere with the activity of these growth factors as well. Specifically, alcohol interferes with growth factor signaling through impaired ligand binding and activation of receptor tyrosine kinases [41]. Ligand binding and tyrosine kinase receptors play a crucial role in the controlled growth and death of cells [119]. The impairment of these mechanisms causes the cells to become more susceptible to intracellular damage [120]. Alcohol interferes with IGF-I receptors and disrupts cell division, which can disrupt the survival of cells and therefore increase inappropriate apoptosis [41]. This prevents the normal function and production of central nervous system cells that are ultimately affected by increased oxidative stress and mitochondrial damage. More research investigating the therapeutic potential of stimulants to natural growth factors that would otherwise be inhibited by alcohol exposure could alleviate the deleterious effects of alcohol on cells during the early development stages.

Effects on Glial Cells

Microglia

Overactivation of neuronal apoptosis by microglia may pose a potential mechanism for decreased brain weight in newborns exposed to alcohol *in utero* [121]. This abnormal neuronal cell loss in the brain due to alcohol exposure during fetal development likely causes irreversible damage on the developing brain. Microglia are the major phagocytic cells (consumers of foreign material) of the central nervous system (CNS) and have been shown to have a significant role in neuronal development in mice by constantly monitoring functional environments of synapses and synaptic pruning [122, 123]. During late fetal and postnatal development, microglia strictly control regulated-cell death of excess neuronal cells via apoptosis throughout the brain of mice, including the hippocampus and cerebellum [124, 125]. Normal microglia function is optimized to minimize inflammation following neuronal apoptosis [124], however, in the presence of ethanol, neuronal apoptosis by microglial cells triggers the release of pro-inflammatory cytokines, including TNF-β, IL-1β, and nitric oxide in third-trimester equivalent postnatal mice [126]. The toll-like receptor 4 (TLR4) pathway, which normally is important in synaptogenesis and synaptic regulation, is one important mediator of this pro-inflammatory cytokine response and the increased apoptosis due to ethanol exposure [127]. A recent study found that TLR4 knockout (KO) mice did not experience increased apoptosis when their neurons were cultured with ethanol, compared to control Wild-type (WT) mice [126]. Further, when compared to WT mice given an equal exposure of ethanol prenatally, KO mice showed significantly lower levels of microglial activation, cytokine release, and synaptic alterations, as well as reduced memory and anxiety impairments [127]. Altogether, this points to the TLR4 pathway being a significant mediator in microglial dysfunction due to prenatal alcohol exposure, resulting in physical malformation of the brain.

Oligodendrocytes

Cognitive and sensory processing deficits are common symptoms in patients with FAS [128]. A 2007 study found clear oculomotor dysfunction and decreased overall executive function in a cohort of children with FASD [129]. Chief among sensory dysfunction in FASD is a high frequency of different visual deficits in FASD patients, including deficits in visual acuity, visual spatial memory, and visual processing (see Chap. 11 for more detail) [130, 131]. Damage from prenatal alcohol exposure targeting oligodendrocytes and oligodendrocyte precursor cells (OPCs) has clear, lasting effects for FASD patients. Oligodendrocytes play an important role in neuronal development and protection, producing the myelin sheath that lines CNS neurons [132]. OPCs myelinate new axons and differentiate into mature oligodendrocytes throughout fetal development and into adulthood, which allows the CNS to actively remodel its infrastructure as needed [133]. This constant development and restructuring suggest that early fetal development can leave a lasting impact on future brain development. Although myelination can still occur following ethanol exposure *in utero*, the existing damage may be irreversible, as observed in FASD patients [134]. Early imaging studies support this, with one study showing decreased myelination and generalized hypoplasia throughout white matter regions of the brain in patients with severe prenatal alcohol exposure [135]. In third-trimester equivalent mice exposed to ethanol vapor, there was a 58% decrease of mature oligodendrocytes and 75% decrease of OPCs in white matter regions of the brain [136]. Because myelination has an essential role in cognition and healthy brain function [137], prenatal alcohol exposure's interaction with oligodendrocytes and OPCs is a likely contributor to the cognitive deficits common in FASD. Further, demyelination of the optic nerve was observed in rats exposed prenatally to alcohol [138], while a clinical study uncovered ~50% prevalence of optic nerve hypoplasia in a group of children in Sweden born to parents with alcohol use disorder [139]. Such high frequency of oligodendrocyte dysfunction poses a possible mechanism for sensory processing deficits in FASD. While the role of oligodendrocytes in FASD symptoms is not yet entirely understood, current evidence strongly points to its strong negative impact on changes in overall executive function seen commonly in patients with FASD.

Astrocytes

Marked neuroinflammation, decreased brain density and cortical development, and even microcephaly are all associated with prenatal alcohol exposure [140]. Astrocytes have an important function of maintaining the integrity of the central nervous system by maintaining homeostasis, which include maintaining the blood–brain barrier, providing neuronal support via reuptake of necessary ions, and many other homeostatic functions [141]. The unique position of astrocytes in many essential brain functions makes them especially susceptible to damage from prenatal alcohol exposure. Alcohol exposure in astrocytes triggers a pro-inflammatory state through activation of the TLR4/IL-1R pathway (14). Ethanol-induced activation of these pathways has been demonstrated to release pro-inflammatory cytokines TNF-β, IL-1β, and COX-2 in cerebral cortex cell cultures of third-trimester-equivalent mice [142]. This is not dissimilar from the role of microglia discussed earlier, and in fact, astrocytes and microglia may have some direct interactions. Microglia may produce ROS following prenatal alcohol exposure in response to TLR4 pathway activation, which may serve as a mechanism for interaction with astrocytes [126]. One study in tadpoles exposed to ethanol prenatally found ROS inhibited Pax6 gene expression [143]. When catalase, the enzyme that breaks down H_2O_2, was overexpressed, it helped to limit microcephaly in the tadpoles [143]. While more research into this systemic pathway is necessary, the crosstalk between astrocytes and microglia likely contributes to a pro-inflammatory state that may negatively affect neurodevelopment.

Alcohol is also linked with decreased proliferation and differentiation of astrocytes, specifically inhibiting muscarinic-induced proliferation of astrocytes in cell cultures of gestational day 21 rat cortices [134]. Furthermore, alcohol decreases the number and density of astrocytes due to apoptosis in the cerebrum and somatosensory cortex of adolescent-equivalent rat pups exposed to ethanol during the late first and second trimester [99]. These effects contribute to the decreased brain density and cortical development attributed with prenatal alcohol exposure. Loss of astrocytes, autoimmune destruction, and astrocyte integrity due to alcohol exposure therefore contribute to the already agitated neuroimmune system in FASD.

Neurotransmitter Signaling

Norepinephrine/Epinephrine

Children and adolescents with FASD are at a significantly higher risk for experiencing developmental delays, mental illness, and substance use disorder [144]. Growing evidence has strongly linked ADHD and FASD as comorbidities in affected populations, with one study reporting that >60% of patients qualified for comorbid diagnoses based on cognitive and emotional tests [145]. Similarly, substance use disorder is more common in those diagnosed with FASD, with one estimate placing the frequency at nearly 40% [146]. The numerous effects of prenatal alcohol exposure on adrenergic systems in the CNS have vast consequences, but the full scope of disturbance is not yet fully understood. Norepinephrine (NE) and epinephrine are catecholamines, produced as hormones by the adrenal glands, and also released as excitatory neurotransmitters in both the central and peripheral sympathetic nervous systems. NE is synthesized by the CNS in the locus coeruleus. NE is an important neuromodulator with a variety of functions—arousal, memory, attention, emotions, and other diverse functions—depending on the brain region in which it acts [147, 148]. During gestation and postnatal development, NE also contributes to synaptic plasticity in a variety of ways. One study in neonatal rats (a model for third-trimester-equivalent exposure in human pregnancy) found that NE acted as a potent neurotrophic factor promoting development of adrenergic pyramidal neurons in the cerebral cortex [149]. NE is also believed to have an important role in infant attachment and sensory processing in the olfactory bulb [150, 151]. Ethanol exposure during pregnancy has been strongly linked to decreased NE levels, particularly within the hypothalamus and corpus striatum of prenatal pups [152]. Further, ethanol exposure during fetal development decreases the stability and number of NE-producing locus coeruleus neurons [153]. Because of the importance of the striatum and hypothalamus in emotional regulation and the brain reward circuit system, deficiencies in NE may mediate increased rates of substance use disorder and other reward seeking behaviors common in FASD. Despite these NE deficiencies, mice exposed to ethanol prenatally (equivalent to the first and second trimester periods of human pregnancy) exhibited marked increase in NE transporters in the striatum, which may be a homeostatic response to decreased NE levels being produced [154]. As NE transporters are a point of interest in ADHD, increases in transporters due to prenatal alcohol exposure may be tied to greater onset of ADHD symptoms. NE's strong relation to attention, arousal, and other executive functions may further underly characteristic symptoms of FASD, however this research is yet underdeveloped.

Dopamine

When measuring executive function using a variety of cognitive tests, children prenatally exposed to alcohol or diagnosed with FAS test significantly lower than alcohol-free controls [155]. With evidence of decreased levels of dopamine in the brains of rat pups exposed to ethanol prenatally [152], dopamine deficits may contribute to common cognitive phenotypes seen in FASD, including increased rates of ADHD and other learning disabilities, as well as substance abuse disorders [144]. Dopamine is an excitatory and inhibitory catecholamine neurotransmitter of the central nervous system. Dopamine has a vast array of functions in the CNS, including motor control, higher cognition, reward systems, and working memory [156]. Dopaminergic neurons originating in the basal ganglia project throughout the brain to areas such as the limbic system and prefrontal cortex. Following normal prefrontal cortex development, dopamine acts as a neuromodulator that enables higher level processing, such as working memory and decision making [157]. In neonatal, third-trimester-equivalent rat pups, prenatal alcohol exposure reduced dendritic spine density and altered dendritic organization in layers II and III of the medial prefrontal cortices [158]. Given the known importance of the prefrontal cortex in decision-making and impulse control functions, these findings likely contribute to the frequent comorbidity of FASD and ADHD [145]. The interaction between dopaminergic neurons and prenatal alcohol exposure has been further investigated in adult rhesus monkeys, that were either exposed to alcohol a) continuously throughout pregnancy, or b) only during the first-early second trimester of pregnancy. Both unique cohorts of rhesus monkeys demonstrated decreased function of their dopamine systems following moderate-to-high levels of ethanol exposure *in utero* [159]. Another study uncovered similarly impaired striatal dopamine system efficiency in rats exposed to ethanol *in utero* [160]. Rats exposed to ethanol prenatally (throughout the first and second trimester- equivalent periods of human pregnancy) exhibited significantly lower levels of dopamine in the striatum. The striatum's reliance on dopamine to regulate many cognitive functions including working memory [161], outlines how serious dopamine deficiencies may impact critical early developmental periods in patients with FASD. Overall, FASD and dopamine are heavily intertwined, and dopaminergic systems are thus susceptible to damage caused by prenatal ethanol exposure. It is likely these effects contribute to the many cognitive symptoms of FASD.

Gamma-Aminobutyric Acid (GABA)

GABA is the main inhibitory neurotransmitter of the adult CNS. Prenatal alcohol exposure likely affects the GABA system of the CNS at many different stages of development, thereby contributing to long-lasting consequences for FASD patients. When heavy prenatal alcohol exposure coincides with GABAergic interneuron development, severe prenatal brain malformations, such as hydrocephalus and then displacement of brain layers, as well as low birth weight can occur [162]. Further, interactions between alcohol and developing GABA systems regulate the development of fine motor skills, with one study finding a significant association between patients with FASD and underdeveloped motor skills, including coordination and balance [163]. In the developing CNS, GABA acts as an autocrine neurotrophic factor, promoting neuronal proliferation/growth in early embryonic chicks [164]. One subtype of GABAergic neurons are uniquely specialized interneurons that begin migrating tangentially and radially from the medial ganglionic eminences during the late-first trimester, and continue thereafter as needed throughout the telencephalon of the brain [165]. This helps to create complex formations of GABA interneurons in the developing brain [166]. In second-trimester equivalent rats exposed to ethanol, there is a marked decrease in neuronal cell proliferation in the medial ganglionic eminence and an increase in premature tangential GABA neuronal migration from the medial ganglionic eminence throughout different ventricular zones [167].

While multiple cells function using GABA neurotransmitters, Purkinje cells, GABAergic projection neurons found in the cerebellum, may be especially vulnerable to damage due to prenatal alcohol exposure [168]. Purkinje cells regulate complex motor function through inhibitory signaling in the CNS. These cells have been shown to be extremely vulnerable to ethanol exposure, with documented and pronounced apoptosis due to a single exposure of ethanol in postnatal day 4 rats, which coincides with the third trimester of human pregnancies [169]. Another study in macaque monkeys suggests that ethanol exposure in the first trimester equivalent or throughout the entire gestational period decreases GABA neuronal density in the somatosensory cortex of the brain, suggesting a more generalized inhibition of GABAergic function [95]. These differences in somatosensory cortex composition may be a result of premature tangential migration discussed earlier. GABA systems in the CNS are a clear target of alcohol's teratogenic effects from conception to birth.

Serotonin

Persons with a diagnosis of FASD are at higher risk for developing disorders of mood and affect, including anxiety, depression, ADHD, substance use disorder, and suicidal ideation [144]. FASD in males is linked with a ~20-fold increase in suicidal ideations and attempted suicide compared to the national average [170]. One postmortem study in humans has found that individuals who committed suicide had marked decreases in Serotonin (5-HT) levels compared to the general population [171]. In the context of FASD, decreased 5-HT levels may be a possible mechanism that leads to increased severe mental illness. 5-HT has been recognized as an important inhibitory neurotransmitter for numerous higher level brain functions, including homeostatic maintenance and behavioral control [172]. Clusters of 5-HT neurons in midbrain and brainstem raphe nuclei, project widely - anteriorly into forebrain and posteriorly into spinal cord - to influence perceptual, cognitive, and affective responses in the mature adult brain [173]. However, during early fetal development, 5-HT, like other neurotransmitters, acts as a neurotrophic factor, and in an explant culture model was shown to promote proliferation, growth, and differentiation of new serotonergic cortical neurons [174]. This 5-HT function is especially important in FASD, because serotonergic neurons are known to begin differentiating and proliferating heavily in the brain stem by the mid-first trimester in human fetuses [175]. The first trimester is also the period of pregnancy with the highest frequency of alcohol use. One study in the United States found that almost 50% of participants consumed alcohol at some point during their early pregnancy [176]. Chronic prenatal alcohol exposure has also been shown to decrease serotonin levels globally in third-trimester rats [177] and diminishes proliferation, maturation, and migration of serotonergic neurons in the forebrain of late prenatally exposed mice [178]. It is likely that these deficits persist well after birth, as a study examining adolescent mice exposed to ethanol during the second trimester reported chronic deficits in 5-HT neurons in the dorsal and medial raphe nuclei due to an increase of caspase-3 [179, 180]. Serotonin deficiency has been strongly implicated in disorders of affect such as depression and anxiety [181] and poses a potential mechanism for the frequency of developing mental illness in FASD. Consequently, serotonergic circuit dysfunction is predicted to constitute an important component of the neurobehavioral disabilities associated with FASD.

Immune Function

Compromised immune function and predisposition to infection have long been reported in the FASD population [182, 183] and have been recapitulated in animal studies [184–186]. Underlying causes of this include:

- *Disruption of normal thymic development from neural crest cells following prenatal alcohol exposure* [187], *which lead to abnormal proportions of T cell subsets* [188, 189] *and T cell dysfunction* [106, 190, 191].
- *Altered interleukin-2 (IL-2)/IL-2 receptor interactions* [106, 192, 193].
- *Perturbed norepinephrine/β-adrenoreceptors regulation of immune cell populations in lymphoid organs* [194].

Innate Immunity

Innate immunity entails nonspecific defense mechanisms that come into play immediately or within hours of an antigen's appearance in the body, and consists of physical, chemical, and cellular defenses against pathogens. In particular, natural killer (NK) cells and myeloid lineage cells (e.g., monocytes, macrophage, dendritic cells, and neutrophils) have a role in innate immunity and are impacted by prenatal alcohol exposure. Basal increases in NK and myeloid lineage cells were observed in secondary lymphoid organs of rats prenatally exposed to ethanol [191]. Furthermore, there is decreased NK cell cytotoxic activity [195] and increased pro-inflammatory myeloid cell-derived cytokines (e.g., TNF and IL-1β) in prenatally-exposed adult rats [196]. This means innate immune cell function is perturbed, in addition to overall population numbers, further disrupting the normally precise balance that is required in immune system regulation. The consequences of this disruption may manifest as adult-onset neuropathic pain [191] or increased risk of respiratory infection in newborns. Specifically, a decrease in the antioxidant glutathione as a result of *in utero* exposure to ethanol leads to impaired differentiation and phagocytic activity of alveolar macrophages in the lungs of rodents [197–199]. This increases subsequent risk for experimentally-induced pneumonia in newborn pups [200]. Potentially exacerbating this alveolar macrophage dysfunction in the lung is a decrease in the surfactant proteins (SP) SP-A and SP-D observed in sheep exposed to ethanol *in utero* [201, 202]. These proteins are essential mediators of the local immune response in the lung, modulating dendritic and T cell function and facilitating removal of pathogens by alveolar macrophages [203]. Taken together, impairment of innate immunity in FASD may contribute to a predisposition for infection.

Adaptive Immunity

In addition to deficits in innate immunity, there is also dysfunction in adaptive immunity. Adaptive immunity, also known as acquired immunity, mobilizes after innate immunity has proven insufficient to remove invading pathogens and consists of humoral (antibody-mediated) and cell-mediated defenses that adapt to the specific pathogen, enhancing the immunological response. In particular, B cell and T cell lineages have proven sensitive to *in utero* ethanol exposure. Impaired B cell function is typically associated with recurrent infections by encapsulated and pyrogenic bacteria, while impaired T cell function is usually associated with recurrent opportunistic infections and viral and fungal infections. All of these types of recurrent infections are common in FASD children [182], indicating that both lymphocyte lineages are impacted.

B Cell Lineage

Reduced numbers of splenic and bone marrow B cells were found in postnatal mice following prenatal alcohol exposure, and this reduction persisted until adolescence [204, 205]. Moreover, isolated B cells showed a weakened proliferative response to lipopolysaccharide (LPS; a bacterial cell wall component) [204]. Following intrauterine alcohol exposure, impaired differentiation into mature B cells has been demonstrated in B lineage cells from liver [206, 207] and in oligoclonal-neonatal-progenitor (ONP) cells [208, 209], which are capable of differentiating into B lymphocytes depending on the cytokines to which they are exposed. Specifically, the ONP cells isolated from prenatal alcohol exposure newborn mice had a greatly reduced capacity to commit to the B cell lineage. Additional investigations have demonstrated that alcohol affects ONP cell differentiation into B cell lineage by downregulating the expression of several transcription factors and cytokine receptors [210].

T Cell Lineage

Prenatal alcohol exposure also impacts thymocyte development. Rodent studies have shown delayed thymic development [211], decreased number of thymocytes, and reduced proliferation response to stimulation by thymocytes isolated from late-second trimester mouse fetuses [212]. This alcohol-associated suppression of proliferative response and cell numbers of thymocytes has been shown to persist through childhood and begin to return to normal or elevated levels by adolescence [189, 190, 213–215]. Although this proliferative capacity may recover by adolescence, the lasting consequences of a perturbed developmental environment on the T cell lineage are persistent, with lasting T cell dysfunction [106, 190, 191] and alterations in T cell numbers [188, 189]. This lasting dysregulation contributes to increased susceptibility to infections across the lifespan [182, 184, 185] and other autoimmune/inflammatory related diseases, such as adjuvant-induced arthritis (a model for rheumatoid arthritis) [216] and adult-onset neuropathic pain resulting from a predisposition for allodynia in FASD individuals [191].

Maternal and Fetal Cytokines as Biomarkers for FASD

Because of the distinct impact alcohol has on the immune system in both adults and in utero, recent studies have examined whether there exists specific immunological biomarkers of FASD. Of primary focus have been cytokines, which are small peptide molecules that are crucial in cell-cell signaling of the immune system. Cytokines are present in all tissues and, most importantly, in circulation, making them readily measurable after a simple blood draw. Prenatal alcohol exposure influences cytokine profiles of both the pregnant individual and child after birth. This provides a unique opportunity to define unique cytokine profiles in pregnant individuals and children that can be used to identify those children at increased risk of neurodevelopmental delays, and to provide a supplemental diagnostic tool to help physicians diagnose FASD [217–219].

Non-Protein-Coding RNAs

Many of the teratogenic consequences of prenatal alcohol exposure may be mediated through non-protein-coding RNAs (ncRNAs), which are distinct from messenger RNA (mRNA) in that they are not translated into protein. They perform a wide variety of regulatory functions, modulating mRNA and protein levels via complex signaling networks of which they are a part. Moreover, these RNA and protein networks play a crucial role in developmental processes [220, 221]. The specific ncRNAs that are key components of these networks are sensitive to environmental changes, such as prenatal alcohol exposure, as discussed below.

microRNAs

MicroRNAs (miRNAs) are a diverse and plentiful class of short ncRNAs (19–25 nucleotides) with tissue-specific expression patterns that vary temporally and spatially [222] and inhibit protein translation by targeting RNA-induced silencing complex (RISC) to the 3′ untranslated region (UTR) of mRNA [223]. miRNAs can be secreted as paracrine or endocrine signals capable of choreographing gene expression and function in recipient cells [224, 225]. Through these mechanisms of action, miRNAs regulate developmental timing and pattern formation, promoting the rapid clearance of transcripts as cells transition from one state to another during development, and fine-tuning gene expression [226].

Research has shown that miRNAs are sensitive to prenatal alcohol exposure. One study of miRNAs was performed using cultured neuroepithelial cells isolated from the mouse fetal cerebral cortex, and revealed several differentially expressed miRNAs in response to ethanol treatment, including the suppression of miR-9, a crucial regulator of neurogenesis [94]. Moreover, genetic inhibition of miR-9 in zebrafish and mice results in morphological features associated with FASD, such as microcephaly [227, 228] and, for zebrafish, results in the same juvenile swimming phenotype as that of alcohol-treated animals [227, 229]. Another study found similar results in primary cultures of cerebellar granule neurons isolated from neonatal mice, identifying miR-9, miR-29a, and miR-29b as decreased after ethanol exposure [230]. This study also showed that miR-29b may mediate ethanol-induced apoptosis during the period of cerebellar sensitivity to alcohol exposure. Moreover, in primary neuronal cells from fetal mice, chronic intermittent ethanol exposure resulted in widespread alterations in miRNA expression profiles [231]. Importantly, this study demonstrated that even after ethanol withdrawal, this altered expression of miRNAs persisted, revealing that alcohol exposure can permanently reprogram the miRNome. Similarly, widespread alterations of miRNA were identified in the brains of adult mice exposed to ethanol prenatally [232], supporting the idea that prenatal alcohol exposure causes long-term reprogramming of ncRNA networks which result in persistent teratogenicity.

Excitingly, circulating miRNAs are being interrogated for use as potential diagnostic biomarkers of FASD because of consistent alterations in the patterns of miRNAs perturbed by developmental ethanol exposure. The first study to address this idea profiled plasma miRNAs in pregnant ewes and newborn lambs exposed to alcohol, identifying miR-9, miR-15b, miR-19b, and miR-20a [233]. Research has progressed to human studies with populations based in Ukraine [92] and South Africa [234], identifying specific miRNA panels in children prenatally exposed to alcohol. Subsequent analyses have identified infant sex as an important factor for consideration when developing more accurate miRNA biomarker panels for diagnosis [235]. As this research progresses, sensitive miRNA panels may be another useful tool in aiding physicians to provide a diagnosis of FASD to their patients.

Long Noncoding RNAs

Long noncoding RNAs (lncRNAs) are >200 nucleotides in size and lack the potential to code for a protein >100 amino acids [236]. lncRNAs play an important role in development, as shown in the developing foregut and lungs [237], brain [238], and adipose [239], and in osteogenic differentiation of mesenchymal stem cells [240]. lncRNAs may carry out their developmental role by binding chromatin modifying complexes such as the histone methyltransferase G9a or the polycomb repressive complex (PRC)2 [241–243]. By interacting with these protein complexes, lncRNAs guide them to either modify or "read" chromatin in the promotion of pluripotency and repression of differentiation signals [244, 245].

The impact of developmental alcohol exposure on lncRNAs remains poorly understood, but is a promising avenue of research for providing epigenetic control during development. To date, there are three studies that directly measure the consequences of developmental alcohol exposure on lncRNA expression. The first identified is linc1354, which is associated with neural stem cell differentiation and interacts with PRC2, and is decreased in fetal mouse neurospheres following ethanol exposure [246]. This decrease in linc1354 may impact downstream targets of PRC2 that are crucial in normal developmental gene regulatory networks, resulting in abnormal differentiation in the fetal brain. A second study identified the lncRNA Oct4 pseudogene on mouse chromosome 9 (*m*Oct4pg9) as being increased following ethanol exposure in fetal mouse neurospheres [247]. Moreover, this study determined that *m*Oct4pg9 is associated with increased cell proliferation and maturation, potentially contributing to the pro-maturation effects of ethanol exposure that result in the loss of neural stem cells and subsequent decrease in brain growth. A third study showed suppression of the lncRNA *Xist* in female mouse fetuses exposed *in utero* to ethanol [248]. Normally, *Xist*, which is located on the X chromosome, inactivates the second X chromosome present in female cells (XX), modulating expression of X-linked genes so that a single copy is expressed in females, similarly to how males (XY) only express one copy. However, in this study, prenatal alcohol exposure resulted in decrease of *Xist* and loss of X-inactivation, with subsequent changes in X-linked genes and gene regulatory networks during neural development. Altogether, these studies support the idea that lncRNA are sensitive to the teratogenic consequences of developmental alcohol exposure, consequently perturbing neurogenesis and organogenesis.

Circular RNAs

Another type of ncRNA that may mediate the consequences of prenatal alcohol exposure is circular RNAs (circRNAs). circRNAs are ncRNAs greater than 200 nucleotides that have circularized by covalently bonding a 3′ downstream donor to a 5′ upstream splice acceptor in a process referred to as "backsplicing" [249]. circRNAs may play a crucial role in ncRNA networks by acting as sponges for miRNAs, as they often contain multiple in-tandem miRNA binding elements, allowing for de-repression of miRNA target genes [250, 251]. Furthermore, circRNAs have been shown to play a role in development in various organs of the body, such as the heart, lungs, and brain, demonstrating spatio-temporal dynamics as development of the embryo progresses [252–254].

Normally, circRNAs are a part of the homeostasis of RNA networks that are finely balanced during development. However, the balance of RNA networks may be disrupted if a teratogenic exposure occurs, a growing area of research in the FASD field with only one study to date. This study found that prenatal alcohol exposure alters circRNA expression in whole brains of second trimester-equivalent mice in a sex-specific manner [255]. The study also found that prenatal alcohol exposed males and females had similarly altered expression of protein-coding mRNAs when compared to their control counterparts. Interestingly, circRNA expression was altered in a sex-specific manner. Prenatal alcohol exposed females had a specific set of upregulated and downregulated circRNAs, and this specific set of circRNAs did not overlap with those altered in prenatal alcohol exposed males. This suggests that though altered mRNA expression may be shared between males and females after prenatal alcohol exposure, the regulatory networks by which they are achieved are sex-dependent. This is an important factor to consider when designing therapeutics targeting similar regulatory networks, because such therapeutics may need to be sex specific.

More studies on the role of circRNAs in the etiology of FASD are needed, particularly because of the significant potential for circRNAs to serve as therapeutic targets. For instance, circRNAs packaged in nanoparticles or extracellular vesicles (EVs) have been used as a therapy in animal models of disease [256–259]. Once inside their target cell, the circRNAs are thought to act as a miRNA sponge, helping to balance the RNA network that was disrupted by a disease state. Alternatively, in diseases characterized by high levels of circRNAs, these circRNAs have been targeted by nanoparticle and EV packaged short interfering RNA (siRNA) or short hairpin RNA (shRNA) that target specific circRNAs for destruction, returning levels to closer to normal [260–262]. This may be a promising therapeutic avenue for complex disorders that result in the dysregulation of entire gene networks.

Teratogenic Consequences of Ethanol-Induced Epigenetic Modifications

Epigenetic modifications (DNA changes that impact gene expression without altering the DNA sequence) are closely associated with early brain development [263], cardiogenesis [264], immune system development [265], and organogenesis in general. Alterations to the normal progression of these modifications, which have been shown to occur following prenatal alcohol exposure, can lead to lasting neurodevelopmental and behavioral consequences [266], congenital heart disease [264], and autoimmune disorders [267] (Fig. 5.4).

DNA Methylation

Ethanol-induced changes in DNA methylation status have several outcomes. On a cellular level, ethanol exposure alters the natural progression of DNA methylation status in rat neural stem cells [268]. This resulted in changes in expression of genes associated with differentiation and in turn, changes in phenotypes, such as delayed neuronal formation, migration, and growth processes. The exact timing of prenatal alcohol exposure during pregnancy (i.e., either first, second, or third trimester exposure) can uniquely perturb DNA methylation status, with each exposure window resulting in its own set of genes altered by ethanol [269]. These methylation

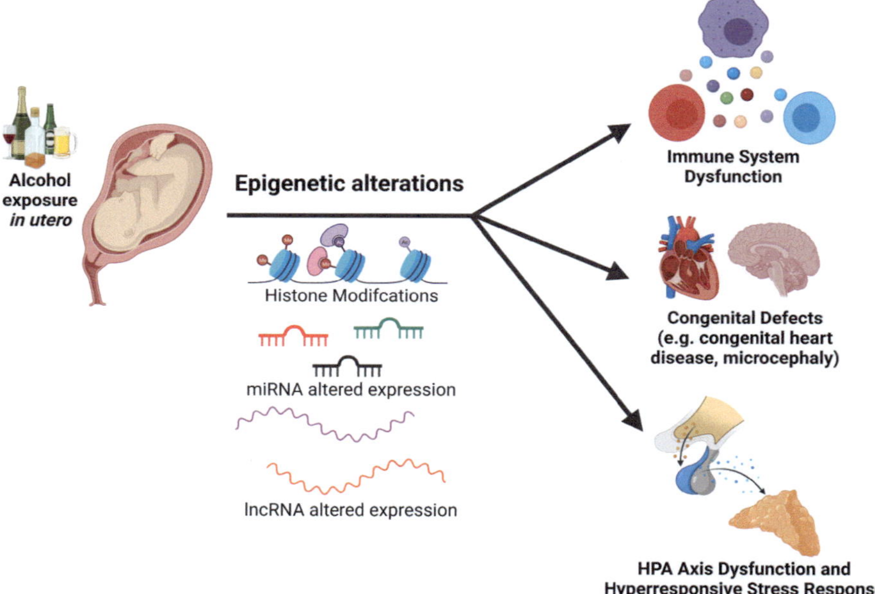

Fig. 5.4 The effects of prenatal alcohol exposure on epigenetic profiles and health outcomes in offspring. Prenatal alcohol exposure induces multiple forms of epigenetic changes, including histone modifications and shifts in expressions of micro(mi)RNA and long noncoding (lnc) RNA. These alcohol-induced alterations have been associated with poor physical and behavioral health outcomes in exposed offspring

perturbations last into adulthood in mice, indicating the life-long consequences of these early life, prenatal alcohol exposure-sensitive changes. While the exact set of changed genes is unique to each exposure window, the overall prenatal alcohol exposure-sensitive pathways and phenotypes overlap (e.g., synaptogenesis, apoptosis, cellular identity, cell–cell adhesion, and signaling), indicating that these developmental pathways are vulnerable to prenatal alcohol exposure throughout pregnancy.

Furthermore, the lasting impact of ethanol exposure on cellular phenotypes also manifests on a larger scale in behavioral phenotypes that last into adulthood. One study found that increased anxiety-like behavior in adult prenatal alcohol exposure rats was associated with increased expression of DNA methyltransferases in the hippocampus [270], an outcome that would presumably lead to increased DNA methylation, and consequently, heterochromatin formation. However, another study documented decreased expression of mRNA transcripts for methyl CpG binding protein 2 (MeCP2, a protein which binds to methylated regions of chromatin to prevent transcription) in the cortex and striatum of adult rodents prenatally exposed to alcohol. Moreover, this decrease in MeCP2 mRNA was associated with the FASD-like phenotypes of increased impulsivity, hyperactivity, and inattention [154]. Altogether, these studies show that prenatal alcohol exposure's effects on the epigenetic landscape are complex, and modifications that occur during development can persist throughout the lifespan.

These lasting methylation changes implicate a possibility of defining an epigenetic profile that serves as a biomarker for prenatal alcohol exposure [271–273]. Genes identified in these studies are implicated in a number of FASD phenotypes, such as cognitive function, anxiety, attention deficit hyperactivity disorder, and mood disorders, revealing a link between altered DNA methylation and observed FASD phenotypes and symptoms. This means that a clearly defined epigenetic profile of prenatal alcohol exposure may potentially serve as a diagnostic tool for identifying individuals with FASDs. One such study has used buccal swabs from children to determine individual DNA methylation profiles [274]. While the study did successfully identify a potential diagnostic profile that could span two different cohorts, the study was limited due to small sample size and a lack of demographic diversity. However, there is a strong potential to develop a more universal diagnostic profile with further investigation.

Histone Modifications

Prenatal alcohol exposure also affects the epigenome via histone modifications. These modifications can either be gene-repressive or gene-activating, and this classification is specific to the histone residue and the precise modification. This means that while there is no generalized rule for histone methylation, the histone methylation code is specific in terms of site and degree of modification for whether gene expression is increased or decreased.

The most studied histone modification after prenatal alcohol exposure is histone H3 lysine 9 acetylation (H3K9ac), which is associated with gene-activation [275, 276]. Of particular interest for prenatal alcohol exposure research has been the role of altered H3K9ac in cardiac development, as prenatal alcohol exposure increases the rate of heart defects [277–280]. This higher rate of congenital heart defects may, in part, be attributed to increased H3K9 acetylation. Studies using culture models of cardiac progenitor cells demonstrate that increased H3K9 acetylation results in increased expression of key cardiac development genes [281, 282]. When continued in a mouse model, increased histone acetyltransferase (HAT) expression and activity coincided with abnormal heart development in the fetal mice, resulting in congenital heart defects similar to those associated with FASDs [283].

Additionally, the effect of prenatal alcohol exposure on histone methylation has been a large focus in prenatal alcohol exposure research. Ethanol exposure in neonatal mouse pups, equivalent to the late pregnancy period in humans, increased methyltransferase expression and activity led to increased dimethylation of histones in the brain [284, 285]. This finding was supported by another study showing a persistent increase in histone dimethylation up to gestational day 17 (GD17) in fetal mice previously exposed to ethanol on GD7 [286]. This increase in histone dimethylation was consistently observed in prenatal alcohol exposed pups with facial dysmorphologies, but largely absent in prenatal alcohol exposed pups without facial dysmorphologies, and was found to robustly occur on genetic loci for a panel of genes associated with normal progression of neural development. Increases in histone dimethylation have also been documented in 2-month-old male rats, i.e., early adulthood, along with additional prenatal alcohol exposure-induced histone modifications, in the arcuate nucleus of the hypothalamus [287, 288]. The lasting consequence was decreased expression of the proopiomelanocortin (Pomc) gene transcript, a precursor for adrenocorticotrophic hormone among other hormones. Interestingly, the inhibition of Pomc was counterintuitively associated with a hyper-responsive adrenal gland, suggesting destabilization of an important neuroendocrine circuit for stress management. In contrast to the observed methylation of the POMC gene locus, other studies have also shown a global decrease in methylation, which is usually attributed to decreased availability of the methyl donor S-adenosylmethionine. One study has shown that an ethanol-induced decrease in histone methylation alters the normal progression of gene expression during neurogenesis [246] while another demonstrated suppression of osteogenesis and adipogenesis in mesenchymal stem cells after ethanol exposure [289]. Taken together, global histone modifications may contribute, in part, to the lifelong repercussions of prenatal alcohol exposure.

Potential Therapeutics Targeting Prenatal Alcohol Exposure-Induced Histone Modifications

Identifying histone modifications as a mediator of the lasting consequences of prenatal alcohol exposure raises the exciting possibility of potential pharmacological and nutritional interventions. There are a number of natural HAT inhibitors, such as turmeric and anacardic acid, that may be able to mitigate the effects of prenatal alcohol exposure. One study demonstrated that use of curcumin, a compound found in turmeric, can reverse increased histone acetylation in the caspase-3 and caspase-8 promoters in cardiocytes, reducing apoptosis after ethanol exposure [290]. Additionally, another group of researchers treated pregnant mice simultaneously with anacardic acid and ethanol and found that co-administration of anacardic acid, a phenolic lipid derived from cashew nut shells, significantly reduced ethanol-induced hyperacetylation of histones in cardiac tissues [281]. The effects of prenatal alcohol exposure could also be mitigated through choline supplementation to increase histone and DNA methylation, as choline can contribute to increased levels of methionine. Choline supplementation has been shown to normalized histone and DNA methylation, *Pomc* expression, and corticosterone levels in offspring of pregnant rats when supplemented concurrently with ethanol exposure [287]. Choline supplementation is currently under clinical investigation as a therapeutic intervention for prenatal alcohol exposure consequences on neurobehavior and growth [291, 292].

Transgenerational Consequences of Prenatal Alcohol Exposure via Genomic Imprinting

Epigenetic modifications extend beyond the direct effects of prenatal alcohol exposure during pregnancy by perturbing genomic imprinting, a form of epigenetic inheritance that causes genes to be expressed in a parent-of-origin-specific manner, prior to conception. This means that preconception ethanol exposure in germ cells (i.e., sperm and oocytes) can contribute to phenotypes typically associated with prenatal alcohol exposure or FASDs. For example, one multigenerational study traced prenatal alcohol exposure-induced increases in *Pomc* promoter methylation through the male germline [288]. Researchers found decreased *Pomc* expression in the hypothalamus and increased adrenocorticotropic hormone (ACTH) and corticosterone levels in the plasma of both male and female offspring of first generation (F1) progeny, but this pattern only persisted in males of the male prenatal alcohol exposure germline in F2 and F3 progeny, pointing to male germline transmission of increased methylation of the *Pomc* promoter. This same group later demonstrated similar findings for interferon-γ (IFN-γ), a cytokine known to regulate both innate and adaptive immunity. Increased methylation for *Ifn-γ* gene promoter and subsequent decrease in *Ifn-γ* mRNA were identified in both F1 males and females [293]. However, this methylation and expression pattern was continued only in the male germline to the F3 generation. The implication of these data is that prenatal alcohol exposure can directly affect the developing fetus at the time of ethanol exposure, but can also impact future progeny of that fetus, thus affecting families across multiple generations.

Looking Forward: Identification of Risk and Resilience Factors

In this chapter, we have addressed a multitude of targeted research avenues that can inform the advancement of treatments for individuals with FASD. As a developmental disorder, FASD poses unique challenges for healthcare professionals and clinicians, including the absence of a definitive diagnostic test to uncover prenatal alcohol exposure in offspring, and social stigmatization which limits accurate self-reports of drinking by pregnant individuals. When considering the complex interactions of exposure variables (including timing during gestation and pattern/repetition of exposure) and subjects (sex, age, species, etc.) on symptom expression, it is perhaps unsurprising that debate exists among medical professionals and the general public about the dangers of alcohol exposure during pregnancy. However, we have aimed to demonstrate through our discussion of alcohol toxicology and teratology, that alcohol alters the fate of numerous intra and intercellular systemic functions that can contribute to the persistent deficits observed in humans with known FASD. By acknowledging alcohol as more than a toxic, poisonous agent, and rather as a highly variable and widespread cellular teratogen, we believe scientists can better refine their research questions and experiments to directly target biochemical systems underlying FASD symptomology. This includes investigating a range of biological and genetic differences between offspring prenatally exposed to alcohol, and associating these innate phenotypes with symptom expression. Such comparisons can facilitate the isolation of factors that lead a child to be "at risk" or "resilient" to a particular symptom of FASD, and subsequently, can pinpoint specific mechanisms of importance for the development of therapeutic interventions for affected individuals.

Glossary

5-HT (Serotonin) A monoamine transmitter with a variety of functions, including emotional and behavioral regulation.

ACTH (Adrenocorticotropic hormone) A pituitary gland hormone that initiates the production of *cortisol*, which is key to the body's response to stress and infection, as well as regulating blood sugar levels and maintaining blood pressure.

ADHD (Attention deficit hyperactivity disorder) A neurodevelopmental disorder characterized by difficulty with focusing, lack of impulse control, and hyperactivity.

Apoptosis Programmed cell death that can occur as a normal, controlled process to eliminate unwanted or damaged cells, but can also be induced inappropriately with the introduction of a toxin or teratogen.

circRNAs (Circular RNA) Noncoding RNAs greater than 200 nucleotides in size, that form a closed loop from linked 5′ and 3′ termini in a process of exon back-splicing.

CNS (Central nervous system) The part of the nervous system consisting of the brain and spinal cord.

COX-2 (Cyclooxygenase 2) An enzyme involved in the inflammatory response, that converts arachidonic acid to prostaglandins.

Epigenetic(s) Modifications in the expression of a gene, rather than changes in the genetic code itself. Without altering the DNA sequence, external factors can change whether a gene is turned "on"—and can interact with other cellular processes, leading to protein transcription- or turned "off."

GABA (Gamma-aminobutyric acid) An amino acid neurotransmitter, and the primary inhibitory neurotransmitter in the adult CNS.

H_2O_2 (Hydrogen peroxide) A reactive oxygen species, broken down in the body by catalase.

HAT (Histone acetyltransferase) An enzyme that catalyzes acetylation of lysine amino acids on histone complexes.

IBA-1 (Ionized calcium-binding adapter molecule 1) An intracellular protein found in microglial cells.

IL-1 (Interleukin-1 beta) A cytokine produced by macrophages that mediates the pro-inflammatory response.

IL-1R (Interleukin 1 receptor) A cytokine receptor involved in the immune response which binds preferentially to IL1.

IL-2 (Interleukin 2) A pro-inflammatory cytokine mainly involved in the acquired immune response.

Interferon (IFN) A cytokine that is critical for innate and adaptive immunity against viral and some bacterial infections. Named for their ability to "interfere" with viral replication by protecting cells from virus infections, IFNs are produced principally by natural killer (NK) cells.

KO (Knockout) Refers to the use of genetic engineering to inactivate or remove one or more specific genes from an organism. Scientists create knockout organisms to study the impact of removing a gene from an organism, and thus learn about that gene's function.

LncRNAs (Long noncoding RNA) Noncoding RNAs of greater than 200 nucleotides in size. LncRNAs primarily interact with mRNA, DNA, protein, and miRNA and consequently regulate gene expression.

LPS (Lipopolysaccharide) A major surface membrane component present in almost all Gram-negative bacteria. It is essential to both the structural integrity and function of the outer membrane.

MeCP2 (Methyl CpG binding protein 2) A protein that binds to methylated regions of chromatin to prevent transcription.

Microglia Immune cells of the central nervous system, capable of interacting with neurons and non-neuronal cells. They account for ~10% of cells in the brain and are first responders in the brain's response to infections and inflammation.

miR-9 (microRNA 9) A microRNA involved in neurogenesis.

miR-29a (microRNA 29a) A microRNA involved in tumor suppression.

miR-29b (microRNA 29b) A microRNA involved in tumor suppression.

miRNAs (microRNAs) Small, non-protein coding RNA involved in tissue-specific gene expression patterns.

miRNome (Micro RNA genome) A complete set of microRNAs in a genome.

mRNA (Messenger RNA) A type of cellular RNA that carries the genetic information needed to make proteins. mRNA carries the information from DNA, located in the nucleus of the cell, to the cytoplasm, where the proteins are created.

ncRNAs (Non-protein-coding RNAs) A type of cellular RNA that cannot be coded into a protein.

NE (Norepinephrine) An excitatory catecholamine neurotransmitter produced in the CNS and PNS with many associated functions, including attention, memory, and emotional regulation.

NK (Natural killer cell) A cytotoxic lymphocyte and type of white blood cell that is essential to the innate immune response.

OPC (Oligodendrocyte precursor cell) A CNS glial cell that myelinates new axons and develops into mature oligodendrocytes.

Pomc (Proopiomelanocortin) A precursor, or prohormone, to hormones such as adrenocorticotropic hormone and beta-endorphin, which are involved in adrenal function and pain regulation.

PRC2 (Polycomb repressive complex 2) A transcription protein that catalyzes repression of histones

RISC (RNA-induced silencing complex) Protein complex involved in translation silencing.

ROS (Reactive oxygen species) A highly reactive chemical formed from oxygen that acts as a cell signaling molecule.

shRNA (Short hairpin RNA) An artificial RNA molecule that is used to silence target gene expression (gene silencing) through RNA interference.

siRNA (Short/small interfering RNA) A class of double-stranded RNA that interferes with the expression of specific genes by degrading mRNA after transcription, thus preventing translation.

SP-A/SP-D (Surfactant protein A/D) Pulmonary collectin proteins involved in the innate immune response.

TLR4 (Toll-like receptor 4) A transmembrane protein involved in the innate immune response, specifically the Nf-Kb intracellular pathway.

TNF-B (Tumor necrosis factor beta) Also known as lymphotoxin alpha, a cytokine produced by different lymphocytes with various immune functions, including the pro-inflammatory response triggered by microglial cells.

UTR (Untranslated region) A sequence on both ends of an mRNA molecule that is not translated into a protein.

WT (Wild-type) A typical phenotype seen in nature/outside of the laboratory.

XX Sex chromosomes pertaining to female cells.

XY Sex chromosomes pertaining to male cells.

References

1. Jones KL, Smith DW. Recognition of the fetal alcohol syndrome in early infancy. Lancet. 1973;302(7836):999–1001.
2. Warner RH, Rosett HL. The effects of drinking on offspring: an historical survey of the American and British literature. J Stud Alcohol. 1975;36(11):1395–420.
3. Brown JM, et al. A brief history of awareness of the link between alcohol and fetal alcohol spectrum disorder. Can J Psychiatry. 2019;64(3):164–8.
4. Sugiyama H, et al. Mortality among individuals exposed to atomic bomb radiation in utero: 1950-2012. Eur J Epidemiol. 2021;36(4):415–28.
5. Kim JH, Scialli AR. Thalidomide: the tragedy of birth defects and the effective treatment of disease. Toxicol Sci. 2011;122(1):1–6.
6. Lemoine P, et al. Children of alcoholic parents—observed anomalies: discussion of 127 cases. Ther Drug Monit. 2003;25(2):132–6.
7. Schneider ML, Moore CF, Adkins MM. The effects of prenatal alcohol exposure on behavior: rodent and primate studies. Neuropsychol Rev. 2011;21(2):186–203.
8. Corrigan PW, et al. The public stigma of birth mothers of children with fetal alcohol spectrum disorders. Alcohol Clin Exp Res. 2017;41(6):1166–73.

9. Cavanaugh SE. A transition in fetal alcohol syndrome research: the shift from animal modeling to human intervention. Alcohol Alcohol. 2015;50(2):251–5.
10. Arzua T, et al. Modeling alcohol-induced neurotoxicity using human induced pluripotent stem cell-derived three-dimensional cerebral organoids. Transl Psychiatry. 2020;10(1):347.
11. Tyler CR, Allan AM. Prenatal alcohol exposure alters expression of neurogenesis-related genes in an ex vivo cell culture model. Alcohol. 2014;48(5):483–92.
12. Jacobson SW, et al. Validity of maternal report of prenatal alcohol, cocaine, and smoking in relation to neurobehavioral outcome. Pediatrics. 2002;109(5):815–25.
13. Lechner WV, et al. Effects of alcohol-induced working memory decline on alcohol consumption and adverse consequences of use. Psychopharmacology (Berl). 2016;233(1):83–8.
14. Sawada Feldman H, et al. Prenatal alcohol exposure patterns and alcohol-related birth defects and growth deficiencies: a prospective study. Alcohol Clin Exp Res. 2012;36(4):670–6.
15. Clarren SK, Bowden DM, Astley SJ. Pregnancy outcomes after weekly oral administration of ethanol during gestation in the pig-tailed macaque (Macaca nemestrina). Teratology. 1987;35(3):345–54.
16. Meyer J, et al. Psychopharmacology. Oxford University Press; 2022.
17. Dasgupta A. Alcohol a double-edged sword: health benefits with moderate consumption but a health hazard with excess alcohol intake. In: Dasgupta A, editor. Alcohol, drugs, genes and the clinical laboratory. Academic Press; 2017. p. 1–21.
18. Savage DD, et al. Dose-dependent effects of prenatal ethanol exposure on synaptic plasticity and learning in mature offspring. Alcohol Clin Exp Res. 2002;26(11):1752–8.
19. Easey KE, et al. Prenatal alcohol exposure and offspring mental health: a systematic review. Drug Alcohol Depend. 2019;197:344–53.
20. Flak AL, et al. The association of mild, moderate, and binge prenatal alcohol exposure and child neuropsychological outcomes: a meta-analysis. Alcohol Clin Exp Res. 2014;38(1):214–26.
21. O'Neil E. Developmental timeline of alcohol-induced birth defects. Embryo Project Encyclopedia; 2012.
22. Ethen MK, et al. Alcohol consumption by women before and during pregnancy. Matern Child Health J. 2009;13(2):274–85.
23. Sulik KK, Johnston MC, Webb MA. Fetal alcohol syndrome: embryogenesis in a mouse model. Science. 1981;214(4523):936–8.
24. Michaelis EK. Fetal alcohol exposure: cellular toxicity and molecular events involved in toxicity. Alcohol Clin Exp Res. 1990;14(6):819–26.
25. Clarren S. In: West JR, editor. Neuropathology in fetal alcohol syndrome in alcohol and brain development. New York: Oxford Press; 1986. p. 158–66.
26. Clarren SK, et al. Cognitive and behavioral deficits in nonhuman primates associated with very early embryonic binge exposures to ethanol. J Pediatr. 1992;121(5 Pt 1):789–96.
27. Bandoli G, et al. Patterns of prenatal alcohol use that predict infant growth and development. Pediatrics. 2019;143(2):e20182399.
28. Mukherjee RA, Hollins S, Turk J. Fetal alcohol spectrum disorder: an overview. J R Soc Med. 2006;99(6):298–302.
29. Sies H. Oxidative stress: from basic research to clinical application. Am J Med. 1991;91(3):S31–8.
30. Smith SM. Alcohol-induced cell death in the embryo. Alcohol Health Res World. 1997;21(4):287–97.
31. Cabiscol E, Tamarit J, Ros J. Oxidative stress in bacteria and protein damage by reactive oxygen species. Int Microbiol. 2000;3(1):3–8.
32. Humphries KM, Szweda LI. Selective inactivation of alpha-ketoglutarate dehydrogenase and pyruvate dehydrogenase: reaction of lipoic acid with 4-hydroxy-2-nonenal. Biochemistry. 1998;37(45):15835–41.
33. Kotch LE, Chen SY, Sulik KK. Ethanol-induced teratogenesis: free radical damage as a possible mechanism. Teratology. 1995;52(3):128–36.

34. Tamarit J, Cabiscol E, Ros J. Identification of the major oxidatively damaged proteins in Escherichia coli cells exposed to oxidative stress. J Biol Chem. 1998;273(5):3027–32.
35. Burton GJ, Jauniaux E. Oxidative stress. Best Pract Res Clin Obstet Gynaecol. 2011;25(3):287–99.
36. Brocardo PS, Gil-Mohapel J, Christie BR. The role of oxidative stress in fetal alcohol spectrum disorders. Brain Res Rev. 2011;67(1–2):209–25.
37. Ledig M, et al. An experimental study of fetal alcohol syndrome in the rat: biochemical modifications in brain and liver. Alcohol Alcohol. 1989;24(3):231–40.
38. Perez-Rodriguez L, et al. Measuring oxidative stress: the confounding effect of lipid concentration in measures of lipid peroxidation. Physiol Biochem Zool. 2015;88(3):345–51.
39. Muralidharan P, et al. Fetal alcohol spectrum disorder (FASD) associated neural defects: complex mechanisms and potential therapeutic targets. Brain Sci. 2013;3(2):964–91.
40. Raijmakers MT, et al. Placental NAD(P)H oxidase mediated superoxide generation in early pregnancy. Placenta. 2006;27(2–3):158–63.
41. Chu J, Tong M, de la Monte SM. Chronic ethanol exposure causes mitochondrial dysfunction and oxidative stress in immature central nervous system neurons. Acta Neuropathol. 2007;113(6):659–73.
42. Yanni PA, Lindsley TA. Ethanol inhibits development of dendrites and synapses in rat hippocampal pyramidal neuron cultures. Brain Res Dev Brain Res. 2000;120(2):233–43.
43. Henderson GI, et al. In utero ethanol exposure elicits oxidative stress in the rat fetus. Alcohol Clin Exp Res. 1995;19(3):714–20.
44. Ramachandran V, et al. Ethanol-induced oxidative stress precedes mitochondrially mediated apoptotic death of cultured fetal cortical neurons. J Neurosci Res. 2003;74(4):577–88.
45. Antonio AM, Druse MJ. Antioxidants prevent ethanol-associated apoptosis in fetal rhombencephalic neurons. Brain Res. 2008;1204:16–23.
46. Bhatia S, et al. Oxidative stress and DNA damage in the mechanism of fetal alcohol spectrum disorders. Birth Defects Res. 2019;111(12):714–48.
47. Kuznetsov AV, Margreiter R. Heterogeneity of mitochondria and mitochondrial function within cells as another level of mitochondrial complexity. Int J Mol Sci. 2009;10(4):1911–29.
48. Bukiya AN. Fetal cerebral artery mitochondrion as target of prenatal alcohol exposure. Int J Environ Res Public Health. 2019;16(9):1586.
49. Romert P, Matthiessen ME. Alcohol-induced injury of mitochondria in hepatocytes of minipig fetuses. Virchows Arch A Pathol Anat Histopathol. 1983;399(3):299–305.
50. Lee S, et al. Mitochondrial fission and fusion mediators, hFis1 and OPA1, modulate cellular senescence. J Biol Chem. 2007;282(31):22977–83.
51. Manzo-Avalos S, Saavedra-Molina A. Cellular and mitochondrial effects of alcohol consumption. Int J Environ Res Public Health. 2010;7(12):4281–304.
52. Thayer WS, Rubin E. Effects of chronic ethanol intoxication on oxidative phosphorylation in rat liver submitochondrial particles. J Biol Chem. 1979;254(16):7717–23.
53. Zhao RZ, et al. Mitochondrial electron transport chain, ROS generation and uncoupling (Review). Int J Mol Med. 2019;44(1):3–15.
54. Poderoso JJ, et al. Nitric oxide regulates oxygen uptake and hydrogen peroxide release by the isolated beating rat heart. Am J Phys. 1998;274(1):C112–9.
55. Mannella CA. Structural diversity of mitochondria: functional implications. Ann N Y Acad Sci. 2008;1147:171–9.
56. Walker DW, Benzer S. Mitochondrial "swirls" induced by oxygen stress and in the Drosophila mutant hyperswirl. Proc Natl Acad Sci U S A. 2004;101(28):10290–5.
57. Devi BG, et al. Effect of ethanol on rat fetal hepatocytes: studies on cell replication, lipid peroxidation and glutathione. Hepatology. 1993;18(3):648–59.
58. Deng Y, Kohlwein SD, Mannella CA. Fasting induces cyanide-resistant respiration and oxidative stress in the amoeba Chaos carolinensis: implications for the cubic structural transition in mitochondrial membranes. Protoplasma. 2002;219(3–4):160–7.

59. Kim WH, et al. Hepatitis B virus X protein sensitizes primary mouse hepatocytes to ethanol- and TNF-alpha-induced apoptosis by a caspase-3-dependent mechanism. Cell Mol Immunol. 2005;2(1):40–8.

60. Liu X, et al. Induction of apoptotic program in cell-free extracts: requirement for dATP and cytochrome c. Cell. 1996;86(1):147–57.

61. Hoek JB, Cahill A, Pastorino JG. Alcohol and mitochondria: a dysfunctional relationship. Gastroenterology. 2002;122(7):2049–63.

62. Cai J, Yang J, Jones DP. Mitochondrial control of apoptosis: the role of cytochrome c. Biochim Biophys Acta. 1998;1366(1–2):139–49.

63. Srinivasula SM, et al. Molecular ordering of the Fas-apoptotic pathway: the Fas/APO-1 protease Mch5 is a CrmA-inhibitable protease that activates multiple Ced-3/ICE-like cysteine proteases. Proc Natl Acad Sci U S A. 1996;93(25):14486–91.

64. Kluck RM, et al. The release of cytochrome c from mitochondria: a primary site for Bcl-2 regulation of apoptosis. Science. 1997;275(5303):1132–6.

65. Cartwright MM, Smith SM. Stage-dependent effects of ethanol on cranial neural crest cell development: partial basis for the phenotypic variations observed in fetal alcohol syndrome. Alcohol Clin Exp Res. 1995;19(6):1454–62.

66. Norton JD, Atherton GT. Coupling of cell growth control and apoptosis functions of Id proteins. Mol Cell Biol. 1998;18(4):2371–81.

67. Qin XQ, et al. Deregulated transcription factor E2F-1 expression leads to S-phase entry and p53-mediated apoptosis. Proc Natl Acad Sci U S A. 1994;91(23):10918–22.

68. Brill A, et al. The role of apoptosis in normal and abnormal embryonic development. J Assist Reprod Genet. 1999;16(10):512–9.

69. Bodey B, Bodey B Jr, Kaiser HE. Apoptosis in the mammalian thymus during normal histogenesis and under various in vitro and in vivo experimental conditions. In Vivo. 1998;12(1):123–33.

70. Collins JA, et al. Major DNA fragmentation is a late event in apoptosis. J Histochem Cytochem. 1997;45(7):923–34.

71. Brison DR, Schultz RM. Apoptosis during mouse blastocyst formation: evidence for a role for survival factors including transforming growth factor alpha. Biol Reprod. 1997;56(5):1088–96.

72. Luo J, et al. Ethanol induces cell death and cell cycle delay in cultures of pheochromocytoma PC12 cells. Alcohol Clin Exp Res. 1999;23(4):644–56.

73. Dunty WC Jr, et al. Selective vulnerability of embryonic cell populations to ethanol-induced apoptosis: implications for alcohol-related birth defects and neurodevelopmental disorder. Alcohol Clin Exp Res. 2001;25(10):1523–35.

74. Grummer MA, Langhough RE, Zachman RD. Maternal ethanol ingestion effects on fetal rat brain vitamin A as a model for fetal alcohol syndrome. Alcohol Clin Exp Res. 1993;17(3):592–7.

75. Slater SJ, et al. Inhibition of protein kinase C by alcohols and anaesthetics. Nature. 1993;364(6432):82–4.

76. Stachecki JJ, et al. Blastocyst cavitation is accelerated by ethanol- or ionophore-induced elevation of intracellular calcium. Biol Reprod. 1994;50(1):1–9.

77. Cartwright MM, Tessmer LL, Smith SM. Ethanol-induced neural crest apoptosis is coincident with their endogenous death, but is mechanistically distinct. Alcohol Clin Exp Res. 1998;22(1):142–9.

78. Schafer KA. The cell cycle: a review. Vet Pathol. 1998;35(6):461–78.

79. White J, Dalton S. Cell cycle control of embryonic stem cells. Stem Cell Rev. 2005;1(2):131–8.

80. Stead E, et al. Pluripotent cell division cycles are driven by ectopic Cdk2, cyclin A/E and E2F activities. Oncogene. 2002;21(54):8320–33.

81. Dannenberg JH, et al. Ablation of the retinoblastoma gene family deregulates G(1) control causing immortalization and increased cell turnover under growth-restricting conditions. Genes Dev. 2000;14(23):3051–64.

82. Anthony B, et al. Alcohol exposure alters cell cycle and apoptotic events during early neurulation. Alcohol Alcohol. 2008;43(3):261–73.

83. Santillano DR, et al. Ethanol induces cell-cycle activity and reduces stem cell diversity to alter both regenerative capacity and differentiation potential of cerebral cortical neuroepithelial precursors. BMC Neurosci. 2005;6:59.

84. Hicks SD, Middleton FA, Miller MW. Ethanol-induced methylation of cell cycle genes in neural stem cells. J Neurochem. 2010;114(6):1767–80.

85. Mikami K, Haseba T, Ohno Y. Ethanol induces transient arrest of cell division (G2 + M block) followed by G0/G1 block: dose effects of short- and longer-term ethanol exposure on cell cycle and cell functions. Alcohol Alcohol. 1997;32(2):145–52.

86. Clemens DL, et al. Ethanol metabolism results in a G2/M cell-cycle arrest in recombinant Hep G2 cells. Hepatology. 2003;38(2):385–93.

87. Messerschmidt DM, Knowles BB, Solter D. DNA methylation dynamics during epigenetic reprogramming in the germline and preimplantation embryos. Genes Dev. 2014;28(8):812–28.

88. Borgel J, et al. Targets and dynamics of promoter DNA methylation during early mouse development. Nat Genet. 2010;42(12):1093–100.

89. He S, Nakada D, Morrison SJ. Mechanisms of stem cell self-renewal. Annu Rev Cell Dev Biol. 2009;25:377–406.

90. Rossi DJ, et al. Deficiencies in DNA damage repair limit the function of haematopoietic stem cells with age. Nature. 2007;447(7145):725–9.

91. Becker KA, et al. Self-renewal of human embryonic stem cells is supported by a shortened G1 cell cycle phase. J Cell Physiol. 2006;209(3):883–93.

92. Balaraman S, et al. Plasma miRNA profiles in pregnant women predict infant outcomes following prenatal alcohol exposure. PLoS One. 2016;11(11):e0165081.

93. Chung DD, et al. Toxic and teratogenic effects of prenatal alcohol exposure on fetal development, adolescence, and adulthood. Int J Mol Sci. 2021;22(16):8785.

94. Sathyan P, Golden HB, Miranda RC. Competing interactions between micro-RNAs determine neural progenitor survival and proliferation after ethanol exposure: evidence from an ex vivo model of the fetal cerebral cortical neuroepithelium. J Neurosci. 2007;27(32):8546–57.

95. Miller MW. Effect of prenatal exposure to ethanol on glutamate and GABA immunoreactivity in macaque somatosensory and motor cortices: critical timing of exposure. Neuroscience. 2006;138(1):97–107.

96. Di Rocco G, et al. Stem cells under the influence of alcohol: effects of ethanol consumption on stem/progenitor cells. Cell Mol Life Sci. 2019;76(2):231–44.

97. Le Belle JE, et al. Proliferative neural stem cells have high endogenous ROS levels that regulate self-renewal and neurogenesis in a PI3K/Akt-dependant manner. Cell Stem Cell. 2011;8(1):59–71.

98. Roitbak T, et al. Moderate fetal alcohol exposure impairs neurogenic capacity of murine neural stem cells isolated from the adult subventricular zone. Exp Neurol. 2011;229(2):522–5.

99. Miller MW, Potempa G. Numbers of neurons and glia in mature rat somatosensory cortex: effects of prenatal exposure to ethanol. J Comp Neurol. 1990;293(1):92–102.

100. Pinson MR, et al. Extracellular vesicles in premature aging and diseases in adulthood due to developmental exposures. Aging Dis. 2021;12(6):1516–35.

101. Tseng AM, et al. Ethanol exposure increases miR-140 in extracellular vesicles: implications for fetal neural stem cell proliferation and maturation. Alcohol Clin Exp Res. 2019;43(7):1414–26.

102. Choi IY, Allan AM, Cunningham LA. Moderate fetal alcohol exposure impairs the neurogenic response to an enriched environment in adult mice. Alcohol Clin Exp Res. 2005;29(11):2053–62.

103. Klintsova AY, et al. Persistent impairment of hippocampal neurogenesis in young adult rats following early postnatal alcohol exposure. Alcohol Clin Exp Res. 2007;31(12):2073–82.
104. Polanco TA, et al. Fetal alcohol exposure increases mammary tumor susceptibility and alters tumor phenotype in rats. Alcohol Clin Exp Res. 2010;34(11):1879–87.
105. Thanh NX, Jonsson E. Life expectancy of people with fetal alcohol syndrome. J Popul Ther Clin Pharmacol. 2016;23(1):e53–9.
106. Weinberg J, Jerrells TR. Suppression of immune responsiveness: sex differences in prenatal ethanol effects. Alcohol Clin Exp Res. 1991;15(3):525–31.
107. Yang J, et al. Prenatal alcohol exposure and congenital heart defects: a meta-analysis. PLoS One. 2015;10(6):e0130681.
108. Aaronson SA. Growth factors and cancer. Science. 1991;254(5035):1146–53.
109. Wolff GS, et al. Epidermal growth factor-like growth factors prevent apoptosis of alcohol-exposed human placental cytotrophoblast cells. Biol Reprod. 2007;77(1):53–60.
110. Boschen KE, et al. Effects of developmental alcohol exposure vs. intubation stress on BDNF and TrkB expression in the hippocampus and frontal cortex of neonatal rats. Int J Dev Neurosci. 2015;43:16–24.
111. Heaton MB, et al. Ethanol-induced alterations in the expression of neurotrophic factors in the developing rat central nervous system. Brain Res Dev Brain Res. 2000;121(1):97–107.
112. Heaton MB, et al. Ethanol effects on neonatal rat cortex: comparative analyses of neurotrophic factors, apoptosis-related proteins, and oxidative processes during vulnerable and resistant periods. Brain Res Dev Brain Res. 2003;145(2):249–62.
113. Antonakopoulos N, et al. Association between brain-derived neurotrophic factor (BDNF) levels in 2(nd) trimester amniotic fluid and fetal development. Mediat Inflamm. 2018;2018:8476217.
114. Paria BC, Dey SK. Preimplantation embryo development in vitro: cooperative interactions among embryos and role of growth factors. Proc Natl Acad Sci U S A. 1990;87(12):4756–60.
115. Heaton MB, et al. Responsiveness of cultured septal and hippocampal neurons to ethanol and neurotrophic substances. J Neurosci Res. 1994;39(3):305–18.
116. Rossant J. Stem cells and lineage development in the mammalian blastocyst. Reprod Fertil Dev. 2007;19(1):111–8.
117. Rossant J. Stem cells from the mammalian blastocyst. Stem Cells. 2001;19(6):477–82.
118. Aros S, et al. Effects of prenatal ethanol exposure on postnatal growth and the insulin-like growth factor axis. Horm Res Paediatr. 2011;75(3):166–73.
119. Xu J, et al. Ethanol impairs insulin-stimulated neuronal survival in the developing brain: role of PTEN phosphatase. J Biol Chem. 2003;278(29):26929–37.
120. Cesen MH, et al. Lysosomal pathways to cell death and their therapeutic applications. Exp Cell Res. 2012;318(11):1245–51.
121. Komada M, et al. Mechanisms underlying neuro-inflammation and neurodevelopmental toxicity in the mouse neocortex following prenatal exposure to ethanol. Sci Rep. 2017;7(1):4934.
122. Wake H, et al. Resting microglia directly monitor the functional state of synapses in vivo and determine the fate of ischemic terminals. J Neurosci. 2009;29(13):3974–80.
123. Paolicelli RC, et al. Synaptic pruning by microglia is necessary for normal brain development. Science. 2011;333(6048):1456–8.
124. Takahashi K, Rochford CD, Neumann H. Clearance of apoptotic neurons without inflammation by microglial triggering receptor expressed on myeloid cells-2. J Exp Med. 2005;201(4):647–57.
125. Marın-Teva JL, et al. Microglia promote the death of developing Purkinje cells. Neuron. 2004;41(4):535–47.
126. Fernandez-Lizarbe S, Montesinos J, Guerri C. Ethanol induces TLR4/TLR2 association, triggering an inflammatory response in microglial cells. J Neurochem. 2013;126(2):261–73.
127. Pascual M, et al. TLR4 response mediates ethanol-induced neurodevelopment alterations in a model of fetal alcohol spectrum disorders. J Neuroinflammation. 2017;14(1):145.

128. Stromland K. Visual impairment and ocular abnormalities in children with fetal alcohol syndrome. Addict Biol. 2004;9(2):153–7; discussion 159–60.
129. Green CR, et al. Deficits in eye movement control in children with fetal alcohol spectrum disorders. Alcohol Clin Exp Res. 2007;31(3):500–11.
130. Streissguth AP, et al. Neurobehavioral effects of prenatal alcohol: Part III. PLS analyses of neuropsychologic tests. Neurotoxicol Teratol. 1989;11(5):493–507.
131. Drover JR, et al. Children with fetal alcohol spectrum disorder show amblyopia-like vision deficits. Invest Ophthalmol Vis Sci. 2009;50(13):2494.
132. McTigue DM, Tripathi RB. The life, death, and replacement of oligodendrocytes in the adult CNS. J Neurochem. 2008;107(1):1–19.
133. Dimou L, et al. Progeny of Olig2-expressing progenitors in the gray and white matter of the adult mouse cerebral cortex. J Neurosci. 2008;28(41):10434–42.
134. Guizzetti M, Costa LG. Inhibition of muscarinic receptor-stimulated glial cell proliferation by ethanol. J Neurochem. 1996;67(6):2236–45.
135. Archibald SL, et al. Brain dysmorphology in individuals with severe prenatal alcohol exposure. Dev Med Child Neurol. 2001;43(3):148–54.
136. Newville J, et al. Acute oligodendrocyte loss with persistent white matter injury in a third trimester equivalent mouse model of fetal alcohol spectrum disorder. Glia. 2017;65(8):1317–32.
137. Filley CM, Fields RD. White matter and cognition: making the connection. J Neurophysiol. 2016;116(5):2093–104.
138. Phillips D, Krueger S. Effects of combined pre-and postnatal ethanol exposure (three trimester equivalency) on glial cell development in rat optic nerve. Int J Dev Neurosci. 1992;10(3):197–206.
139. Pinazo-Duran MD, et al. Optic nerve hypoplasia in fetal alcohol syndrome: an update. Eur J Ophthalmol. 1997;7(3):262–70.
140. Streissguth AP, et al. Fetal alcohol syndrome in adolescents and adults. JAMA. 1991;265(15):1961–7.
141. Kim Y, Park J, Choi YK. The role of astrocytes in the central nervous system focused on BK channel and heme oxygenase metabolites: a review. Antioxidants (Basel). 2019;8(5):121.
142. Blanco AM, et al. Involvement of TLR4/type I IL-1 receptor signaling in the induction of inflammatory mediators and cell death induced by ethanol in cultured astrocytes. J Immunol. 2005;175(10):6893–9.
143. Peng Y, et al. A critical role of Pax6 in alcohol-induced fetal microcephaly. Neurobiol Dis. 2004;16(2):370–6.
144. Pei J, et al. Mental health issues in fetal alcohol spectrum disorder. J Ment Health. 2011;20(5):473–83.
145. Rasmussen C, et al. The impact of an ADHD co-morbidity on the diagnosis of FASD. J Popul Ther Clin Pharmacol. 2010;17(1):e165.
146. Popova S, et al. Cost of specialized addiction treatment of clients with fetal alcohol spectrum disorder in Canada. BMC Public Health. 2013;13:570.
147. Hansen N, Manahan-Vaughan D. Locus coeruleus stimulation facilitates long-term depression in the dentate gyrus that requires activation of β-adrenergic receptors. Cerebral Cortex (New York, N.Y.: 1991). 2015;25(7):1889–96.
148. Borodovitsyna O, Flamini M, Chandler D. Noradrenergic modulation of cognition in health and disease. Neural Plast. 2017;2017:6031478.
149. Felten DL, Hallman H, Jonsson G. Evidence for a neurotropic role of noradrenaline neurons in the postnatal development of rat cerebral cortex. J Neurocytol. 1982;11(1):119–35.
150. Landers MS, Sullivan RM. The development and neurobiology of infant attachment and fear. Dev Neurosci. 2012;34(2–3):101–14.
151. Sullivan RM. Unique characteristics of neonatal classical conditioning: the role of the amygdala and locus coeruleus. Integr Physiol Behav Sci. 2001;36(4):293–307.
152. Detering N, et al. Comparative effects of ethanol and malnutrition on the development of catecholamine neurons: changes in neurotransmitter levels. J Neurochem. 1980;34(6):1587–93.

153. Srivastava N, Backman C. Effects of ethanol on development of locus coeruleus brain stem transplants in oculo. Exp Neurol. 1998;149(1):139–50.
154. Kim P, et al. Effects of ethanol exposure during early pregnancy in hyperactive, inattentive and impulsive behaviors and MeCP2 expression in rodent offspring. Neurochem Res. 2013;38(3):620–31.
155. Mattson SN, et al. Executive functioning in children with heavy prenatal alcohol exposure. Alcohol Clin Exp Res. 1999;23(11):1808–15.
156. Chinta SJ, Andersen JK. Dopaminergic neurons. Int J Biochem Cell Biol. 2005;37(5):942–6.
157. Ott T, Nieder A. Dopamine and cognitive control in prefrontal cortex. Trends Cogn Sci. 2019;23(3):213–34.
158. Lawrence RC, Otero NKH, Kelly SJ. Selective effects of perinatal ethanol exposure in medial prefrontal cortex and nucleus accumbens. Neurotoxicol Teratol. 2012;34(1):128–35.
159. Schneider ML, et al. Moderate-level prenatal alcohol exposure alters striatal dopamine system function in rhesus monkeys. Alcohol Clin Exp Res. 2005;29(9):1685–97.
160. Druse MJ, et al. Effects of in utero ethanol exposure on the developing dopaminergic system in rats. J Neurosci Res. 1990;27(2):233–40.
161. Landau SM, et al. Striatal dopamine and working memory. Cereb Cortex. 2008;19(2):445–54.
162. Kotkoskie LA, Norton S. Prenatal brain malformations following acute ethanol exposure in the rat. Alcohol Clin Exp Res. 1988;12(6):831–6.
163. Lucas BR, et al. Gross motor deficits in children prenatally exposed to alcohol: a meta-analysis. Pediatrics. 2014;134(1):e192–209.
164. Spoerri PE. Neurotrophic effects of GABA in cultures of embryonic chick brain and retina. Synapse. 1988;2(1):11–22.
165. De Carlos J, López-Mascaraque L, Valverde F. Dynamics of cell migration from the lateral ganglionic eminence in the rat. J Neurosci. 1996;16(19):6146–56.
166. Marin O, Rubenstein JL. A long, remarkable journey: tangential migration in the telencephalon. Nat Rev Neurosci. 2001;2(11):780–90.
167. Cuzon VC, et al. Ethanol consumption during early pregnancy alters the disposition of tangentially migrating GABAergic interneurons in the fetal cortex. J Neurosci. 2008;28(8):1854–64.
168. Pierce DR, Goodlett CR, West JR. Differential neuronal loss following early postnatal alcohol exposure. Teratology. 1989;40(2):113–26.
169. Light K, Belcher S, Pierce D. Time course and manner of Purkinje neuron death following a single ethanol exposure on postnatal day 4 in the developing rat. Neuroscience. 2002;114(2):327–37.
170. O'Connor MJ, et al. Suicide risk in adolescents with fetal alcohol spectrum disorders. Birth Defects Res. 2019;111(12):822–8.
171. Roy A, Linnoila M. Suicidal behavior, impulsiveness and serotonin. Acta Psychiatr Scand. 1988;78(5):529–35.
172. Berger M, Gray JA, Roth BL. The expanded biology of serotonin. Annu Rev Med. 2009;60:355–66.
173. Lesch K-P, Waider J. Serotonin in the modulation of neural plasticity and networks: implications for neurodevelopmental disorders. Neuron. 2012;76(1):175–91.
174. Chubakov AR, et al. The effects of serotonin on the morpho-functional development of rat cerebral neocortex in tissue culture. Brain Res. 1986;369(1):285–97.
175. Sundström E, et al. Neurochemical differentiation of human bulbospinal monoaminergic neurons during the first trimester. Brain Res Dev Brain Res. 1993;75(1):1–12.
176. Sundermann AC, et al. Week-by-week alcohol consumption in early pregnancy and spontaneous abortion risk: a prospective cohort study. Am J Obstet Gynecol. 2021;224(1):97.e1–97.e16.
177. Druse MJ, Kuo A, Tajuddin N. Effects of in utero ethanol exposure on the developing serotonergic system. Alcohol Clin Exp Res. 1991;15(4):678–84.

178. Zhou FC, et al. Prenatal alcohol exposure retards the migration and development of serotonin neurons in fetal C57BL mice. Brain Res Dev Brain Res. 2001;126(2):147–55.
179. Zhou FC, Sari Y, Powrozek TA. Fetal alcohol exposure reduces serotonin innervation and compromises development of the forebrain along the serotonergic pathway. Alcohol Clin Exp Res. 2005;29(1):141–9.
180. Sari Y, Zhou FC. Prenatal alcohol exposure causes long-term serotonin neuron deficit in mice. Alcohol Clin Exp Res. 2004;28(6):941–8.
181. Baldwin D, Rudge S. The role of serotonin in depression and anxiety. Int Clin Psychopharmacol. 1995;9:41.
182. Johnson S, et al. Immune deficiency in fetal alcohol syndrome. Pediatr Res. 1981;15(6):908–11.
183. Church MW, Gerkin KP. Hearing disorders in children with fetal alcohol syndrome: findings from case reports. Pediatrics. 1988;82(2):147–54.
184. Seelig LL Jr, Steven WM, Stewart GL. Effects of maternal ethanol consumption on the subsequent development of immunity to Trichinella spiralis in rat neonates. Alcohol Clin Exp Res. 1996;20(3):514–22.
185. McGill J, et al. Fetal exposure to ethanol has long-term effects on the severity of influenza virus infections. J Immunol. 2009;182(12):7803–8.
186. Grossmann A, et al. Immune function in offspring of nonhuman primates (macaca nemestrina) exposed weekly to 1.8 g/kg ethanol during pregnancy: preliminary observations. Alcohol Clin Exp Res. 1993;17(4):822–7.
187. Sulik KK, et al. Fetal alcohol syndrome and DiGeorge anomaly: critical ethanol exposure periods for craniofacial malformations as illustrated in an animal model. Am J Med Genet Suppl. 1986;2:97–112.
188. Bray LA, Shao H, Ewald SJ. Effect of ethanol on development of fetal mouse thymocytes in organ culture. Cell Immunol. 1993;151(1):12–23.
189. Taylor AN, Tio DL, Chiappelli F. Thymocyte development in male fetal alcohol-exposed rats. Alcohol Clin Exp Res. 1999;23(3):465–70.
190. Ewald SJ. T lymphocyte populations in fetal alcohol syndrome. Alcohol Clin Exp Res. 1989;13(4):485–9.
191. Sanchez JJ, et al. Prenatal alcohol exposure is a risk factor for adult neuropathic pain via aberrant neuroimmune function. J Neuroinflammation. 2017;14(1):254.
192. Mei-Ping C, et al. Mechanism of the impaired T-cell proliferation in adult rats exposed to alcohol in utero. Int J Immunopharmacol. 1994;16(4):345–57.
193. Taylor AN, et al. Actions of alcohol on immunity and neoplasia in fetal alcohol exposed and adult rats. Alcohol Alcohol·Suppl. 1993;2:69–74.
194. Gottesfeld Z, et al. Prenatal ethanol exposure alters immune capacity and noradrenergic synaptic transmission in lymphoid organs of the adult mouse. Neuroscience. 1990;35(1):185–94.
195. Arjona A, et al. Fetal ethanol exposure disrupts the daily rhythms of splenic granzyme B, IFN-gamma, and NK cell cytotoxicity in adulthood. Alcohol Clin Exp Res. 2006;30(6):1039–44.
196. Noor S, et al. The LFA-1 antagonist BIRT377 reverses neuropathic pain in prenatal alcohol-exposed female rats via actions on peripheral and central neuroimmune function in discrete pain-relevant tissue regions. Brain Behav Immun. 2020;87:339–58.
197. Gauthier TW, et al. Fetal alcohol exposure impairs alveolar macrophage function via decreased glutathione availability. Pediatr Res. 2005;57(1):76–81.
198. Ping XD, et al. In vivo dysfunction of the term alveolar macrophage after in utero ethanol exposure. Alcohol Clin Exp Res. 2007;31(2):308–16.
199. Gauthier TW, et al. Delayed neonatal lung macrophage differentiation in a mouse model of in utero ethanol exposure. Am J Physiol Lung Cell Mol Physiol. 2010;299(1):L8–L16.
200. Gauthier TW, et al. In utero ethanol exposure impairs defenses against experimental group B streptococcus in the term Guinea pig lung. Alcohol Clin Exp Res. 2009;33(2):300–6.
201. Sozo F, et al. Repeated ethanol exposure during late gestation alters the maturation and innate immune status of the ovine fetal lung. Am J Physiol Lung Cell Mol Physiol. 2009;296(3):L510–8.

202. Lazic T, et al. Maternal alcohol ingestion reduces surfactant protein A expression by preterm fetal lung epithelia. Alcohol. 2007;41(5):347–55.
203. Sorensen GL, Husby S, Holmskov U. Surfactant protein A and surfactant protein D variation in pulmonary disease. Immunobiology. 2007;212(4–5):381–416.
204. Wolcott RM, Jennings SR, Chervenak R. In utero exposure to ethanol affects postnatal development of T- and B-lymphocytes, but not natural killer cells. Alcohol Clin Exp Res. 1995;19(1):170–6.
205. Moscatello KM, et al. Effects of in utero alcohol exposure on B cell development in neonatal spleen and bone marrow. Cell Immunol. 1999;191(2):124–30.
206. Robinson RS, Seelig LL. Effects of maternal ethanol consumption on hematopoietic cells in the rat fetal liver. Alcohol. 2002;28(3):151–6.
207. Biber KL, et al. Effects of in utero alcohol exposure on B-cell development in the murine fetal liver. Alcohol Clin Exp Res. 1998;22(8):1706–12.
208. Wang H, et al. In utero exposure to alcohol alters cell fate decisions by hematopoietic progenitors in the bone marrow of offspring mice during neonatal development. Cell Immunol. 2006;239(1):75–85.
209. Wang H, et al. Alcohol affects the late differentiation of progenitor B cells. Alcohol Alcohol. 2011;46(1):26–32.
210. Wang H, et al. Ethanol exhibits specificity in its effects on differentiation of hematopoietic progenitors. Cell Immunol. 2009;255(1–2):1–7.
211. Ewald SJ, Walden SM. Flow cytometric and histological analysis of mouse thymus in fetal alcohol syndrome. J Leukoc Biol. 1988;44(5):434–40.
212. Ewald SJ, Frost WW. Effect of prenatal exposure to ethanol on development of the thymus. Thymus. 1987;9(4):211–5.
213. Zhu X, Seelig LL Jr. Developmental aspects of intestinal intraepithelial and lamina propria lymphocytes in the rat following placental and lactational exposure to ethanol. Alcohol Alcohol. 2000;35(1):25–30.
214. Chiappelli F, et al. Selective effects of fetal alcohol exposure on rat thymocyte development. Alcohol. 1992;9(6):481–7.
215. Carol MKW, et al. Prenatal exposure to alcohol enhances thymocyte mitogenic responses postnatally. Int J Immunopharmacol. 1992;14(2):303–9.
216. Zhang X, et al. Prenatal alcohol exposure alters the course and severity of adjuvant-induced arthritis in female rats. Brain Behav Immun. 2012;26(3):439–50.
217. Sowell KD, et al. Implications of altered maternal cytokine concentrations on infant outcomes in children with prenatal alcohol exposure. Alcohol. 2018;68:49–58.
218. Bodnar TS, et al. Altered maternal immune networks are associated with adverse child neurodevelopment: impact of alcohol consumption during pregnancy. Brain Behav Immun. 2018;73:205–15.
219. Bodnar TS, et al. Immune network dysregulation associated with child neurodevelopmental delay: modulatory role of prenatal alcohol exposure. J Neuroinflammation. 2020;17(1):39.
220. Statello L, et al. Gene regulation by long non-coding RNAs and its biological functions. Nat Rev Mol Cell Biol. 2021;22(2):96–118.
221. Herranz H, Cohen SM. MicroRNAs and gene regulatory networks: managing the impact of noise in biological systems. Genes Dev. 2010;24(13):1339–44.
222. Miranda RC. Chapter 7: MicroRNAs and ethanol toxicity. In: Pandey SC, editor. International review of neurobiology. Academic Press; 2014. p. 245–84.
223. Meister G, et al. Human Argonaute2 mediates RNA cleavage targeted by miRNAs and siRNAs. Mol Cell. 2004;15(2):185–97.
224. Mittelbrunn M, et al. Unidirectional transfer of microRNA-loaded exosomes from T cells to antigen-presenting cells. Nat Commun. 2011;2:282.
225. Zhang Y, et al. Secreted monocytic miR-150 enhances targeted endothelial cell migration. Mol Cell. 2010;39(1):133–44.

226. Perera RJ, Ray A. MicroRNAs in the search for understanding human diseases. BioDrugs. 2007;21(2):97–104.
227. Pappalardo-Carter DL, et al. Suppression and epigenetic regulation of MiR-9 contributes to ethanol teratology: evidence from zebrafish and murine fetal neural stem cell models. Alcohol Clin Exp Res. 2013;37(10):1657–67.
228. Shibata M, et al. MicroRNA-9 regulates neurogenesis in mouse telencephalon by targeting multiple transcription factors. J Neurosci. 2011;31(9):3407–22.
229. Tal TL, et al. MicroRNAs control neurobehavioral development and function in zebrafish. FASEB J. 2012;26(4):1452–61.
230. Qi Y, et al. MicroRNA-29b regulates ethanol-induced neuronal apoptosis in the developing cerebellum through SP1/RAX/PKR cascade. J Biol Chem. 2014;289(14):10201–10.
231. Guo Y, et al. Chronic intermittent ethanol exposure and its removal induce a different miRNA expression pattern in primary cortical neuronal cultures. Alcohol Clin Exp Res. 2012;36(6):1058–66.
232. Mantha K, Laufer BI, Singh SM. Molecular changes during neurodevelopment following second-trimester binge ethanol exposure in a mouse model of fetal alcohol spectrum disorder: from immediate effects to long-term adaptation. Dev Neurosci. 2014;36(1):29–43.
233. Balaraman S, et al. Maternal and neonatal plasma microRNA biomarkers for fetal alcohol exposure in an ovine model. Alcohol Clin Exp Res. 2014;38(5):1390–400.
234. Mahnke AH, et al. Infant circulating MicroRNAs as biomarkers of effect in fetal alcohol spectrum disorders. Sci Rep. 2021;11(1):1429.
235. Salem NA, et al. Association between fetal sex and maternal plasma microRNA responses to prenatal alcohol exposure: evidence from a birth outcome-stratified cohort. Biol Sex Differ. 2020;11(1):51.
236. Guttman M, et al. Chromatin signature reveals over a thousand highly conserved large noncoding RNAs in mammals. Nature. 2009;458:223.
237. Herriges MJ, et al. Long noncoding RNAs are spatially correlated with transcription factors and regulate lung development. Genes Dev. 2014;28(12):1363–79.
238. Ng S-Y, et al. The long noncoding RNA RMST interacts with SOX2 to regulate neurogenesis. Mol Cell. 2013;51(3):349–59.
239. Sun L, et al. Long noncoding RNAs regulate adipogenesis. Proc Natl Acad Sci. 2013;110(9):3387–92.
240. Feng L, et al. Linc-ROR promotes osteogenic differentiation of mesenchymal stem cells by functioning as a competing endogenous RNA for miR-138 and miR-145. Mol Ther Nucleic Acids. 2018;11:345–53.
241. Khalil AM, et al. Many human large intergenic noncoding RNAs associate with chromatin-modifying complexes and affect gene expression. Proc Natl Acad Sci U S A. 2009;106(28):11667–72.
242. Lyle R, et al. The imprinted antisense RNA at the Igf2r locus overlaps but does not imprint Mas1. Nat Genet. 2000;25(1):19–21.
243. Rinn JL, et al. Functional demarcation of active and silent chromatin domains in human HOX loci by noncoding RNAs. Cell. 2007;129(7):1311–23.
244. Guttman M, et al. lincRNAs act in the circuitry controlling pluripotency and differentiation. Nature. 2011;477(7364):295–300.
245. Pandey RR, et al. Kcnq1ot1 antisense noncoding RNA mediates lineage-specific transcriptional silencing through chromatin-level regulation. Mol Cell. 2008;32(2):232–46.
246. Veazey KJ, et al. Alcohol-induced epigenetic alterations to developmentally crucial genes regulating neural stemness and differentiation. Alcohol Clin Exp Res. 2013;37(7):1111–22.
247. Salem NA, et al. A novel Oct4/Pou5f1-like non-coding RNA controls neural maturation and mediates developmental effects of ethanol. Neurotoxicol Teratol. 2021;83:106943.
248. Salem NA, et al. Cell-type and fetal-sex-specific targets of prenatal alcohol exposure in developing mouse cerebral cortex. iScience. 2021;24(5):-102439.
249. Barrett SP, Salzman J. Circular RNAs: analysis, expression and potential functions. Development. 2016;143(11):1838–47.

250. Jeck WR, et al. Circular RNAs are abundant, conserved, and associated with ALU repeats. RNA. 2013;19(2):141–57.
251. Hansen TB, et al. Natural RNA circles function as efficient microRNA sponges. Nature. 2013;495:384.
252. Szabo L, et al. Statistically based splicing detection reveals neural enrichment and tissue-specific induction of circular RNA during human fetal development. Genome Biol. 2015;16(1):126.
253. Venø MT, et al. Spatio-temporal regulation of circular RNA expression during porcine embryonic brain development. Genome Biol. 2015;16(1):245.
254. Memczak S, et al. Circular RNAs are a large class of animal RNAs with regulatory potency. Nature. 2013;495:333.
255. Paudel P, et al. Prenatal alcohol exposure results in sex-specific alterations in circular RNA expression in the developing mouse brain. Front Neurosci. 2020;14(1165):581895.
256. Wu N, et al. YAP circular RNA, circYap, attenuates cardiac fibrosis via binding with tropomyosin-4 and gamma-actin decreasing actin polymerization. Mol Ther. 2021;29(3):1138–50.
257. Yang Z-G, et al. The circular RNA interacts with STAT3, increasing its nuclear translocation and wound repair by modulating Dnmt3a and miR-17 function. Mol Ther. 2017;25(9):2062–74.
258. Du WW, et al. Induction of tumor apoptosis through a circular RNA enhancing Foxo3 activity. Cell Death Differ. 2017;24(2):357–70.
259. Yang L, et al. Extracellular vesicle-mediated delivery of circular RNA SCMH1 promotes functional recovery in rodent and nonhuman primate ischemic stroke models. Circulation. 2020;142(6):556–74.
260. Du WW, et al. A circular RNA circ-DNMT1 enhances breast cancer progression by activating autophagy. Oncogene. 2018;37(44):5829–42.
261. Fang L, et al. The circular RNA circ-Ccnb1 dissociates Ccnb1/Cdk1 complex suppressing cell invasion and tumorigenesis. Cancer Lett. 2019;459:216–26.
262. Wang X, et al. Exosome-delivered circRNA promotes glycolysis to induce chemoresistance through the miR-122-PKM2 axis in colorectal cancer. Mol Oncol. 2020;14(3):539–55.
263. Keverne EB, Pfaff DW, Tabansky I. Epigenetic changes in the developing brain: effects on behavior. Proc Natl Acad Sci. 2015;112(22):6789–95.
264. Moore-Morris T, et al. Role of epigenetics in cardiac development and congenital diseases. Physiol Rev. 2018;98(4):2453–75.
265. Madhok A, deSouza A, Galande S. Chapter 3: Understanding immune system development: an epigenetic perspective. In: Kabelitz D, Bhat J, editors. Epigenetics of the immune system. Academic Press; 2020. p. 39–76.
266. Resendiz M, et al. Epigenetic regulation of the neural transcriptome and alcohol interference during development. Front Genet. 2014;5:285.
267. Mazzone R, et al. The emerging role of epigenetics in human autoimmune disorders. Clin Epigenetics. 2019;11(1):34.
268. Zhou FC, et al. Alcohol alters DNA methylation patterns and inhibits neural stem cell differentiation. Alcohol Clin Exp Res. 2011;35(4):735–46.
269. Kleiber ML, et al. Neurodevelopmental alcohol exposure elicits long-term changes to gene expression that alter distinct molecular pathways dependent on timing of exposure. J Neurodev Disord. 2013;5(1):6.
270. Lucia D, et al. Periconceptional maternal alcohol consumption leads to behavioural changes in adult and aged offspring and alters the expression of hippocampal genes associated with learning and memory and regulators of the epigenome. Behav Brain Res. 2019;362:249–57.
271. Kleiber ML, et al. Long-term alterations to the brain transcriptome in a maternal voluntary consumption model of fetal alcohol spectrum disorders. Brain Res. 2012;1458:18–33.
272. Laufer BI, et al. Long-lasting alterations to DNA methylation and ncRNAs could underlie the effects of fetal alcohol exposure in mice. Dis Models Mech. 2013;6(4):977–92.

273. Stringer RL, et al. Reduced expression of brain cannabinoid receptor 1 (Cnr1) is coupled with an increased complementary micro-RNA (miR-26b) in a mouse model of fetal alcohol spectrum disorders. Clin Epigenetics. 2013;5(1):14.

274. Laufer BI, et al. Associative DNA methylation changes in children with prenatal alcohol exposure. Epigenomics. 2015;7(8):1259–74.

275. Gates LA, Foulds CE, O'Malley BW. Histone marks in the 'Driver's Seat': functional roles in steering the transcription cycle. Trends Biochem Sci. 2017;42(12):977–89.

276. Gates LA, et al. Acetylation on histone H3 lysine 9 mediates a switch from transcription initiation to elongation. J Biol Chem. 2017;292(35):14456–72.

277. Burd L, et al. Congenital heart defects and fetal alcohol spectrum disorders. Congenit Heart Dis. 2007;2(4):250–5.

278. Löser H, Majewski F. Type and frequency of cardiac defects in embryofetal alcohol syndrome. Report of 16 cases. Br Heart J. 1977;39(12):1374–9.

279. Sandor GGS, Smith DF, MacLeod PM. Cardiac malformations in the fetal alcohol syndrome. J Pediatr. 1981;98(5):771–3.

280. Steeg CN, Woolf P. Cardiovascular malformations in the fetal alcohol syndrome. Am Heart J. 1979;98(5):635–7.

281. Peng C, et al. Inhibition of histone H3K9 acetylation by anacardic acid can correct the overexpression of Gata4 in the hearts of fetal mice exposed to alcohol during pregnancy. PLoS One. 2014;9(8):e104135.

282. Zhong L, et al. Ethanol and its metabolites induce histone lysine 9 acetylation and an alteration of the expression of heart development-related genes in cardiac progenitor cells. Cardiovasc Toxicol. 2010;10(4):268–74.

283. Pan B, et al. Alcohol consumption during gestation causes Histone3 Lysine9 hyperacetylation and an alternation of expression of heart development-related genes in mice. Alcohol Clin Exp Res. 2014;38(9):2396–402.

284. Subbanna S, et al. G9a-mediated histone methylation regulates ethanol-induced neurodegeneration in the neonatal mouse brain. Neurobiol Dis. 2013;54:475–85.

285. Subbanna S, et al. Ethanol induced acetylation of histone at G9a exon1 and G9a-mediated histone H3 dimethylation leads to neurodegeneration in neonatal mice. Neuroscience. 2014;258:422–32.

286. Veazey KJ, et al. Dose-dependent alcohol-induced alterations in chromatin structure persist beyond the window of exposure and correlate with fetal alcohol syndrome birth defects. Epigenetics Chromatin. 2015;8(1):39.

287. Bekdash RA, Zhang C, Sarkar DK. Gestational choline supplementation normalized fetal alcohol-induced alterations in histone modifications, DNA methylation, and proopiomelanocortin (POMC) gene expression in β-endorphin-producing POMC neurons of the hypothalamus. Alcohol Clin Exp Res. 2013;37(7):1133–42.

288. Govorko D, et al. Male germline transmits fetal alcohol adverse effect on hypothalamic proopiomelanocortin gene across generations. Biol Psychiatry. 2012;72(5):378–88.

289. Leu Y-W, et al. Early life ethanol exposure causes long-lasting disturbances in rat mesenchymal stem cells via epigenetic modifications. Biochem Biophys Res Commun. 2014;453(3):338–44.

290. Yan X, et al. Inhibition of histone acetylation by curcumin reduces alcohol-induced fetal cardiac apoptosis. J Biomed Sci. 2017;24(1):1.

291. Jacobson SW, et al. Efficacy of maternal choline supplementation during pregnancy in mitigating adverse effects of prenatal alcohol exposure on growth and cognitive function: a randomized, double-blind, placebo-controlled clinical trial. Alcohol Clin Exp Res. 2018;42(7):1327–41.

292. Wozniak JR, et al. Four-year follow-up of a randomized controlled trial of choline for neurodevelopment in fetal alcohol spectrum disorder. J Neurodev Disord. 2020;12(1):9.

293. Gangisetty O, Palagani A, Sarkar DK. Transgenerational inheritance of fetal alcohol exposure adverse effects on immune gene interferon-Υ. Clin Epigenetics. 2020;12(1):70.

Chapter 6
Alcohol and Embryology

Scott E. Parnell and Johann K. Eberhart

Overview of Embryological Development

No discussion on the effects of alcohol during early embryological development would be complete without at least a brief description of the key developmental events occurring during these critical periods of early life. While this section could not possibly provide a complete education on embryology, it will detail enough for a basic understanding of early developmental events that are impacted by prenatal alcohol exposure. It is fortunate that many aspects of development discussed here are conserved across many vertebrates; so we are able to use mouse and zebrafish models of fetal alcohol spectrum disorders (FASD) to rather accurately predict what might occur in humans.

In any discussion comparing embryological development across species, it is important to recognize that clinicians and developmental biologists often count the beginning of development differently. In rodents and fish, it is possible to know the exact timing of fertilization, down to the exact day, or even in some cases, to the exact hour, particularly in fish, which are fertilized externally to the mother. In humans, outside of in vitro fertilization cases, it is often difficult to know exactly when fertilization occurred, and clinicians usually count from the first day of the

S. E. Parnell (✉)
Department of Cell Biology and Physiology, Bowles Center for Alcohol Studies, Carolina Institute for Developmental Disabilities, University of North Carolina at Chapel Hill, Chapel Hill, NC, USA
e-mail: sparnell@med.unc.edu

J. K. Eberhart
Department of Molecular Biosciences, Waggoner Center for Alcohol and Addiction Research, Institute for Neuroscience, University of Texas at Austin, Austin, TX, USA
e-mail: eberhart@austin.utexas.edu

women's last menstrual period. This typically adds 2 weeks to the actual stage of human development. For the sake of comparison, we will count development from the day/hour of fertilization.

Gastrulation

Most animal species are triploblastic with adult tissues arising from three germ layers: ectoderm, mesoderm, and endoderm. The ectoderm is the outermost germ layer and will generate structures such as the epidermis, central nervous system, cranial placodes, and the neural crest. Endoderm is the innermost layer and generates the gastrointestinal tract and internal organs including the lungs, liver, pancreas, thyroid, and parathyroid. The middle layer, mesoderm, generates muscle, skeletal elements of the body and parts of the head, and blood vessels.

These germ layers arise through the process of gastrulation. While there are differences between species, the evolutionarily conserved process of gastrulation requires cell rearrangements to position the mesoderm between the ectoderm and endoderm. Generally, in vertebrate species, following fertilization and the subsequent series of cell division, the developing embryo forms a bilaminar disk, the dorsal epiblast and ventral hypoblast that will begin to undergo the process of gastrulation. Starting roughly in the middle of the cranial (rostral)-caudal axis of the embryo, the epiblast cells will proliferate and migrate ventrally through the midline-situated primitive node as the primitive node progresses toward the caudal end of the embryo creating the primitive streak. The first wave of migrating cells will join the cells of the hypoblast to form the endoderm. The next wave of cells to migrate through the node and subsequent primitive streak will form the mesoderm, the middle layer of cells in the embryo. The rest of the epiblast cells that did not migrate into one of the other layers will remain dorsal to form the ectoderm. These three layers of cells will make up all of the structures in our body. The endoderm will become the lining of the gastrointestinal system and parts of the liver and respiratory system. The mesoderm will form the majority of the musculoskeletal system, while the caudal part of the ectoderm will form the spinal cord and skin. The cranial portion of the ectoderm will proliferate and generate ectodermal tissue that will form the cranial portion of the neural plate and will develop into the brain and neural crest cells that go on to form many structures of the head, face, and neck.

Neurulation

The vertebrate central nervous system (CNS) is a hollow structure with the central canal of the spinal cord and the ventricles of the brain filled with cerebrospinal fluid that supports the function of the CNS. Neurulation is the process by which ectoderm is shaped into this hollow structure. There are two general types of neurulation. In primary neurulation, a flat sheet of cells is folded into a hollow tube while in secondary neurulation a solid rod of cells undergoes cavitation to hollow out. Individual species may use both types of neurulation, frequently with just the most posterior region of the embryo using secondary neurulation. For this reason, here we focus on primary neurulation.

In vertebrate species, neural ectoderm is generated in the dorsal midline of the embryo and is induced by signals from adjacent tissues. Following its induction, the neural ectoderm is distinctive as a thickening, along its apical/basal (outside/inside) axis, relative to the adjacent non-neural ectoderm and is termed the neural plate. Cells within the neural plate are highly proliferative and will form all of the cells within the CNS, as well as cell types that emigrate away from the CNS, such as the neural crest. As the neural plate proliferates, cell shape changes in the midline of the neural plate cause the right and left halves to bend dorsally to form the neural folds. Similar shape changes in the lateral aspect of these neural folds cause them to begin to bend back toward the midline and approximate each other. Cell adhesion differences between cells in the neural ectoderm versus the non-neural ectoderm enable fusion of the two sides closing the neural tube and separating it from the overlying surface ectoderm.

Neural tube closure initiates in the middle of the embryo around the region that will eventually become the junction between the brainstem and spinal cord. After this initial fusion event, the neural folds fuse together in a "zipper-like fashion" progressing both rostrally and caudally simultaneously. The anterior neuropore closes first in the region of the neural tube that will eventually become forebrain tissue. The posterior neuropore closes shortly thereafter. This basic process of forming the neural tube from the neural plate is very highly conserved across vertebrate species, although it should be noted that some of the basic cellular mechanisms involved in neurulation and the relative utilization of primary versus secondary neurulation may vary.

As the neural tube is closing, it is already beginning to segment itself into vesicles, with the neural tube first developing three vesicles, represented by the prosencephalon (forebrain), mesencephalon (midbrain), and rhombencephalon (hindbrain). Prior to closure of the anterior neural tube, the optic cups are already beginning to evaginate out of the neural folds that will form the prosencephalon. Following the formation of the prosencephalic vesicle, it is already possible to distinguish between the caudal part of the prosencephalon that will form the diencephalon and the more rostral telencephalon. Similarly, the rhombencephalon subdivides into the metencephalon and the myelencephalon. Following the formation of this five-vesicle brain massive waves of neurogenesis begin in earnest to form the mature brain. The myelencephalon will generate the medulla oblongata and the metencephalon will generate the cerebellum. The majority of the diencephalon will form the thalamus and associated structures. The ventral telencephalon will form the hypothalamus (from which the optic primordia are evaginating) and the dorsal telencephalon will form two additional vesicles that will be the cerebral cortices.

Neural Crest Cells

As mentioned previously, after the ectoderm is formed during gastrulation, the midline portion begins to differentiate into neuroectoderm that will form the neural plate, while the lateral edge of the ectoderm will differentiate into surface ectoderm. At the border of the neural plate ectoderm and surface ectoderm, cells will differentiate into neural crest cells (NCCs; Fig. 6.1). NCCs are a vertebrate-specific cell type that are migratory, multi-potent cells and will form diverse structures within the embryo. Distinct subpopulations of NCCs are distributed along the anterior-posterior axis of the embryo. In posterior regions of the embryo, trunk NCCs will generate cell types such as melanocytes, sensory neurons of the dorsal root ganglia, and sympathetic neurons. Vagal and sacral NCCs flank the trunk NCCs, anteriorly and posteriorly, respectively. These NCCs will generate structures including enteric ganglia lining the gastrointestinal track. Cardiac NCCs reside toward the anterior end of the embryo and will contribute to the outflow tract of the heart. Cranial NCCs reside most anteriorly in the embryo and generate the vast majority of the craniofacial skeleton and its associated connective tissue among other cell types. Because of their lineage, cranial NCCs are particularly important in the genesis of FASD.

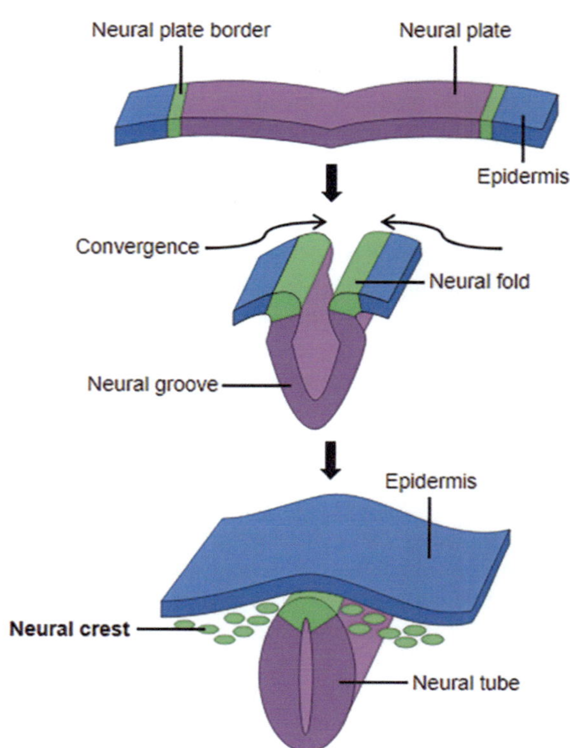

Fig. 6.1 Generation of neural crest cells from the dorsal neural tube

In all vertebrate species, cranial NCCs migrate away from the neural tube in three migratory streams. Cells within these streams will populate transient reiterated embryonic structures termed pharyngeal (or branchial) arches. The total number of pharyngeal arches varies by species (e.g., 4 in human and mouse or 7 in zebrafish). Across species, the first and second neural crest streams populate the first and second pharyngeal arches, respectively. The third stream populates all of the remaining arches. Ectoderm and pharyngeal endoderm bound the NCCs and provide signals that support their survival, proliferation, and differentiation, as well as the subsequent shaping of the resultant skeletal elements.

The first pharyngeal arch is of particular importance to our understanding of FASD as it generates the facial skeleton. As NCCs proliferate within the first pharyngeal arch three swellings (prominences) form that will generate the skeletal elements of distinct regions of the face. The mandibular prominence is located adjacent to the floor of the oral ectoderm and will generate the lower jaw. The maxillary prominence rests on the roof of the oral ectoderm and generates the upper jaw and the secondary palate. The frontonasal prominence is medial to the maxillary prominence spanning the midline of the embryo. It will generate the midfacial skeleton, including the primary palate. Interestingly, fate mapping experiments have demonstrated a correlation between the location of a NCC along the anterior-posterior axis and the skeletal elements that it will populate [1, 2]. For example, NCCs from the most anterior part of the neural tube will develop into the midface, while NCCs that arise from hindbrain neural tube will go on to form part of the lower jaw. This information can be extremely useful in identifying to where NCCs will migrate, as well as the future potential abnormalities that may develop following an insult to a specific part of the dorsal neural tube. Thus, as NCCs arise from the dorsal neural tube, they migrate to form structures in a pattern consistent with where they originated from in the neural tube.

Comparative Developmental Timing

While the processes of gastrulation, neurulation and initial neural crest formation are complex, involve substantial cell proliferation and movement, and are vital to embryonic development, the actual timing of these events is quite short relative to the rest of development. In humans, from the beginning of gastrulation to the end of neural tube closure is just over 10 days, beginning about embryonic day 16 (E16) and ending about E28. In mice these events occur in just over 3 days from about E6.5 to E10 and in zebrafish it is less than a day, beginning about 6 h post-fertilization (HPF) to about 20 HPF. Gastrulation and neurulation are often described as sequential events and indeed, within a given part of the embryo, they are. However, it must be recognized that within the entire embryo, one part may be undergoing gastrulation while another part of the neural plate is beginning to fold. For example, in humans, gastrulation occurs from about E16–E20, while neurulation spans

E18–E28. This information is critical in modeling and comparing specific developmental events among various species.

Methods for Studying the Effects of Prenatal Alcohol Exposure on Embryologic Development

Vertebrate embryologic development has been studied in many different species including the frog, chicken, zebrafish, and mouse. The use of these varied species to model human diseases is facilitated by the fact that, as mentioned previously, much of embryological development is fairly similar across vertebrate species. The same is true of early prenatal alcohol exposure. The effects of alcohol on gastrulation, neurulation, and neural crest cell development have been studied in the chicken, zebrafish, and mouse. Each species has its advantages and disadvantages. Zebrafish and chicken have the advantage that developmental events can be imaged in real time. This is especially true of the zebrafish which has a clear chorion surrounding the embryo. Chickens are a bit more limited as a window can be cut into the shell, but only in certain locations. Mice have the advantage that like humans they are placental mammals with a maternal-fetal interface and fully subject to maternal physiological changes, which could be an important factor in examining the effects of environmental agents. However, in utero development largely precludes real time imaging, particularly of younger embryos, which are too small for even the most advanced in vivo imaging options, such as high-resolution MRI or ultrasound. Mouse embryos can be cultured during some of these early stages, which can be very useful, but only for a short amount of time, and this takes away the maternal component, which is one of the strengths of the mouse model.

One of the advantages of animal model systems is that developmental staging can be quite precise. Because we can control the timing of fertilization and we know the relative rates of development we can study precise periods of alcohol exposure. For example, if we only wanted to expose the embryos to alcohol during gastrulation, we can simply administer the alcohol at the appropriate times. However, this highlights some of the methodological differences between species and some of their relative strengths and weaknesses. Pregnant mice can be administered alcohol via the drinking water, through a liquid diet containing alcohol, by intragastric (IG) intubation, by intraperitoneal (IP) injection, or even inhaled via vapor. Each has its advantages, with drinking being the most similar to human consumption, and IG and IP the most amenable to precise control of exposure timing. However, relying on mice to drink alcohol does not lend itself to accurate control of alcohol dosage or timing and is extremely variable among the many different mouse strains. Regardless of the manner of alcohol administration, in the end, mouse embryos still receive alcohol in a similar manner, i.e., placental transfer from maternal blood via the uterine arteries. In contrast to the myriad different ways to expose developing rodents to alcohol, developing zebrafish are simply immersed into their normal water containing the pre-determined concentration of alcohol. The tissue levels of alcohol equilibrate within 5 min, with a majority of studies showing that these levels are roughly one fourth to one-third of the level in the water [3]. Alcohol is equally rapidly eliminated from the zebrafish embryo following wash out. This demonstrates one of the advantages of the zebrafish model in that both the beginning and ending of the alcohol exposure can be tightly controlled.

Findings on Timing and Pattern of Alcohol Exposure on Development

The effects of prenatal alcohol exposure vary greatly across individuals. This variability is due to many different factors including genetics, amount of alcohol exposure, nutrition, and the timing and pattern of alcohol exposure. For example, the characteristic craniofacial features of FAS are largely caused by alcohol exposure during the periods of gastrulation and early neurulation [4]. These periods, particularly gastrulation, are also particularly vulnerable to the most severe alcohol-induced brain defects, those within the holoprosencephaly (HPE) spectrum [5]. These developmental defects include varying amounts of growth delays and fusion of the cerebral cortices, as well as dysgenesis or agenesis of the corpus callosum as has often been observed in genetic holoprosencephaly cases. In the most severe cases, a complete absence of the cortices has been observed. Although less well characterized clinically, gastrulation-stage alcohol exposure can also induce defects of the ventral midline brain, particularly involving the septal region, striatum, and hypothalamus. Concomitant with these effects in the brain, a gastrulation-stage exposure can also significantly affect the face, especially the philtrum, upper lip, and eyes (reduced palpebral fissure length/microphthalmia). These brain and craniofacial effects lie within the HPE spectrum and are believed to be a result of alcohol-induced apoptotic cell death within the part of the mid-gastrulation-stage embryo that will form the anterior neural ridge [6]. In turn, the anterior neural ridge will give rise to much of the neural plate that will form the forebrain (cortex and anterior ventral midline subcortical regions), as well as the neural crest cells that will develop into midline structures of the face.

The period of neurulation is longer than that of gastrulation, and the effects of alcohol are more subtle, but still quite impactful. During this stage, alcohol typically has much less impact on craniofacial development, but in both mice and fish is capable of inducing major brain and ocular abnormalities [2, 7–10]. While both types of defects are typically less severe during this developmental period relative to those occurring following a gastrulation-stage exposure, they are still quite dysmorphic. In addition to microphthalmia, a neurulation stage exposure has been shown to induce defects in midline subcortical brain regions, the cerebellum, and midbrain areas in mice, as well as midbrain/hindbrain junction abnormalities in zebrafish. Finally, a consistent finding, particularly in mice across the different days of neurulation, is that of hydrocephalus, or enlarged ventricles, although it is unclear if this is due to an obstructive hydrocephalus, versus a general trend toward microencephaly following alcohol exposure at this stage. Finally, as neurulation nears completion, the effects of alcohol on gross ocular dysmorphology wanes, although research at later periods of development has clearly shown that the retina remains sensitive to alcohol's effects for quite some time [11, 12]. Similarly, while not discussed here, as the gross dysmorphic effects on the brain seem to diminish as the end of neurulation is reached, it should be stressed that the brain remains sensitive to alcohol throughout the rest of development, including the rest of gestation and through adolescence [13, 14]. Together, these studies demonstrate that even small differences in developmental timing during early embryogenesis gradually alter different aspects of the brain and face generally progressing from anterior to posterior as development proceeds.

While this short summary of alcohol's stage-dependent effects has focused largely on early development, it demonstrates the basic idea that the effects of alcohol on the developing embryo and fetus can vary largely depending on the timing of exposure. This factor is one of many that explains the large variability present in FASD populations. Of course, adding to the complexity of FASD presentations is that some children are exposed nearly continuously throughout pregnancy. These children are likely to be most severely affected. However, all other elements being equal, embryos exposed to binge alcohol sessions at different periods of time will likely manifest with different phenotypes, particularly those involving the brain and face. Of course, as discussed in the next section, there are numerous other factors to consider, not the least of which is genetic variation.

Historical and Future Trends

In the nearly 50 years since FAS was first diagnosed, the field has changed dramatically. Over the years, we have come to realize that FAS is just the tip of the iceberg, and that alcohol can disrupt many developmental processes without inducing the distinctive craniofacial characteristics of FAS. This led to the development of the umbrella term FASD to encompass the wider range of effects of prenatal alcohol exposure, including individuals without the effects on the face, but still possessing significant neurobehavioral and cognitive issues. Over the years we have also discovered many of the confounding variables that can alter susceptibility to prenatal alcohol exposure. For example, preclinical work has demonstrated that peak blood alcohol concentration (BAC) is a critical factor that can determine the amount and extent of alcohol-induced damage at any given point in development [15, 16]. Likewise, nutritional factors have also been shown to dramatically influence how alcohol affects development. We have discovered that many drugs, legal and non-legal, prescription and non-prescription, can interact with alcohol to disrupt normal development [17–21]. Finally, there are genetic factors that can also modify susceptibility to prenatal alcohol exposure.

It has long been recognized that there is a genetic component to FAS and FASD. Almost 30 years ago, it was observed that monozygotic twins had a significantly higher concordance of being diagnosed with FAS as compared to dizygotic twins, despite the same intrauterine environment [22]. Not surprisingly, it has also been noted that allelic variations in alcohol metabolism genes alter susceptibility to prenatal alcohol exposure [23]. Likewise, several genes related to the Sonic hedgehog (Shh) pathway and other growth factors have been identified to be either protective or associated with greater susceptibility to prenatal alcohol exposure in various animal model systems of FASD [24–26]. Human and animal studies investigating the genetics of FASD have been discussed in great detail elsewhere [27]. More recently, it has been demonstrated that numerous genes involved in apoptosis, reactive oxygen species (ROS) homeostasis, and immune signaling can also alter susceptibility to prenatal alcohol exposure, with some gene variants making an individual more susceptible to alcohol while other variants confer resistance [26, 28–32]. While only a small percentage of the total number of genes have been explored in terms of their interaction with prenatal alcohol exposure, this area of the FASD field has improved our understanding of the pathogenesis involved in alcohol's mechanisms of action during development. This has remained one of the most elusive areas of research as we still know very little about the mechanisms as to how alcohol affects the developing brain. Understanding even the basic pathogenic mechanisms has the significant potential to enhance future therapeutic and/or preventative studies designed to lessen the burden of FASD. Our pace of knowledge regarding all of these variables that contribute to FASD continues to grow; however, there are still many gaps in our knowledge that require extensive further investigation.

Glossary

Agenesis Complete absence of an organ or structure due to a failure to form.

Anterior neural ridge The most anterior (cranial) portion of the neural plate that will go on the form a significant portion of the telencephalon.

Anterior neuropore The most anterior (cranial) closure point of the neural tube.

Caudal Direction toward the tail.

Cranial placodes Specialized regions of the embryonic ectoderm that will give rise to structures in the head and neck such as sensory ganglia. They also contribute to many of the special sensory organs.

Cranial Direction toward the head.

Diencephalon Posterior portion of the prosencephalon which will generate the thalamus, subthalamus, epithalamus, and in some literature the hypothalamus.

Dysgenesis Abnormal formation of an organ.

Epiblast Primitive ectoderm in the inner cell mass. During gastrulation, the epiblast will proliferate and give rise to more ectodermal cells, and cells of the mesoderm and endoderm.

Forebrain (prosencephalon) Most cranial (rostral) primary vesicle of the developing neural tube. Will develop into the telencephalon and diencephalon.

Frontonasal prominence Region of the developing embryo that will generate the midface, the primary palate, and anterior skull.

Gastrulation Early developmental process in which the three germ layers (endoderm, mesoderm, and ectoderm) are generated and organized relative to one another.

Hindbrain (rhombencephalon) Most caudal of the three primary brain vesicles. Will develop into the metencephalon and myelencephalon.

Holoprosencephaly Failure of the two cerebral cortices to separate from each other forming one continuous structure with a continuous ventricle. The resulting defect in the brain also causes defects in the midline of the face and skull.

Hypoblast Layer of cells in the inner cell mass that sits beneath the epiblast. In mammals and birds, the hypoblast contributes to the chorion, while in fish it also contributes to the endoderm and mesoderm.

Mandibular prominence Region of the developing head that will form the lower jaw and associated structures.

Maxillary prominence Region of the developing head that will form the upper jaw, the secondary palate, and sides of the face.

Metencephalon Brain vesicle that will form the pons and cerebellum.

Microphthalmia Abnormally small eye.

Midbrain (mesencephalon) Middle primary vesicle of the brain.

Myelencephalon Brain vesicle that will generate the medulla oblongata.

Neural crest Cells derived from the dorsal neural tube that will migrate to develop into a wide variety of cell types including most of the craniofacial skeleton.

Neural plate Neuroectoderm that will proliferate and bend into the neural tube during neurulation.

Neurulation The process of generating a hollow neural tube that will go on to form the entire central nervous system.

Optic cups Evaginations of the prosencephalon that will form most of the future eye.

Pharyngeal (branchial) arches Transient, serially reiterated embryonic structures made up of endoderm, mesoderm, ectoderm, and neural crest cells that will generate hard and soft tissues in the head and neck. In fish, they also go on to form the gills.

Posterior neuropore Most posterior (caudal) point of closure of the neural tube. In normal development, this is the last part of the neural tube to close and becomes the most caudal part of the spinal cord. Failure to close the posterior neuropore is one of the most common neural tube closure defects and causes spina bifida.

Primitive node Gastrulation organizing center through which proliferating epiblast cells will migrate ventrally to form the mesoderm and endoderm. As gastrulation progresses, the node migrates caudally.

Primitive streak Midline streak formed from the caudal progression of the primitive node. Both the primitive node and subsequent primitive streak will help set up bilateral (left-right) asymmetry.

Rostral During embryogenesis, the direction toward the most anterior aspect of the neural tube. Later in development, it is defined as toward the nose, or the most anterior aspect of the frontal lobe.

Telencephalon Cerebral hemispheres and basal ganglia. Some literature also includes the hypothalamus.

References

1. Zhang C, Frazier JM, Chen H, Liu Y, Lee JA, Cole GJ. Molecular and morphological changes in zebrafish following transient ethanol exposure during defined developmental stages. Neurotoxicol Teratol. 2014;44:70–80.
2. Köntges G, Lumsden A. Rhombencephalic neural crest segmentation is preserved throughout craniofacial ontogeny. Development. 1996;122(10):3229–42.
3. Lovely CB, Nobles RD, Eberhart JK. Developmental age strengthens barriers to ethanol accumulation in zebrafish. Alcohol. 2014;48(6):595–602.
4. Sulik KK, Johnston MC, Webb MA. Fetal alcohol syndrome: embryogenesis in a mouse model. Science. 1981;214(4523):936–8.
5. Godin EA, O'Leary-Moore SK, Khan AA, Parnell SE, Ament JJ, Dehart DB, Johnson BW, Allan Johnson G, Styner MA, Sulik KK. Magnetic resonance microscopy defines ethanol-induced brain abnormalities in prenatal mice: effects of acute insult on gestational day 7. Alcohol Clin Exp Res. 2010;34(1):98–111.
6. Dunty WC Jr, Chen SY, Zucker RM, Dehart DB, Sulik KK. Selective vulnerability of embryonic cell populations to ethanol-induced apoptosis: implications for alcohol-related birth defects and neurodevelopmental disorder. Alcohol Clin Exp Res. 2001;25(10):1523–35.
7. Parnell SE, O'Leary-Moore SK, Godin EA, Dehart DB, Johnson BW, Allan Johnson G, Styner MA, Sulik KK. Magnetic resonance microscopy defines ethanol-induced brain abnormalities in prenatal mice: effects of acute insult on gestational day 8. Alcohol Clin Exp Res. 2009;33(6):1001–11.
8. Parnell SE, Johnson GA, Sulik KK. Brain abnormalities resulting from gestational day nine ethanol exposure in the mouse: a study utilizing high-resolution MRI. Alcohol Clin Exp Res. 2008;773:204A.
9. Bilotta J, Saszik S, Givin CM, Hardesty HR, Sutherland SE. Effects of embryonic exposure to ethanol on zebrafish visual function. Neurotoxicol Teratol. 2002;24(6):759–66.
10. Kashyap B, Frederickson LC, Stenkamp DL. Mechanisms for persistent microphthalmia following ethanol exposure during retinal neurogenesis in zebrafish embryos. Vis Neurosci. 2007;24(3):409–21.
11. O'Leary-Moore SK, Parnell SE, Lipinski RJ, Sulik KK. Magnetic resonance-based imaging in animal models of fetal alcohol spectrum disorder. Neuropsychol Rev. 2011;21(2):167–85.
12. O'Leary-Moore SK, Parnell SE, Godin EA, Dehart DB, Ament JJ, Khan AA, Johnson GA, Styner MA, Sulik KK. Magnetic resonance microscopy-based analyses of the brains of normal and ethanol-exposed fetal mice. Birth Defects Res A Clin Mol Teratol. 2010;88(11):953–64.
13. West JR, Hodges CA, Black AC Jr. Prenatal exposure to ethanol alters the organization of hippocampal mossy fibers in rats. Science. 1981;211(4485):957–9.
14. Pascual M, Boix J, Felipo V, Guerri C. Repeated alcohol administration during adolescence causes changes in the mesolimbic dopaminergic and glutamatergic systems and promotes alcohol intake in the adult rat. J Neurochem. 2009;108(4):920–31.
15. Bonthius DJ, Goodlett CR, West JR. Blood alcohol concentration and severity of microencephaly in neonatal rats depend on the pattern of alcohol administration. Alcohol. 1988;5(3):209–14.
16. Bonthius DJ, West JR. Blood alcohol concentration and microencephaly: a dose-response study in the neonatal rat. Teratology. 1988;37(3):223–31.

17. Fish EW, Murdaugh LB, Zhang C, Boschen KE, Boa-Amponsem O, Mendoza-Romero HN, Tarpley M, Chdid L, Mukhopadhyay S, Cole GJ, Williams KP, Parnell SE. Cannabinoids exacerbate alcohol teratogenesis by a CB1-hedgehog interaction. Sci Rep. 2019;9(1):16057.
18. Gilbert MT, Sulik KK, Fish EW, Baker LK, Dehart DB, Parnell SE. Dose-dependent teratogenicity of the synthetic cannabinoid CP-55,940 in mice. Neurotoxicol Teratol. 2016;58:15–22.
19. Barr HM, Streissguth AP. Caffeine use during pregnancy and child outcome: a 7-year prospective study. Neurotoxicol Teratol. 1991;13(4):441–8.
20. Streissguth AP, Grant TM, Barr HM, Brown ZA, Martin JC, Mayock DE, Ramey SL, Moore L. Cocaine and the use of alcohol and other drugs during pregnancy. Am J Obstet Gynecol. 1991;164(5 Pt 1):1239–43.
21. Streissguth AP, Barr HM, Martin DC, Herman CS. Effects of maternal alcohol, nicotine, and caffeine use during pregnancy on infant mental and motor development at eight months. Alcohol Clin Exp Res. 1980;4(2):152–64.
22. Streissguth AP, Dehaene P. Fetal alcohol syndrome in twins of alcoholic mothers: concordance of diagnosis and IQ. Am J Med Genet. 1993;47(6):857–61.
23. Viljoen DL, Carr LG, Foroud TM, Brooke L, Ramsay M, Li TK. Alcohol dehydrogenase-2*2 allele is associated with decreased prevalence of fetal alcohol syndrome in the mixed-ancestry population of the Western Cape Province, South Africa. Alcohol Clin Exp Res. 2001;25(12):1719–22.
24. Kietzman HW, Everson JL, Sulik KK, Lipinski RJ. The teratogenic effects of prenatal ethanol exposure are exacerbated by Sonic Hedgehog or GLI2 haploinsufficiency in the mouse. PLoS One. 2014;9(2):e89448.
25. Hong M, Krauss RS. Cdon mutation and fetal ethanol exposure synergize to produce midline signaling defects and holoprosencephaly spectrum disorders in mice. PLoS Genet. 2012;8(10):e1002999.
26. McCarthy N, Wetherill L, Lovely CB, Swartz ME, Foroud TM, Eberhart JK. Pdgfra protects against ethanol-induced craniofacial defects in a zebrafish model of FASD. Development. 2013;140(15):3254–65.
27. Eberhart JK, Parnell SE. The genetics of fetal alcohol spectrum disorders. Alcohol Clin Exp Res. 2016;40:1154.
28. Fish EW, Mendoza-Romero HN, Love CA, Dragicevich CJ, Cannizzo MD, Boschen KE, Hepperla A, Simon JM, Parnell SE. The pro-apoptotic Bax gene modifies susceptibility to craniofacial dysmorphology following gastrulation-stage alcohol exposure. Birth Defects Res. 2022;114:1229.
29. Fish EW, Tucker SK, Peterson RL, Eberhart JK, Parnell SE. Loss of tumor protein 53 protects against alcohol-induced facial malformations in mice and zebrafish. Alcohol Clin Exp Res. 2021;45(10):1965–79.
30. Boschen KE, Ptacek TS, Berginski ME, Simon JM, Parnell SE. Transcriptomic analyses of gastrulation-stage mouse embryos with differential susceptibility to alcohol. Dis Model Mech. 2021;14(6):dmm049012.
31. Boschen KE, Gong H, Murdaugh LB, Parnell SE. Knockdown of Mns1 increases susceptibility to craniofacial defects following gastrulation-stage alcohol exposure in mice. Alcohol Clin Exp Res. 2018;42(11):2136–43.
32. Swartz ME, Wells MB, Griffin M, McCarthy N, Lovely CB, McGurk P, Rozacky J, Eberhart JK. A screen of zebrafish mutants identifies ethanol-sensitive genetic loci. Alcohol Clin Exp Res. 2014;38(3):694–703.

Chapter 7
Care During the Newborn Period

Vincent C. Smith

Prenatal Alcohol Exposure

The American Academy of Pediatrics (AAP) has stated that there is no amount of alcohol known to be safe to drink during pregnancy [1]. Alcohol is a known teratogen (i.e., an agent or factor which causes malformation of a developing fetus), so all drinks that contain alcohol have the potential to harm a developing fetus [2]. Although not all individuals who have prenatal alcohol exposure (PAE) develop a Fetal Alcohol Spectrum Disorder (FASD), all those with an FASD had PAE. The effects of PAE vary by pregnancy and fetus, making it difficult to know which fetuses will be affected and to what degree [2]. A twin study confirms virtually identical PAE can lead to markedly different FASD outcomes [3]. Therefore, the AAP [1] concludes the following:

- During pregnancy, there is no risk-free amount of alcohol consumption.
- During pregnancy, there is no risk-free kind of alcohol consumption.
- During pregnancy, there is no risk-free time to consume alcohol.

Although no amount of alcohol should be considered safe during pregnancy, the more alcohol a fetus is exposed to the higher likelihood of it developing an FASD. PAE of one or more drinks per day is associated with reduced birth weight and intrauterine growth retardation, spontaneous abortion, preterm delivery, and stillbirth [4]. Binge drinking patterns (the consumption of 12 oz of beer or wine cooler, 5 oz of wine, or 1.5 oz of liquor four or more times on one occasion) while pregnant results in a high peak blood alcohol level and poses the greatest risk to the developing fetus [4, 5].

V. C. Smith (✉)
Division of Newborn Medicine, Department of Pediatrics, Boston Medical Center, Boston University Medical School, Boston, MA, USA
e-mail: Vincent.smith@bmc.org

Screening for Prenatal Alcohol Exposure

Screening for PAE is an early step toward diagnosing an FASD [2]. Lack of documentation of PAE is often one of the greatest barriers to diagnosis of a child with an FASD [1]. The most direct way to obtain information about PAE is to ask the birth mother. Asking for a self-report works best when normalized to all patients. This "universal screening" approach to screening for PAE helps decrease stigmatization [1].

The AAP recommends that screening for PAE be incorporated into a standard script during birth history, anticipatory guidance, or any other appropriate portion of the parent interview, after asking standard guidance questions (e.g., about medications, tobacco, home environment) [1]. Please see Chap. 4 for a much more detailed discussion of screening tools. The following are examples from the AAP of questions that could be used to screen for PAE [1]:

- How far along were you before you found out you were pregnant?
- Before you knew you were pregnant, how much alcohol (beer, wine, or liquor) did you drink?
- After you found out you were pregnant, how much alcohol did you drink?

Any acknowledgment of alcohol consumption during pregnancy counts as a positive screen [1]. It important that pediatricians document the results of their screening of all patients for future reference, but there is no uniformly accepted practice regarding documenting PAE screening results. That means each pediatric practice will have to determine for themselves where in the medical record they document the results of screening for PAE, how they phrase the results, and who has access to the information. Pediatricians can also advocate for standardization of PAE documentation.

Once a child screens positive for PAE, there is no need to continue to screen that individual [1]. After documenting the positive results of the screening in the medical record, the pediatrician will monitor the child for developmental delays, behavior problems, social challenges, cognitive deficits, learning difficulties, and other potential signs of an FASD [1]. Since many systems of care can be involved with some individuals with an FASD, there is potential for PAE screening information to get lost. Without a standardized method of documentation of PAE, screening needed to aid in transitions from one system to another may not be readily available and precipitate the need for repeat PAE screening. It is possible that improved documentation and more effective communication between providers could help decrease the amount of information lost.

In addition to maternal self-report, there are some other ways to indirectly note potential PAE. This includes social or legal problems in proximity to (before or during) the index pregnancy [6]. For example, a history of citation(s) for driving while intoxicated or history of treatment of an alcohol-related condition during the pregnancy could count as prenatal alcohol exposure [6]. Another example could be certification of intoxication during pregnancy by blood, breath, or urine alcohol content testing [6]. Another option could be direct eye-witnessed accounts of alcohol use while pregnant from creditable witnesses. Recall that second hand and/or anecdotal accounts alone are insufficient. Still it can be challenging to get exact and correct data about the quantity and frequency of PAE [7]. In the future, alcohol biomarkers may be used to assess PAE.

Biomarkers for Prenatal Alcohol Exposure

There is not a currently accepted gold standard biomarker for PAE. There have been a number of promising human and animal studies, but more work is required before any of them will be helpful clinically [8]. Measurement of blood alcohol or its metabolite acetaldehyde are not ideal biomarkers given they are only useful for recent exposure given the relatively rapid metabolism and lack of appreciable accumulation for long time periods [8]. Some alcohol-exposure biomarkers during pregnancy or at birth include analysis of fatty acid ethyl esters, phosphatidylethanol, and/or ethyl glucuronide in maternal hair, fingernails, urine, or blood, or placenta, or meconium [6]. Some promising research has studied long-term alterations to DNA methylation as a biomarker of PAE [9], but the research is not yet ready for clinical use. Also some low-molecular weight markers such as the plasma ratio of 5-hydroxytryptophol to 5-hydroxyindolylacetic acid measured in either plasma or serum have been used to diagnose chronic maternal alcohol consumption, but vary based on age and non-alcohol related diseases [8]. Differential methylation may be used as a biomarker for PAE [10]. Because it is known that PAE during all trimesters of pregnancy can impact the presence and severity of FASD, it is unlikely that one or even two biomarkers could be used to address these points [8]. Goldberg et al. present a full discussion of some of the potential biomarker and their usefulness [8]. Please also see Chap. 4 for a much more detailed discussion of biomarkers.

Etiology and Contributing Factors to Developing an FASD

Approximately 45% of pregnancies are unplanned, and it may take 6–8 weeks after a missed period for the pregnancy to be recognized [11]. PAE can occur before the pregnancy is recognized, during the days after the first missed menstrual period [11]. During the early stage of development, PAE may disrupt gastrulation and neurulation, resulting in the characteristic cranial dysmorphology seen in some FASDs [11].

Being exposed to alcohol in the first trimester can lead to malformation of major structures. Although the first trimester is considered to be the most vulnerable period for the fetus, it is now understood that PAE throughout the entire gestational period may cause permanent damage [4, 8]. Second trimester exposure may lead to spontaneous abortion [4]. Third trimester exposure has the highest impact on height, weight, and brain growth [4]. Because the fetal brain is growing and evolving throughout the entire pregnancy, the fetal brain can be affected by PAE from any trimester.

The effects of fetal exposure to alcohol vary and are hard to predict. There are genetic differences in how women and their fetuses metabolize alcohol that make it different for each pregnancy [4]. Genetic variations are largely responsible for one mother's propensity to, despite similar patterns of alcohol consumption, give birth to a child with an FASD from one pregnancy but having a child without an FASD from another pregnancy [3, 8]. Also, fetus has limited ability to metabolize alcohol and fetal alcohol levels may be higher or present for a prolonged period comparted to maternal blood alcohol levels [4].

Newborn Exam

Overview of a Newborn Exam

The newborn exam generally begins with the general observation or gestalt that a clinician obtains by simply watching a baby before the start of a physical exam [12]. When observing the general appearance, make note of normal and dysmorphic features (especially of the face) [13]. When awake, the baby should be vigorous and alert as well as energetic and strong when crying [12].

Evaluate the overall head size and shape should for asymmetry or gross structural abnormalities, and the fontanelles and sutures should be palpated with the newborn in the upright position [12, 13]. Microcephaly is isolated asymmetrically small head (i.e., Occipital Frontal Circumference or OFC), less than the 10th percentile or two standard deviations below the mean for age and sex [13].

The eyes need to be assessed for the red reflex, extraocular movements, palpebral fissure length, and pupillary size and shape [12]. The eye evaluation also includes noting eye color; appearance of the conjunctiva, sclera, and eyelid; eye movement; and spacing between the eyes [13]. Ears are assessed for size, shape, positioning, anomalies, and tags [12, 13]. Ears are considered low-set when the helix of the ear meets the cranium at a level below that of a horizontal plane through both inner canthi [13]. Nose checked for nasal patency [12]. To assess patency of the nostrils, a small-caliber catheter can be passed through the nasal passages [13]. The mouth should have the palate and dentition assessed [12]. The maxilla and mandible should fit together well and open at equal angles [13]. Neck should be inspected for full range of motion, swelling and cysts [12, 13].

Chest examined for symmetric chest rise with respirations and lack of retractions or accessory respiratory muscle use [12]. Chest movement should be symmetric [14]. Lungs should have symmetric aeration and bilateral clear breath sounds [12]. Heart exam upon auscultation of the heart in the standard four locations (right upper sternal border, left upper sternal border, left lower sternal border, and between the fifth and sixth intercostal space in the midclavicular line), the first heart sound should be single and the second heart sound split [13]. Heart must be assessed its rate and rhythm [12]. The presences of murmurs, gallops, or rubs should be noted and evaluated as clinically indicated.

The abdomen exam includes reviewing the size and shape and checking for hepatosplenomegaly and cord vessels at birth [12]. When examining the abdomen, it may be beneficial to use the one hand to hold the legs with the hips and knees flexed to help relax the newborn, and use the other hand to palpate the abdomen [14]. Genital exam includes review for inguinal masses, testicular/scrotal asymmetry (for male infants), genital hypertrophy, or lesions [12]. Rectal should be examined for normal placement and patency [12, 14]. A sacral dimple is considered simple if it is less than 0.5 cm in diameter, is located within 2.5 cm of the anal verge, and is not associated with cutaneous stigmata [14].

The hands and feet should be inspected for range of motion, tenderness, syndactyly and polydactyly, skin tag [12, 14]. Hips are examined for stability, range of motion, and clicks [12]. Neurological exam includes assessing overall tone and movement as well as reflexes (i.e., suck, palmar and plantar grasp, root, primitive stepping, and Moro) [12, 14].

Another important component of the newborn assessment is the infant's birth weight, length, and head circumference or OFC [12]. Infants are considered appropriate for gestational age (AGA) if their birth weight is within two standard deviations from the mean [12]. A newborn is considered small for gestational age if birth weight is below the 10th percentile. Intrauterine growth restriction occurs when the baby's growth during pregnancy is poor compared with norms [13].

Review of Literature on Birth Defects Seen with Prenatal Alcohol Exposure

Physical finding may be present at birth, but sometimes are harder to recognize until the individual is older (i.e., early childhood). Therefore, it is important the physical exam be repeated as the individual ages because some things like lip, philtrum, and eyes may be more apparent in older children than in newborns. In this section, we discuss how the physical exam may be altered when there is PAE. A more detailed discussion about diagnostic criteria and timing of diagnosis (e.g., newborn versus early childhood) is in Chap. 9.

Cardinal Features of Fetal Alcohol Syndrome

The cardinal facial features of fetal alcohol syndrome (i.e., required for a diagnosis) are short palpebral fissures ($\leq$10th centile), a smooth philtrum (rank 4 or 5 on a racially normed lip/philtrum guide), and a thin vermillion border of the upper lip (rank 4 or 5 on a racially normed lip/philtrum guide) [2, 6, 11, 15, 16]. Fetal alcohol syndrome is only one of the conditions in the FASD spectrum [2]. The cardinal features of fetal alcohol syndrome are not exclusive to fetal alcohol syndrome and may be present other FASDs.

Growth Deficits

Growth deficits are common and sometime the only signs of PAE seen in the newborn period. There can be prenatal and/or postnatal growth deficiency with height, weight, and/or head circumference [2, 11]. Weight, height, and head circumference should be measured and plotted by using population-specific growth curves [6]. Growth deficiency could be defined as weight, head circumference, and/or height ≤10th centile (plotted on a racially or ethnically as well as gestational age appropriate growth curve) [6]. Microcephaly (e.g., OFC <10th centile) may result from PAE [6, 15, 17]. If an infant is born SGA, PAE should be considered in differential diagnosis and screened for as part of the diagnostic process.

Other anomalies that are not diagnostic of an FASD, but are associated with PAE. It has been reported that the number of minor physical anomalies correlates with the magnitude of prenatal alcohol exposure [11].

Facial

In addition to the cardinal facial features of fetal alcohol syndrome mentioned above, there can be other facial anomalies associated with PAE. Some will have ptosis of the eyelids (i.e., droopy eyelids) and/or epicanthal folds (i.e., a skin fold of the upper eyelid covering the inner corner of the eye) [11, 15]. The can also be a short inner canthal distance (i.e., distance between the medial angles of the palpebral fissures), inter-pupillary distance (i.e., distance between the centers of the eyes), anteverted nares (i.e., upturned nose), underdevelopment of the midface [11, 16]. The ears can have a railroad track configuration (i.e., a prominent horizontal crus of the helix in combination with a prominent and parallel inferior crus of the antihelix) [11, 15]. These include cleft lip/palate, maxillary hypoplasia (i.e., underdevelopment of bones in the upper jaw), or micrognathia (i.e., smaller than normal lower jaw) [2, 11, 16].

Heart Defects

PAE could result in congenital heart disease including atrial and ventricular septal defects, other defects, or unspecified congenital heart disease [18].

Musculoskeletal

PAE may result in some musculoskeletal anomalies. There can be a lack of complete extension of one or more digits known as camptodactyly [15] as well as clinodactyly (i.e., an abnormal bend or curvature of the finger) [11, 15, 16]. There can also be decreased supination/pronation at the elbows [15]. There can be joint contractures including inability to completely extend and/or contract at the hips, knees, and ankles [11, 15]. On the hands, there can be a "hockey stick" palmar crease and other palmar crease abnormalities [11, 15].

Brain Anomalies

Because the fetal brain is growing and evolving throughout the entire pregnancy, the fetal brain can be affected by PAE from any trimester. Although no specific anatomic region of the brain is preferentially affected, structural abnormalities secondary to PAE are widespread and have been reported in almost every brain structure and region [6, 7, 11, 17]. This may result in uniformly small brain volumes including total brain volume, cerebellum, and corpus callosum [7, 17]. The corpus callosum, the largest white matter tract in the human brain, appears to be especially vulnerable with abnormalities ranging from complete absence to malformations after PAE [7, 11]. Malformations resulting from migration abnormalities, cavum septum pellucidum, cerebellar vermis underdevelopment or incomplete development, and underdevelopment or incomplete development of the basal ganglia and hippocampus have been documented after PAE [6]. PAE has an effect on frontal, parietal, temporal, occipital, and limbic/deep gray matter regions [7]. Furthermore, white matter and gray matter volumes are also typically smaller and the gyral pattern can be simplified [7, 11]. All parts of brain development have potential to be altered by PAE including neurogenesis, neuronal growth and differentiation, neuronal migration, synaptogenesis, apoptosis, plasticity, cortical synaptogenesis, development of cortical gray matter, myelination of sensory pathways, myelination of motor pathways, and maturation of the limbic system [6]. Chapter 10 contains a more detailed discussion of the neuroimaging finding seen in individuals with an FASD.

Lacking accurate and precise information about PAE makes it challenging to make exact correlations between PAE and the patterns of brain anomalies noted [7]. However, magnetic resonance imaging (MRI) studies from Astley et al. [17] support that the size of various brain regions decreased significantly and incrementally with increasing frequency, quantity, and/or duration of reported PAE. They noted that in general the greater the PAE the smaller the brain regions [17]. They also note that a binge drinking pattern [5] was the most damaging for the developing fetal brain [17]. Finally, loss of brain volume worsening with longer exposure to PAE meaning exposure in all three trimesters was worse than exposure in the first trimester alone [17].

Behavioral Newborn Conditions Potentially Seen with Prenatal Alcohol Exposure

The most common manifestations of PAE are behavioral issues and learning disabilities that may not be apparent in the newborn period. The domains affected including neurocognitive functioning, self-regulation, adaptation, and executive function are discussed in more detail in Chap. 11. In infants and young children 3 years old or younger, there can be cognitive delays that range from mild developmental delays or learning disabilities to global developmental delay [4, 6, 17]. Some self-regulation issues include tremulousness, persistent startle, feeding difficulties, poor habituation/disordered state regulation, impaired emotional regulation, and infant emotional withdrawal [4]. Adaptation issues include both gross and fine motor delays [4, 6]. Because executive functioning involves planning, self-control, working memory, adaptation, organization, and similar skills, deficits in this area are often not noted until early childhood. There are some reports that suggest deficits in executive functioning could be recognized earlier [19].

Care and Management for Newborns and Family Considerations

There is no cure for FASD and treatment is targeted on symptoms [2, 4]. Still, affected individuals may experience improved outcomes through intervention over a period of time and treatment that maximize protective factors and build capacity in identified strengths [2]. In the newborn period, there is rarely a need for pharmacologic treatment. Most of the care is supportive for the infant, education for the family about the effects of PAE as well as parenting strategies, environmental modifications, social support, and developmental interventions [2, 4]. It is important to keep in mind that no two individuals with FASD will have the exact same pattern of impairment [2, 4, 20].

Physicians are mandated reporters of any suspicion of child abuse or neglect to the relevant authorities. Federal law called CAPTA (Child Abuse Prevention and Treatment Act) from 2017 51061(b)(2)(B)(ii) states the following:

> Infants born with and identified as being affected by substance use or withdrawal symptoms resulting from prenatal substance exposure or who are diagnosed with an Fetal Alcohol Spectrum Disorder at less than the age of three require reporting to child protective services (https://www.govinfo.gov/content/pkg/USCODE-2017-title42/html/USCODE-2017-title42-chap67.htm)

The report is not intended to be punitive for the family, but rather to help connect the family to resources hopefully improving the overall outcome for the child and family.

Future Trends

Despite the prevalence and burden to society, the effects of PAE and FASD remain under-recognized and under-diagnosed [11]. A future trend will be to raise awareness about the teratogenic effects of alcohol on a developing fetus and improve recognition and management of FASDs. The diagnosis of an FASD may be impeded by the lack of a universally accepted diagnostic schema [11]. A future trend may be toward using the most recent FASD research and clinical data to extensively assess FASD diagnostic schema and potentially settle on a universally accepted approach.

Self-reports of alcohol consumption during pregnancy can be unreliable [8]. The lack of documentation of PAE is one of the most common reasons for not being able to make an FASD diagnosis [2, 8], having a more robust biomarker of PAE would be very helpful. Given the interest in PAE-associated biomarker [8–11], a future trend may be toward identifying a biomarker for PAE that could aid in the diagnosis of an FASD. There are some ongoing studies that could aid in this challenge including current studies that focus on microRNAs and facial imaging technology. Independent of the diagnostic dilemma, ascertaining the diagnosis remains challenging. A future trend could be toward developing a global reporting system.

Given that PAE often occurs with polysubstance use, the diagnostic picture can be complicated [11]. A future direction may continue to focus on the isolated effects of PAE and to help decipher the effects of PAE in conjunction with other substances. Finally, future trends may accommodate internationally accepted diagnostic criteria and a global reporting system, diagnosis that is consistent, biomarkers to make the diagnosis less subjective, and quantification of prenatal alcohol exposure with risk for FASD.

References

1. AAP. Screening for prenatal alcohol exposure: an implementation guide for primary care pediatric providers, 14 Nov 2018. https://www.aap.org/en-us/Documents/FASD_PAE_Implementation_Guide_FINAL.pdf. Accessed 25 Jun 2021.
2. Williams JF, Smith VC, Committee on Substance Abuse. Fetal alcohol spectrum disorders. Pediatrics. 2015;136(5):e1395–406.
3. Hemingway SJ, Bledsoe JM, Brooks A, Davies JK, Jirikowic T, Olson EM, Thorne JC. Twin study confirms virtually identical prenatal alcohol exposures can lead to markedly different fetal alcohol spectrum disorder outcomes—fetal genetics influences fetal vulnerability. Adv Pediatr Res. 2018;5(3):23.
4. Senturias YS, Weitzman CC, Amgott R. Fetal alcohol spectrum disorders. In: Augustyn M, Zuckerman B, editors. Zuckerman Parker handbook of developmental and behavioral pediatrics for primary care. 4th ed. Philadelphia: Wolters Kluwer; 2019. p. 242.
5. Siqueira L, Smith VC, Committee on Substance Abuse. Binge drinking. Pediatrics. 2015;136(3):e718–26.
6. Hoyme HE, Kalberg WO, Elliott AJ, Blankenship J, Buckley D, Marais AS, Manning MA, Robinson LK, Adam MP, Abdul-Rahman O, Jewett T. Updated clinical guidelines for diagnosing fetal alcohol spectrum disorders. Pediatrics. 2016;138(2):e20154256.

7. Lebel C, Roussotte F, Sowell ER. Imaging the impact of prenatal alcohol exposure on the structure of the developing human brain. Neuropsychol Rev. 2011;21(2):102–18.

8. Goldberg EM, Aliani M. Metabolomics and fetal alcohol spectrum disorder. Biochem Cell Biol. 2018;96(2):198–203.

9. Laufer BI, Chater-Diehl EJ, Kapalanga J, Singh SM. Long-term alterations to DNA methylation as a biomarker of prenatal alcohol exposure: from mouse models to human children with fetal alcohol spectrum disorders. Alcohol. 2017;60:67–75.

10. Cobben JM, Krzyzewska IM, Venema A, Mul AN, Polstra A, Postma AV, Smigiel R, Pesz K, Niklinski J, Chomczyk MA, Henneman P. DNA methylation abundantly associates with fetal alcohol spectrum disorder and its subphenotypes. Epigenomics. 2018;11(7):767–85.

11. Wozniak JR, Riley EP, Charness ME. Clinical presentation, diagnosis, and management of fetal alcohol spectrum disorder. Lancet Neurol. 2019;18(8):760–70.

12. Lowe MC Jr, Woolridge DP. The normal newborn exam, or is it? Emerg Med Clin North Am. 2007;25(4):921–46.

13. Lewis ML. A comprehensive newborn exam: part I. General, head and neck, cardiopulmonary. Am Fam Physician. 2014;90(5):289–96.

14. Lewis ML. A comprehensive newborn exam: part II. Skin, trunk, extremities, neurologic. Am Fam Physician. 2014;90(5):297–302.

15. Jones KL, Hoyme HE, Robinson LK, Del Campo M, Manning MA, Prewitt LM, Chambers CD. Fetal alcohol spectrum disorders: extending the range of structural defects. Am J Med Genet A. 2010;152(11):2731–5.

16. May PA, Baete A, Russo J, Elliott AJ, Blankenship J, Kalberg WO, Buckley D, Brooks M, Hasken J, Abdul-Rahman O, Adam MP. Prevalence and characteristics of fetal alcohol spectrum disorders. Pediatrics. 2014;134(5):855–66.

17. Astley SJ, Aylward EH, Olson HC, Kerns K, Brooks A, Coggins TE, Davies J, Dorn S, Gendler B, Jirikowic T, Kraegel P. Magnetic resonance imaging outcomes from a comprehensive magnetic resonance study of children with fetal alcohol spectrum disorders. Alcohol Clin Exp Res. 2009;33(10):1671–89.

18. Burd L, Deal E, Rios R, Adickes E, Wynne J, Klug MG. Congenital heart defects and fetal alcohol spectrum disorders. Congenit Heart Dis. 2007;2(4):250–5.

19. Fuglestad AJ, Whitley ML, Carlson SM, Boys CJ, Eckerle JK, Fink BA, Wozniak JR. Executive functioning deficits in preschool children with fetal alcohol spectrum disorders. Child Neuropsychol. 2015;21(6):716–31.

20. Astley SJ, Olson HC, Kerns K, Brooks A, Aylward EH, Coggins TE, Davies J, Dorn S, Gendler B, Jirikowic T, Kraegel P. Neuropsychological and behavioral outcomes from a comprehensive magnetic resonance study of children with fetal alcohol spectrum disorders. J Can Pharmacol Clin. 2009;16(1):e178.

Chapter 8
Evolution of Diagnostic Systems

Diego A. Gomez and H. Eugene Hoyme

Brief Historical Context on Medical System Views of Prenatal Alcohol Exposure Prior to Formal Diagnostic Systems

The link between alcohol use and its harmful effects on the developing fetus is well established in the scientific literature. However, alcohol's teratogenic effects went largely unnoticed prior to the twentieth century. Until then, beliefs that alcohol posed no risk to either the mother or fetus were widespread. Despite such common thinking in the medical community, historical references to the negative effect of alcohol during pregnancy exist. Among the first admonitions about drinking in pregnancy are those found in the Old Testament. The *Book of Judges* (13:3–4) describes an angel warning a woman about her preparation for pregnancy: "Now see to it that you drink no wine or other fermented drink and that you do not eat anything unclean." The Ancient Greeks and Romans may have also been aware of alcohol's effects on reproduction. Aristotle's *Problemata* declares "foolish, drunken, or haire-brain women [for the] most part bring forth children like unto themselves, morose and feeble" [1, 2]. While these historical references present a link between maternal alcohol consumption and birth defects, for hundreds of years the medical community and the general public were largely unaware of the risks posed by prenatal alcohol consumption.

D. A. Gomez (✉)
Mayo Clinic Alix School of Medicine, Scottsdale, AZ, USA
e-mail: Gomez.diego@mayo.edu

H. E. Hoyme
Department of Pediatrics, University of South Dakota Sanford School of Medicine, Sioux Falls, SD, USA

Sanford Children's Genomic Medicine Consortium, Sanford Health, Sioux Falls, SD, USA
e-mail: gene.hoyme@sanfordhealth.org

O. A. Abdul-Rahman, C. L. M. Petrenko (eds.), *Fetal Alcohol Spectrum Disorders*,
https://doi.org/10.1007/978-3-031-32386-7_8

A few centuries ago, the attitude of physicians toward the use of alcohol began to change. In the late seventeenth century, the English Government passed a range of legislation that lifted distilling restrictions, resulting in an increased production of gin. This ready availability, along with the low cost of gin, led to a massive rise in consumption, commonly known as the Gin Craze. By 1743, the average person in England was drinking 2.2 gallons of gin per year [3]. During that time, several physician groups in England described impairments in children born to alcoholic mothers. The Royal College of Physicians of London blamed gin consumption for "weak, feeble, and distempered" children who were "born weak and silly... shriveled and old, as though they had numbered many years" [4]. Similarly, English writer Daniel Defoe complained that drunken mothers were threatening to produce a "fine spindle-shanked generation" of children [5]. Public awareness of the possible link between alcohol and birth defects proliferated. The efforts of anti-gin campaigners resulted in the passing of the Gin Act in 1751, which aided in the reduction of gin consumption. However, for the next century and a half the medical literature remained quiet on the risks of prenatal alcohol consumption, perhaps due to this decrease in alcohol use.

More than a century passed before the connection between prenatal drinking and birth defects became a cause for scientific study. In the 1820s, a period known as the Victorian era, alcohol consumption made a resurgence through the appearance of "Gin Palaces." These venues proliferated in England and catered to both men and women, reviving the consumption of cheap gin. In the late 1800s, Dr. William Sullivan, a physician in the Liverpool prison system, conducted the first scientific study of children born after prenatal alcohol exposure. His 1899 article concluded that children prenatally exposed to alcohol were characterized by a pattern of birth defects of increasing severity. Higher rates of miscarriage amongst this population were also reported. Dr. Sullivan found that mothers who were unable to access alcohol due to their imprisonment tended to have healthier children. Furthermore, he observed that paternal alcohol consumption did not have a considerable effect on the offspring, concluding that alcohol appeared to have a "direct toxic action on the embryo" [6].

More recently, in 1968, Paul Lemoine published a report on 127 children born in France to alcoholic mothers [7]. His report detailed both physical and behavioral patterns among these children, including growth restriction, neurodevelopmental alterations, distinct facial features, and structural birth defects. However, the article did not include any diagnostic criteria for this condition and, unfortunately, received very little attention from the broader scientific community.

Initial Criteria and Formal Diagnostic Domains Through the 1980s

The first detailed report describing the pattern of malformation seen in children with prenatal alcohol exposure was published in *The Lancet* in June of 1973. The authors, Kenneth Lyons Jones and David Smith, dysmorphologists from the University of Washington School of Medicine, along with pediatrician Christy Ulleland and psychologist Ann Streissguth, described findings in eight children born to "mothers who were chronic alcoholics during pregnancy" [8]. The work of Christy Ulleland and Ann Stresissguth played an instrumental role in this publication. As a chief resident in pediatrics in 1968, Ulleland noticed a few infants in the high-risk maternal infant clinic with low birth weight, who were delayed in growth and development, and whose mothers consumed alcohol during pregnancy. A subsequent study led by Ulleland identified 12 infants from the clinic with prenatal alcohol exposure who had similar patterns of growth deficiency and developmental delay, prompting Kenneth Lyons Jones and David Smith to seek out and identify children from their own records with similar characteristics. Subsequently, psychologist Ann Streissguth conducted psychological testing on eight of these children, characterizing their neuropsychological findings.

Later, in November of 1973, a groundbreaking publication by Jones and Smith coined the term fetal alcohol syndrome (FAS). The authors defined FAS as "a constellation of abnormalities resulting from in utero alcohol exposure resulting in growth deficiency that persisted postnatally, microcephaly, developmental delay, and distinct facial characteristics, including short palpebral fissures, maxillary hypoplasia with relative prognathism, and epicanthal folds." The diagnostic criteria for FAS also required confirmation of maternal alcohol use during pregnancy, which in turn required a diagnosis of chronic alcoholism using National Institutes of Health (NIH) criteria [9].

The 1973 *Lancet* papers garnered more attention than Lemoine's report and stimulated further research on the teratogenicity of alcohol. The National Institute on Alcohol Abuse and Alcoholism (NIAAA), which had been established in 1971, subsequently funded many animal and epidemiological studies in this field, finding clear evidence for alcohol's teratogenic effects. Clinicians quickly began to recognize that children with prenatal alcohol exposure did not always present with the same classical signs of FAS. Therefore, the term fetal alcohol effects (FAE) began to be employed in the literature to describe less severe phenotypes, such as those seen in children without distinct facial features. This term was not intended to be a formal diagnosis, but rather an indicator that the abnormalities seen in the child were compatible with those caused by prenatal alcohol exposure, even though the pattern did not conform to all the classical signs and symptoms of FAS.

In 1980, the Fetal Alcohol Study Group of the Research Society on Alcoholism proposed the use of FAE to encompass "any conditions thought to be secondary to alcohol exposure *in utero*" in an effort to capture children in the FAS clinical spectrum who did not meet criteria for full FAS [10]. Unfortunately, the term FAE was thereupon applied too broadly to include any child with growth deficiency and developmental delays in whom a maternal history of drinking could be identified or was suspected. Some clinicians, educators, and social workers began employing this term in order to help a child qualify for financial assistance and educational intervention. In this context, several researchers started questioning the clinical validity of the term FAE and advocated for its abandonment in favor of employing solely the term "full" fetal alcohol syndrome [11]. They argued that each component of the FAS diagnosis was too nonspecific on its own, and that only the combination of all components allowed the definition of FAS.

Despite the lack of consensus regarding diagnostic guidelines for FAS, the scientific community was beginning to realize that any amount of alcohol consumption during pregnancy could lead to a plethora of birth defects. On July 18, 1981, the United States Surgeon General's office issued a statement that "Pregnant women should drink absolutely no alcohol because they may be endangering the health of their unborn children." This was the first time the general public had been advised that there was no known safe level of alcohol during pregnancy. Subsequently, in 1989, the U.S. Congress mandated that language warning of the consequences of drinking during pregnancy be included on all alcoholic beverage labels.

Established Diagnostic Systems After 1990

Increased awareness and recognition of FAS as a public health issue soon led the U.S. Congress to mandate that the Institute of Medicine (IOM) of the National Academy of Sciences conduct a study of FAS and related birth defects. In 1996, the IOM produced a report aimed at improving the tools and approaches for diagnosing FAS, as well as making key recommendations on prevalence studies, surveillance systems, and treatment programs for this condition [12]. The IOM report acknowledged that prenatal alcohol exposure resulted in a spectrum of adverse effects, necessitating several diagnostic categories to define these effects. The committee delineated five diagnostic categories within fetal alcohol spectrum disorders (FASD): FAS with a history of maternal alcohol exposure, FAS without a history of maternal alcohol exposure, partial FAS with a history of maternal alcohol exposure, alcohol-related birth defects (ARBD), and alcohol-related neurodevelopmental disorder (ARND). The report also included diagnostic guidelines for each diagnostic category, requiring the assessment of prenatal alcohol exposure, facial anomalies, growth anomalies, and CNS neurodevelopmental abnormalities. The IOM report was seminal in FAS research as it not only acknowledged that maternal alcohol consumption resulted in a spectrum of disorders, but also delineated criteria to diagnose each condition.

Additionally, the IOM report allowed for a more nuanced view of FASD by recognizing that the amount of alcohol exposure could vary greatly in each pregnancy, resulting in a wide phenotypic range. Further, the ability to diagnose FAS without confirmation of maternal alcohol exposure allowed for recognition of cases for whom a reliable exposure history could not be obtained. This was especially useful for children who were adopted or were in the foster care system, or for individuals diagnosed in adulthood and adolescence whose parents were deceased or otherwise unavailable to provide information on prenatal alcohol exposure. Although the IOM report set forth a scheme for classification and diagnosis for each category, the authors did not provide criteria to define pertinent physical and neurodevelopmental findings. For example, it was up to the clinician to determine what "low birth weight" or "decreased cranial size at birth" meant. Similarly, the report did not include a quantifiable definition of prenatal alcohol exposure, thus leaving this to the interpretation of the clinician. Furthermore, although the criteria recognized that neurobehavioral impairments commonly result from prenatal alcohol exposure, it did not establish criteria for determining such deficits. The IOM report required "evidence of a complex pattern of behavior or cognitive abnormalities that are inconsistent with developmental level and cannot be explained by familial background or environment alone, such as learning difficulties; deficits in school performance; poor impulse control; problems in social perception; deficits in higher level receptive and expressive language; poor capacity for abstraction or metacognition; specific deficits in mathematical skills; or problems in memory, attention, or judgment."

In 2000, Susan Astley and Sterling Clarren developed the 4-Digit Diagnostic Code based on analysis of the records of 1014 patients in the FAS Diagnostic and Prevention Network (DPN) at the University of Washington. This system was based on assigning a series of Likert-scaled numerical codes to a child with a potential FASD based on the independent assessment of four key diagnostic features: (1) growth deficiency, (2) facial phenotype, (3) brain damage/dysfunction, and (4) gestational alcohol exposure. Their work recognized several limitations in the diagnostic systems of the time, such as those published by the Institute of Medicine. The authors argued that the current guidelines were not sufficiently specific to assure diagnostic accuracy and precision, leading physicians to often perform a "gestalt" approach to diagnosis. Further, Astley and Clarren argued for nomenclature that conveyed the diversity of outcomes among individuals with prenatal exposure on the basis that no two individuals with FAS presented with precisely the same constellation of anomalies and disabilities. Perhaps most importantly, these authors recognized the lack of objective, quantitative scales to measure and report the magnitude of expression of key diagnostic features. Although a thin upper lip and smooth philtrum had been widely recognized as key diagnostic features of FAS, quantitative scales had never been used to objectively measure these features [13].

The 4-Digit Diagnostic Code introduced new ways of objectively assessing the facial phenotype of children prenatally exposed to alcohol, including anthropometric charts and a pictorial lip and philtrum guide. The lip and philtrum guide comprised a scale for ranking lip thinness and philtrum smoothness, each coded independently on a 5-point Likert scale. Higher scores corresponded to a greater upper lip circularity, which in turn represented a thinner upper lip. Palpebral fissure lengths were ranked according to their corresponding z-scores (standard deviations above or below the mean), with higher scores representing measurements 2 or greater standard deviations below the mean. After assigning a ranking score of 1–4 to each of the four diagnostic domains, 256 possible Diagnostic Code combinations resulted, ranging from 1111 to 4444. In addition, each diagnostic code fell into one of 22 unique clinical diagnostic categories. The 22 diagnostic categories translated to four main diagnoses with different specifiers: fetal alcohol syndrome, partial fetal alcohol syndrome, static encephalopathy, and neurobehavioral disorder. Distinct categories existed for FAS with alcohol exposure and with unknown alcohol exposure, while a diagnosis of partial FAS could only be made with knowledge of alcohol exposure. The static encephalopathy and neurobehavioral disorder diagnoses could be specified based on the presence of alcohol exposure, unknown alcohol exposure, or no alcohol exposure.

More than 10,000 professionals have been trained in the use of the 4-Digit Diagnostic Code since its inception, resulting in widespread use across the globe [14]. This diagnostic system captures a wide continuum of FAS features through objective measurements. However, the large number of diagnostic code combinations and the perceived complexity of the diagnostic algorithm may limit its use by providers who are less knowledgeable with the diagnosis of FASD or who do not have access to a multidisciplinary team. Importantly, the first iteration of the lip and philtrum guide was based on a primarily US population, and thus could not be generalized to other countries or populations.

In 2002, the U.S. Congress directed the Centers for Disease Control (CDC) to develop guidelines for diagnosing FAS. Through a scientific working committee, the CDC established three criteria for the diagnosis of FAS: (1) all three dysmorphic facial features (smooth philtrum, thin vermillion border, and short palpebral fissures), (2) prenatal or postnatal growth deficit in height or weight, and (3) CNS abnormalities. The criteria did not require confirmation of prenatal alcohol exposure. The threshold for growth deficit was below the 10th percentile, while the criteria for CNS abnormality could be met through either a head circumference below the 10th percentile or either a global or specific functional deficit below the 16th percentile. These guidelines only captured forms of FASD that present with more physical and cognitive symptoms, recognizing that the majority of persons with prenatal alcohol exposure did not express all features necessary for an FAS diagnosis. The CDC cited a lack of available scientific evidence needed to develop guidelines for the diagnosis of ARND, ARBD, and partial FAS [15]. Although a later consensus statement by the NIAAA in 2011 [16] indicated sufficient evidence for the existence of ARND, diagnostic criteria were not pursued at that time [17].

In an effort to harmonize the Institute of Medicine and 4-Digit Diagnostic Code approaches, a subcommittee of the Public Health Agency of Canada's National Advisory Council on FASD developed the 2005 Canadian guidelines for diagnosis. Similar to previous criteria, the Canadian diagnostic guide recognized three characteristic facial features: short palpebral fissures, smooth or flattened philtrum, and a thin vermilion border of the upper lip [18]. A philtrum and thin vermilion border were considered to be positive if rated at a 4 or 5 on the 5-point lip-philtrum guide developed by Astley and Clarren; whereas, palpebral fissure length was determined to be abnormally short when it was measured at or below the 3rd centile. The Canadian guidelines described three diagnostic categories: FAS, partial FAS, and ARND, while stating that the ARBD category had limited utility in the diagnosis of FASD. A diagnosis of FAS required all three cardinal facial features, while a diagnosis of partial FAS required only two cardinal facial features. Evidence of growth deficiency was also required for the diagnosis, determined by a height or weight at or below the 10th centile. The Canadian guidelines did not recognize microcephaly as a single, sufficient marker to establish neurobehavioral impairment. Rather, neurobehavioral impairment required evidence of impairment (defined as two standard deviations or more below the mean) in at least three cognitive domains. The Canadian guidelines recommended taking a thorough history of maternal alcohol consumption to confirm prenatal alcohol exposure, documenting the number and types of beverages, as well as patterns of drinking when available. Though they did not set forth specific criteria for confirmation of prenatal alcohol use, the guidelines employed IOM criteria to define significant alcohol exposure, requiring "a pattern of excessive intake characterized by substantial, regular intake or heavy episodic drinking" [12].

Concurrent to the development of the Canadian guidelines in 2005, a group of researchers in the United States led by Dr. Eugene Hoyme set out to establish clear guidelines for the diagnosis of FASD. This group acknowledged the limitations found in the initial IOM criteria and proposed changes that would allow for a more practical diagnostic algorithm. Among the obstacles identified in the IOM report, Hoyme et al. noted a lack of specificity in the parameters being used to measure growth, facial dysmorphic features, and behavioral and cognitive impairments. Another deficiency noted was the lack of a clinical definition of alcohol-related birth defects (ARBD) and alcohol-related neurodevelopmental disorder (ARND) [19].

At the time, the 4-digit diagnostic system, also known as the Washington criteria, had gained popularity among providers in North America. This system set clear standards for classification of each of the four key diagnostic features of FAS: growth deficiency, characteristic FAS facial features, central nervous system dysfunction, and alcohol exposure in utero. Yet, its perceived complexity resulting from a multitude of diagnostic categories were criticized by Hoyme et al., who described the system as "complex and confusing."

The perceived drawbacks in both the IOM and Washington criteria led Hoyme et al. to develop a classification system for FASD that would allow accurate diagnoses of affected individuals. The team evaluated 1500 children in the United States and South Africa using the IOM diagnostic criteria during a period of 5 years. Each child was assessed in three domains: (1) growth and structural development, (2) neuropsychological development, and (3) maternal risk factors. For the dysmorphology assessment, the researchers employed Astley and Clarren's lip and philtrum guide to evaluate facial phenotypic features. After assigning each child and their age-matched controls a diagnosis of FAS, not FAS, or deferred diagnosis, the group proposed revisions for the IOM diagnostic categorizations. First, the diagnosis of FAS, which could be made with or without confirmed maternal alcohol exposure, required abnormalities in all three assessed domains. Second, the diagnosis of partial FAS (with or without confirmed maternal alcohol exposure) required the presence of the typical FAS facial dysmorphic features and abnormalities in *one* of the other two domains. The guidelines also proposed clarifications for the diagnoses of ARBD and ARND. Diagnosis of ARBD required confirmed maternal alcohol exposure, a characteristic pattern of minor facial anomalies, and the presence of congenital structural defects that had previously been associated with prenatal alcohol exposure. A diagnosis of ARND also required confirmation of maternal alcohol exposure and either evidence of deficient brain growth or evidence of a complex pattern of behavioral or cognitive abnormalities. Importantly, the team noted that complex tests of executive functioning were needed to capture the neurobehavioral impairments seen in ARND.

Hoyme et al. addressed most of the ambiguity seen in the IOM criteria by establishing cutoffs for the assessment of facial phenotype and growth deficiency, allowing for ease of clinical application. Evidence of prenatal and/or postnatal growth deficiency required a height and/or weight below the 10th percentile on racially normed scales. The three key facial features assessed included short palpebral fissures (below the 10th percentile), thin vermilion border of the upper lip (scored as 4 or 5 on the lip/philtrum guide), and a smooth philtrum (scored as 4 or 5 on the lip/philtrum guide). Key differences in facial phenotype were described among diagnostic groups: for diagnoses of FAS or PFAS, two of the three cardinal facial anomalies were required; whereas, for diagnoses of ARND or ARBD, no specific facial phenotype was required. Evidence of deficient brain growth required a head circumference at or below the 10th percentile or a structural brain abnormality. Maternal alcohol exposure was assessed via a maternal interview or reliable collateral sources. Following the IOM guidelines, Hoyme et al. defined confirmed maternal alcohol exposure as "a pattern of excessive intake characterized by substantial regular intake or heavy episodic drinking." Thus, the Hoyme criteria, comparable to the Canadian criteria, continued to be ambiguous in regard to maternal alcohol consumption, leaving room for interpretation by the clinician.

A noted limitation of the IOM update was the ambiguity in the definition of behavioral and cognitive abnormalities. Although Hoyme et al. defined the domains which were impaired in FASD (complex task solving, higher level receptive and expressive language deficits, and disordered behavior), they did not establish cutoffs for practical neuropsychologic testing and diagnosis, partially due to a lack of concrete knowledge regarding the exact neurobehavioral characteristics of children with FASD at the time. Furthermore, a subsequent study comparing the performance of the Washington criteria and the Hoyme guidelines found that these systems diagnosed different individuals with FASD, with little overlap between both populations [20]. The marked differences between the patients identified under both systems highlighted the need for further refinement of these diagnostic guidelines.

Recent Developments in Diagnostic Systems

The fifth edition of the Diagnostic and Statistical Manual of Mental Disorders (DSM-5), published in 2013 [21], captured the range of developmental disabilities caused by prenatal alcohol exposure under the diagnosis "Neurodevelopmental Disorder Associated with Prenatal Alcohol Exposure" (ND-PAE; coded 315.8 under Other Specified Neurodevelopmental Disorder) (American Psychiatric Association [22]). This represented the first time that a diagnosis along the FASD continuum was incorporated into the DSM-5 manual. The recognition of the effects of prenatal alcohol exposure by a major professional organization in behavioral health helped shed light on the importance of this disorder.

In order to help healthcare professionals identify and diagnose children with prenatal alcohol exposure, the DSM-5 appendix defined diagnostic criteria for ND-PAE. These included: (1) a history of more than minimal alcohol exposure during gestation; (2) impaired neurocognitive functioning; (3) impaired self-regulation; and (4) impaired adaptive functioning. Importantly, these criteria required that the symptoms could not be better explained by another genetic or teratogenic condition. Unfortunately, these guidelines did not contain specific cutoffs that could be employed by clinicians to determine a diagnosis. Later studies provided practical guidelines for the neuropsychological assessment based on the DSM-5 ND-PAE guidelines [23, 24].

As the field of FASD continued to evolve, a need to revise current guidelines was recognized. In 2016, the Canada Fetal Alcohol Spectrum Disorder Research Network revised their 2005 guidelines. These guidelines were established based on literature reviews, consultation with local clinics, and focus groups. An initial key change was the use of fetal alcohol spectrum disorder (FASD) as a unitary diagnostic term. The team classified the three facial features associated with FASD as "sentinel facial features" (SFF), arguing that all three must be present because of their specificity to prenatal alcohol exposure. Furthermore, growth deficiency was removed as a diagnostic criterion on the basis that it was not a sufficiently specific feature of FASD, given that growth could be influenced by many factors. Two diagnostic categories were recognized: FASD without SFF and FASD with SFF. Individuals who presented with some of the diagnostic features but not enough to qualify for diagnosis of FASD could be classified as at risk. FASD without SFF required confirmation of prenatal alcohol exposure along with a CNS impairment. On the other hand, a diagnosis of FASD with SFF could be made in two ways. First, the presence of all three facial features and CNS impairment, with confirmation or an unknown status of prenatal alcohol exposure was sufficient for this diagnosis. In the absence of CNS impairment, microcephaly in a child younger than 6 years of age, with all three facial features and confirmation or an unknown status of prenatal alcohol exposure would result in a diagnosis of FASD with SFF [25].

In 2016, a working group in the U.S. led by Dr. Eugene Hoyme also published a revision of their 2005 guidelines in order to reflect updated research on FASD. The group comprised investigators in the NIAAA-funded multi-site "Collaboration on FASD Prevalence" (CoFASP) [26]. The authors convened over a 12-month period to revisit three key components of the previous Hoyme et al. diagnostic criteria: dysmorphology evaluation, neurobehavioral assessment, and the definition of significant documented prenatal alcohol exposure. In the realm of dysmorphology, the authors recognized that both major and minor anomalies could result from prenatal alcohol exposure. While evaluation of the face and the three cardinal facial features associated with FASD continued to be imperative in a diagnostic assessment of FASD, the importance of other associated minor anomalies was stressed. In this vein, the group further clarified a previously published "dysmorphology score" [27] based on objective observations of growth and minor anomalies in 370 children with FAS, thus allowing for a quantitative objective comparison of growth and dysmorphology among groups of children with FASD. The expert dysmorphologists also further specified diagnostic differences between the two categories within PFAS: PFAS with and without confirmed alcohol exposure. The updated guidelines required evidence of neurobehavioral impairment for FAS, partial FAS, and ARND, but evidence of neurobehavioral impairment was not a diagnostic requirement for ARBD. Neurobehavioral impairment was updated to encompass global intellectual ability, specific cognitive areas, and behavioral regulation. Adaptive skills were also noted to be commonly impaired in FASD, although specific cutoffs and adaptive requirements were not included. The neurobehavioral criteria revision represented a significant improvement from the 2005 guidelines due to the delineation of specific domains within cognitive and behavioral skills, as well as the definition of neurobehavioral impairment as equal or greater than 1.5 Standard Deviations below the mean.

The seminal 2016 publication included a definition of documented prenatal alcohol exposure. Documentation of alcohol exposure involved a maternal interview to obtain information on quantity, frequency, and timing of alcohol consumed during pregnancy as well as during the 3 months before pregnancy recognition or a positive pregnancy test. If the number of standard drinks consumed per week during pregnancy was unavailable, other sources could be employed, such as documentation of intoxication, positive testing with established alcohol-exposure biomarkers, or increased risk demonstrated by a validated screening tool [26]. The use of reliable informants or collateral sources of information was considered key to obtaining a prenatal alcohol exposure history during routine FASD evaluations. Under these updated guidelines, confirmed prenatal alcohol exposure was required for the diagnosis of ARND and ARBD; whereas, a diagnosis of FAS or partial FAS could be made in the absence of confirmed prenatal alcohol exposure.

In the same year as the Canadian and Hoyme guidelines were updated, a team of Australian researchers developed guidelines for the diagnosis of FASD, which closely resembled the Canadian guidelines [28]. The Australian guidelines, updated in 2020, recognized two diagnostic categories: FASD with three sentinel facial features and FASD with less than three sentinel facial features. Three areas were assessed in an FASD evaluation: prenatal alcohol exposure, neurodevelopmental domains, and the presence of sentinel facial features. Similar to the Canadian guidelines, a diagnosis of FASD could be made if prenatal alcohol exposure was confirmed or "unknown." Confirmation of prenatal alcohol exposure was based on the validated Alcohol Use Disorders Identification Test (AUDIT-C) to capture risk exposure, or other reliable evidence of high consumption. See Table 8.1 for a comparison of the different diagnostic systems, and Table 8.2 for a comparison of definitions of prenatal alcohol exposure.

Table 8.1 Comparison of six clinical diagnostic systems for FASD

	4-Digit code	CDC	DSM-5	Hoyme guidelines	Canadian guidelines	Australian guidelines
Year published	2004	2005	2013	2016	2016	2020
Dataset employed	1014 patients	Panel Consensus	Panel Consensus	Adaptation of IOM Criteria and panel consensus	AGREE II Framework meta-analysis and panel consensus	Literature review and panel consensus
Diagnostic categories	• Fetal alcohol syndrome (FAS) • Partial fetal alcohol syndrome (PFAS) • Sentinel physical findings • Static encephalopathy • Neurobehavioral disorder	• Fetal alcohol syndrome (FAS)	• Neurobehavioral disorder associated with prenatal alcohol exposure (ND-PAE)	• Fetal alcohol syndrome (FAS) • Partial fetal alcohol syndrome (PFAS) • Alcohol-related neurodevelopmental disorder (ARND) • Alcohol-related birth defects (ARBD)	• FAS with sentinel facial features (SFF) • FAS without SFF • At risk for neurodevelopmental disorder and FASD	• FASD with three sentinel facial features • FASD with less than three sentinel facial features
Features assessed	• Growth deficiency • Three facial features • CNS structural and functional anomalies • Prenatal alcohol exposure	• Growth deficiency • Three facial features • CNS structural and functional anomalies • Prenatal alcohol exposure	• Three functional domains (self-regulation, neurocognitive, adaptive functioning)	• Growth deficiency • Three facial features • CNS structural and functional anomalies • Prenatal alcohol exposure	• Three facial features • CNS structural and functional anomalies • Prenatal alcohol exposure	• Growth deficiency • Three facial features • CNS structural and functional anomalies • Prenatal alcohol exposure (with or without confirmation)

Benefits	• Structured assessment of the lip and philtrum through the lip and philtrum guide • Reduces the subjectivity in diagnosis of many features	• Established parameters for growth and CNS abnormalities	• Creates a system for the evaluation of ND-PAE within the mental health setting, which most people with FASD come in contact with • Focuses on neurobehavioral functioning, which commonly guides treatment for children with FASD	• Establishes clear definition of prenatal alcohol exposure	• Simplifies guidelines by establishing two diagnoses	• Simplifies guidelines by establishing two diagnoses
Limitations	• Yields 256 possible combinations	• No structured assessment of cardinal facial features • No recognition of milder forms of FASD	• Does not consider physical features		• Growth is not assessed • May not capture full spectrum of impairments	• Growth is not assessed • May not capture full spectrum of impairments

Table 8.2 Definition of prenatal alcohol exposure in \six clinical FASD diagnostic systems

	4-Digit code (2004)	CDC (2005)	DSM-5 (2013)	Hoyme guidelines (2016)	Canadian guidelines (2016)	Australian guidelines (2020)
Definition of standard drink	Not specified	Not specified	Not specified	14 g of pure alcohol	Not specified	10 g of pure alcohol
Criteria for prenatal alcohol exposure	Four possible scores: 1. No risk (confirmed absent exposure) 2. Unknown risk (exposure is not known or information is of questionable reliability 3. Some risk (alcohol use confirmed) 4. High risk (high peak blood-alcohol concentrations delivered at least weekly in early pregnancy)	Two possible categories: • Confirmed prenatal alcohol exposure (based on clinical observation or self-reports, reliable informants, medical records, or social, legal, or medical problems related to drinking) • Unknown prenatal alcohol exposure	Proposed criteria in appendix require confirmation from maternal self-report of alcohol use during pregnancy, medical or other records, or clinical observation	One or more of the following: – $\geq$6 drinks per week for $\geq$2 week during pregnancy – $\geq$3 drinks per occasion on $\geq$2 occasions during pregnancy – Documentation of alcohol-related social or legal problems in proximity to (before or during) the index pregnancy (e.g., history of citation[s] for driving while intoxicated or history of treatment of an alcohol-related codition) – Documentation of intoxication during pregnancy by blood, breath, or urine alcohol content testing – Positive testing with established alcohol-exposure biomarker(s) during pregnancy or at birth (e.g., analysis of fatty acid ethyl esters, phosphatidylethanol, and/or ethyl glucuronide in maternal hair, fingernails, urine, or blood, or placenta, or meconium) – Increased prenatal risk associated with drinking during pregnancy as assessed by a validated screening tool of, for example, T-ACE (tolerance, annoyance, cut down, eye-opener) or AUDIT (alcohol use disorders identification test)	Requires documentation that the biological mother consumed alcohol during the index pregnancy based on reliable clinical observation; self-report; reports by a reliable source; medical records documenting positive blood-alcohol concentrations; alcohol treatment; or other social, legal or medical problems related to drinking during the pregnancy	Four possible scores: 1. No exposure (confirmed absence), no risk of FASD 2. Unknown exposure (alcohol use is unknown) 3. Confirmed exposure (AUDIT-C score = 1–4; or confirmed use, but exposure less than high-risk level for FASD; or confirmed use, but not known if exposed at a high-risk level for FASD) 4. Confirmed-high-risk exposure (AUDIT-C score = 5+; confirmed use, exposure at high-risk level for FASD)

| Is PAE required for diagnostic classification? | Required for partial FAS. Not required for FAS, sentinel physical findings, static encephalopathy, or neurobehavioral disorder. | Not required | Required for ND-PAE | Confirmed prenatal alcohol exposure is required for diagnosis of ARND and ARBD. Not required for FAS and PFAS. | Required for FASD without SFF. Not required for FASD with SFF | Required for FASD with <3 SFF. Not required for FASD with 3 SFF |

ARND alcohol-related neurodevelopmental disorder, *ARBD* alcohol-related birth defects, *SFF* sentinel facial features, *AUDIT* alcohol use disorders identification test

Questions and Further Study

Since the first description in the literature of the effects of prenatal alcohol exposure on the developing fetus, many scientific groups have set forth guidelines for the diagnosis of this continuum of disabilities. In most classification systems, FASD is recognized as a spectrum of conditions resulting from maternal alcohol consumption. However, debate is ongoing regarding which diagnostic system most accurately captures the spectrum of disabilities resulting from prenatal alcohol exposure, and there continues to be no international consensus on diagnostic criteria for FASD. This lack of standardization of diagnosis has been analyzed objectively in the literature [29]. A recent study found at best only moderate agreement in the diagnostic classification of alcohol-exposed children among the five major diagnostic systems applied [29]. The authors concluded: "Substantial agreement among systems would have inspired confidence that all systems accurately identify a similar, underlying condition, or set of relationships, and that the methods recommended were appropriate for such identification. Given these results, however, we cannot be comfortable making these assumptions without further evaluation. In addition, in the absence of an external standard, despite the obvious discrepancy among systems, we cannot say that one system is better or worse in identifying the effects of prenatal alcohol exposure."

Certain aspects of the current diagnostic criteria are up for debate. For example, should two or three of the "cardinal" facial features be required for a diagnosis of FAS or PFAS? The current Canadian guidelines require all three sentinel facial features, while the updated Hoyme guidelines allow for the presence of two out of the three facial features. Another debate relates to whether the 3rd or the 10th centile should constitute the cutoff for head circumference, height, weight, and palpebral fissure length in FASD. While the 4-digit code and Canadian guidelines require palpebral fissure length to be at or below the 3rd centile, the CDC and Hoyme criteria establish their cutoff at the 10th centile. Some guidelines, such as the Canadian and Australian criteria, do not include growth in their diagnostic parameters. Similarly, while most systems recognize a neurobehavioral impairment resulting from prenatal alcohol exposure, the specific neurobehavioral profile and its integration into the diagnostic criteria are up for debate. In particular, the number and type of neurobehavioral domains, as well as standard cutoffs (1.5 SD or 2 SD below the mean) differ between the major diagnostic systems.

Another highly debated question is whether the diagnosis of partial FAS should be made with or without confirmation of maternal drinking. As has been discussed, each diagnostic system requires different thresholds of prenatal alcohol consumption. Although all systems recognize that there is no safe amount of alcohol that can be consumed during the prenatal period, disagreement remains around the definition and criteria for confirmation of prenatal alcohol exposure. Finally, regarding the continuum of disorders seen in FASD, should FAS, partial FAS, ARND, and ARBD be the terms used to classify the broad array of symptoms that define this spectrum? Prenatal alcohol exposure results in a wide variety of symptoms that differ in severity, making it challenging to reach a diagnostic classification. The 4-digit system allows for this variability by independently ranking key features; other systems, such as the Hoyme guidelines, consider the presence of minor anomalies that have been observed consistently in children with FASD.

Despite the contested aspects of current diagnostic criteria, research and clinical efforts should be geared toward developing commonly accepted international guidelines that are able to capture this spectrum of related conditions. Recently, the NIAAA has convened a group of international experts representing all of the current diagnostic systems for FASD whose goal is to come to a consensus and formulate common data-driven diagnostic guidelines. The complexity of this diagnostic spectrum requires a multidisciplinary team approach for the FASD diagnostic evaluation, and accurate diagnostic systems are essential for early diagnosis and treatment. Furthermore, they are a necessary, critical tool which can be used to help determine the prevalence and economic burden of this condition, which in turn can guide policy and support funding for the numerous services needed by those affected by FASD. Future research is required in order to establish practical, evidence-based guidelines that can bring consensus to this rapidly evolving field.

References

1. Abel EL. Was the fetal alcohol syndrome recognized by the Greeks and Romans? Alcohol Alcohol. 1999;34(6):868–72.
2. Burton R, et al. The Anatomy of Melancholy. Clarendon Press; Oxford University Press. 1989.
3. Dillon P. Gin: the much-lamented death of madam Geneva: the eighteenth-century gin craze. London: Review; 2002. p. 228.
4. Goodacre K. Guide to the Middlesex sessions records 1549–1889: prepared for the Standin. London: Greater London Records Office; 1965. p. 785.
5. Defoe D. A brief case of the distillers, and of the distilling trade in England, shewing how far it is the interest of England to encourage the said trade… Humbly recommended to the Lords and Commons of Great Britain, in the present parliament assembled, T. Warner; 1725.
6. Sullivan WC. A note on the influence of maternal inebriety on the offspring. J Ment Sci. 1899;45(190):489–503.
7. Lemoine P, Harousseau H, Borteyru JP, Menuet JC. Les enfants des parents alcooliques: anomalies observees apropos de 127 cas. Ouest Med. 1968;21:476–82.
8. Jones KL, Smith DW, Ulleland CN, Streissguth P. Pattern of malformation in offspring of chronic alcoholic mothers. Lancet. 1973;1(7815):1267–71. https://doi.org/10.1016/s0140-6736(73)91291-9.
9. Jones KL, Smith DW. Recognition of the fetal alcohol syndrome in early infancy. Lancet. 1973;302(7836):999–1001. https://doi.org/10.1016/s0140-6736(73)91092-1.
10. Rosett HL. A clinical perspective of the fetal alcohol syndrome. Alcohol Clin Exp Res. 1980;4(2):119–22. https://doi.org/10.1111/j.1530-0277.1980.tb05626.x.
11. Aase JM, Jones KL, Clarren SK. Do we need the term 'FAE'? Pediatrics. 1995;95(3):428–30.
12. Stratton K, Howe C, Battaglia F, editors. Institute of Medicine. Fetal alcohol syndrome: diagnosis, epidemiology, prevention, and treatment. Washington, DC: National Academies Press; 1996.
13. Astley SJ, Clarren SK. Diagnosing the full spectrum of fetal alcohol-exposed individuals: introducing the 4-digit diagnostic code. Alcohol Alcohol. 2000;35(4):400–10.

14. Astley SJ. Validation of the fetal alcohol spectrum disorder (FASD) 4-digit diagnostic code. J Popul Ther Clin Pharmacol. 2013;20(3):e416–67.
15. Bertrand J, Floyd LL, Weber MK, Fetal Alcohol Syndrome Prevention Team, Division of Birth Defects and Developmental Disabilities, National Center on Birth Defects and Developmental Disabilities, Centers for Disease Control and Prevention (CDC). Guidelines for identifying and referring persons with fetal alcohol syndrome [published correction appears in MMWR Morb Mortal Wkly Rep. 2006 May 26;55(20):568]. MMWR Recomm Rep. 2005;54(RR-11):1–14.
16. Interagency Coordinating Committee on Fetal Alcohol Spectrum Disorders. Consensus statement recognizing alcohol-related neurodevelopmental disorder (ARND) in primary health care of children. Rockville, MD: National Institute on Alcohol Abuse and Alcoholism; 2011.
17. Warren KR, et al. Recognizing alcohol-related neurodevelopmental disorder (ARND) in primary health care of children; 2011. Obtained from: https://www.niaaa.nih.gov/sites/default/files/ARNDConferenceConsensusStatementBooklet_Complete.pdf.
18. Chudley AE, Conry J, Cook JL, et al. Fetal alcohol spectrum disorder: Canadian guidelines for diagnosis. CMAJ. 2005;172(5 Suppl):S1–S21. https://doi.org/10.1503/cmaj.1040302.
19. Hoyme HE, May PA, Kalberg WO, Piyadasa Kodituwakku J, Gossage P, Trujillo PM, Buckley DG, Miller JH, Aragon AS, Khaole N, Viljoen DL, Jones KL, Robinson LK. A practical clinical approach to diagnosis of fetal alcohol spectrum disorders: clarification of the 1996 Institute of Medicine criteria. Pediatrics. 2005;115(1):39–47.
20. Astley SJ. Comparison of the 4-digit diagnostic code and the Hoyme diagnostic guidelines for fetal alcohol spectrum disorders [published correction appears in Pediatrics. 2007 Jan;119(1):227]. Pediatrics. 2006;118(4):1532–45.
21. American Psychiatric Association. Diagnostic and statistical manual of mental disorders. 5th ed. Washington, DC: American Psychiatric Publishing; 2013.
22. American Psychiatric Association. Diagnostic and statistical manual of mental disorders (5th ed.). 2013. https://doi.org/10.1176/appi.books.9780890425596.
23. Doyle LR, Mattson SN. Neurobehavioral disorder associated with prenatal alcohol exposure (ND-PAE): review of evidence and guidelines for assessment. Curr Dev Disord Rep. 2015;2(3):175–86. https://doi.org/10.1007/s40474-015-0054-6.
24. Hagan JF Jr, Balachova T, Bertrand J, et al. Neurobehavioral disorder associated with prenatal alcohol exposure. Pediatrics. 2016;138(4):e20151553. https://doi.org/10.1542/peds.2015-1553.
25. Cook JL, Green CR, Lilley CM, et al. Fetal alcohol spectrum disorder: a guideline for diagnosis across the lifespan. CMAJ. 2016;188(3):191–7. https://doi.org/10.1503/cmaj.141593.
26. Hoyme HE, Kalberg WO, Elliott AJ, Blankenship J, Buckley D, Marais AS, Manning MA, Robinson LK, Adam MP, Abdul-Rahman O, Jewett T, Coles CD, Chambers C, Jones KL, Adnams CM, Shah PE, Riley EP, Charness ME, Warren KR, May PA. Updated clinical guidelines for diagnosing fetal alcohol spectrum disorders. Pediatrics. 2016;138(2):e20154256. https://doi.org/10.1542/peds.2015-4256. Epub 2016 Jul 27.
27. Ervalahti N, Korkman M, Fagerlund A, Autti-Rämö I, Loimu L, Hoyme HE. Relationship between dysmorphic features and general cognitive function in children with fetal alcohol spectrum disorders. Am J Med Genet A. 2007;143A(24):2916–23. https://doi.org/10.1002/ajmg.a.32009.
28. Bower C, Elliott EJ. Australian guide to the diagnosis of fetal alcohol spectrum disorder (FASD). Perth: Telethon Kids Institute; 2016. p. 85–103.
29. Coles CD, Gailey AR, Mulle JG, Kable JA, Lynch ME, Jones KL. A comparison among 5 methods for the clinical diagnosis of fetal alcohol spectrum disorders. Alcohol Clin Exp Res. 2016;40(5):1000–9.

Chapter 9
The Diagnostic Process

Omar A. Abdul-Rahman, Christie L. M. Petrenko, and Lynn L. Cole

In the previous chapter, various clinical criteria for fetal alcohol spectrum disorders (FASD) were reviewed, each having been proposed based upon data from different populations. Given the benefits and limitations of each of the diagnostic systems that have been published, the Hoyme 2016 guidelines [1] were selected for this chapter based on two factors. First, the Hoyme guidelines have the greatest sensitivity in diagnosing FASD as noted in the previous chapter [2]. Second, the specific criteria utilized in the Hoyme guidelines (e.g., facial features, neurobehavioral impairment, etc.) are shared among many of the other diagnostic systems with some minor differences in the nature of the thresholds used. Finally, the Hoyme guidelines have strong clinical utility. Therefore, the points discussed in this chapter will be broadly applicable for the diagnostician regardless of which criteria they choose to apply in practice.

FASD diagnostic evaluations can be accomplished in both clinical and research settings, though there are significant differences in the methodology applied depending on the nature of the assessment. The research setting may be more flexible in allotting significantly more time in collecting data such as maternal interviews, anthropometric measurements, and extensive neuropsychological batteries. In the clinical setting, where there may be more limitations related to clinician availability,

O. A. Abdul-Rahman (✉)
Division of Medical Genetics, Department of Pediatrics, Weill Cornell Medicine,
New York, USA
e-mail: oma4009@med.cornell.edu

C. L. M. Petrenko
Mt. Hope Family Center, University of Rochester, Rochester, NY, USA
e-mail: christie.petrenko@rochester.edu

L. L. Cole
Division of Developmental and Behavioral Pediatrics, University of Rochester Medical Center, Rochester, NY, USA
e-mail: lynn_cole@urmc.rochester.edu

time allocation, and financial reimbursement, a more targeted approach may be utilized. For example, diagnostic clinics may utilize substantial pre-appointment chart and document review, including prenatal exposure history, medical history, and parent and teacher assessments that are completed ahead of the appointment in order to maximize efficiency within the clinic. The time spent in clinic may be focused on clarifying exposure and medical history information, conducting a physical examination, reviewing psychoeducational or neuropsychological assessment results, and discussion of the final diagnosis. Although a multidisciplinary evaluation has been suggested in the literature as the gold standard, the benefits of this model over a single-discipline model for straight forward cases has not been established. In determining a model, it is critical that factors such as diagnostic capacity in the region and system of health care finances be taken into account. A tiered clinic model may be beneficial to best manage allocation of limited resources, reserving multidisciplinary for more complex cases where neurobehavioral assessment or more involved differential diagnostic consideration is needed. A tiered model can reduce waitlists and get patients into earlier intervention.

Most FASD clinics will have a medical and psychological provider and may include other types of expertise, such as a genetic counselor, social worker, occupational therapist, physical therapist, speech therapist, parent resource coordinator, patient navigator, school advocate, and/or case manager, among others. Telemedicine platforms have also been utilized to expand access to diagnostic services but will typically require some type of field training for staff who are present on the patient side to obtain the anthropometric measurements. Field staff have been shown to be reliably trained in this manner [3]. Other application-based systems have also been deployed including the 4-digit diagnostic code [4] and facial recognition analyses utilizing both 2-D and 3-D imaging [5, 6] the latter not being currently used in the clinical setting since validation studies are still required.

All current diagnostic guidelines that are in widespread use continue to be based on assessment of several of five primary domains, which remain consistent since the initial description of fetal alcohol syndrome by Jones and Smith [7]. The original definition was based on confirmation of significant alcohol exposure, a specific facial phenotype, growth restriction of prenatal onset with persistence postnatally, and neurocognitive deficits. The domains that are currently in use have separated the neurocognitive deficits into abnormalities of the neurological system and neurobehavioral impairment. Therefore, the domains that will be discussed individually in this chapter are (1) prenatal alcohol exposure; (2) cardinal facial features; (3) growth deficiency; (4) abnormality of neurological structure/function; and (5) neurobehavioral impairment.

Figure 9.1 illustrates how these criteria map on to the individual FASD diagnoses within the Hoyme 2016 criteria, including fetal alcohol syndrome (FAS), partial fetal alcohol syndrome (pFAS), and alcohol-related neurodevelopmental disorder (ARND). After reviewing criterion for each domain, considerations for how to integrate this information to render a diagnosis will be discussed.

One final point to make is that providers are often concerned about the stigma associated with an FASD diagnosis. Often if a child is receiving school services, the

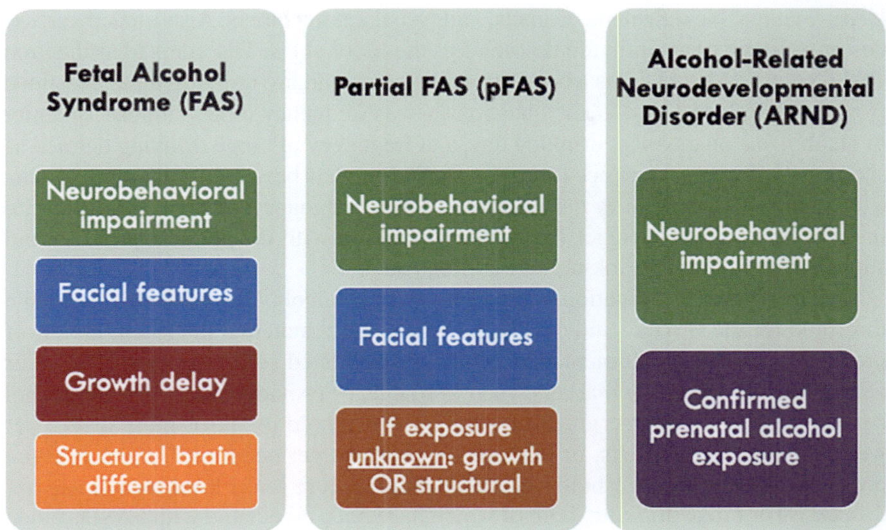

Fig. 9.1 Illustration of various domains affected by PAE and how they map against Hoyme et al. (2016) diagnostic categories

provider may not be clear on the benefits of making such a stigmatizing diagnosis. While some of the school services for children affected with FASD may not be altered by a diagnosis, knowing the etiology of the symptoms can offer power of understanding for the individual and their family, lead to reframing and more appropriate accommodations, and help guide services and long-term planning.

Assessing Prenatal Alcohol Exposure

The ideal time to obtain information about prenatal alcohol exposure is during pregnancy. Interviewing pregnant individuals should be conducted in a way so as to build rapport and encourage candid responses. Normalizing the behavior of alcohol intake is often helpful, particularly when discussing the period prior to recognition of the pregnancy. Baseline alcohol intake in the preconception period is correlated to PAE during the first few weeks of a pregnancy [8]. Additionally, many prenatal settings have integrated some type of screening, frequently based on instruments initially developed for the general population. Some of these instruments have been validated in the prenatal population, and others have been modified to target pregnant individuals. Frequently used measures in the United States have included the T-ACE and TWEAK (see Chap. 4 for further discussion of these tools), with similar sensitivity and specificity for pregnancy risk drinking. The Alcohol Use Disorders Identification Test (AUDIT) [9] involves ten items and has been validated in several countries outside the US including Finland, Chile, Korea, Sweden, Germany, the

UAE, Uganda, New Zealand, Canada, and Nepal among others. A shortened version designed for pregnant individuals known as the Alcohol Use Disorders Identification Test-Concise (AUDIT-C) is a brief screening questionnaire utilizing three questions from the lengthier AUDIT. The questions assess frequency of alcohol use, quantity of alcohol use on a typical drinking day, and frequency of binge drinking defined as six or more drinks on one occasion. Although there has been some attempt to define a threshold score to identify risky drinking during pregnancy, most of these tools are intended to serve as a trigger for further discussion with the prenatal provider and support a reduction in drinking during pregnancy.

During an FASD evaluation, identifying prenatal alcohol exposure that meets the threshold for the Hoyme guidelines can involve direct maternal interview, review of prenatal records for documentation of either a validated screening tool, relative or other observer report, biomarkers when available, or provider discussion of alcohol consumption. The Hoyme guidelines utilize a threshold of six or more drinks per week for 2 or more weeks, or three or more drinks per occasion for two or more occasions. These two thresholds are designed to capture lower level regular use (~1 drink/day) or binge drinking, both of which have been associated with FASD. When possible, direct maternal interviews should be structured to reduce stigma and facilitate a non-judgmental discussion of pre-pregnancy and pregnancy behaviors. Normalizing drinking behavior and focusing initially on drinking outside of a recognized pregnancy is frequently an effective means to determine baseline drinking patterns. Specifically asking about the 3 months prior to recognition of the pregnancy is highly correlated with prenatal alcohol exposure, particularly as the mean time to pregnancy awareness is 5.5 weeks of gestation [10]. See Box 9.1 for examples of how to ask about PAE.

Box 9.1 Examples of How to Ask About Prenatal Alcohol Exposure
- Normalize the behavior and use passive instead of active verbs

  - "Many individuals report having a beer or a glass of wine when pregnant. Do you recall anything like this happening to you?"

- Destigmatize the behavior by asking about the preconception period

  - "Before you became pregnant, what would be an average number of drinks you might have per week?"

- Embed questions regarding PAE with other nutritional assessments

  - "What types of foods did you consume during your pregnancy? Did you restrict or were unable to tolerate any of them? What types of drinks did you consume during your pregnancy? Did you restrict or were unable to tolerate any of them?"

Many children who present for assessment will not be in the care of their biological parent, and so alternative sources of information will need to be considered to document prenatal alcohol exposure. Direct observation by relatives or friends with details regarding the type of alcohol consumed, frequency, and quantity during pregnancy including any negative outcomes such as loss of consciousness, hospitalization, admission to rehabilitation facilities, legal ramifications (e.g., citation for driving under the influence (DUI), or known medical complications of alcohol use such as cirrhosis provide strong support for sufficient prenatal alcohol exposure to result in FASD. In situations in which child protective services or other child social services agencies are involved, staff observations during the pregnancy or documentation of interviews with the biological parent documenting alcohol use may be considered as confirmatory. Concomitant use of other substances such as marijuana or opiates is not uncommon, but care must be taken during the assessment to differentiate actual evidence of alcohol use during the target pregnancy from assumptions others may have about alcohol use in the context of other drug use. In the authors experience, it is very common for families with complex dynamics to extrapolate one set of negative behaviors such as marijuana or opioid use to various other substances, including alcohol. In addition to causing inaccurate reporting of prenatal exposure, it can also create a negative impression of and stigma against the biological parent.

Measuring Facial Features

The initial Jones and Smith report identified a number of facial features observed in fetal alcohol syndrome, including short palpebral fissures when plotted against normative values, epicanthal folds, and midfacial hypoplasia with relative prognathism [7]. Images from the report demonstrated a thin upper lip and smooth philtrum that are now recognized as hallmarks of the condition. They also identified several anomalies of the limbs including reduction in elbow extension, supination, and pronation along with crease alterations of the hands. The facial features are understood to be the result of alcohol's effect on the neural crest cells that migrate to form the affected parts of the face. Work by Astley and Clarren in 1995 identified three discriminating features that are now known to be the cardinal facial findings, these being short palpebral fissures, thin upper lip, and smooth philtrum [11]. Through their development of the 4-digit diagnostic code, Astley and Clarren developed a scoring system for assessment of the lip and philtrum individually on a 5-point scale [4] which is now widely used across the majority of diagnostic systems.

The optic vesicles begin at the end of the fourth week of gestation as outpouchings of the developing forebrain and extend to the surface ectoderm to induce development of the eye [3]. The palpebral fissure length is correlated to the size of the globe and hence is influenced by changes in forebrain development that can be the result of prenatal alcohol exposure. In addition to their correlation with underlying forebrain anomalies, palpebral fissure measurements are clearly the most objective of the three facial features to obtain and require a direct measurement using a clear plastic ruler. The left palpebral fissure is ideally suited for this measurement because the 0-point on the ruler can be placed directly over the inner canthus. The ruler must be placed as close to the eye as possible to reduce the parallax error, without touching the globe or the eyelashes to prevent blinking (Fig. 9.2). Parallax error occurs when the viewer is attempting to align the two canthi along the scale of a ruler placed too anterior to the subject resulting in a falsely enlarged palpebral fissure length. The subject is asked to look in an upward gaze to elevate the lateral portion of the upper eyelid revealing the outer canthus, and the palpebral fissure is measured with the ruler following the natural posterior cant of the face from the inner to the outer canthus. It is best performed with the posterior aspect of the examiner's hand pressed against the zygomatic arch of the patient for better stability of the ruler, and the examiner's eye positioned perpendicular to the midpoint of the palpebral fissure measurement (Fig. 9.3). The measurement should then be plotted on a curve based on age, ideally in a population that matches the racial and ethnic background of the patient. A palpebral fissure measurement that falls at or below the 10th percentile is considered abnormal.

The philtrum and upper lip are derived from neural crest cells that migrate ventrally from the boundaries of the oral cavity and form the medial nasal and maxillary

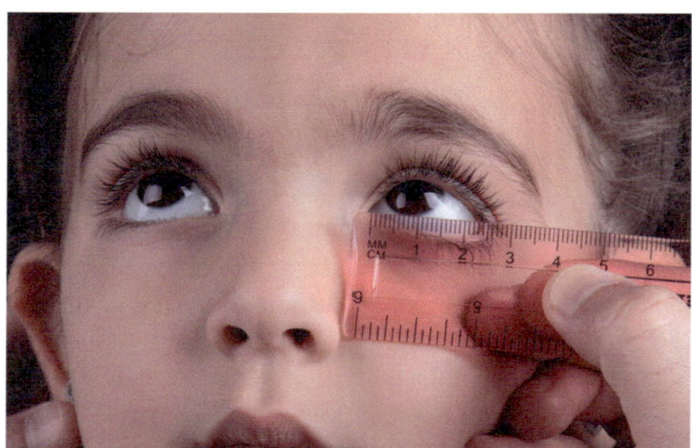

Fig. 9.2 Ruler placed as close to the eye as possible following the natural curve of the face

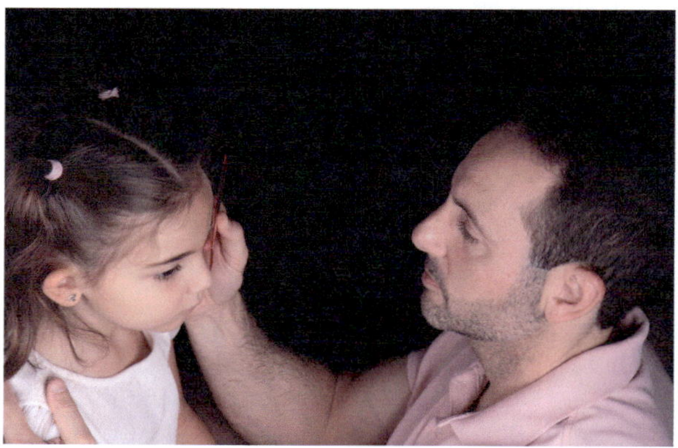

Fig. 9.3 Examiner at same level as subject viewing eye perpendicular to palpebral fissure

prominences [12]. The site of fusion of these two structures gives rise to the philtral columns with an intervening philtral groove (or dimple). The philtral columns represent the insertion site of the superficial fibers of the orbicularis oris muscle, with both ipsilateral and contralateral fibers creating tension and elevation of the columns. The upper lip has a similar underlying structure and is shaped like a cupid's bow, the peaks of which connect to the base of the philtral columns (Fig. 9.4). The lip and philtrum are individually assessed using a lip-philtrum guide (Fig. 9.5). The subject should be asked to provide a neutral expression, as smiling can cause flattening of the philtrum and thinning of the upper lip (Fig. 9.6). Several lip-philtrum guides have been developed for various populations, including Caucasian, African-American, and South African. The assessment should be performed in a well-lit location, but care must be taken to avoid bright lights aimed directly at the patient's face that can wash out the shadowing created by the philtral columns. Some lip-philtrum guides have provided a view of the face at a 45° angle to allow for appreciation of the elevation of the philtral columns, an important feature that provides additional cues to the examiner when scoring the philtrum (Fig. 9.7). A score of 1–5 is given depending on the elevation of the columns, how far they extend from the

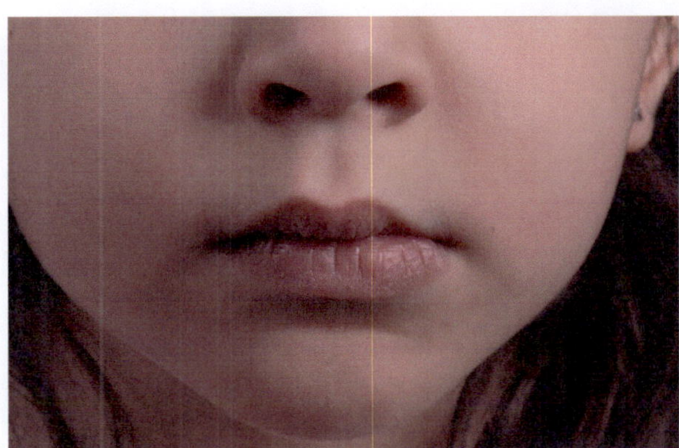

Fig. 9.4 Lip and philtrum observed in a subject with a neutral expression

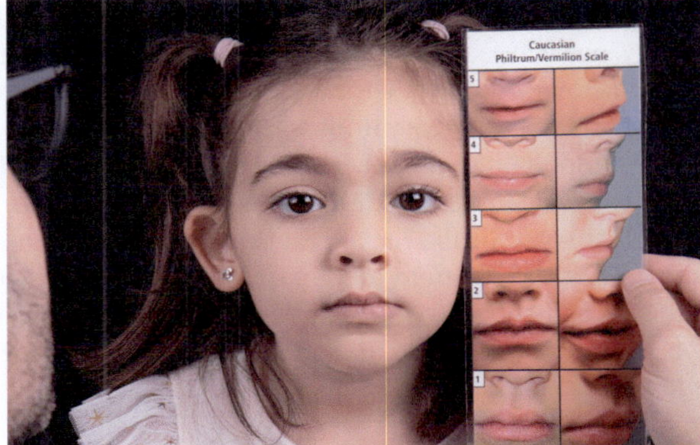

Fig. 9.5 Lip-philtrum guide placed alongside face for comparison and scoring

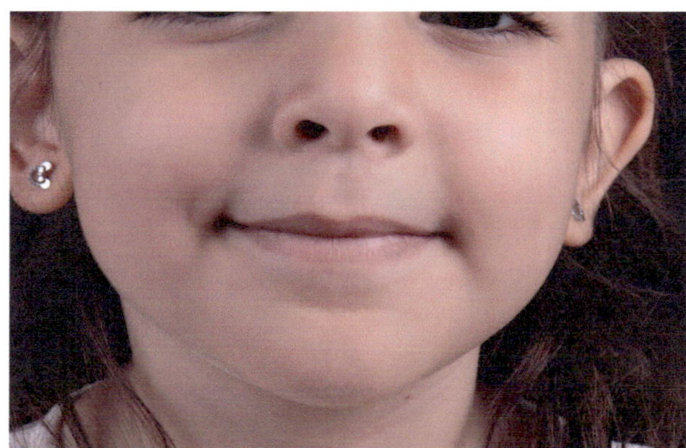

Fig. 9.6 Lip and philtrum observed in a smiling subject causing an increase in lip and philtrum scores

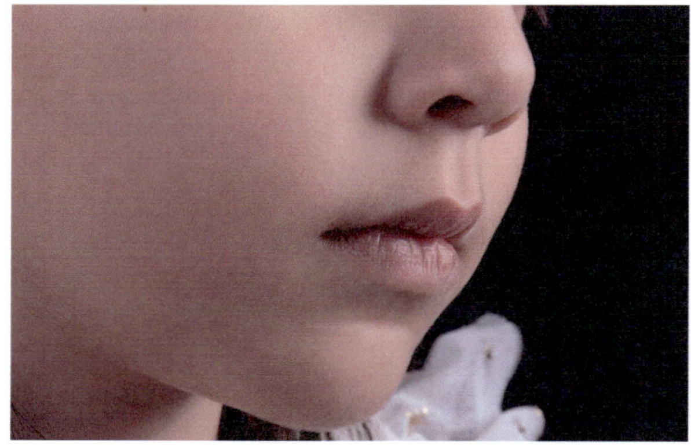

Fig. 9.7 Lip and philtrum viewed from a 45° angle to provide additional reference points for scoring

cupid's bow to the nasion, and how deep the philtral groove appears to be. The upper lip is then assessed separately, with considerations given for the volume of the upper lip, the height of the peaks of the cupid's bow, and the angle created between the two peaks of the cupid's bow. Again, a score of 1–5 is given for the upper lip. Generally, because the philtrum and upper lip are derived from similar embryonic origins, the score for the lip and philtrum will not differ by more than one point. Rarely, one can see a difference of 2 scores for the two structures, but these are often associated with some other malformation of the lip and/or philtrum such as significant shortening of the philtrum.

It is important to note that while school age is the ideal time to assess for facial features, evaluations in adulthood are not uncommon. Preliminary evidence suggests that some of the facial features can evolve with age [13]. For example, it is known that the philtrum and upper lip can elongate, creating less defined philtral columns and cupid's bow. Therefore, photographs taken of the individual at an earlier age may be useful to determine if the findings were present early on or may be age-related.

Measuring Growth

Growth in FASD was initially observed as uniformly impacted in all the early FAS cases. The growth pattern was noted to be of prenatal onset, but without any evidence of catch-up growth after birth. Additionally, the pattern of growth deficiency appeared to be greatest for length when compared to weight, an atypical finding if the mechanism is related to placental insufficiency [14]. Several animal models demonstrated the effect of alcohol exposure on epigenetic programming as a possible explanation for preferential length reduction. And the impact of alcohol on imprinted gene expression in placental samples has demonstrated alterations that correlate statistically with a reduction in length [15]. Although some of the recent guidelines (e.g., Canadian) have eliminated growth as a criterion due to studies showing that the effect of alcohol on growth is attenuated when adjusted for other factors [16], evidence remains that growth restriction of prenatal onset persisting into postnatal life is highly correlated with the degree of alcohol exposure and cognitive impairment [17].The Hoyme 2016 guidelines continue to use growth as an essential criterion for the diagnosis of fetal alcohol syndrome, and as a method of confirmation of partial fetal alcohol syndrome when prenatal alcohol exposure cannot be confirmed. Of note, given the population changes with weight over the last several decades, prenatal growth deficiency that improves after birth may be more representative of the effects of PAE with current nutritional status.

Use of population-specific growth charts is necessary to assess for deficiency in either height or weight. In the United States, WHO growth charts are recommended for use up to age 2 years for breastfed infants since the normative values were obtained in a primarily breastfed population. CDC growth charts are then recommended for use in children 2–18 years of age. The CDC growth charts in the first 2 years are based on a primarily formula-fed population; therefore, formula-fed children should be plotted on CDC growth charts throughout life. In other populations, country-specific normative values should be used when available. In the absence of population-specific data, WHO growth charts can be used.

Preterm birth is a known complication of prenatal alcohol exposure, and so growth deficiency in premature infants can only be determined by using appropriate growth charts. Previously, growth of premature infants was expected to follow the same trajectory as fetuses that remain in utero. It is now clear that the growth pattern for premature infants is different until 6 months corrected age, after which the infant can be tracked on growth charts for term newborns [18]. The International Fetal and Newborn Growth Consortium for the 21st Century (INTERGROWTH-21st) has developed growth charts beginning at 27 weeks postmenstrual age for preterm infants that should be used to assess for growth deficiency in this population.

Assessing the Neurological System

The earliest recognition of neurological abnormalities was presented by Sullivan in 1900 when he recognized that epilepsy occurred after prenatal alcohol exposure [19]. Specific malformations of the brain were first described by Smith and Jones in 1973 on a necropsy of an infant with FAS who died at 5 days of age [14]. The brain was small and demonstrated abnormal neuronal migration, lissencephaly, and absence of the corpus callosum. Early guidelines proposed by the IOM, the Canadian guidelines, and the Hoyme 2005 guidelines suggested including several findings reflective of the impact of alcohol on the brain, such as hard and soft neurological signs, microcephaly, agenesis of the corpus callosum, and cerebellar hypoplasia. Over the next decade, many of these findings were eliminated from various guidelines as the focus shifted to neurobehavioral impairment. However, the literature is consistent that findings within the central nervous system (CNS) remain a feature of FASD, and so the Hoyme 2016 guidelines continue to incorporate this as one of the criteria as part of the diagnosis of fetal alcohol syndrome or to make a diagnosis of partial fetal alcohol syndrome when prenatal alcohol exposure cannot be confirmed. In these guidelines, microcephaly, afebrile seizures, and structural brain malformations are considered as findings that would meet this criterion. It should be noted that in the absence of specific neurologic indications, neuroimaging is not routinely recommended in patients with suspected FASD as management is not likely to be altered based upon the findings. For a detailed review of the structural and functional imaging findings associated with FASD from group-based research studies, please see Chap. 10.

Neurobehavioral Impairment

Considerable research has documented neurobehavioral impairment associated with prenatal alcohol exposure over the last 40 years, as reviewed in Chap. 11. In 1973, the initial report described general developmental delay across all initial eight cases [14]. Subsequent criteria have elaborated more specific domains impacted showing more variability across children and adults with an FASD diagnosis. FASD diagnostic criterion for CNS or neurobehavioral impairment have become better specified over time as our knowledge of neuropsychological outcomes in this population has advanced. The prior iteration of the Hoyme criteria (2005) recognized that individuals with FASD often show a complex pattern of behavioral and cognitive abnormalities, often including difficulties with tasks requiring executive skills (e.g., problem solving, planning, judgment, arithmetic), higher-level receptive and expressive language, and disordered behavior (e.g., emotional dysregulation, social skills, academic performance) [20]. However, the number of domains or degree of impairment required to meet this criterion was not yet specified.

In the Hoyme 2016 criteria, neurobehavioral impairment is defined as functioning 1.5 standard deviations below the mean on standardized assessments (see Table 9.1 for examples to assess domains). For individuals 3 years and older, neurobehavioral impairment criterion can be met in one or of the following ways:

1. Evidence of global impairment: includes general conceptual ability, performance IQ, verbal IQ, and/or spatial IQ. Only one area is needed to meet criterion.
2. Evidence of specific cognitive deficit(s): domains include executive functioning, specific learning impairment, memory impairment, and/or visual-spatial impairment. For FAS and pFAS, only one domain is needed. For ARND, at least two domains are required.
3. Evidence of behavioral deficit(s) in self-regulation: domains include mood or behavioral regulation impairment, attention deficit, and/or impulse control. For FAS and pFAS, only one domain is needed. For ARND, at least two domains are required. Note that for many standardized measures of behavioral impairment, greater difficulties are reflected by higher scores, which would translate to scores 1.5 standard deviations above the mean.

Table 9.1 List of example standardized tests that can be used to assess neurobehavioral impairment in identified domains for fetal alcohol spectrum disorders

Domain	Example standardized tests
General cognitive ability	Wechsler Preschool and Primary Scale of Intelligence Wechsler Intelligence Scale for Children Differential Ability Scales
Memory	California Verbal Learning Test, Children's Edition Children's Memory Scale Wide Range Assessment of Memory and Learning NEPSY-II, Memory Subtests Rey Complex Figure Test
Executive functioning	Delis-Kaplan Executive Function System NEPSY-II, Executive Function Subtests Wisconsin Card Sorting Test WISC-V Working Memory Index
Visual-spatial	NEPSY-II, Visual-Spatial Subtests Developmental Test of Visual Motor Integration Rey Complex Figure Test
Learning	Wechsler Individual Achievement Test Woodcock Johnson Tests of Achievement
Attention, behavior regulation, impulse control	Conners Continuous Performance Test Test of Variables of Attention Child Behavior Checklist/Teacher Report Form Conners Third Edition Behavior Assessment System for Children Behavior Rating Inventory of Executive Function
Development (under 3 years; FAS/pFAS only)	Bayley Scales of Infant and Toddler Development

For children under 3 years of age, neurobehavioral impairment criterion can be met with evidence of developmental delay (1.5 standard deviations below the mean) for FAS or pFAS only. Children with documented prenatal alcohol exposure who do not meet criteria for FAS or pFAS should be monitored and additional assessments can be completed after age 3 to determine if they meet criteria for ARND.

A comprehensive neuropsychological assessment with adequate coverage of the above domains is optimal for FASD diagnosis and guiding recommendations and treatment planning for the individual and family. Selecting assessment tools that were developed and standardized with individuals of similar background (e.g., culture, language, geography) to the person being assessed facilitates norm-referenced decision-making about the degree of impairment. Clinical judgment is needed when the individual varies significantly from the normative sample. Incorporating multiple sources of information (e.g., parent and teacher report measures, observational data, clinical interviews) can complement 1:1 standardized testing and guide treatment planning.

In clinical settings when neuropsychological assessment is limited or not possible to obtain, psychoeducational and behavior assessments completed through the school district or other settings can sometimes yield sufficient evidence of neurobehavioral impairment for an FASD.

Putting It All Together to Render Diagnosis

Once all the data has been collected regarding prenatal alcohol exposure, growth, facial features, neurologic findings, and neurobehavioral impairment, the Hoyme guidelines can be applied to render a diagnosis (see decision tree in Hoyme 2016 guidelines). Although the individual features of FASD (e.g., short stature, developmental delay, microcephaly) are relatively common and can be attributed to a variety of medical, genetic, and developmental conditions, the *pattern* of findings is specific for FASD. When a multidisciplinary evaluation has been completed, a case conference is an ideal opportunity for full discussion of the case and determination of the presence or absence of a FASD diagnosis as well as alternate diagnoses or co-occurring diagnoses. When multidisciplinary conferencing is not possible or practical, a clinician with expertise in both FASD diagnoses and other genetic and developmental disorders who can effectively evaluate data in the five domains should lead the process of diagnostic determination by applying the diagnostic criteria to the patient-specific signs and symptoms.

The process of ruling in or ruling out a FASD diagnosis must include evaluation of both alternate explanations for symptomology (i.e., genetic disorder, hereditary short stature), as well as for the presence of conditions that may co-occur with FASD (i.e., anxiety, sleep, or trauma and stressor-related disorders), and would be important in treatment planning. Although the three cardinal facial features of FAS are most commonly associated with prenatal alcohol exposure, isolated overlapping features and other dysmorphology can also be seen in a variety of genetic and teratologic conditions (Hoyme 2005), necessitating consideration of additional genetic testing. The presence of co-occurring trauma- or anxiety-related disorders may result in overlapping neurobehavioral features, but are commonly seen in individuals with FASD, so should not be considered exclusionary.

There are a number of both major and minor anomalies (birth defects) that have been associated with PAE involving the cardiac, skeletal, renal, ocular, and auditory systems. A separate diagnostic category called alcohol-related birth defects (ARBD) was created to capture patients who have PAE and one or more of these birth defects. However, it is rarely used primarily because many patients who have PAE and a resulting birth defect typically meet one of the other diagnostic categories (FAS, PFAS, or ARND).

The role of genetic testing in individuals with suspected FASD is determined based on the clinical suspicion of the evaluator. The presence of both major and minor anomalies (birth defects) that have not been reported with PAE are an indicator that genetic testing may be indicated. Chromosomal microarray analysis is the predominant first-tier test that is most often covered by third-party payors. However, recent evidence suggests that whole exome sequencing and whole genome sequencing may now supplant the microarray giving data regarding both sequence changes in addition to chromosomal deletions or duplications. Consulting with a clinical geneticist on cases that have features atypical for FASD could be helpful in guiding genetic testing.

Giving Feedback to Families

Sharing the diagnosis with the individual with FASD and with parents, caregivers, or important support people is an important part of the evaluation process. It has been noted in a variety of diagnoses that the moment of sharing the diagnosis presents a key opportunity to affect the individual's (and likely the family's) perceptions of the disorder [21]. Feedback that utilizes a strengths-focused approach while avoiding stigma or shame provides a critical opening to facilitate diagnostic understanding, treatment planning, and positive developmental trajectories.

In FASD, the first challenge of feedback is determining to whom the feedback is being provided. For very young children, information about diagnosis is generally provided to the parents or caregivers, though caseworkers or others may be involved, depending upon circumstances. For school-aged children, many parents and caregivers prefer to receive diagnostic information first and then discuss strategies for sharing information, in a developmentally appropriate manner, with the child. For older school-age children and adolescents, it may be appropriate to allow the youth the option to participate in hearing feedback and diagnosis directly or to have their parents get the information and share it with them at another time. Adults should be provided the diagnosis directly, though should be encouraged to have a support person accompany them to assist with comprehension, asking follow-up questions, and recording information. The willingness of adolescents and young adults to be part of the feedback process, and the supports that may be required, will likely depend on factors such as attention, memory, processing speed, anxiety, and level of comfort and perceived support during the process.

There is a rich body of literature on sharing difficult news in medicine. Although the majority of the literature describes studies of physicians sharing life-limiting diagnoses with adult patients, many findings are relevant to sharing information about a developmental disability diagnosis with the affected individual or a parent or caregiver. Multiple different frameworks for sharing difficult news have been described, all with common features pertinent to FASD diagnosis, including (a) setting, (b) perceptions/understanding, (c) rapport-building, (d) clear communication of the important information, (e) empathy, and (f) summary/plan [21–23].

In the context of FASD, the setting may be considered to be the family context. A clear understanding of the family make-up, relationship between the individual with FASD and caregiver (i.e., biological parent, relative, foster/adoptive parent), as well as any family stressors such as parental incarceration or involvement of child protective services will allow the provider of feedback to do so in a way that is sensitive and non-stigmatizing. Next, the person providing feedback must have an understanding of the caregivers' perceptions of the child's problems. Many families enter the evaluation process with a belief or perception about the etiology of the child's difficulties that may or may not be accurate. Understanding this as well as the family's pre-evaluation beliefs and knowledge about PAE provides an important starting point for feedback.

In many situations, rapport may be established during the process of gathering history and completing the physical exam. Rapport can often be strengthened in a manner that supports the strengths-based approach to feedback by commenting on strengths of the individual, or positive aspects of the relationship between the individual and caregiver or family member. Once these factors are attended to, information about the FASD diagnosis can be provided. Provision of information can be aided by starting at the level of comprehension and vocabulary of the individual or caregiver, use of non-technical words, giving information in small chunks, and checking periodically for understanding [23]. For some families, talking through the five symptom areas (exposure itself, facial, growth, neurologic, and learning and behavior), and how they apply to the individual using a visual representation can facilitate understanding of the specific diagnosis.

After provision of information, it is critical that the provider check in on the emotional response of the individual and family and provide an empathetic response. Even for families who entered the evaluation process suspecting or expecting a FASD diagnosis, the provision of this information may lead to emotional reactions that may vary from silence to feeling overwhelmed, crying or anger. The act of observing and naming the emotion or use of open-ended questions to query the patient as to what they are thinking or feeling can be supportive to the family [23]. Finally, completing the session with a plan for next steps will allow the family to begin to move from their emotional response to the diagnosis toward some practical changes. It is important to remember that, following provision of diagnostic information, the ability of individuals and families to process and recall a significant amount of additional information may be limited, so clinicians may wish to use strategies such as giving a limited number of high priority recommendations, or providing families with initial recommendations in writing.

Barriers to Diagnosis

There are many barriers to diagnosis. The first barrier to diagnosis experienced by many individuals is the lack of information about prenatal alcohol exposure. Although it is possible to receive an FAS or pFAS diagnosis without confirmation of prenatal alcohol exposure when facial features and growth criteria are present, the majority of individuals do not present with these characteristics. Thus, many people with PAE go undiagnosed because PAE was never asked about or documented appropriately. There are several components to this challenge, starting in the preconception and the prenatal period. Despite guidelines recommending that all child-bearing-aged women be screened for alcohol use and provided brief interventions during the course of primary care [24], just one half to 2/3 of women in this age range receive routine preventative visits, and of those, only 70% report discussion of alcohol or drug use [25].

Similarly, during the prenatal and perinatal period, prenatal alcohol exposure may not be asked about at all, may be asked about in a manner that does not support accurate reporting, and/or may not be documented [26]. In fact, the evidence shows that accurate documentation of other substances such as cocaine, opiates, or marijuana is much more likely than documentation of alcohol use [27]. Finally, for children with FASD who are not in the care of a biological family member, access to information about health history and prenatal exposures can be particularly challenging, and this challenge increases incrementally with the number of different home placements [27]. Children in foster or adoptive care disproportionately lack confirmation of PAE required for diagnosing pFAS and ARND and have been noted to have a high rate of experiencing multiple different home placements when in care, which further compromises access to health information [27, 28].

Lack of awareness about FASD in health and social services settings is a second barrier that has been noted internationally, and across multiple studies [29, 30]. Lack of professional awareness can contribute to an inaccurate or missed diagnosis in a variety of ways. For example, clinicians may fail to recognize an individual's symptoms as atypical (for example, when a parent reports severe tantrums in a toddler or preschooler). Alternately, when concerning symptoms are recognized, clinicians may fail to recognize the pattern as being suggestive of an over-arching and diagnosable disorder or may mis-diagnose symptoms as a disorder they are more familiar with. Others may fail to appreciate the benefits of having a FASD diagnosis, so may not adequately consider this possibility [31–33].

Even when a FASD is suspected, affected individuals experience barriers in accessing diagnostic services due to a shortage of trained clinicians as well as financial and geographic barriers. Studies of diagnostic capacity in the U.S., Canada, and internationally show wide variability in access to diagnostic clinics in different regions with none having sufficient capacity to meet estimated need. For example, Clarren, Lutke, and Sherbuck described diagnostic capacity across Canada in 2011, estimating the national capacity for diagnosis of 2288 evaluations per year, with 0.21–5.85 diagnostic slots per 10,000 people per year. In the United States, many states lack even a single diagnostic center while prevalence rates have been estimated in the 1.1–5% range among first graders [34].

Funding represents an additional barrier. In a descriptive report of 14 clinics in 11 U.S. states, most sites relied on research grants or state/federal funding to operate, while other sources included fee for service and insurance. Insurance coverage of services including neuropsychological testing required to establish a diagnosis represents an additional barrier.

Stigma, the final barrier to diagnosis described herein, could be considered a barrier by itself, but could also be considered as a contributing factor to all the previously described barriers. Stigma about FASD and about alcohol use in general leads people to avoid talking with family, friends, and health care providers about prenatal alcohol exposure. Stigma causes clinicians to avoid discussion of alcohol use with their patients. Stigma contributes to general low community awareness about PAE and FASD in health and human services fields that interact with pregnant or potentially pregnant people, or children and adults who may be affected by FASD. In pediatric care, stigma deters pediatric health care providers from asking parents about PAE. Clinicians may also avoid giving a FASD diagnosis due to the stigma associated with the diagnosis itself. Once a diagnosis is established, caregivers (especially birth parents) may avoid sharing the diagnosis with others supporting the child due to the stigma.

Practical Suggestions for Providers

Clinicians of all disciplines can contribute to improving access to diagnosis and care for individuals affected by FASD by activities such as increasing awareness in one's organization, increasing one's own knowledge about FASD and skills in diagnostic assessment, and by connecting with others engaged in FASD work. The following resources are suggested for clinicians interested in this work:

Diagnostic curricula
Pan American Health Organization. (2020). *Assessment of Fetal Alcohol Spectrum Disorders: A Training Workbook*. Washington, DC. License: CC BY-NC-SA 3.9 IGO. Available at: https://iris.paho.org/handle/10665.2/52216
FASD Regional Training Centers Curriculum Development Team. (2015). *Fetal Alcohol Spectrum Disorders Competency-based curriculum development guide for medical and allied health education and practice*. Retrieved from Centers for Disease Control and Prevention website: https://www.cdc.gov/ncbddd/fasd/curriculum/index.html
Tools for diagnosis

Ordering lip-philtrum guide and ruler for measurement of palpebral fissure length: https://depts.washington.edu/fasdpn/htmls/order-forms.htm Also available in the Hoyme 2016 updated clinical guidelines.
Facial measurement training tools: https://depts.washington.edu/fasdpn/htmls/photo-face.htm
Screening, diagnosis and health care
American Academy of Pediatrics FASD Toolkit: https://www.aap.org/fasd
Centers for Disease Control online trainings: https://www.cdc.gov/ncbddd/fasd/index.html
SAMHSA Treatment Improvement Protocol (TIP #58) Fetal Alcohol Spectrum Disorders: https://www.samhsa.gov/resource/ebp/tip-58-addressing-fetal-alcohol-spectrum-disorders-fasd
Expand awareness and knowledge about FASD
FASD United (Formerly NOFAS) and affiliates: https://fasdunited.org/
National Institute on Alcohol Abuse and Alcoholism: https://www.niaaa.nih.gov/
Collaborative Initiative on Fetal Alcohol Spectrum Disorders (CIFASD): https://cifasd.org
Canadian Fetal Alcohol Spectrum Disorder Network (CanFASD): https://canfasd.ca/
National Organization for Fetal Alcohol Spectrum Disorder (NOFASD) Australia: https://www.nofasd.org.au/
National FASD (UK): https://nationalfasd.org.uk/
FASD Ireland: https://www.fasdireland.ie/
FASD Collaborative: https://www.fasdcollaborative.com/

Future Directions

There are a number of advances that have been made to solve several issues around the evaluation of patients for FASD given the many barriers that exist today. Firstly, there is a concerted effort funded by the National Institutes on Alcohol Abuse and Alcoholism (NIAAA) to harmonize all of the various diagnostic criteria through the Collaborative Initiate on Fetal Alcohol Spectrum Disorders (CIFASD). There are a number of projects underway to increase the limited capacity for centers to screen and evaluate individuals for FASD. One such project that is part of CIFASD is centered around the development of an electronic version of the FASD decision tree (known as eTree) in a web-based format that can be used to screen lower risk populations and measure domains known to be affected in FASD [35, 36]. The goal of eTree is to identify at-risk individuals who require further diagnostic assessment. Telemedicine has been deployed to expand the reach of various centers that have expertise in FASD [37]. Alternatively, Project ECHO (Extension for Community Healthcare Outcomes) is a well-known innovative training and mentoring model that has been used to increase competence of community providers in the care of people with various common but complex chronic conditions. The model uses secure, low-cost, and widely available videoconferencing to link clinicians in underserved communities with an interdisciplinary team of specialists at academic medical centers during virtual *"teleECHO"* sessions where case-based learning and co-management are utilized to provide education in best-practice assessment and treatment protocols [38]. Several groups are currently testing the use of ECHO for improving awareness, screening, and diagnosis of FASD. Recently, Project ECHO has been used successfully by the authors to expand capacity of FASD diagnostics in both the US [39] and in South America.

Assessment of prenatal alcohol exposure continues to involve biomarker investigation discussed in Chaps. 4 and 5, though none is routinely used on a clinical basis at the current time. Given the challenges of making an ARND diagnosis (requiring both confirmation of PAE and extensive neurodevelopmental testing), artificial intelligence has been deployed in facial image analysis of both two- and three-dimensional images. The literature suggests there is significant success of these systems to recognize sub-clinical features of ARND that have not been previously identified [5, 6, 40]. It is expected that technology will continue to find novel ways of evaluating patients and improving access on a global scale.

References

1. Hoyme HE, Kalberg WO, Elliott AJ, Blankenship J, Buckley D, Marais AS, et al. Updated clinical guidelines for diagnosing fetal alcohol spectrum disorders. Pediatrics. 2016;138(2):e20154256.
2. Coles CD, Gailey AR, Mulle JG, Kable JA, Lynch ME, Jones KL. A comparison among 5 methods for the clinical diagnosis of fetal alcohol spectrum disorders. Alcohol Clin Exp Res. 2016;40(5):1000–9.
3. Jones KL, Hoyme HE, Robinson LK, del Campo M, Manning MA, Bakhireva LN, et al. Developmental pathogenesis of short palpebral fissure length in children with fetal alcohol syndrome. Birt Defects Res A Clin Mol Teratol. 2009;85(8):695–9.
4. Astley SJ, Clarren SK. Diagnosing the full spectrum of fetal alcohol-exposed individuals: introducing the 4-digit diagnostic code. Alcohol Alcohol. 2000;35(4):400–10.
5. Valentine M, Bihm DCJ, Wolf L, Hoyme HE, May PA, Buckley D, et al. Computer-aided recognition of facial attributes for fetal alcohol spectrum disorders. Pediatrics. 2017;140(6):e20162028.
6. Suttie M, Wozniak JR, Parnell SE, Wetherill L, Mattson SN, Sowell ER, et al. Combined face–brain morphology and associated neurocognitive correlates in fetal alcohol spectrum disorders. Alcohol Clin Exp Res. 2018;42(9):1769–82.
7. Jones KL, Smith DW. The fetal alcohol syndrome. Teratology. 1975;12(1):1–10.
8. Skagerström J, Alehagen S, Häggström-Nordin E, Årestedt K, Nilsen P. Prevalence of alcohol use before and during pregnancy and predictors of drinking during pregnancy: a cross sectional study in Sweden. BMC Public Health. 2013;13(1):780.
9. Saunders JB, Aasland OG, Babor TF, de la Fuente JR, Grant M. Development of the Alcohol Use Disorders Identification Test (AUDIT): WHO Collaborative Project on early detection of persons with harmful alcohol consumption—II. Addiction (Abingdon, England). 1993;88(6):791–804.
10. Branum AM, Ahrens KA. Trends in timing of pregnancy awareness among US women. Matern Child Health J. 2017;21(4):715–26.
11. Astley SJ, Clarren SK. A fetal alcohol syndrome screening tool. Alcohol Clin Exp Res. 1995;19(6):1565–71.
12. Jiang R, Bush JO, Lidral AC. Development of the upper lip: morphogenetic and molecular mechanisms. Dev Dyn. 2006;235(5):1152–66.

13. Jacobson SW, Hoyme HE, Carter RC, Dodge NC, Molteno CD, Meintjes EM, et al. Evolution of the physical phenotype of fetal alcohol spectrum disorders from childhood through adolescence. Alcohol Clin Exp Res. 2021;45(2):395–408.
14. Jones KL, Smith DW. Recognition of the fetal alcohol syndrome in early infancy. Lancet (London, England). 1973;302(7836):999–1001.
15. Carter RC, Chen J, Li Q, Deyssenroth M, Dodge NC, Wainwright HC, et al. Alcohol-related alterations in placental imprinted gene expression in humans mediate effects of prenatal alcohol exposure on postnatal growth. Alcohol Clin Exp Res. 2018;42:1431.
16. O'Leary CM, Nassar N, Kurinczuk JJ, Bower C. The effect of maternal alcohol consumption on fetal growth and preterm birth. BJOG Int J Obstet Gynaecol. 2009;116(3):390–400.
17. Carter RC, Jacobson JL, Molteno CD, Dodge NC, Meintjes EM, Jacobson SW. Fetal alcohol growth restriction and cognitive impairment. Pediatrics. 2016;138(2):e20160775.
18. Villar J, Giuliani F, Barros F, Roggero P, Coronado Zarco IA, Rego MAS, et al. Monitoring the postnatal growth of preterm infants: a paradigm change. Pediatrics. 2018;141(2):e20172467.
19. Sullivan WC. A note on the influence of maternal inebriety on the offspring. 1899. Int J Epidemiol. 2011;40(2):278–82.
20. Hoyme HE, May PA, Kalberg WO, Kodituwakku P, Gossage JP, Trujillo PM, et al. A practical clinical approach to diagnosis of fetal alcohol spectrum disorders: clarification of the 1996 institute of medicine criteria. Pediatrics. 2005;115(1):39–47.
21. Ledford CJW, Seehusen DA, Cafferty LA, Rider HA, Rogers T, Fulleborn S, et al. Diabetes ROADMAP: teaching guideline use, communication, and documentation when delivering the diagnosis of diabetes. MedEdPORTAL. 2020;16:10959.
22. Edwards WF, Malik S, Peters J, Chippendale I, Ravits J. Delivering bad news in amyotrophic lateral sclerosis: proposal of specific technique ALS ALLOW. Neurol Clin Pract. 2021;11(6):521–6.
23. Baile WF, Buckman R, Lenzi R, Glober G, Beale EA, Kudelka AP. SPIKES—a six-step protocol for delivering bad news: application to the patient with cancer. Oncologist. 2000;5(4):302–11.
24. Floyd RL, Jack BW, Cefalo R, Atrash H, Mahoney J, Herron A, et al. The clinical content of preconception care: alcohol, tobacco, and illicit drug exposures. Am J Obstet Gynecol. 2008;199(6 Suppl B):S333–9.
25. Long M, Frederiksen B, Ranji U. Women's health care utilization and costs: findings from the 2020 KFF Women's Health Survey. KFF; 2021 [cited 2022 Jul 11]. Available from: https://www.kff.org/womens-health-policy/issue-brief/womens-health-care-utilization-and-costs-findings-from-the-2020-kff-womens-health-survey/.
26. Chiodo LM, Cosmian C, Pereira K, Kent N, Sokol RJ, Hannigan JH. Prenatal alcohol screening during pregnancy by midwives and nurses. Alcohol Clin Exp Res. 2019;43(8):1747–58.
27. Astley SJ. Profile of the first 1,400 patients receiving diagnostic evaluations for fetal alcohol spectrum disorder at the Washington State Fetal Alcohol Syndrome Diagnostic & Prevention Network. Can J Clin Pharmacol. 2010;17(1):e132–64.
28. Bakhireva LN, Garrison L, Shrestha S, Sharkis J, Miranda R, Rogers K. Challenges of diagnosing fetal alcohol spectrum disorders in foster and adopted children. Alcohol. 2018;67:37–43.
29. Lange S, Shield K, Rehm J, Popova S. Prevalence of fetal alcohol spectrum disorders in child care settings: a meta-analysis. Pediatrics. 2013;132(4):e980–95.
30. Salmon J. Fetal alcohol spectrum disorder: New Zealand birth mothers' experiences. J Popul Ther Clin Pharmacol. 2008;15(2) [cited 2022 Jul 11]. Available from: https://www.jptcp.com.
31. Chasnoff IJ, Wells AM, King L. Misdiagnosis and missed diagnoses in foster and adopted children with prenatal alcohol exposure. Pediatrics. 2015;135(2):264–70.
32. O'Connor MJ, Best A. Under recognition of prenatal alcohol exposure in a child inpatient psychiatric setting. Ment Health Asp Dev Disabil. 2006;9(4):5.
33. Petrenko CLM, Tahir N, Mahoney EC, Chin NP. Prevention of secondary conditions in fetal alcohol spectrum disorders: identification of systems-level barriers. Matern Child Health J. 2014;18(6):1496–505.

34. May PA, Chambers CD, Kalberg WO, Zellner J, Feldman H, Buckley D, et al. Prevalence of fetal alcohol Spectrum disorders in 4 US communities. JAMA. 2018;319(5):474–82.
35. Goh PK, Doyle LR, Glass L, Jones KL, Riley EP, Coles CD, et al. A decision tree to identify children affected by prenatal alcohol exposure. J Pediatr. 2016;177:121–127.e1.
36. Bernes GA, Courchesne-Krak NS, Hyland MT, Villodas MT, Coles CD, Kable JA, et al. Development and validation of a postnatal risk score that identifies children with prenatal alcohol exposure. Alcohol Clin Exp Res. 2022;46(1):52–65.
37. Del Campo M, Beach D, Wells A, Jones KL. Use of telemedicine for the physical examination of children with fetal alcohol spectrum disorders. Alcohol Clin Exp Res. 2021;45(2):409–17.
38. Arora S, Kalishman S, Thornton K, Dion D, Murata G, Deming P, et al. Expanding access to hepatitis C virus treatment—Extension for Community Healthcare Outcomes (ECHO) project: disruptive innovation in specialty care. Hepatology. 2010;52(3):1124–33.
39. Cole L. ECHO FASD: tele-mentoring program to increase healthcare capacity for fetal alcohol Spectrum disorder (FASD) diagnosis. Rochester, NY: University of Rochester School of Nursing; 2021.
40. Suttie M, Foroud T, Wetherill L, Jacobson JL, Molteno CD, Meintjes EM, et al. Facial dysmorphism across the fetal alcohol spectrum. Pediatrics. 2013;131(3):e779–88.

Chapter 10
Neuroimaging Findings in FASD Across the Lifespan

Madeline N. Rockhold, Kirsten A. Donald, Carson Kautz-Turnbull, and Christie L. M. Petrenko

Introduction

Prenatal alcohol exposure (PAE) has a wide range of effects on the developing embryo and fetus, including changes in brain structure and function. Over the last three decades, an increasing literature has described changes in more traditional metrics of structure and brain volume as well as alterations in the connections between regions, structural and resting-state functional networks, and differences in regional recruitment during specific task based functional outcomes in children and adolescents exposed to alcohol prenatally. These unique changes in the brain can lead to cognitive, behavioral, and adaptive functioning differences across development [1]. Fetal alcohol spectrum disorders (FASD) includes a range of specifically defined conditions that can include facial characteristics, neurological effects, and neurobehavioral impairment following PAE. Depending on the constellation of symptoms present, FASD encompasses fetal alcohol syndrome (FAS), partial FAS (pFAS), and alcohol-related neurodevelopmental disorder (ARND) [2]. Individuals with FASD exhibit important strengths including social motivation, self-awareness, perseverance, and hope, among many others [3]. FASD is one of the most common neurodevelopmental disorders in the United States, affecting 2–5% of the population [4]. The global prevalence rate of FASD is 7.7 per 1000 children, with the prevalence in special populations (children in care, corrections, special education,

M. N. Rockhold · C. Kautz-Turnbull · C. L. M. Petrenko (✉)
Mt. Hope Family Center, University of Rochester, Rochester, NY, USA
e-mail: mrockhol@ur.rochester.edu; ckautz@ur.rochester.edu;
christie.petrenko@rochester.edu

K. A. Donald
Division of Developmental Paediatrics, Department of Paediatrics and Child Health, Red Cross War Memorial Children's Hospital, Cape Town, South Africa

Neuroscience Institute, University of Cape Town, Cape Town, South Africa
e-mail: Kirsty.donald@uct.ac.za

© The Author(s), under exclusive license to Springer Nature Switzerland AG 2023
O. A. Abdul-Rahman, C. L. M. Petrenko (eds.), *Fetal Alcohol Spectrum Disorders*,
https://doi.org/10.1007/978-3-031-32386-7_10

specialized clinical, and other communities with increased risk for PAE) globally being 10–40 times higher [5]. PAE is therefore a significant global public health problem. Given this impact of PAE, understanding the range of structural and functional brain alterations associated with this exposure across the life-course, and in different cultures and geographies, remains an important area of research.

The first glimpse into the inner workings of the brain of individuals with FASD occurred in the mid-1970s with the original autopsy studies showing abnormalities (including agenesis) of the corpus callosum, incomplete development of the cerebral cortex, and microcephaly [6–8]. The advent of non-invasive neuroimaging techniques in the 1970s and 1980s allowed for a greater depth of understanding and a deeper look into brain–behavior relationships. The first case reports and studies including MRIs of children with FASD were published in the early- to mid-1990s and reflected the findings of the original autopsy studies while also demonstrating smaller volumes in the basal ganglia, cerebral vault, brain stem, and thalamus [9–13]. Since that time and with wider access to and large advances in MRI technology, the breadth and knowledge of neuroimaging have expanded immensely, and the field has been able to reach a deeper understanding of the neuropsychological underpinnings of FASD. This review will demonstrate those findings and show the impressive work done globally to reach a better understanding of the inner workings of the prenatally exposed brain.

Methods

A literature search was conducted in both PsycINFO and PubMed databases to identify published studies. Combinations of the following keywords were utilized: fetal alcohol spectrum disorders, prenatal alcohol exposure, FAS, FASD, PAE, neuroimaging, MRI, fMRI, DTI, MRS, infant, child, adolescent, adult. Search criteria were limited to the abstract and title. All abstracts were screened for relevance. Inclusion criteria were met if the article was published in a peer-reviewed journal, was published in English, stated confirmed PAE or FASD diagnosis, and focused on neuroimaging. Articles were excluded for a focus on animal research or a lack of a control group comparison. The search included all articles published before September 8, 2021. In the original search, 102 articles were identified. After duplicates and those not meeting inclusion criteria were removed, a total of 85 articles were utilized for this review.

The majority of the studies originated in the US, with clusters of studies in the Western Cape of South Africa and Europe. There are large portions of the globe that are not represented in literature on FASD imaging (see Fig. 10.1). The range of ages studied in these samples spanned from infancy to young adulthood. Articles were divided into four different sections, based on either findings within certain types of brain matter (white matter, cortex/deep gray matter, cerebellum) or modality (functional imaging). These findings are shown in Tables 10.1, 10.2, 10.3, and 10.4. In sections where there was enough literature available for meaningful examination by developmental stage, the section was further subdivided based on the mean age of study participants. For those articles with a wide age range, the mean age of the PAE group was used for categorization. For a list of commonly used abbreviations and their accompanying meanings, see Table 10.5.

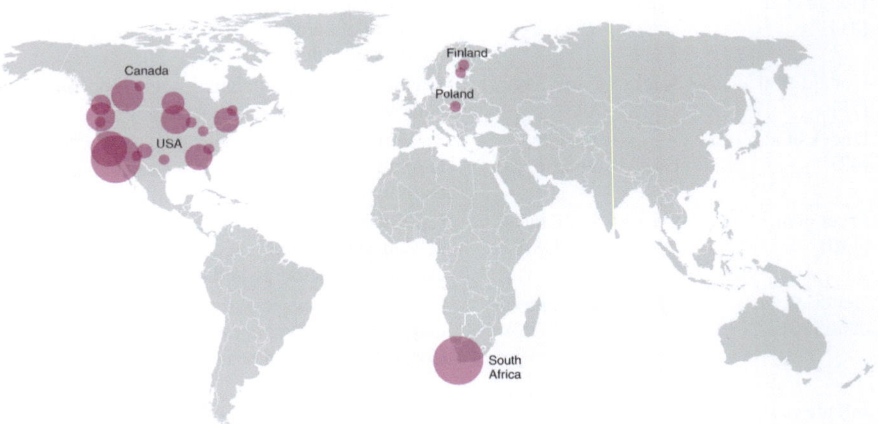

Fig. 10.1 Locations of FASD imaging studies across the globe, with the size of the circle indicating the number of studies originating from the area indicated. (Courtesy of James A. Perkins)

Table 10.1 Cortex and deep gray matter imaging findings in FASD

Reference	Age	Location	Main finding
Archibald et al. [18]	7–24 years	San Diego, CA USA	Parietal volume more affected than temporal and occipital volumes Reduced volume in basal ganglia, caudate nucleus Hippocampus mainly unaffected
Astley et al. [23]	8–16 years	Seattle, WA, USA	Smaller total brain volume Smaller frontal lobe Smaller caudate, putamen, hippocampus
Chen et al. [19]	23 years[a]	Atlanta, GA, USA	Smaller occipital and temporal region volumes
De Guio et al. [32]	9 years	Cape Town, SA	Reduction in cortical folding related to increase in PAE
de Water et al. [21]	8–16 years	Minneapolis, MN, USA	Smaller precuneus and lateral orbitofrontal cortex volumes
Dodge et al. [41]	9–10 years	Cape Town, SA	Smaller hippocampal volumes Smaller volumes associated with spatial navigation deficits
Donald et al. [33]	2–4 weeks	Cape Town, SA	Smaller amygdala, thalamus, and hippocampal volumes
Dudek et al. [42]	11–14 years	Toronto, Ontario, CA	Smaller hippocampal volumes Hippocampal volume reduction related to memory challenges
Fryer et al. [110]	9–21 years	San Diego, CA, USA	Caudate volume best predictor of neuropsychological functioning, specifically executive functioning and learning ability
Hendrickson et al. [30]	9–16 years	Multiple sites in the USA	Significantly lower cortical gyrification across majority of cerebral cortex Cortical gyrification positively correlated with IQ scores
Infante et al. [31]	12–16 years	San Diego, CA, USA	Reduce gyrification in various areas of the cortex including parietal, postcentral, precentral, and lateral occipital regions
Joseph et al. [38]	11 years[a]	Cape Town, SA	Left hippocampus and bilateral caudate volume reduced Significant shape differences in hippocampus and caudate nucleus
Krueger et al. [34]	8–16 years	Minneapolis, MN, USA	Smaller volumes in the caudate, hippocampus, and putamen
Little et al. [48]	5–18 years	Alberta, CA	Developed a multivariate model to distinguish FASD from control groups based on volumetric imaging data and reached 77% accuracy
Mattson et al. [36]	8–19 years	San Diego, CA, USA	Volume reductions in the basal ganglia, caudate nucleus, and diencephalon
Meintjes et al. [46]	9–11 years	Cape Town, SA	All significant volumetric decrease findings lost when controlling for total intercranial volume (thalamus, cerebellum, midbrain, frontal lobe, occipital lobe, parietal lobe)

Table 10.1 (continued)

Reference	Age	Location	Main finding
Migliorini et al. [24]	15 years[a]	San Diego, CA, USA	Surface area reductions in anterior cingulate cortex related to performance on inhibition tasks
Miles et al. [20]	9–14 years	Cape Town, SA	Reductions in the left interparietal sulcus associated with reductions in arithmetic skills
Nardelli et al. [15]	6–17 years	Alberta, CA	Overall deep gray matter structures show a 13% reduction in volume No significant volumetric differences in the amygdala Caudate, global pallidus, hippocampus, putamen all have significant volume reductions
Rajaprakash et al. [47]	8–15 years	Toronto, Ontario, CA	All significant volume reductions lost when controlling for total intercranial volume (frontal lobe, left parietal lobe, right temporal lobe)
Roediger et al. [43]	8–16 years	Minneapolis, MN, USA	Reductions in volume of multiple subfields in the hippocampus (CA1, CA4, presubiculum, subiculum, hippocampal tail)
Roussotte et al. [16]	12 years[a]	Los Angeles, CA, USA	Reduced volume in the global pallidus, diencephalon, overall gray matter Smaller palpebral fissure length associated with smaller diencephalon
Sowell et al. [27]	8–22 years	San Diego, CA, USA	Increase in cortical thickness in lateral surface of all four lobes that can be as large as 1.2 mm This difference is associated with palpebral fissure length Thinner prefrontal gray matter associated with learning difficulties
Sowell et al. [26]	8–22 years	San Diego, CA, USA	Significant volume decreases in parietal, frontal, temporal lobes
Sowell et al. [29]	8–22 years	San Diego, CA, USA	Cortical surface gray matter hemispheric asymmetry most pronounced in temporal lobe
Willoughby et al. [44]	9–15 years	Ontario, CA	Significant volume reduction in left hippocampus Hippocampal volume reductions associated with memory difficulties
Yang et al. [28]	13 years[a]	Cape Town, CA	Significant increase in cortical thickness Increased cortical thickness associated with smaller palpebral fissure length
Zhou et al. [17]	5–18 years	Multiple sites in CA	Significant volume reductions in overall gray matter volume Significant reductions in frontal, parietal, occipital, and temporal lobe areas
Zhou et al. [25]	5–18 years	Multiple sites in CA	Significant volume reductions in total gray matter volume, bilateral cortical gray matter, and cerebellum Significant reductions in cortical thickness in frontal, parietal, occipital, and temporal areas

FASD fetal alcohol spectrum disorder; *PAE* prenatal alcohol exposure
[a] Age range not given, mean age noted

Table 10.2 White matter imaging findings in FASD

Reference	Age	Location	Main finding
Anna Dylaq et al. [59]	8 years[a]	Krakow, Poland	Corpus callosum significantly more narrow Narrowing 20.7% more
Bookstein et al. [71]	18+ years[a]	Seattle, WA, USA	Callosal midline shape has more variability
Bookstein et al. [49]	14–37 years[a]	Seattle, WA, USA	Shape and location of corpus callosum more variable in adolescents Same result found in adults, indicating a "permanent" record of prenatal alcohol exposure
Bookstein et al. [51]	<17 weeks	Seattle, WA, USA	Angle between terminal bulb of splenium and the long axis of callosal outline were different in 4/7ths of the exposed infants compared to unexposed infants
Bookstein et al. [52]	1.4–16.7 weeks	Seattle, WA, USA	Presence of a "hook" in between the splenium and the arch of the corpus callosum
Candelaria-Cook et al. [61]	8–12 years	Albuquerque, NM, USA	Overall reduction in corpus callosum connectivity
Donald et al. [54]	2–4 weeks	Cape Town, SA	Presence of altered microstructure in the right inferior cerebellar peduncle This alteration is associated with infant neurobehavioral outcomes in the first week of life
Fan et al. [62]	9–11 years	Cape Town, SA	Lower FA in left and right inferior longitudinal fasciculi, splenium, and isthmus of corpus callosum Higher MD in a multitude of white matter regions White matter damage mediated effects of PAE on information processing speed and eyeblink conditions
Fryer et al. [68]	8–18 years	San Diego, CA, USA	Lower FA in multiple areas Less group differences in mean diffusivity Higher MD in right temporo-parieto-occipital junction and left superior frontal lobe
Gautam et al. [57]	6–17 years	Cape Town, SA	Significantly smaller volumes in corpus callosum and overall white matter An increase in white matter volumes over time is associated with an increase of executive functioning ability
Green et al. [67]	6–40 days	Edmonton, Alberta, CA	Altered white matter brain regions related to oculomotor control problems
Jacobson et al. [50]	2–7 years	Cape Town, SA	Significantly smaller corpus callosum
Kar et al. [63]	23 years[a]	Alberta, CA	FA higher in the genus of the corpus callosum MD lower in bilateral uncinate fasciculus

Table 10.2 (continued)

Reference	Age	Location	Main finding
Li et al. [69]	18–25 years	Atlanta, GA, USA	Significant decrease in FA at isthmus of the corpus callosum
Ma et al. [70]	5–18 years	Atlanta, GA, USA	Decreased FA in genu and splenium of corpus callosum
Paolozza et al. [64]	8–18 years	Multiple sites in CA	Significantly higher MD in splenium
Paolozza et al. [65]	2–3 years	Multiple sites in CA	Decreased FA in genu, body, splenium of corpus callosum, right corticospinal tract, and three left hemisphere tracts connecting to the frontal lobe
Riley et al. [12]	9–14 years	San Diego, CA, USA	Reduced corpus callosum area
Roos et al. [55]	6–17 years	Cape Town, SA	Lower FA in uncinate fasciculus
Schneble et al. [60]	0–44 years	Multiple sites in USA	No significant difference in corpus callosum notches
Taylor et al. [53]	36–44 weeks	Cape Town, SA	Lower MD and AD in R-ASSOC, L-ASSOC, L-PROJ, R-PROJ, and corona radiata Lower FA in R-ASSOC
Wozniak et al. [58]	10–13 years	Minneapolis, MN, USA	No significant difference in white matter volume Significantly higher MD in isthmus of corpus callosum
Yang et al. [56]	8–16 years	Cape Town, SA	Significant reductions in overall white matter volumes, callosal thickness, and corpus callosum area

FASD fetal alcohol spectrum disorder, *FA* fractional anisotropy, *MD* medial diffusivity, *AD* axial diffusivity, *R-ASSOC* right hemisphere association fibers, *L-ASSOC* left hemisphere association fibers, *R-PROJ* right hemisphere projection fibers, *L-PROJ* left hemisphere projection fibers
[a] Age range not given, mean age noted

Table 10.3 Cerebellum imaging findings in FASD

Reference	Age	Location	Main finding
Fan et al. [80]	10 years[a]	Cape Town, SA	Lower FA in superior cerebellar peduncles Higher MD in left middle peduncle Both lower FA and higher MD associated with poorer eyeblink conditioning performance
Inkelis et al. [75]	13–30 years	Seattle, WA, USA	Smaller cerebellar volume Males show larger volumes than females
O'Hare et al. [77]	8–22 years	Multiple sites in USA	Significantly reduced area of anterior vermis Vermal displacement correlated with learning ability
Sowell et al. [78]	8–22 years	San Diego, CA, USA	Significant reduction in anterior region of the vermis No significant differences in posterior vermis
Spottiswoode et al. [79]	11 years[a]	Cape Town, SA	Lower FA in left middle cerebellar peduncle Performance on trace conditioning task related to higher FA and perpendicular diffusivity Higher FA and lower PD related to performance on trace conditioning tasks
Sullivan et al. [76]	20 years[a]	Seattle, WA, USA	Significantly smaller cerebellum white and gray matter volume

FASD fetal alcohol spectrum disorder, *FA* fractional anisotropy, *PD* perpendicular diffusivity, *MD* mean diffusivity

[a] Age range not given, mean age noted

Table 10.4 Functional imaging findings in FASD

Reference	Age	Location	Main finding
Astley et al. [106]	8–15 years	Seattle, WA, USA	Choline concentration in frontal/parietal white matter lower Choline decreased as white matter volume and corpus callosum length decreased Choline decreased with increased facial phenotype severity
Cheng et al. [103]	10 years[a]	Cape Town, SA	Abnormalities in connectivity are associated with difficulty in behavioral conditioning (eyeblink conditioning)
Cortese et al. [107]	9–12 years	Detroit, MI, USA	Higher NAA/Cr in left caudate nucleus
Diwadkar et al. [94]	8–10 years	Cape Town, SA	Different regions activated in PAE v. control during working memory tasks PAE group activated crus I/lobule VI and lobule VIIB/VIIIA, and inferior parietal cortex
Donald et al. [83]	2–4 weeks	Cape Town, SA	Increased connectivity between the brainstem, motor, somatosensory, and striatal intrinsic networks Significant difference in connectivity between networks for motor behavior

Table 10.4 (continued)

Reference	Age	Location	Main finding
Du Plessis et al. [105]	8–12 years	Cape Town, SA	Alcohol consumption at conception and throughout pregnancy related to level of glutamate plus glutamine Lower levels of NAA in deep nuclei
Fagerlund et al. [108]	14–21 years	Multiple sites in FI	Lower levels of NAA/Cho and/or NAA/Cr found in parietal and frontal cortex, frontal white matter, corpus callosum, thalamus, and cerebellar dentate nucleus No group differences in Cho/Cr
Fan et al. [84]	11 years[a]	Cape Town, SA	Alcohol dose-dependent reductions in connectivity in the anterior default mode, ventral attention, and dorsal attention networks
Fryer et al. [98]	8–18 years	San Diego, CA, USA	Greater BOLD activation during an inhibition task in prefrontal cortex Lower BOLD activation during an inhibition task in right caudate nucleus Similar task performance across all groups
Gautam et al. [101]	7–14 years	Los Angeles, CA, USA	Significant decreases in activation over time during a visuo-spatial attention task in superior and inferior parietal cortices, lingual gyrus, and right cerebellum Activated similar brain regions to controls during task
Kodali et al. [100]	8–12 years	Cape Town, SA	PAE and control groups activate different regions during inhibition tasks PAE group showed greater activation in the lateral middle and left superior frontal cortex
Lewis et al. [97]	10–14 years	Cape Town, SA	Additional activation in various regions during a memory task Additional regions activated varied by FASD diagnosis
Li et al. [102]	18–24 years	Atlanta, GA, USA	More widespread activation of networks during sustained attention tasks, specifically in the temporal-occipital regions
Lindinger et al. [104]	9–14 years	Cape Town, SA	Higher BOLD signals for neutral faces over pixelated images in left fusiform gyrus and right posterior superior temporal sulcus Weaker BOLD signal for processing angry faces in left posterior superior temporal sulcus and right nucleus accumbens
Little et al. [85]	5–18 years	Multiple sites in CA	Lower connectivity for salience, executive functioning, and language networks
Long et al. [91]	2–7 years	Alberta, CA	More variability in brain connectivity in children with PAE across age-groups

(continued)

Table 10.4 (continued)

Reference	Age	Location	Main finding
Norman et al. [93]	15 years[a]	San Diego, CA, USA	Fewer regions of activity during working memory tasks Significantly greater activation in a wide range of frontal area
Riikonen et al. [109]	5–16 years	Kotka, FI	SPECT imaging demonstrating reduced serotonin in medial frontal cortex and increased dopamine binding in basal ganglia
Rodriguez et al. [89]	16 years[a]	Albuquerque, NM, USA	Lower global efficiency Lower characteristic path lengths for individuals with ARND compared to FAS/pFAS and controls
Roussotte et al. [95]	7–15 years	Los Angeles, CA, USA	Increased activation in right cerebellum, lateral occipital cortex, left dorsolateral prefrontal cortex during working memory tasks
Roussotte et al. [96]	7–15 years	Los Angeles, CA, USA	Decreased connectivity in frontal regions, caudate, and putamen during working memory task
Santhanam et al. [86]	23 years[a]	Atlanta, GA, USA	Less activation of the default mode network, specifically the prefrontal cortex and posterior cingulate cortex
Spadoni et al. [92]	10–18 years	San Diego, CA, USA	Greater BOLD activation during working memory tasks across cortical regions, insulate, claustra, globus pallidum, and putamen
Ware et al. [99]	13–16 years	San Diego, CA, USA	Greater BOLD response in frontal, striatal, and cingulate regions during response inhibition task (no-go/go task) The harder the inhibition task, the greater the BOLD activation
Wozniak et al. [87]	10–17 years	Minneapolis, MN, USA	Paracentral regions show lower functional connectivity
Wozniak et al. [88]	10–17 years	Minneapolis, MN, USA	Significantly lower global efficiency Significantly higher characteristic path length
Wozniak et al. [90]	7–17 years	Multiple sites in USA	Atypical connectivity associated with lower cognitive abilities No significant difference in characteristic path length

FASD fetal alcohol spectrum disorder, *BOLD* blood oxygenation level dependent, *PAE* prenatal alcohol exposure, *ARND* alcohol-related neurodevelopmental disorder, *FAS* fetal alcohol syndrome, *pFAS* partial FAS

[a] Age range not given, mean age noted

Table 10.5 Abbreviations

Abbreviation	Meaning
FASD	*Fetal alcohol spectrum disorder*
PAE	Prenatal alcohol exposure
FAS	Fetal alcohol syndrome
pFAS	Partial fetal alcohol syndrome
ARND	Alcohol-related neurodevelopmental disorder
PFL	Palpebral fissure length
GM	*Gray matter*
TIV	Total intracranial volume
WM	*White matter*
CC	Corpus callosum
L-ASSOC	Left hemisphere association network
R-ASSOC	Right hemisphere association network
L-PROJ	Left hemisphere projection network
R-PROJ	Right hemisphere projection network
Imaging modalities and terms	
MRI	Magnetic resonance imaging
DTI	Diffusion tensor imaging
FA	Fractional anisotropy
MD	Mean diffusivity
AD	Axial diffusivity
fMRI	Functional magnetic resonance imaging
CPL	Characteristic path length
MRS	Magnetic resonance spectroscopy
NAA	*N*-acetylaspartate
Cr	Creatine
Cho	Choline
SPECT	Single-photon emission computerized tomography

Results and Discussion

Cortex and Deep Gray Matter

The brain can be divided into cortical and subcortical regions. The cortex is the outer part of the brain that contains the four lobes (frontal, temporal, occipital, parietal) that are involved in many of the higher order thinking processes. These processes can include language, motor function, organization, and decision-making. Beneath the cortex (subcortical) are those regions which have been typically understood to be involved in functions which include movement, emotions, learning, and bodily functions. The two divisions (cortical and subcortical) are not independent but rather interconnected and interacting constantly. The subcortical gray matter also serves as a critical hub within the central nervous system, relaying and modulating information passing to different regions of the brain. Both cortical and subcortical areas are made up largely of gray matter, which contains neuronal cell bodies, dendrites, and axon terminals [14]. Structural magnetic resonance imaging is the most commonly used modality for gray matter metrics. Outcome measures of

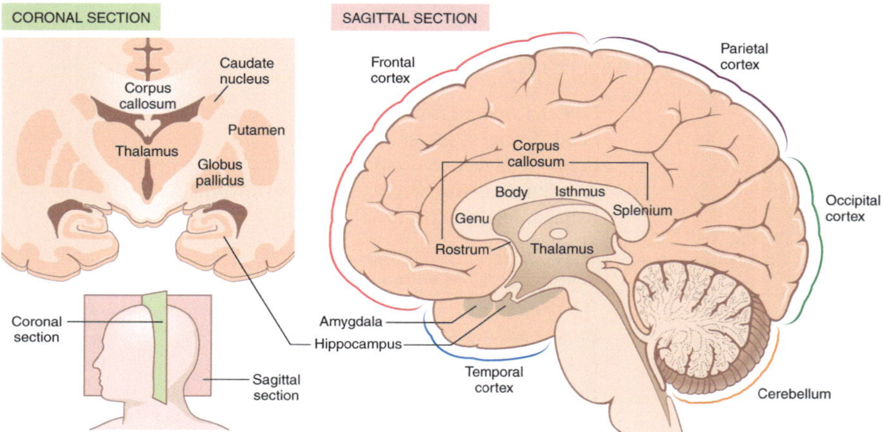

Fig. 10.2 An overview of the gray matter regions affected by prenatal alcohol exposure. (Courtesy of James A. Perkins)

gray matter imaging can include volumetric, surface area, and thickness data regarding specific regions of interest, specific lobes, or the entire cortex.

The cortex and deep gray matter regions of the brain are the most studied areas in FASD imaging research. Nearly all of the current research is centered around middle childhood and early teen years, with sparse literature on either end of that age range. With the advancements made in structural magnetic imaging, from the improvement of magnet strength to the accessibility of imaging, this modality has become crucial in better understanding the neurological differences in the gray matter of individuals with PAE. Across studies, results show reductions in overall gray matter volume, both at the cortical and deep gray matter level, in children with PAE [15–17] (see Fig. 10.2).

Cortical

Looking at overall gray matter in the cerebral cortex, children with PAE ages 6–17 show a 7.8% reduction in volume compared to their peers without exposure [15]. Each of the four lobes of the cortex is affected differently by PAE. The parietal lobe volume tends to be more affected than temporal and occipital regions in both children and young adults [18]. In young adults, the temporal and occipital regions do still show significant decreases [19]. These parietal lobe differences, specifically with the left intraparietal sulcus (LIPS), have been associated with arithmetic challenges, with individuals with PAE demonstrating lower arithmetic scores associated with lower LIPS volumes [20]. It has also been demonstrated that the precuneus, an area in the superior parietal lobe involved in memory, is also volumetrically smaller in children with PAE [21]. Additionally, the largest amount of asymmetry in children with PAE is found in the temporal lobe compared to control groups [22]. PAE also impacts the gray matter in the frontal lobe, with smaller volumes reported across various regions [21, 23]. The impact of PAE on the frontal lobe has shown behavioral associations as well, with a smaller anterior cingulate cortex surface area associated with poor performance on inhibition tasks in children with PAE [24].

Results on cortical thickness in FASD have been shown to vary across studies and across age-points. Cortical thickness refers to the width of the gray matter within the cortex. It should be noted that there are different windows for maximal growth and volume, as well as variations in the growth curve itself, for different areas of the brain. As PAE impacts some regions more than others, there is a level of complexity associated with assessing whether smaller or larger cortical thickness is analytically advantageous at any one age in any one area. Abnormality in the cortical width, either thicker or thinner, is an indicator of abnormal neuropathology and affected gray matter. While volume tends to represent the density of gray matter in a certain area, thickness may be an indication of how cortical neurons are arranged within that gray matter [22]. A portion of this research in children and adolescents shows that individuals with PAE demonstrate reduced cortical gray matter thickness. In all four lobes, there has been evidence that children with PAE show decreased cortical gray matter thickness [17, 25, 26]. Thinner dorsal prefrontal gray matter is also associated with poorer performance on verbal learning tasks in one FASD cohort [27]. Additional results in adolescent studies have shown an increase in cortical thickness in the lateral brain surfaces in all four lobes compared to controls [28]. This difference can be as large as 1.2 mm in individuals with an FASD [27]. This increase is associated with a reduction in palpebral fissure length (PFL), a facial characteristic of individuals with FASD [28]. Additionally, there is more hemispheric asymmetry in the temporal lobe in individuals with PAE compared to control samples [29].

Cortical gyrification, or the folds found on the surface of the brain, is also measurements of interest in gray matter analyses. Cortical gyrification allows for a larger surface area of the cortex in relation to total brain volume. Individuals with PAE have generally been reported to have lower cortical gyrification across the majority of the cerebral cortex. Cortical gyrification reductions in PAE may be related to age as older age is correlated with a decrease in gyrification in the PAE group while controls demonstrated an increase in gyrification as they aged. Additionally, a smoother cortex, which has been previously associated with neuro-developmental impairment, is related to lower IQ scores [30, 31]. Cortical gyrification (or folding) can be quantified using a global sulcal index. The relationship between global sulcal index and PAE appears to be dose dependent. Those with higher levels of alcohol exposure experienced lower global sulcal indices. This relationship is maintained even when there is not an overall reduction in brain volume [32].

As evidenced by the above discussion on the cortex, there are a variety of gray matter regions that are impacted by alcohol exposure prenatally. The impacted regions not only show abnormal brain development, but also relate to delays in IQ, verbal learning, and arithmetic skills [20, 27, 30].

Subcortical

Subcortical gray matter structures, or those found below the cerebral cortex, are involved in more complex processes ranging from emotion, to memory, to various facets of behavior. Like the cortex, even though these structures are parceled apart for imaging analysis purposes, they are all interconnected and represent important hubs for information transfer in many networks. This will become more evident in the functional imaging section below. Overall, deep gray matter structures in children with PAE (ages 6–17) show a 13% lower volume compared to their similar aged peers without PAE [15]. Specific regions of interest that seem to produce the most consistent findings in children with PAE are the caudate and putamen of the basal ganglia and the hippocampus. Findings within specific structures are detailed below.

Amygdala

The amygdala is the structure most strongly associated with emotion regulation. Gray matter analyses involving the effects of PAE on the amygdala report mixed findings. The volumetric results of this region appear to be based on age. Research on infants with PAE has shown smaller bilateral volumes in the amygdala [33]. In children ages 6–9, no significant differences were found volumetrically in this region [15]. There are contradictory findings for ages 9–17, with studies reporting both smaller volumes or no change compared to similar aged control groups [15, 34].

Basal Ganglia

The basal ganglia, encompassing the caudate, putamen, and globus pallidus, is a deep gray structure related to a multitude of human functions, including behavior, executive functioning, motor learning, and emotions [35]. This region is one of the most conclusive in regard to MRI findings of children with PAE. When accounting for the entire basal ganglia, children with PAE have reduced gray matter volumes [16, 18, 36]. Findings within specific substructures are as follows.

Caudate nucleus: The caudate is a structure involved in executing movement, learning, and executive functioning. It is divided into three parts, the head, body, and tail [37]. The caudate shows clear findings of abnormalities in individuals with PAE. In line with the findings that the overall basal ganglia has reduced volume, the caudate also appears smaller [15, 23, 34, 36, 38]. There are also significant shape differences in the caudate nucleus between controls and those with a FAS/pFAS diagnosis, with the tail and the head showing more abnormalities than the body. These differences in shape were related to the amount of alcohol exposure, with larger amounts of alcohol exposure associated with abnormalities in the tail of the right caudate nucleus [38]. Additionally, the caudate is found to be the most consistent predictor of performance on measures of neuropsychological functioning, specifically measures of executive functioning and learning, even above that of total intracranial volume (TIV) [38].

Putamen: The putamen is also a structure involved in movement and learning. This structure, coupled with the caudate nucleus discussed above, make up the striatum [39]. Putamen volumetric data in children with PAE has consistently reported smaller volumes [15, 23, 34]. Lower volume in the putamen is associated with lower Full-Scale IQ (FSIQ) scores in children with PAE [15].

Globus pallidus: The globus pallidus also assists in movement [39]. There is less research on this specific area of the basal ganglia. The one study with a matched control population that did analyze this region showed, parallel to the above findings, reduced volumes in children with PAE [16].

Diencephalon

The diencephalon is found between the midbrain and the forebrain and contains the thalamus. The diencephalon is involved in a variety of functions, including processing sensory information, regulating alertness, and coordinating the production of hormones. The diencephalon has shown a reduction in gray matter volume in children with PAE [16, 36]. Additionally, the ventral diencephalon is related to facial dysmorphology in children with FASD, as smaller PFL are associated with smaller volumes in this region [16].

Thalamus: A specific area of focus for PAE imaging research within the diencephalon is the thalamus. The thalamus plays a critical role in alertness and sleep/wake cycles [40]. In infants with PAE, the left hemisphere showed significantly smaller thalamus volumes [33]. Additionally, facial characteristics are associated with thalamus volume. Higher lipometer scores are associated with lower thalamus volumes, although this significance is reduced to a trend-level association when controlling for TIV [16].

Hippocampus

The hippocampus is another widely studied region with regard to gray matter imaging research in children with PAE. There are two hippocampi in the brain, one in each hemisphere. These hippocampi can be divided into subfields, all of which contribute to one's memory and learning ability. In children and adolescents with PAE, the hippocampus demonstrates smaller volume overall [15, 34, 41, 42]. Not only is the overall volume reduced, but there is also smaller volume across multiple hippocampal subfields in both hemispheres [43]. Conflicting results have only found this to be true in the left hemisphere hippocampus in children with PAE [44]. This aligns well with some infant imaging research, which has also only found significantly smaller volumes in the left hippocampus [33]. Volumetric differences are accompanied by shape abnormalities in the body and tail of the hippocampus when comparing controls to those with PAE [38]. A reduction in hippocampal volume has been associated with both spatial navigation deficits [41] and memory challenges in children with PAE [42, 44].

In summary, it is evident that infants and children with PAE demonstrate smaller gray matter volumes across cortical and subcortical levels; there is a large gap in this literature involving adult samples to date. It should be noted that many studies that have shown significant regional gray matter volume differences do lose significance when controlling for TIV [45–47]. TIV is often controlled for in FASD imaging research, as the overall volume of the brain is typically smaller as a result of the PAE [22]. Gray matter volume reduction has been linked to a variety of deficits including executive functioning, memory, learning, spatial navigation, arithmetic, and FSIQ.

The degree of structural abnormalities in cortical and subcortical regions have also been tied to diagnosis. Individuals with FAS/pFAS diagnoses tend to have a greater degree of abnormalities than alcohol-exposed individuals without facial dysmorphology, who also show abnormalities relative to non-exposed controls [23]. Additionally, there are results suggesting that facial characteristics (PFL, philtrum) of FASD are related to gray matter volumes [16, 28]. With the depth of research in deep gray matter imaging, the question has been proposed as to whether this data could be used to distinguish individuals who have had PAE from those who have not. To investigate this, Little et al. developed a multivariate model that could discriminate a control group from an FASD group with 77% accuracy based on brain imaging volumetrics [48].

White Matter

White matter is found in the subcortical, or deeper, regions of the brain and refers to tissue that is made up of myelinated nerve fibers. The myelin is what gives white matter its different color. This myelination helps to speed up the signal between cells and allows for the brain to quickly send and receive information from one area to the next. The corpus callosum, which is a collection of white matter tracts connecting the left and right hemispheres, is one of the most studied white matter areas of the brain in FASD. The corpus callosum can be split into five distinct parts, listed here from the front of the brain to back: the rostrum, genu, body, isthmus, and splenium. Two white matter tracts disproportionately affected in the FASD literature are the superior longitudinal and uncinate fasciculus. The superior longitudinal fasciculus helps connect the four lobes (frontal, temporal, occipital, parietal) of the cortex (see Fig. 10.3). The uncinate fasciculus connects the orbitofrontal cortex to the anterior temporal lobe [45]. Both of these tracts are considered association fibers, present in both the left and right hemispheres (L-ASSOC, R-ASSOC), which connect cortical regions. There are also projection fibers (L-PROJ, R-PROJ) that connect the cortex to other parts of the central nervous system (CNS), such as the spinal cord and brainstem [14].

The historical progression of white matter imaging techniques has evolved from basic volumetric measurements and region-of-interest tracing through traditional MRI to much more novel analyses techniques such as diffusion tensor imaging (DTI), which came into play in the mid-1990s [49] (see Table 10.6 for explanation). DTI outcome measures include fractional anisotropy (FA), mean diffusivity (MD), and axial diffusivity (AD). These broadly measure white matter integrity, membrane density, and the diffusion of water molecules, respectively. In infants, transfontanelle ultrasound can also be utilized to capture white matter measurements (see Table 10.6).

White matter literature in FASD largely focuses on the corpus callosum, as it is the largest white matter tract and a midline structure. DTI methodologies are the most commonly reported. White matter volumes are often more affected than gray matter volumes in reported studies of children with PAE, with parietal regions generally showing larger effects compared to temporal or occipital areas [18]. Below, the teratogenic effects of PAE on white matter is explained by age-group (infant and toddler: 0–3 year, early/middle childhood: 4–12 years, teenage: 13–17 years, and adult: 18+ years). In general, studies of individuals with PAE across different developmental stages have reported smaller and/or unique shaping of the corpus callosum and lower overall white matter volumes, especially in areas closer to the midline of the brain. Mixed findings have been reported with regard to metrics of white matter microstructural integrity. It is evident that PAE damages the integrity of white matter in the developing brain in various ways and this finding is present throughout the lifespan. The bulk of white matter research involves the early/middle childhood age-group, with small but evolving research in the younger and older age categories.

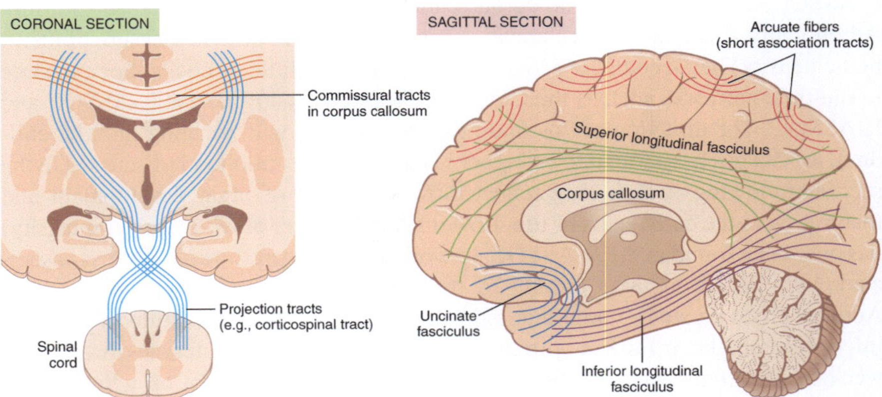

Fig. 10.3 An overview of the white matter regions and tracts affected by prenatal alcohol exposure. (Courtesy of James A. Perkins)

Table 10.6 Imaging techniques

Modality	Definition
MRI	A method of structural imaging utilizing strong magnetic fields
DTI	A form of MRI measuring the motion of water molecules in white matter through the following outcomes: Fractional anisotropy: a summary measure of white matter microstructural integrity Medial diffusivity: an inverse measure of membrane density Axial diffusivity: the mean diffusion of water molecules parallel to fiber tracts
Transfontanelle ultrasound	A form of brain imaging used in infant research that assesses cerebral blood flow through sound waves
fMRI	A form of MRI that demonstrates functional connectivity between regions of the brain through examination of blood-oxygenation levels
MRS	A form of MRI that measures the composition of chemicals in various areas of brain tissue utilizing the follow outcomes: Cho: Choline NAA: *N*-acetylaspartate Cr: Creatine
SPECT	A nuclear form of MRI that uses a gamma scanner to measure blood flow in the brain

Infant and Toddler

Infant and toddler research has reported a significantly smaller corpus callosum in those prenatally exposed to alcohol compared to those who were not exposed [50]. There are also slight reported differences in the splenium angle of the corpus callosum, whether that be a larger angle or the appearance of a "hook" in this region [51, 52]. DTI findings show that infants have altered AD (a measure of the diffusion of water molecules parallel to white matter tracts) in a variety of white matter networks, including the right superior longitudinal fasciculus, L-PROJ, R-PROJ, L-ASSOC, R-ASSOC, and the corpus callosum corona radiata (CCCR) [33, 53]. Additionally, there have been changes reported in MD (an inverse measure of membrane density) between those with PAE and those with little or no alcohol exposure in multiple networks such as the CCCR, L-PROJ and R-PROJ, and L-ASSOC and R-ASSOC. The direction of this finding does not align with imaging in older children, as MD has been found to be higher in early/middle childhood (discussed in the section following) which may reflect different stages of brain development and maturation in the early years of life. Lower FA (a measure of white matter integrity) has only been found in the R-ASSOC network and has been shown to be less associated with PAE than MD or AD in this region in the infant age-group [53]. Additionally, one study found that indicators of altered microstructure in the right inferior cerebellar peduncle correlate with neurobehavioral outcomes in the first week of life, suggesting that the brain-altering effects of alcohol on white matter structures may impact an infant's irritability, cry, alertness, consolability, visual orientation, and/or auditory orientation [54]. Toddlers (ages 2–3) demonstrate similar widespread alterations in white matter integrity compared to infants, such as lower FA in the uncinate fasciculus and lower MD in the corticospinal tract and fornix stria terminalis [55].

Early/Middle Childhood

Early/middle childhood brain imaging research is the most robust of any age-group. Aligning with the infant literature, research on early/middle childhood has shown significantly smaller white matter volumes overall in children ranging from ages 8 to 16 [56, 57]. There is one contradictory finding in the literature that indicated no significant differences in white matter volumes in children ages 10–13, which could be a result of a narrow age range and a smaller sample size in this study [58]. The corpus callosum has widely been demonstrated to be both significantly smaller in volume and area, coupled with unique shaping of the structure, including narrowing/reduced thickness [56, 57, 59]. An area of the corpus callosum that appears to be unaffected by thinning in PAE at this age is the dorsal surface, as there are no differences in thinning in this region compared to controls [60]. Additionally, an overall reduction in corpus callosum connectivity has been reported at his age [61].

DTI techniques have demonstrated a variety of results regarding FA and MD metrics within various white matter regions. Following on from the initial volumetric work in this region, FA has been shown to be lower in the body, splenium, and isthmus of the corpus callosum [62]. Findings reported in the genus of the corpus callosum are less consistent due to age differences in samples studied. One study demonstrated increased FA in individuals ages 2–7, while others demonstrated decreased FA in this specific area in children ages 9–11 [62, 63]. In the mid-childhood age-group results reporting MD generally suggest higher diffusion in PAE groups, specifically in the left uncinate fasciculus, splenium, isthmus, left inferior longitudinal fasciculus, right superior longitudinal fasciculus, and the bilateral corticospinal tracts [64–66], suggesting damage to the white matter in these areas. There is one contradictory finding within the bilateral uncinate fasciculus showing lower MD [63]. These altered white matter regions have been shown to be associated with challenges in oculomotor control, demonstrated by eye movement tasks [65, 67].

The white matter alterations demonstrated here, in a variety of regions, appear to be correlated with both cognitive and motor processes. White matter differences partially mediate the effects of PAE on both information processing speed tasks and eyeblink conditioning [65]. Longitudinal research has shown that in FASD, an increase in white matter volumes over time is associated with an increase of executive functioning ability. This indicates that individuals with FASD show a degree of white matter plasticity that, if targeted through intervention, could result in positive cognitive outcomes [57].

Adolescence

The imaging research within adolescents and adults is somewhat sparse but as the focus on this key life stage has increased, an emerging literature has become available. Consistent with other age-groups, the corpus callosum in the teenage brain is significantly smaller than those of individuals without PAE [12]. The shape and location of the corpus callosum are reported to be more variable in the brains of adolescents with PAE, with this abnormality persisting into adulthood [49]. Additionally, adolescents with PAE exhibit lower FA in multiple areas across the front, parietal, and occipital lobes, specifically the right superior longitudinal fasciculus, with fewer group differences reported in MD [68].

Adults

Adults with PAE show very similar white matter inconsistencies as do adolescents, with a decrease in FA reported in the isthmus, genu, and splenium of the corpus callosum and the connected callosal fibers [69, 70]. The callosal midline shape also shows more variability in adults with PAE compared to those without [71]. Also similar to findings in teenage imaging studies, abnormalities in white matter structures appear to be associated with both executive functioning and motor difficulties. A thicker corpus callosum is associated with executive functioning deficits in adults prenatally exposed to alcohol, with a thinner corpus callosum associated with motor deficits.

Cerebellum

Cerebellum development is extensive during the prenatal period. The cerebellum is one of the first regions to differentiate in utero, but also one of the last to fully mature, making the development period of this structure relatively long [72]. This means that the region is particularly vulnerable to the impact of exposure to external substances, such as alcohol, potentially leading to long-term motor and cognitive difficulties [73, 74]. Similar to other areas of the brain in individuals with PAE, the cerebellum is relatively smaller [25, 75, 76]. Individuals with a FAS diagnosis have smaller cerebellum volumes compared to alcohol-exposed individuals without facial dysmorphology, and individuals without PAE having the largest volumes [76]. There are alterations throughout all areas of the cerebellum (gray matter, white matter, cerebral spinal fluid, and total volumes) in individuals with FAS, while those with non-dysmorphic PAE show only reductions in gray matter and total overall volume of the cerebellum [76]. Gender differences are also reported within the cerebellum in the context of PAE, with males showing larger volumes than females with PAE [75].

Aligning with consistently reported differences in midline regions of the brain of individuals with PAE, the cerebellar vermis has demonstrated similar effects. The anterior region of the cerebellar vermis is significantly smaller in individuals prenatally exposed to alcohol while the posterior region shows little to no significant difference [77, 78]. Additionally, displacement of the cerebellar vermis has shown to be related to learning and memory. Those with a smaller vermis score lower on a measure of learning and memory [77]. Studies using DTI techniques have further demonstrated lower levels of FA and higher levels of perpendicular diffusivity (PD) in the left middle cerebellar peduncle. FA is found to mediate the effect of PAE on trace conditioning, a task associated with associative learning ability [79]. Similar findings regarding eyeblink conditioning tasks have shown lower FA and higher MD in the cerebellar peduncle to be associated with poorer performance, with both mediating the relationship between PAE and task performance. This could be an indication of poorer myelination in the cerebellar nerve fibers due to the teratogenic effects of alcohol exposure [80].

Functional Imaging

Functional imaging can refer to the measurement of real-time brain oxygenation and activity, such as with functional magnetic resonance imaging (fMRI), or to neurochemistry, as seen in magnetic resonance spectroscopy (MRS) and single-photon emission computerized tomography (SPECT). The subtypes of functional imaging utilized in this review include resting-state fMRI, task-specific fMRI, MRS, and SPECT. All of these are described in their respective sections below and included in Table 10.6. fMRI is the most common technique utilized in FASD functional imaging. fMRI is a newer technique, compared to traditional structural technology, with its conception in the 1990s [81]. fMRI is based on the blood-oxygen-level dependent (BOLD) theory that states that BOLD signals demonstrate changes in brain blood oxygenation. These measures are commonly used as an indicator of brain activity [82].

fMRI in FASD has been utilized since the early 2000s, with an increase in publications with this modality starting in the mid-2010s. Like structural imaging, nearly all of these studies focus on children, adolescents, and teens with PAE. There is a clear gap in the research involving younger children and adult populations. The following summation of fMRI findings in FASD is divided by subtype of functional imaging.

Resting-State fMRI

Resting-state fMRI (RS-fMRI) aims to assess the interconnectedness of brain regions/networks while an individual is inactive, or at rest. While in the scanner, individuals are asked to remain still and not attend to anything in particular, as the goal is to better understand the connectedness of networks without the presence of a task or stimulus. The main outcome measure is connectivity, or a significant relationship between measures of activity between two spatially distinct regions.

Aligning with all other areas of imaging research in FASD, the majority of studies in resting-state fMRI literature utilize child and adolescent samples. It should be noted that there is little known about whether an increase or decrease in connectivity at young ages is better or worse in terms of typical development. The network findings presented here may need to be replicated for confirmation and there is a need for longitudinal studies to better understand connectivity in FASD in children. There is a single study on resting-state measures of the infant brain, which found an increase in connectivity between the brainstem, motor, somatosensory, and striatal intrinsic networks in infants with PAE when compared to controls. This finding indicates that alcohol exposure may alter connectivity networks related to motor control in infancy [83].

Child studies have demonstrated connectivity reductions in a variety of networks including the anterior default mode, salience, ventral attention, dorsal attention, and executive control networks [84, 85]. As stated previously, although these findings differ from the findings in infancy above, preliminary connectivity findings have not shown a clear indication of whether increased or decreased connectivity is a better or worse sign for brain development. The anterior default mode network, a network primarily activated while an individual is at rest and involved in internal cognition, as well as the ventral and dorsal attentional networks, has reduced connectivity in alcohol-exposed individuals without facial dysmorphology compared to those with both PAE and facial dysmorphology and non-exposed controls [84]. There is a single young adult study in this area with findings indicating that adults with PAE also have significantly reduced default mode network activation, specifically between the medial prefrontal cortex and the posterior cingulate cortex [86]. Many paracentral regions, which encompass areas of both the parietal and frontal areas and are connected by posterior callosal fibers, have also shown lower functional connectivity in children, paralleling the findings that paracentral regions of the brain also show structural abnormalities [87].

In addition to examining connectivity within and across various regions or networks, resting-state fMRI can also examine global efficiency, or the overall connectivity and ability to transfer information within a network. In general, findings of global efficiency show that individuals with PAE experience lower global efficiency than those without [88, 89]. Global efficiency can be determined by calculating the inverse of the harmonic mean of the shortest paths in a specific network. Characteristic path length (CPL) is used to determine the shortest path in a specific network, as shorter paths indicate a high integration across the network of various nodes. This is another way to measure connectivity. There are mixed findings regarding CPL, or the average shortest path between all pairs of nodes in a specific network, in children with PAE. A study looking at CPL in children and adolescents with PAE ages 10–17 found higher CPL, indicating less integration across networks. Another study found no significant difference in CPL compared to controls [90]. Lastly, a similar study looking at adolescents and young adults ages 12–22 found the ARND group to have lower CPL compared to individuals with both FAS and controls [89]. The latter findings do not align with most FASD research, in that the ARND group showed the best measures of connectivity above those who were controls and those with FAS. The team of Rodriguez et al. (2021) point to the oddity in this finding and note that this may be a reason why studies that combine all FASD diagnoses under one category may not find significant results when comparing the entire spectrum to a control group [89]. They did not believe the finding to be age related, as CPL has been shown to be consistent throughout the lifespan. Additionally, atypical connectivity, as demonstrated here as present in children with PAE, is associated with lower cognitive ability scores [90].

The team of Long et al. (2019) aimed to examine the "functional connectome" of children ages 2–7 with PAE by measuring the stability of the brain's connectivity [91]. Inter-participant stability of connectivity did increase in controls with age, while there is no such relationship found in the PAE group. This indicates there is more variability in brain connectivity in children with PAE across age-groups. This could indicate that the variability in functional connectivity found in multiple older child studies could originate in early childhood.

Task-Specific fMRI

In contrast to resting-state fMRI, task-specific fMRI requires the completion of various tasks in order to measure brain activation during tests of cognitive ability, making this a more targeted modality for investigating quite specific questions. The following sections are sorted by type of cognitive task administered.

Working Memory Tasks

Working memory, or one's ability to hold and manipulate information briefly in mind to complete a task, is an area that is often underdeveloped in children with PAE. An example of a working memory task administered during fMRI would be identifying when a specific shape appeared in the same location on a screen more than once in a sequence of various shapes and locations. When given a task of working memory during fMRI, children and adolescents with PAE show areas of both increased and decreased activity. For most studies of working memory, there is an increase in activity in the PAE group compared to the control group within parts of all four lobes (frontal, temporal, occipital, parietal) and a variety of subcortical regions [92–95]. With task accuracy being equivalent among groups, this is generally interpreted as individuals with FASD having to engage more brain areas to complete a task relative to non-exposed peers. Other findings within similar age ranges have indicated opposite levels of activation, with decreased brain activity within regions of the frontal cortex, the caudate, and the putamen even when task performance between PAE group and control group did not differ [96]. This could indicate that structural damage caused by PAE leads to a decrease of recruitment in these specific areas. As stated previously, further research into the implications of higher or lower activity or connectivity is necessary to reach a conclusion on the implications of the above findings.

Memory Tasks

There is a single study focusing on longer-term memory, utilizing a recognition task. In this study, individuals with FAS/pFAS demonstrated more activation in several additional regions compared to alcohol-exposed individuals without facial dysmorphology and controls. Similar to the working memory tasks above, the FAS/pFAS group had to engage additional brain areas to complete the memory task to the same degree of accuracy as non-exposed controls and non-dysmorphic PAE [97].

Response Inhibition Tasks

Response inhibition, or the ability to stop one's thoughts and actions when necessary, can be a challenge for individuals with FASD. A common response inhibition test is a go/no-go task, in which individuals are asked to respond to certain stimuli (go) and not to respond to other stimuli (no-go). When this task is administered during fMRI, children with PAE show greater BOLD activation in prefrontal regions [98, 99] compared to similar aged controls. The more difficult the no-go/go task, the greater BOLD response in FAS groups [99]. As with the working memory tasks above, the PAE groups and control groups do not tend to differ significantly on task performance, however the PAE groups demonstrated higher activation in certain regions [98–100]. Less activation is shown in the right caudate nucleus, anterior cingulate, temporal lobe, areas of the frontal lobe, and insula [98, 99]. In summation, this may imply that even though the outcome on the cognitive task is the same, children with FASD must use more mental effort to reach the same goal. Those brain regions involved in inhibition need to be more greatly activated, while other regions not involved in the task at hand do not need to be activated to the same degree.

Attention Tasks

Attention is a common area of investigation in FASD, given frequent difficulties in this domain. The team of Gautam et al., looked at visuo-spatial attention tasks over the span of 2 years in children and adolescents with PAE. They found that while FASD groups and control groups tended to activate similar brain regions during attention tasks, the alcohol-exposed individuals without facial dysmorphology showed decreases in activation of these regions over time while the control group saw increases in activation [101]. This indicates that the effects of PAE on regions of the brain involved in visual-spatial attention may be long-lasting. In young adults with FASD, sustained attention tasks showed more widespread activation in the occipital-temporal areas compared to non-exposed individuals [102]. The more diffuse recruitment of brain regions in PAE may represent less efficiency for a given task.

Other Tasks

There are two recent studies that have examined other areas of functioning. The first area involves eyeblink conditioning and the cerebellum. Eyeblink conditioning involves pairings of a conditioned stimulus (such as an auditory noise) with an unconditioned stimulus (such as a puff of air in the eye) that results in the conditioned stimulus (noise) eliciting a conditioned response (eye blink). The ability to condition eye blinking depends completely on the activation of the cerebellum. On an eyeblink classical conditioning task done in an MRI scanner with 10 year olds, only the control group demonstrated significant cerebellar activation. The PAE group showed less conditioned responses overall, in addition to less activation. The abnormalities in brain functioning in the PAE group is associated with behavioral conditioning deficits in PAE [103].

Additionally, on a task of affective appraisal for faces, children with FAS/pFAS demonstrated lower activation for processing angry faces in networks involving facial identity/expression and recognition of aggressive behavior compared to controls and non-dysmorphic PAE. The FAS/pFAS group also demonstrated higher activation for neutral faces over pixelated images in visual sensory social brain related networks [104]. This suggests that individuals with FAS/pFAS demonstrate less efficient processing of more subtle emotions and different processing of angry faces compared to those without PAE and those with non-dysmorphic PAE [104].

MRS

Magnetic Resonance Spectroscopy, or MRS, is an imaging technique that measures the composition of chemicals in various areas of brain tissue. Further detail on the modality and accompanying outcome measures can be found in Table 10.6. Similar to fMRI findings, there has not been enough replication of results to paint a clear picture as to what levels of different concentrations reflect better or worse brain development and functioning. Different levels of the chemicals examined may mean various things in different regions of the brain and at different stages of the lifespan. In early to mid-childhood, MRS research suggests that alcohol consumption at conception and throughout pregnancy is related to levels of glutamate plus glutamine [105]. Additionally, Choline (Cho) concentration in the frontal and parietal white matter is lower in children with PAE, with Cho levels decreasing as both white matter volume and corpus callosum length decreased [106]. Higher *N*-acetylaspartate/Creatine (NAA/Cr) levels are found in the left caudate nucleus in those with FAS [107], with lower NAA levels found in the deep nuclei [105]. In early adulthood, lower levels of NAA/Cho and/or NAA/Cr are found in the following regions:

parietal and frontal cortex, frontal white matter, corpus callosum, thalamus, and the cerebellar dentate nucleus [108]. There were no differences found in Cho/Cr levels when comparing adults with PAE to control groups [108]. Even though findings utilizing MRS technologies cannot draw conclusive evidence at this time, many of the unique findings found in the PAE groups match the regions of structural abnormality discussed earlier.

SPECT

Single-photon emission computerized tomography (SPECT) is a nuclear imaging modality that uses a gamma scanner to measure blood flow in the brain. There has been a single study with a comparison control group in children and adolescents ages 5–16 utilizing this technique. This study demonstrated reduced serotonin binding in the medial frontal cortex and increased striatal dopamine transporter binding in the basal ganglia for those with FAS [109].

Conclusion

The breadth of knowledge demonstrating the teratogenic effects of PAE on the human brain has grown significantly over the last few decades. With the advancement of magnetic resonance technology, and the expansion of access to different and complementary imaging modalities, the field of FASD neuroimaging has been able to draw strong conclusions on anomalies within white matter, gray matter, and functional connectivity. There is substantial agreement surrounding findings of malformation in the size of regions such as the corpus callosum, basal ganglia, hippocampus, as well as smaller overall brain volume. DTI has demonstrated alterations in a variety of white matter tracts, with a large emphasis on the corpus callosum and other large central and association tracts. Abnormal increases and decreases in functional connectivity are present throughout various regions, aligning with underlying structural abnormalities. In other areas where findings are inconclusive, further research is necessary to better understand the potential heterogeneity of these areas among individuals with PAE or to reach consensus. FASD research in the past decade has placed an added emphasis on the tie between the brain and behavior, as studies are beginning to pair cognitive and imaging data. This allows for a better understanding of the behavioral difficulties of children and adults with FASD in the context of this neurodevelopmental disorder.

While the field has exhibited great progress in imaging research, there is still room for growth. There is currently a lack of research in infant, toddler, and adult samples. Research into these samples, as well as the accompanying contextual information related to findings, would address a large gap in the literature. We also know little about the impact of polysubstance exposures on neuroimaging, which are common in individuals with FASD. Longitudinal research would also be beneficial in order to better understand the developmental trajectories of various brain regions and tracts. Additionally, there is a need for more nuanced consideration of trauma and other risk/protective factors that may be affecting brain development. There is an area for growth in better understanding the effect of FASD interventions on the potential for neuroplasticity. Lastly, as detailed in Fig. 10.1 above, many regions of the globe have yet to research the long-lasting effects of prenatal exposure. There is a need for a global effort to further advance the understanding of neurodevelopment in FASD.

References

1. Riley EP, Infante MA, Warren KR. Fetal alcohol spectrum disorders: an overview. Neuropsychol Rev. 2011;21(2):73–80.
2. Hoyme HE, Kalberg WO, Elliott AJ, Blankenship J, Buckley D, Marais A-S, et al. Updated clinical guidelines for diagnosing fetal alcohol spectrum disorders. Pediatrics. 2016 [cited 2021 Feb 25];138(2). Available from: https://www.ncbi.nlm.nih.gov/pmc/articles/PMC4960726/.
3. Flannigan K, Wrath A, Ritter C, McLachlan K, Harding KD, Campbell A, et al. Balancing the story of fetal alcohol spectrum disorder: A narrative review of the literature on strengths. Alcohol Clin Exp Res. 2021 [cited 2021 Nov 24]. Available from: https://onlinelibrary.wiley.com/doi/abs/10.1111/acer.14733.
4. May PA, Gossage JP, Kalberg WO, Robinson LK, Buckley D, Manning M, et al. Prevalence and epidemiologic characteristics of FASD from various research methods with an emphasis on recent in-school studies. Dev Disabil Res Rev. 2009;15(3):176–92.
5. Popova S, Lange S, Shield K, Burd L, Rehm J. Prevalence of fetal alcohol spectrum disorder among special subpopulations: a systematic review and meta-analysis. Addiction. 2019;114(7):1150–72.
6. Jones KL, Smith DW. The fetal alcohol syndrome. Teratology. 1975;12(1):1–10.
7. Jones KL, Smith DW. Recognition of the fetal alcohol syndrome in early infancy. Lancet (London, England). 1973;302(7836):999–1001.
8. Coulter CL, Leech RW, Schaefer GB, Scheithauer BW, Brumback RA. Midline cerebral dysgenesis, dysfunction of the hypothalamic-pituitary axis, and fetal alcohol effects. Arch Neurol. 1993;50(7):771–5.
9. Mattson SN, Riley EP, Jernigan TL, Garcia A, Kaneko WM, Ehlers CL, et al. A decrease in the size of the basal ganglia following prenatal alcohol exposure: a preliminary report. Neurotoxicol Teratol. 1994;16(3):283–9.
10. Mattson SN, Jernigan TL, Riley EP. MRI and prenatal alcohol exposure. Alcohol Health Res World. 1994;18(1):49–52.
11. Mattson SN, Riley EP, Jernigan TL, Ehlers CL, Delis DC, Jones KL, et al. Fetal alcohol syndrome: a case report of neuropsychological, MRI, and EEG assessment of two children. Alcohol Clin Exp Res. 1992;16(5):1001–3.
12. Riley EP, Mattson SN, Sowell ER, Jernigan TL, Sobel DF, Jones KL. Abnormalities of the corpus callosum in children prenatally exposed to alcohol. Alcohol Clin Exp Res. 1995;19(5):1198–202.
13. Johnson VP, Swayze VW II, Sato Y, Andreasen NC. Fetal alcohol syndrome: craniofacial and central nervous system manifestations. Am J Med Genet. 1996;61(4):329–39.
14. Hansen J. Netter's clinical anatomy. 4th ed. Elsevier; 2017. [cited 2021 Nov 3]. Available from: https://www.elsevier.com/books/netters-clinical-anatomy/hansen/978-0-323-53188-7.

15. Nardelli A, Lebel C, Rasmussen C, Andrew G, Beaulieu C. Extensive deep gray matter volume reductions in children and adolescents with fetal alcohol spectrum disorders. Alcohol Clin Exp Res. 2011;35(8):1404–17.
16. Roussotte FF, Sulik KK, Mattson SN, Riley EP, Jones KL, Adnams CM, et al. Regional brain volume reductions relate to facial dysmorphology and neurocognitive function in fetal alcohol spectrum disorders. Hum Brain Mapp. 2012;33(4):920–37.
17. Zhou D, Lebel C, Lepage C, Rasmussen C, Evans A, Wyper K, et al. Developmental cortical thinning in fetal alcohol spectrum disorders. NeuroImage. 2011;58(1):16–25.
18. Archibald SL, Fennema-Notestine C, Gamst A, Riley EP, Mattson SN, Jernigan TL. Brain dysmorphology in individuals with severe prenatal alcohol exposure. Dev Med Child Neurol. 2001;43(3):148–54.
19. Chen X, Coles CD, Lynch ME, Hu X. Understanding specific effects of prenatal alcohol exposure on brain structure in young adults. Hum Brain Mapp. 2012;33(7):1663–76.
20. Miles M, Warton FL, Meintjes EM, Molteno CD, Jacobson JL, Jacobson SW, et al. Effects of prenatal alcohol exposure on the volumes of the lateral and medial walls of the intraparietal sulcus. Front Neuroanat. 2021;15:639800.
21. de Water E, Rockhold MN, Roediger DJ, Krueger AM, Mueller BA, Boys CJ, et al. Social behaviors and gray matter volumes of brain areas supporting social cognition in children and adolescents with prenatal alcohol exposure. Brain Res. 2021;147388:147388.
22. Menary K, Collins PF, Porter JN, Muetzel R, Olson EA, Kumar V, et al. Associations between cortical thickness and general intelligence in children, adolescents and young adults. Intelligence. 2013;41(5):597–606.
23. Astley SJ, Aylward EH, Olson HC, Kerns K, Brooks A, Coggins TE, et al. Magnetic resonance imaging outcomes from a comprehensive magnetic resonance study of children with fetal alcohol spectrum disorders. Alcohol Clin Exp Res. 2009;33(10):1671–89.
24. Migliorini R, Moore EM, Glass L, Infante MA, Tapert SF, Jones KL, et al. Anterior cingulate cortex surface area relates to behavioral inhibition in adolescents with and without heavy prenatal alcohol exposure. Behav Brain Res. 2015;292:26–35.
25. Zhou D, Rasmussen C, Pei J, Andrew G, Reynolds JN, Beaulieu C. Preserved cortical asymmetry despite thinner cortex in children and adolescents with prenatal alcohol exposure and associated conditions. Hum Brain Mapp. 2018;39(1):72–88.
26. Sowell ER, Thompson PM, Mattson SN, Tessner KD, Jernigan TL, Riley EP, et al. Regional brain shape abnormalities persist into adolescence after heavy prenatal alcohol exposure. Cereb Cortex. 2002;12(8):856–65.
27. Sowell ER, Mattson SN, Kan E, Thompson PM, Riley EP, Toga AW. Abnormal cortical thickness and brain–behavior correlation patterns in individuals with heavy prenatal alcohol exposure. Cereb Cortex. 2008;18(1):136–44.
28. Yang Y, Roussotte F, Kan E, Sulik KK, Mattson SN, Riley EP, et al. Abnormal cortical thickness alterations in fetal alcohol spectrum disorders and their relationships with facial dysmorphology. Cereb Cortex (New York, N.Y.: 1991). 2012;22(5):1170–9.
29. Sowell ER, Thompson PM, Peterson BS, Mattson SN, Welcome SE, Henkenius AL, et al. Mapping cortical gray matter asymmetry patterns in adolescents with heavy prenatal alcohol exposure. Neuroimage. 2002;17(4):1807–19.
30. Hendrickson TJ, Mueller BA, Sowell ER, Mattson SN, Coles CD, Kable JA, et al. Cortical gyrification is abnormal in children with prenatal alcohol exposure. Neuroimage Clin. 2017;15:391–400.
31. Infante MA, Moore EM, Bischoff-Grethe A, Migliorini R, Mattson SN, Riley EP. Atypical cortical gyrification in adolescents with histories of heavy prenatal alcohol exposure. Brain Res. 2015;1624:446–54.
32. De Guio F, Mangin J-F, Rivière D, Perrot M, Molteno CD, Jacobson SW, et al. A study of cortical morphology in children with fetal alcohol spectrum disorders. Hum Brain Mapp. 2014;35(5):2285–96.

33. Donald KA, Fouche JP, Roos A, Koen N, Howells FM, Riley EP, et al. Alcohol exposure in utero is associated with decreased gray matter volume in neonates. Metab Brain Dis. 2016;31(1):81–91.

34. Krueger AM, Roediger DJ, Mueller BA, Boys CA, Hendrickson TJ, Schumacher MJ, et al. Para-limbic structural abnormalities are associated with internalizing symptoms in children with prenatal alcohol exposure. Alcohol Clin Exp Res. 2020 [cited 2020 Jul 8]. Available from: https://onlinelibrary.wiley.com/doi/abs/10.1111/acer.14390.

35. Lanciego JL, Luquin N, Obeso JA. Functional neuroanatomy of the basal ganglia. Cold Spring Harb Perspect Med. 2012;2(12):a009621.

36. Mattson SN, Riley EP, Sowell ER, Jernigan TL, Sobel DF, Jones KL. A decrease in the size of the basal ganglia in children with fetal alcohol syndrome. Alcohol Clin Exp Res. 1996;20(6):1088–93.

37. Driscoll ME, Bollu PC, Tadi P. Neuroanatomy, nucleus caudate. In: StatPearls. Treasure Island, FL: StatPearls Publishing; 2021 [cited 2021 Oct 30]. Available from: http://www.ncbi.nlm.nih.gov/books/NBK557407/.

38. Joseph J, Warton C, Jacobson SW, Jacobson JL, Molteno CD, Eicher A, et al. Three-dimensional surface deformation-based shape analysis of hippocampus and caudate nucleus in children with fetal alcohol spectrum disorders. Hum Brain Mapp. 2014;35(2):659–72.

39. Ghandili M, Munakomi S. Neuroanatomy, putamen. In: StatPearls. Treasure Island, FL: StatPearls Publishing; 2021 [cited 2021 Oct 30]. Available from: http://www.ncbi.nlm.nih.gov/books/NBK542170/.

40. Torrico TJ, Munakomi S. Neuroanatomy, thalamus. In: StatPearls. Treasure Island, FL: StatPearls Publishing; 2021 [cited 2021 Oct 30]. Available from: http://www.ncbi.nlm.nih.gov/books/NBK542184/.

41. Dodge NC, Thomas KGF, Meintjes EM, Molteno CD, Jacobson JL, Jacobson SW. Reduced hippocampal volumes partially mediate effects of prenatal alcohol exposure on spatial navigation on a virtual water maze task in children. Alcohol Clin Exp Res. 2020;44(4):844–55.

42. Dudek J, Skocic J, Sheard E, Rovet J. Hippocampal abnormalities in youth with alcohol-related neurodevelopmental disorder. J Int Neuropsychol Soc. 2014;20(2):181–91.

43. Roediger DJ, Krueger AM, de Water E, Mueller BA, Boys CA, Hendrickson TJ, et al. Hippocampal subfield abnormalities and memory functioning in children with fetal alcohol spectrum disorders. Neurotoxicol Teratol. 2021;83:106944.

44. Willoughby KA, Sheard ED, Nash K, Rovet J. Effects of prenatal alcohol exposure on hippocampal volume, verbal learning, and verbal and spatial recall in late childhood. J Int Neuropsychol Soc. 2008;14(6):1022–33.

45. Von Der Heide RJ, Skipper LM, Klobusicky E, Olson IR. Dissecting the uncinate fasciculus: disorders, controversies and a hypothesis. Brain. 2013;136(6):1692–707.

46. Meintjes EM, Narr KL, van der Kouwe AJW, Molteno CD, Pirnia T, Gutman B, et al. A tensor-based morphometry analysis of regional differences in brain volume in relation to prenatal alcohol exposure. Neuroimage Clin. 2014;5:152–60.

47. Rajaprakash M, Chakravarty MM, Lerch JP, Rovet J. Cortical morphology in children with alcohol-related neurodevelopmental disorder. Brain Behav. 2014;4(1):41–50.

48. Little G, Beaulieu C. Multivariate models of brain volume for identification of children and adolescents with fetal alcohol spectrum disorder. Hum Brain Mapp. 2020;41(5):1181–94.

49. Bookstein FL, Sampson PD, Connor PD, Streissguth AP. Midline corpus callosum is a neuroanatomical focus of fetal alcohol damage. Anat Rec. 2002;269(3):162–74.

50. Jacobson SW, Jacobson JL, Molteno CD, Warton CMR, Wintermark P, Hoyme HE, et al. Heavy prenatal alcohol exposure is related to smaller corpus callosum in newborn MRI scans. Alcohol Clin Exp Res. 2017;41(5):965–75.

51. Bookstein FL, Connor PD, Covell KD, Barr HM, Gleason CA, Sze RW, et al. Preliminary evidence that prenatal alcohol damage may be visible in averaged ultrasound images of the neonatal human corpus callosum. Alcohol (Fayettev, NY). 2005;36(3):151–60.

52. Bookstein FL, Connor PD, Huggins JE, Barr HM, Pimentel KD, Streissguth AP. Many infants prenatally exposed to high levels of alcohol show one particular anomaly of the corpus callosum. Alcohol Clin Exp Res. 2007;31(5):868–79.

53. Taylor PA, Jacobson SW, van der Kouwe A, Molteno CD, Chen G, Wintermark P, et al. A DTI-based tractography study of effects on brain structure associated with prenatal alcohol exposure in newborns. Hum Brain Mapp. 2015;36(1):170–86.

54. Donald KA, Roos A, Fouche J-P, Koen N, Howells FM, Woods RP, et al. A study of the effects of prenatal alcohol exposure on white matter microstructural integrity at birth. Acta Neuropsychiatr. 2015;27(4):197–205.

55. Roos A, Wedderburn CJ, Fouche J-P, Subramoney S, Joshi SH, Woods RP, et al. Central white matter integrity alterations in 2-3-year-old children following prenatal alcohol exposure. Drug Alcohol Depend. 2021;225:108826.

56. Yang Y, Phillips OR, Kan E, Sulik KK, Mattson SN, Riley EP, et al. Callosal thickness reductions relate to facial dysmorphology in fetal alcohol spectrum disorders. Alcohol Clin Exp Res. 2012;36(5):798–806.

57. Gautam P, Nuñez SC, Narr KL, Kan EC, Sowell ER. Effects of prenatal alcohol exposure on the development of white matter volume and change in executive function. Neuroimage Clin. 2014;5:19–27.

58. Wozniak JR, Muetzel RL. What does diffusion tensor imaging reveal about the brain and cognition in fetal alcohol spectrum disorders? Neuropsychol Rev. 2011;21(2):133–47.

59. Anna Dyląg K, Sikora-Sporek A, Bańdo B, Boroń-Zyss J, Drożdż D, Dumnicka P, et al. Magnetic resonance imaging (MRI) findings among children with fetal alcohol syndrome (FAS), partial fetal alcohol syndrome (pFAS) and alcohol related neurodevelopmental disorders (ARND). Przegl Lek. 2016;73(9):605–9.

60. Schneble E, Lack C, Zapadka M, Pfeifer CM, Bardo DME, Cagley J, et al. Increased notching of the corpus callosum in fetal alcohol spectrum disorder: a Callosal misunderstanding? AJNR Am J Neuroradiol. 2020;41(4):725–8.

61. Candelaria-Cook FT, Schendel ME, Flynn L, Hill DE, Stephen JM. Altered resting-state neural oscillations and spectral power in children with fetal alcohol spectrum disorder. Alcohol Clin Exp Res. 2021;45(1):117–30.

62. Fan J, Jacobson SW, Taylor PA, Molteno CD, Dodge NC, Stanton ME, et al. White matter deficits mediate effects of prenatal alcohol exposure on cognitive development in childhood. Hum Brain Mapp. 2016;37(8):2943–58.

63. Kar P, Reynolds JE, Grohs MN, Gibbard WB, McMorris C, Tortorelli C, et al. White matter alterations in young children with prenatal alcohol exposure. Dev Neurobiol. 2021;81(4):400–10.

64. Paolozza A, Treit S, Beaulieu C, Reynolds JN. Response inhibition deficits in children with fetal alcohol spectrum disorder: relationship between diffusion tensor imaging of the corpus callosum and eye movement control. Neuroimage Clin. 2014;5:53–61.

65. Paolozza A, Treit S, Beaulieu C, Reynolds JN. Diffusion tensor imaging of white matter and correlates to eye movement control and psychometric testing in children with prenatal alcohol exposure. Hum Brain Mapp. 2016;38(1):444–56.

66. Wozniak JR, Mueller BA, Chang P-N, Muetzel RL, Caros L, Lim KO. Diffusion tensor imaging in children with fetal alcohol spectrum disorders. Alcohol Clin Exp Res. 2006;30(10):1799–806.

67. Green CR, Lebel C, Rasmussen C, Beaulieu C, Reynolds JN. Diffusion tensor imaging correlates of saccadic reaction time in children with fetal alcohol spectrum disorder. Alcohol Clin Exp Res. 2013;37(9):1499–507.

68. Fryer SL, Schweinsburg BC, Bjorkquist OA, Frank LR, Mattson SN, Spadoni AD, et al. Characterization of white matter microstructure in fetal alcohol spectrum disorders. Alcohol Clin Exp Res. 2009;33(3):514–21.

69. Li L, Coles CD, Lynch ME, Hu X. Voxelwise and skeleton-based region of interest analysis of fetal alcohol syndrome and fetal alcohol spectrum disorders in young adults. Hum Brain Mapp. 2009;30(10):3265–74.
70. Ma X, Coles CD, Lynch ME, Laconte SM, Zurkiya O, Wang D, et al. Evaluation of corpus callosum anisotropy in young adults with fetal alcohol syndrome according to diffusion tensor imaging. Alcohol Clin Exp Res. 2005;29(7):1214–22.
71. Bookstein FL, Streissguth AP, Sampson PD, Connor PD, Barr HM. Corpus callosum shape and neuropsychological deficits in adult males with heavy fetal alcohol exposure. NeuroImage. 2002;15(1):233–51.
72. Liu F, Zhang Z, Lin X, Teng G, Meng H, Yu T, et al. Development of the human fetal cerebellum in the second trimester: a post mortem magnetic resonance imaging evaluation. J Anat. 2011;219(5):582–8.
73. Lerman-Sagie T, Prayer D, Stöcklein S, Malinger G. Fetal cerebellar disorders. Handb Clin Neurol. 2018;155:3–23.
74. Haldipur P, Aldinger KA, Bernardo S, Deng M, Timms AE, Overman LM, et al. Spatiotemporal expansion of primary progenitor zones in the developing human cerebellum. Science. 2019;366(6464):454–60.
75. Inkelis SM, Moore EM, Bischoff-Grethe A, Riley EP. Neurodevelopment in adolescents and adults with fetal alcohol spectrum disorders (FASD): a magnetic resonance region of interest analysis. Brain Res. 2020;1732:146654.
76. Sullivan EV, Moore EM, Lane B, Pohl KM, Riley EP, Pfefferbaum A. Graded cerebellar lobular volume deficits in adolescents and young adults with fetal alcohol spectrum disorders (FASD). Cereb Cortex (New York, N.Y.: 1991). 2020; https://doi.org/10.1093/cercor/bhaa020.
77. O'Hare ED, Kan E, Yoshii J, Mattson SN, Riley EP, Thompson PM, et al. Mapping cerebellar vermal morphology and cognitive correlates in prenatal alcohol exposure. Neuroreport. 2005;16(12):1285–90.
78. Sowell ER, Jernigan TL, Mattson SN, Riley EP, Sobel DF, Jones KL. Abnormal development of the cerebellar vermis in children prenatally exposed to alcohol: size reduction in lobules I-V. Alcohol Clin Exp Res. 1996;20(1):31–4.
79. Spottiswoode BS, Meintjes EM, Anderson AW, Molteno CD, Stanton ME, Dodge NC, et al. Diffusion tensor imaging of the cerebellum and eyeblink conditioning in fetal alcohol spectrum disorder. Alcohol Clin Exp Res. 2011;35(12):2174–83.
80. Fan J, Meintjes EM, Molteno CD, Spottiswoode BS, Dodge NC, Alhamud AA, et al. White matter integrity of the cerebellar peduncles as a mediator of effects of prenatal alcohol exposure on eyeblink conditioning. Hum Brain Mapp. 2015;36(7):2470–82.
81. Pillai JJ. The evolution of clinical functional imaging during the past 2 decades and its current impact on neurosurgical planning. Am J Neuroradiol. 2010;31(2):219–25.
82. Hall CN, Howarth C, Kurth-Nelson Z, Mishra A. Interpreting BOLD: towards a dialogue between cognitive and cellular neuroscience. Philos Trans R Soc B Biol Sci. 2016;371(1705):20150348.
83. Donald KA, Ipser JC, Howells FM, Roos A, Fouche J-P, Riley EP, et al. Interhemispheric functional brain connectivity in neonates with prenatal alcohol exposure: preliminary findings. Alcohol Clin Exp Res. 2016;40(1):113–21.
84. Fan J, Taylor PA, Jacobson SW, Molteno CD, Gohel S, Biswal BB, et al. Localized reductions in resting-state functional connectivity in children with prenatal alcohol exposure. Hum Brain Mapp. 2017;38(10):5217–33.
85. Little G, Reynolds J, Beaulieu C. Altered functional connectivity observed at rest in children and adolescents prenatally exposed to alcohol. Brain Connect. 2018;8(8):503–15.
86. Santhanam P, Coles CD, Li Z, Li L, Lynch ME, Hu X. Default mode network dysfunction in adults with prenatal alcohol exposure. Psychiatry Res. 2011;194(3):354–62.

87. Wozniak JR, Mueller BA, Muetzel RL, Bell CJ, Hoecker HL, Nelson ML, et al. Inter-hemispheric functional connectivity disruption in children with prenatal alcohol exposure. Alcohol Clin Exp Res. 2011;35(5):849–61.
88. Wozniak JR, Mueller BA, Bell CJ, Muetzel RL, Hoecker HL, Boys CJ, et al. Global functional connectivity abnormalities in children with fetal alcohol spectrum disorders. Alcohol Clin Exp Res. 2013;37(5):748–56.
89. Rodriguez CI, Vergara VM, Davies S, Calhoun VD, Savage DD, Hamilton DA. Detection of prenatal alcohol exposure using machine learning classification of resting-state functional network connectivity data. Alcohol (Fayettev, NY). 2021;93:25–34.
90. Wozniak JR, Mueller BA, Mattson SN, Coles CD, Kable JA, Jones KL, et al. Functional connectivity abnormalities and associated cognitive deficits in fetal alcohol spectrum disorders (FASD). Brain Imaging Behav. 2017;11(5):1432–45.
91. Long X, Kar P, Gibbard B, Tortorelli C, Lebel C. The brain's functional connectome in young children with prenatal alcohol exposure. Neuroimage Clin. 2019;24:102082.
92. Spadoni AD, Bazinet AD, Fryer SL, Tapert SF, Mattson SN, Riley EP. BOLD response during spatial working memory in youth with heavy prenatal alcohol exposure. Alcohol Clin Exp Res. 2009;33(12):2067–76.
93. Norman AL, O'Brien JW, Spadoni AD, Tapert SF, Jones KL, Riley EP, et al. A functional magnetic resonance imaging study of spatial working memory in children with prenatal alcohol exposure: contribution of familial history of alcohol use disorders. Alcohol Clin Exp Res. 2013;37(1):132–40.
94. Diwadkar VA, Meintjes EM, Goradia D, Dodge NC, Warton C, Molteno CD, et al. Differences in cortico-striatal-cerebellar activation during working memory in syndromal and nonsyndromal children with prenatal alcohol exposure. Hum Brain Mapp. 2012;34(8):1931–45.
95. Roussotte FF, Bramen JE, Nunez SC, Quandt LC, Smith L, O'Connor MJ, et al. Abnormal brain activation during working memory in children with prenatal exposure to drugs of abuse: the effects of methamphetamine, alcohol, and polydrug exposure. NeuroImage. 2011;54(4):3067–75.
96. Roussotte FF, Rudie JD, Smith L, O'Connor MJ, Bookheimer SY, Narr KL, et al. Frontostriatal connectivity in children during working memory and the effects of prenatal methamphetamine, alcohol, and polydrug exposure. Dev Neurosci. 2012;34(1):43–57.
97. Lewis CE, Thomas KGF, Ofen N, Warton CMR, Robertson F, Lindinger NM, et al. An fMRI investigation of neural activation predicting memory formation in children with fetal alcohol spectrum disorders. Neuroimage Clin. 2021;30:102532.
98. Fryer SL, Tapert SF, Mattson SN, Paulus MP, Spadoni AD, Riley EP. Prenatal alcohol exposure affects frontal-striatal BOLD response during inhibitory control. Alcohol Clin Exp Res. 2007;31(8):1415–24.
99. Ware AL, Infante MA, O'Brien JW, Tapert SF, Jones KL, Riley EP, et al. An fMRI study of behavioral response inhibition in adolescents with and without histories of heavy prenatal alcohol exposure. Behav Brain Res. 2015;278:137–46.
100. Kodali VN, Jacobson JL, Lindinger NM, Dodge NC, Molteno CD, Meintjes EM, et al. Differential recruitment of brain regions during response inhibition in children prenatally exposed to alcohol. Alcohol Clin Exp Res. 2017;41(2):334–44.
101. Gautam P, Nuñez SC, Narr KL, Mattson SN, May PA, Adnams CM, et al. Developmental trajectories for visuo-spatial attention are altered by prenatal alcohol exposure: a longitudinal FMRI study. Cereb Cortex. 2015;25(12):4761–71.
102. Li Z, Ma X, Peltier S, Hu X, Coles CD, Lynch ME. Occipital-temporal reduction and sustained visual attention deficit in prenatal alcohol exposed adults. Brain Imaging Behav. 2008;2(1):39–48.
103. Cheng DT, Meintjes EM, Stanton ME, Dodge NC, Pienaar M, Warton CMR, et al. Functional MRI of human eyeblink classical conditioning in children with fetal alcohol spectrum disorders. Cereb Cortex (New York, N.Y.: 1991). 2017;27(7):3752–67.

104. Lindinger NM, Jacobson JL, Warton CMR, Malcolm-Smith S, Molteno CD, Dodge NC, et al. Fetal alcohol exposure alters BOLD activation patterns in brain regions mediating the interpretation of facial affect. Alcohol Clin Exp Res. 2021;45(1):140–52.
105. du Plessis L, Jacobson JL, Jacobson SW, Hess AT, van der Kouwe A, Avison MJ, et al. An in vivo 1H magnetic resonance spectroscopy study of the deep cerebellar nuclei in children with fetal alcohol spectrum disorders. Alcohol Clin Exp Res. 2014;38(5):1330–8.
106. Astley SJ, Richards T, Aylward EH, Olson HC, Kerns K, Brooks A, et al. Magnetic resonance spectroscopy outcomes from a comprehensive magnetic resonance study of children with fetal alcohol spectrum disorders. Magn Reson Imaging. 2009;27(6):760–78.
107. Cortese BM, Moore GJ, Bailey BA, Jacobson SW, Delaney-Black V, Hannigan JH. Magnetic resonance and spectroscopic imaging in prenatal alcohol-exposed children: preliminary findings in the caudate nucleus. Neurotoxicol Teratol. 2006;28(5):597–606.
108. Fagerlund Å, Heikkinen S, Autti-Rämö I, Korkman M, Timonen M, Kuusi T, et al. Brain metabolic alterations in adolescents and young adults with fetal alcohol spectrum disorders. Alcohol Clin Exp Res. 2006;30(12):2097–104.
109. Riikonen RS, Nokelainen P, Valkonen K, Kolehmainen AI, Kumpulainen KI, Könönen M, et al. Deep serotonergic and dopaminergic structures in fetal alcoholic syndrome: a study with nor-beta-CIT-single-photon emission computed tomography and magnetic resonance imaging volumetry. Biol Psychiatry. 2005;57(12):1565–72.
110. Fryer SL, Mattson SN, Jernigan TL, Archibald SL, Jones KL, Riley EP. Caudate volume predicts neurocognitive performance in youth with heavy prenatal alcohol exposure. Alcohol Clin Exp Res. 2012;36(11):1932–41.

Chapter 11
Neuropsychological Outcomes in FASD Across the Lifespan

Matthew T. Hyland, Natasia S. Courchesne-Krak, Chloe M. Sobolewski, Carissa Zambrano, and Sarah N. Mattson

Introduction

Although the exact mechanisms are not completely understood, the teratogenic effect of alcohol on development has been well described by researchers and clinicians. Prenatal alcohol exposure impacts physical, cognitive, and behavioral development and can cause lifelong impairment. Among these effects are a collection of neuropsychological abnormalities that disrupt the cognitive function of individuals with prenatal alcohol exposure, termed fetal alcohol spectrum disorder (FASD). Children and adults living with FASD display deficits in areas including general cognitive function, attention, executive function, learning and memory, language, visuospatial abilities, academic performance, and motor skills [1, 2]. Although individuals with prenatal alcohol exposure may also display some relative strengths in these domains, few studies have explored these strengths. The majority of those that have described strengths focus on character strengths, such as perseverance and compassion, without discussing how these may affect neuropsychological outcomes [3]. Furthermore, while some studies do mention relative strengths within neuropsychological domains, these often seem inconsistent across studies.

Given that children with FASD are often overlooked or misdiagnosed [4], it is imperative that clinicians who evaluate children for developmental disorders are aware of the many neuropsychological and behavioral symptoms associated with prenatal alcohol exposure, including various strengths and weaknesses, so they can more readily identify affected individuals and provide appropriate and effective interventions to both mitigate hardship and maximize strengths. This chapter aims

M. T. Hyland · N. S. Courchesne-Krak · C. M. Sobolewski
C. Zambrano · S. N. Mattson (✉)
Center for Behavioral Teratology and Department of Psychology, San Diego State University, San Diego, CA, USA
e-mail: mthyland@sdsu.edu; nscourchesne@sdsu.edu; csobolewski7107@sdsu.edu; czambrano2@sdsu.edu; sarah.mattson@sdsu.edu

to summarize neuropsychological findings throughout the lifespan. Key terms and phrases are defined in Glossary.

Overall Cognitive Ability

The overall cognitive ability (i.e., general intellectual function) of children and adults with FASD is often impaired in comparison with typically developing individuals. Intellectual disability, defined as having an IQ score <70 and adaptive disability, is 23 times more prevalent in those with FASD than in the general population [2, 5]. However, IQ scores vary widely, both in the population as a whole and within diagnostic categories. For example, it is possible for someone with prenatal alcohol exposure, but none of the associated morphological symptoms, to have more severe impairments than someone with all the features of fetal alcohol syndrome (FAS), and intellectual disability is not required for an FASD diagnosis. In fact, most individuals with FASD do not experience deficits severe enough to qualify as having an intellectual disability [2, 6–8], though average cognitive function is lower when compared to children with other neuropsychological disorders (e.g., attention-deficit/hyperactivity disorder [ADHD], autism spectrum disorder [ASD], receptive and expressive language disorders, and a variety of learning disabilities) [1, 9].

Prenatal alcohol exposure is the most common preventable cause of intellectual impairment [10]. Deficits exist in many components of intellectual functioning, such as lower scores on assessments of perceptual reasoning, processing speed, verbal comprehension, and working memory [11]. Although the majority of studies have recorded lower intellectual functioning (i.e., IQ scores) in this population, some have found no effect of prenatal alcohol exposure on general ability [12, 13].

Both children and adults with FASD display a range of ability levels, as measured by IQ scores, which correlate with levels of prenatal alcohol exposure [13]. A linear dose–response relationship has been observed between exposure levels and IQ test performance, such that greater exposure is associated with lower IQ scores [2, 13]. On the FASD diagnostic spectrum (see Chap. 9), intellectual functioning is, on average, most impaired in individuals with FAS, followed by partial fetal alcohol syndrome (PFAS) and alcohol-related neurodevelopmental disorder (ARND; [1, 13]). Though as mentioned, overall level of function is not strictly related to diagnosis.

One study by Ervalahti and colleagues [14] identified a significant relationship between the severity of physical dysmorphology and the level of cognitive functioning in children with FASD. However, in general, intellectual disability is not dependent on the presence or absence of facial dysmorphology [7, 9]. Physiological and environmental factors associated with FASD can also impact intellectual functioning. Loss of white matter integrity, which can result from prenatal alcohol exposure, negatively affects intelligence and cognitive capability in children and adolescents [15]. Early adverse life experience and trauma may negatively impact neuropsychological outcomes, though research is limited. In one dissertation study, general cognitive ability was affected in children with FASD and histories of trauma but not more than in children with FASD alone. The same results were found using an functional magnetic resonance imaging (fMRI) task involving the prefrontal cortex [16]. Thus, in this singular study, the history of trauma did not exacerbate the effects of prenatal alcohol exposure. However, it may be difficult to disentangle these two critical early life experiences and additional research is needed.

Scores from IQ tests often show significant differences between verbal and nonverbal intelligence, though the direction of these differences is inconsistent between studies [2, 12]. Higher IQ scores have been identified as a protective factor against poor language skills, adaptive functioning, and academic performance in individuals with FASD. Alternatively, lower IQ scores are often predictive of negative educational, occupational, physical, and mental health outcomes. Thus, lower intellectual functioning may play a detrimental and lifelong role in individuals living with FASD [2], though another study conflicts with this idea. Streissguth et al. [17] found that individuals with prenatal alcohol exposure who had lower IQ scores actually had fewer adverse life outcomes. However, it is likely that this is, at least in part, due to the fact that individuals with lower IQ, especially those with a diagnosis of FAS, are more likely to qualify for support due to developmental disabilities.

The effects of prenatal alcohol exposure on general intelligence are largely permanent rather than a developmental delay [2, 18]. In fact, intellectual and cognitive abilities of those with prenatal alcohol exposure may become further impacted with age and greater expectations of independence [18], which likely equates to executive function and complex information processing domains. For example, a study of adolescents, transition-aged youth, and adults with FASD compared difficulties in nine daily living skill domains, including suspension or expulsion from school, employment problems, needing help to live independently, needing assisted or sheltered housing, legal problems including both victimization and offending, incarceration, and misuse of alcohol and other substances. Collectively, transition-aged youth and adults showed significantly more difficulty in these domains [18]. Although daily living skills are not a traditional measure of intellectual impairment, some researchers have indicated that everyday problem-solving skills are a more ecologically valid measure of intellectual ability than IQ scores [19, 20]. Thus, while additional study is needed, it is likely that difficulties in general cognitive function persist beyond adolescence.

Attention

Attentional deficits are one of the most common and persistent neurobehavioral consequences of prenatal alcohol exposure [21, 22]. Various components of attention, both visual and auditory, are impaired in children with heavy prenatal alcohol exposure or FASD, though visual attention deficits seem to be more extreme than those in auditory attention [1, 23, 24]. Attention deficits in children with FASD have been associated with areas of the occipital-temporal region and regions of the frontal lobe, cingulate gyrus, thalamus, corpus striatum, and reticular formation [25, 26].

In a study of both visual and auditory attention, Mattson and colleagues [23] found that children with FASD had trouble maintaining attention in both domains over increasing intertrial intervals. However, while reaction times for children with FASD were slower, no significant differences were found in the children's ability to accurately shift between visual and auditory attention compared to typically developing controls. Another study reported that deficits in sustaining attention were present in preschool-aged children but were not observed in 14-year-old children [24]. Others still have demonstrated that, while deficits in visual attention have been found in children with FASD, these deficits were not observed when compared with typically developing children with similar IQ scores [27].

Many individuals living with FASD also have diagnoses of ADHD [5]. Several studies have directly compared FASD to ADHD while other studies indirectly describe similarities and differences between these two groups (for review, see [2]). These comparisons will be described in the relevant sections below. In terms of attention, although both FASD and ADHD involve attention deficits, the specific aspects of attention deficits vary between the groups. Although deficits in establishing and sustaining attention have been associated with prenatal alcohol exposure [1], Coles et al. [28] reported that children with FASD demonstrated stronger impairments in the ability to shift attentional sets and encode information, while children with ADHD had more trouble focusing and sustaining attention [28]. This may point to sustained attention being a relative strength of individuals with FASD where this domain is concerned.

Adults with histories of prenatal alcohol exposure also show signs of impaired attention, both in self-report and performance-based measures [29]. One study of young adults with prenatal alcohol exposure found that exposed participants performed significantly worse than control participants on measures of auditory and visual attention, although auditory attention seemed to be more impaired. The group with prenatal alcohol exposure had difficulty focusing, sustaining, and shifting attention in auditory tasks and focusing and sustaining attention in the visual tasks [26]. While the pattern of deficits differs slightly from studies of children, these results show that attention deficits persist into adulthood in alcohol-exposed individuals.

Executive Function

Executive function refers to a number of cognitive processes which are used in conjunction with one another to drive goal-related behavior [30]. These processes have been related to regions of the frontal lobe, especially the dorsolateral prefrontal cortex, as well as subcortical circuits [2, 31]. Individuals with FASD exhibit global deficits in executive function, including difficulties in planning and problem solving, concept formation, set-shifting, fluency, response inhibition, working memory, and emotional regulation. Performance on tests of executive function effectively differentiates children with histories of prenatal alcohol exposure from those without exposure [1]. Furthermore, these impairments cannot be explained by deficits in underlying component skills such as reading and motor skills [32].

Additionally, these deficits seem to be independent of comorbidities, such as ADHD, that are so often found in those with FASD. Many studies have explored the differences and similarities between the executive functioning capabilities between children and adolescents with FASD and ADHD (for review, see [1]). For example, Nguyen and colleagues [33] used both performance-based measures and parent ratings to examine executive functioning. In both ratings from parents and performance on cognitive tasks, there were main effects of alcohol exposure and ADHD. This indicates that children with histories of exposure showed more executive function deficits than non-exposed children, regardless of ADHD diagnosis. Likewise, when children living with ADHD with or without prenatal alcohol exposure were grouped together, they displayed more impairment than those without an ADHD diagnosis. The interaction between alcohol exposure and ADHD was not significant, suggesting independent effects on performance-based tasks. On the parent report, however, an interaction was observed between alcohol exposure and ADHD in addition to the main effects. Follow-up analyses indicated that children with both ADHD and a history of prenatal alcohol exposure exhibited significantly greater deficits than children who only had ADHD or prenatal alcohol exposure [33]. Furthermore, in a meta-analysis of 15 studies, children and adolescents with FASD exhibited significantly greater executive dysfunction than those with ADHD and typically developing individuals, though the strength of this difference was small and IQ and socioeconomic status were both significant moderating factors [34].

Impairments in executive function do not fully retreat with age. In fact, Kingdon et al. [35] found that, across a number of studies, overall deficits in executive function seemed to increase from the age of 5–12, and then level off in adolescence, and other studies have found difficulties in adults with prenatal alcohol exposure similar to those in children [36–38].

Planning/Organizing and Problem Solving

Individuals with prenatal alcohol exposure display marked difficulties in their ability to plan and organize future events and solve complex problems [1, 2]. A meta-analysis of 65 studies of executive function found that children and adolescents with FASD consistently showed large deficits in this domain [35]. On tasks assessing planning and problem solving, these children made more errors, completed fewer problems, spent less time planning, and seemed to employ less effective strategies for completing the tasks than typically developing children, especially as the tasks become more complex [1].

In a study of children and adolescents with FASD (FAS and PFAS), participants were asked to perform a variety of cognitive tasks including the progressive planning test, an assessment that contains increasingly complex puzzles. Participants in the FASD group performed comparably to typically developing participants on simpler trials, however, on more complex trials they demonstrated significant difficulty in planning. No differences were observed between participants with FAS and PFAS on either simple or complex trials, supporting previous findings [39]. Mattson et al. [32] found no difference in performance on the Tower of California Test, an assessment of planning, between prenatally exposed children with and without FAS. In order to explore the impact of IQ on planning, Olson and colleagues [40] compared adolescents with FAS to a typically developing group as well as a group without prenatal alcohol exposure matching the mean IQ of the FAS participants. Adolescents with FAS performed worse than both comparison groups on a Stepping Stone Maze test, a task of visual-spatial memory which is also sensitive to planning ability [40].

Planning and organizing impairments are also evident on parent and teacher ratings of children with FASD in comparison to typically developing samples and population norms [33]. They are also sometimes rated as having difficulty with organizing materials and spaces, such as an area of work or play [41]. While children and adolescents with FASD routinely show deficits in planning and organizing in both rating scales and performance-based measures, it is important to note that the two do not always capture impairments in the same domains, suggesting that the different types of measures may be capturing different aspects of executive functioning [33, 42].

Adults with prenatal alcohol exposure also have difficulties in planning, although research is limited. Rangmar et al. [43] found that adults with FAS took significantly more steps to solve an assessment of planning similar to the Tower of California, Tower of Hanoi, compared to controls.

Concept Formation and Set-Shifting

Concept formation, the ability to develop abstract concepts, and set-shifting, switching from one such concept to another, are also impaired in individuals with FASD [28, 44]. Although many aspects of executive function were found to be impaired in the meta-analysis conducted by Kingdon et al. [35], set-shifting was a relative weakness in children with FASD, along with planning. Performance-based measures and rating scales regularly show deficits in both concept formation and set-shifting in this population [28, 33, 41, 45].

In one study, two similar assessments, the Wisconsin Card Sorting Test (WCST) and the California Card Sorting Test (CST), were used to examine concept formation in children and adolescents with prenatal exposure. Participants in the exposed group scored lower than controls on both measures indicating that these individuals had a difficult time finding similarities between the stimuli and making higher order inferences [44]. Mattson and colleagues [32] found difficulties in shifting in a similar population using the California Trail Making Test and California Stroop Test. However, differences between the alcohol-exposed children and typically developing children were only found in the higher-order switching condition (i.e., switching between numbers and letters) and not the lower-level component tasks (e.g., connecting letters only) suggesting that these impairments do not come from simple skills required in the task [32]. Additionally, a few differences between exposed children with and without FAS were present in both studies. In the study conducted by McGee et al. [44], children with FAS tended to perform worse on the WCST than alcohol-exposed participants without the diagnosis. Similarly, Mattson et al. [32] found that only the FAS group differed from controls in the switching condition, but exposed participants without FAS did not, indicating that, while alcohol has an impact on this domain, severity of the condition is related to greater dysfunction [32, 44]. Other studies have sought to determine whether impairments are related to an indicator of general severity (i.e., IQ scores). One study found that adolescents with FAS committed more errors and completed fewer problems in the WCST than IQ-matched controls [40].

Adults with prenatal alcohol exposure also demonstrate difficulties with concept formation and set-shifting. Connor et al. [36] conducted a study of prenatally exposed adults, both with and without a diagnosis of FAS. Individuals with prenatal alcohol exposure performed worse than controls on a Trail Making Test and the WCST, suggesting that these impairments persist well into adulthood. Furthermore, while some aspects of these tests correlated with IQ (Trail Making error scores), most did not, indicating that the deficits in this in concept formation and set-shifting are beyond the impact of general intelligence [36].

Fluency

The ability to produce multiple responses in both verbal and nonverbal domains within time constraints is also hindered in individuals with FASD [1]. This impairment has also been observed in parent and teacher ratings in which alcohol-exposed children are described as having more difficulty initiating tasks and generating ideas [33, 41]. In the meta-analysis conducted by Kingdon and colleagues [35], fluency was named as a third relative weakness across studies of executive function in the FASD population. Moreover, one study showed that IQ was not a significant predictor of performance in children with FASD on either verbal or nonverbal assessments of fluency, indicating that deficits in fluency are independent of general intelligence [45].

Exposed participants have greater difficulty in tests of letter fluency than in category fluency, which is a less complex task of verbal fluency [1, 2]. In addition to these traditional assessments of verbal fluency, some studies also include a category switching test, which is similar to category fluency tasks; however, it requires the participant to switch back and forth between two categories. Two such studies found that alcohol-exposed children performed worse on these fluency tasks compared to controls [39, 45]. However, Schonfeld et al. [45] found that component tasks (more simple verbal fluency) only accounted for 14.6% of the overall variance in the more complex verbal fluency switching task and group membership only accounted for 2%, suggesting there are likely other components at play (e.g., attention, verbal ability).

Nonverbal fluency is less well studied. Deficits were noted on simple and switching conditions of a design fluency task [45] when compared to controls but not in comparison to normative data [46]. Thus, deficits in this area may not be as prominent as in the verbal fluency domain although additional study may be needed.

Impairment in fluency also seems to continue into adulthood. Using a nonverbal assessment of fluency, the Ruff Figural Fluency Test (RFF), Kerns and colleagues [37] found that young adults who had previously been diagnosed with FAS showed deficits compared to norms. Interestingly this study reported both the number of unique designs and perseverations and, although no control group was included, reported results in relation to overall IQ scores. Young adults with FAS and average IQ scores created an average number of unique designs but significantly more perseverative designs than would be expected for their overall ability level. However, participants with FAS and below average IQ scores created fewer unique designs and had more perseverations than predicted by their IQ [37]. Another study using the same task [36], found that adults with prenatal alcohol exposure created fewer unique designs and had higher rates of perseverative, or repeated, designs than would be expected based on general intelligence. Perseveration, but not overall production, was highly correlated with IQ, supporting the notion that deficits in fluency, even those in adults, are beyond the impact of IQ.

Inhibition

Response inhibition is another area where individuals with FASD show impairment, both in performance-based measure and rating scales [1, 2, 33, 41]. Mattson et al. [32] used the Color–Word Interference Test to assess inhibition in children and adolescents with prenatal alcohol exposure and controls. There were no group differences in performance on the first two conditions of the test (word reading and color naming). However, the exposed participants performed significantly worse in the third (interference) condition, which required them to identify the color of the ink a word was printed in, instead of reading the word itself (which was also a color). Hierarchical regression analysis revealed the first two conditions, along with age, accounted for 63% of the variance in the interference condition. Group accounted for an additional 8% of the variance which was significant. This implies that the alcohol-exposed group had deficits in inhibition, which were not completely explained by difficulties with lower-order component skills used in the first two conditions. Additionally, this measure of inhibition was not correlated with IQ in the alcohol-exposed group. While other deficits in executive function were found in the other three tasks employed in this study, components of impaired inhibition were noted in all of them, providing support for the idea of inhibition as a primary deficit in this population [32].

In contrast, the meta-analysis conducted by Kingdon et al. [35] indicated that deficits in inhibition may relate to the degree of FASD-related dysmorphology. Moderate inhibition deficits were identified when comparing dysmorphic FASD participants with typically developing controls but only small, statistically insignificant deficits were observed when comparing non-dysmorphic participants to typically developing controls. The effect size for both comparisons of inhibition was the smallest out of the five domains of executive function examined (i.e., planning, set-shifting, fluency, working memory, and inhibition). Although dysmorphology is not a direct indicator of cognitive dysfunction, future studies should consider severity of alcohol exposure as well as domain of executive function in order to determine whether these results can be replicated.

A study using fMRI and a visual Go/No-Go test indicated group differences in functional activation even when task performance was not impaired [47]. Results suggested that the alcohol-exposed participants displayed an increased recruitment of regions in order to overcome a less efficient executive function network. Additionally, researchers in this study speculated that, since activation associated with inhibition in these regions have been known to become more focused with age, this could indicate an underdeveloped pattern of cortical activation [47]. This study found no correlation between activation and age in participants with prenatal alcohol exposure, nor did they find any difference between exposed participants with and without FAS, suggesting that the physiological response underlying impairment in inhibition persists, at least into late adolescence, and is independent of diagnosis [47].

Working Memory

Working memory is the process by which information can be held and manipulated in the mind for a short period of time. Information in working memory can also be associated with long-term memory, perceptions, and actions [48]. Parents and teachers frequently rate children with FASD as having more problem behaviors related to impaired working memory [33, 41], and they perform more poorly than typically developing children on tasks that involve this domain, although additional study is needed [1, 2].

One study used a principal component analysis to determine which components from attention and executive function tests were impacted by prenatal alcohol exposure [49]. Tests involving aspects of working memory, including Digit Cancellation, Digit Span, Tower of London, Arithmetic, Corsi, and Seashore Rhythm, seemed to be the most directly impacted. Moreover, the working memory component was still significant when IQ was controlled for and there seemed to be no differences between alcohol-exposed children with and without FAS [49]. Compared with controls, individuals with prenatal alcohol exposure also display deficits in the manipulation of information in working memory as the difficulty of the task being performed increases [1].

Verbal and spatial working memory are both affected by prenatal alcohol exposure, and atypical neurodevelopment is observed in brain regions that are essential for spatial working memory performance [50]. fMRI studies have also been used to analyze the physiological aspects of working memory dysfunction in the FASD population and have shown that these deficits are especially linked to frontoparietal regions [1]. In one study [51], children and adolescents completed a verbal Sternberg working memory task while undergoing fMRI. Participants were shown an array of letters and symbols and instructed to remember the numbers. Then, after a short delay, a probe letter was shown and participants were asked to identify whether or not it had been present in the array. Trials varied in working memory load based on the number of letters in the array. Although children with FASD performed similarly on trials with medium and high working memory loads, researchers observed that, even after controlling for IQ differences, the alcohol-exposed group displayed increased functional activation in working memory-related regions compared to controls. Specifically, increased activity was observed in the left dorsolateral prefrontal cortex, left inferior parietal cortex, and bilateral posterior temporal regions. The increase of activity in these regions paired with similar performance in the behavioral measure implies that children and adolescents with FASD utilize a larger cortical network, suggesting less efficient processing when performing tasks requiring verbal working memory [51].

Working memory impairment in individuals with prenatal alcohol exposure seems to increase as children age and extends into adulthood. Research has found that prenatal alcohol exposure showed similar spatial working memory performance at younger ages compared to controls [52]. However, larger group differences were observed as children aged. Adults with prenatal alcohol exposure perform worse on digit span tasks, both forward and backward conditions [43]. In addition, Connor et al. [36] tested adults on a number of executive function tests, including the Consonant Trigrams Test, a task evaluating working memory. Prenatally exposed adults showed consistent deficits on this task compared to typical controls [36]. Another fMRI study compared functional activation during working memory in children and adults with and without histories of prenatal alcohol exposure. This study used an n-back task, which assesses spatial working memory. Overall activation was not the same between groups; both children and adults demonstrated increases in activity in the inferior-middle frontal lobe compared to controls, especially during simpler conditions. Control participants also showed increased frontal lobe activity with an increase in task difficulty, but this was not always observed in adults with FASD and children with FASD showed the opposite [38]. While interpretation of this study is limited by group differences in task performance, it supports other fMRI studies and indicates that the physiological underpinnings of working memory dysfunction continue well into adulthood for individuals prenatally exposed to alcohol.

Learning and Memory

Prenatal alcohol exposure has been shown to disrupt learning and memory in humans; these effects are seen across exposure levels and on multiple tasks [1]. Generally, persistent effects are seen in learning new information while effects on retention are more variable. In most cases children with FASD have difficulties learning new verbal information and recalling that information. However, they do benefit from repeated exposure and are able to retain learned information. Results in tests of nonverbal learning and memory are less consistent. In some studies, it appears that both learning and retention are affected [12, 53, 54]; however, others have found no differences in spatial memory ability once visuospatial abilities were accounted for, indicating a mediated relationship between visuospatial abilities and deficits in observed spatial memory [1].

Studies of moderate exposure have mixed results. In one study [55], children with moderate prenatal alcohol exposure demonstrated deficits in immediate and delayed recall for word pairs on the Children's Memory Scale (CMS) [55]. However, the impact of prenatal alcohol exposure on verbal recall in the same sample was mediated by their performance on the verbal learning assessments. Specifically, larger deficits in verbal recall were observed in children with poorer acquisition of new information. Another study of moderate exposure [56], however, did not support the role of encoding in retention of verbal information.

In those with heavy exposure or FASD, commonly identified neuropsychological deficits include impaired learning and memory, particularly deficits in verbal learning and verbal and spatial recall [53, 57]. A study on the effects of heavy prenatal alcohol exposure in late childhood and early adolescence (ages 9–15) found that smaller left hippocampi, which is essential in memory consolidation and retrieval, correlated with a decrease in verbal learning skills (e.g., memory encoding, storage, retrieval abilities) and spatial memory performance (e.g., "getting lost where he/she has often been before"). In those with FASD, the size of the hippocampus positively correlated with performance on short- and long-term delayed verbal recall [58]. Caudate volume, which is consistently affected in FASD and is the optimal predictor of neuropsychological performance for children prenatally exposed to alcohol, correlated with verbal learning, cognitive control, and recall skills [59]. Altered brain activation patterns during verbal learning, response inhibition, visual attention, and working memory tasks have been observed in children with FASD using functional neuroimaging [1]. Collectively, these results suggest that children with FASD have difficulty acquiring new information, which in turn appears to impact other aspects of their memory function.

Adults with prenatal alcohol exposure display deficits in learning and memory as well. Coles et al. [60] used a Verbal Selective Reminding Memory Test and a Nonverbal Selective Reminding Memory Test to assess both dysmorphic and non-dysmorphic young adults with prenatal alcohol exposure. Participants with histories of prenatal alcohol exposure performed significantly worse on measures of verbal and nonverbal memory than controls. Similar to results often found in children with FASD, memory deficits in these young adults appeared to be due to difficulties in encoding information. Furthermore, there seemed to be a relationship between severity of diagnosis and performance, as those in the dysmorphic group generally performed worse than the non-dysmorphic alcohol-exposed group who performed worse than controls [60].

Language and Communication

Despite descriptions of language difficulties in early case reports of the FASD community, there is relatively little information on the subject and current research has shown mixed results [2]. Some studies have found that children with heavy prenatal alcohol exposure have both expressive and receptive language impairment, with no differences between the two [1, 61]. Others have shown evidence that these children have stronger receptive than expressive skills [1]. Still other studies have found little to no language impairments at all in relation to prenatal alcohol exposure. In a study of children with FAS conducted by Greene et al. [62], only 2 out of 27 measures of language ability met nominal significance after controlling for the effects of the home environment, though the children in this study were very young.

Some of the differences in language among individuals with FASD have been attributed to physical components of hearing and speech. The majority of FAS patients tested by Church and colleagues [63], ranging from 3 to 26 years old, had some form of hearing loss and clinically significant speech disorder. Hearing loss was determined to be a result of recurrent serous otitis media or sensorineural hearing loss, and these disorders may have exacerbated language deficits. However, children with FASD diagnoses other than FAS are no more likely to have physical hearing problems than the general population, and yet often display atypical auditory behaviors. This indicates that poor auditory filtering ability may be mediated by more cognitive factors [64]. Another study of children with FAS concluded that speech deficits were likely due to a combination of central nervous system dysfunction, hearing impairment, oral-motor ability, and structural abnormalities [65].

Language impairments due to prenatal alcohol exposure seem to begin early, as they have been found in children at the ages of 2 and 3 years. Yet, these same children did not exhibit language difficulties at ages 4, 5, or 6 years [2]. Studies that have observed differences in language ability in older children with FASD suggest that, while young children seem to display more global language deficits, older children have more trouble with syntactic and grammatical constructs and are less affected in semantic performance [1]. Notably, children with FASD perform worse on measures of semantic elaboration than typically developing children. Thorne et al. [66] demonstrated that a sample of children with FASD were significantly more likely to use ambiguous references during a narrative, and a measure of semantic elaboration was able to distinguish these children with a high rate of accuracy.

Although there are fewer studies of language including adults with histories of prenatal alcohol exposure, one study discovered that exposed adults had difficulty comprehending affective prosody. In fact, on an assessment of affective prosodic comprehension, prenatally exposed adults performed worse than age-matched controls and recovering alcoholics and had indistinct results from patients with brain damage. Although these participants did not differ from controls on verbal skills, vocabulary, or abstract reasoning, this outcome suggests that some aspects of receptive language impairment may persist into adulthood in individuals with prenatal alcohol exposure [67].

Visuospatial Abilities

Visuospatial ability is measured by the ability to imagine objects, to make global shapes, or to comprehend differences and similarities between objects. Research on the impact of prenatal alcohol exposure on visuospatial abilities is limited. When compared to typically developing controls, impairments in visual perception and construction tasks have been identified in children with prenatal alcohol exposure [68]. In another study, difficulties in other domains such as visual memory in children appear to be related to visuospatial ability [69]. Specifically, a significant difference in spatial memory was not observed once performance on tasks related to perceptual and verbal memory were taken into account. In comparison with children with ADHD, children with prenatal alcohol exposure exhibit greater deficits in visuospatial ability [1]. In a systematic review of motor skills, children ages 12 years or older with prenatal alcohol exposure demonstrated difficulties with visual-motor integration along with fine motor skills and balance skills [70].

Children with prenatal alcohol exposure also exhibit impairments on visual construction tasks that require copying and remembering geometric drawings [57]. On a global-local (i.e., hierarchical) task, children with histories of prenatal alcohol exposure exhibit deficits in the reproduction and recall of local (smaller) features but not global (larger) features [68]. Control conditions indicated that the selective local deficit was not due to the size of the stimuli or to memory.

A study investigating the visuospatial abilities related to mathematics achievement in children with heavy prenatal alcohol exposure identified deficits on spatial span forward (i.e., a measure of spatial attention) and spatial recognition memory (i.e., a measure of spatial memory) among those with FASD compared to controls [71]. Results from the aforementioned study suggest that impairments in mathematics in those with FASD may be related to deficits in spatial processing.

Academic Performance

The aforementioned deficits in broad neuropsychological domains impact everyday life for children and adults living with an FASD [11, 72]. One important domain is academic function. Individuals with FASD have demonstrated poor competency in multiple academic domains including verbal (e.g., reading and spelling) and mathematical skills, even when controlling for global intelligence [1–3].

Marked difficulty in mathematical reasoning is common in both children and adults with FASD [1–3]. Children with prenatal alcohol exposure frequently score lower on tests of global mathematic achievement and particularly struggle in areas of basic numerical processing skills (e.g., estimation), units of measurement (e.g., time and date, length and width, weight), and currency-related calculations [1–3]. A study conducted by Goldschmidt and colleagues [73] found a linear dose–response relationship between prenatal alcohol exposure and poor academic achievement in mathematics. Additionally, heavy prenatal alcohol exposure has been noted to cause greater overall academic impairment than lesser exposure [1, 73]. Recently, multiple neuroimaging studies have indicated a number of brain regions associated with mathematical reasoning deficits in this population, including the medial frontal gyrus and bilateral parietal regions [2]. Difficulty in spelling, reading, and verbal comprehension are also commonly observed in the FASD population. Differing slightly from mathematical impairments, the relationship between deficits in the verbal domains seems to be represented as threshold effects [2].

Deficits in other areas, especially working memory and spatial processing, as described above, contribute to the mathematical difficulties experienced by individuals with FASD [1]. Similarly, poor reading and spelling have been linked to difficulties in working memory [1] and impairment in verbal comprehension, written communication, and following instructions can result from delayed language development [3]. Other aspects of prenatal alcohol exposure can indirectly impact academic performance. Sleep disturbances and sensory-motor deficits, which have been observed in individuals with FASD, likely contribute to poor overall academic performance [3], as do many socio-environmental factors that are associated with the disorders [13].

Motor Skills

Over the years, there has been little research regarding motor impairments in individuals with FASD, likely because it is less frequently assessed by clinicians evaluating children for these disorders [74]. Prenatal alcohol exposure has been known to impact areas of the brain associated with motor skills including the regions of the cerebellum, the basal ganglia, the corpus callosum, and the hippocampus [70, 75]. Deficits in both fine (e.g., precision, dexterity, visual-motor integration, isotonic force, and upper limb coordination) and gross (e.g., general body movements, balance, strength, and coordination) motor skills have been observed in those with prenatal alcohol exposure [74, 76]. However, there is evidence that fine motor skills are significantly more delayed than gross motor skills in young children with FAS. Kalberg et al. [77] found that, in a sample of children with FAS, 43% demonstrated average gross motor abilities while only 7% had average fine motor skills. Exposed children without an FAS diagnosis also had lower mean scores in gross and fine motor assessments, though these differences were not significant [77].

In one longitudinal study, fine motor skills and reaction time at age 4 were related to the amount of alcohol reported during pregnancy [78]. Children exposed to greater than 0.5 ounces of alcohol per day on average during early pregnancy made significantly more errors during tasks of fine motor skills than those who were not exposed [78].

Although they may be a relative strength compared to fine motor skills, impairments in gross motor skills have also been identified in those with prenatal alcohol exposure. One meta-analysis found that children with moderate to heavy prenatal alcohol exposure show significant impairment in gross motor skills [79]. Increased consumption of alcohol during pregnancy has also been correlated with poorer performance on gross motor balance and fine motor ratings and these skills showed negative linear relationships with alcohol intake before pregnancy recognition [76, 78, 80]. Moreover, children and adolescents with high levels of prenatal alcohol exposure were 2.9 times more likely to demonstrate gross motor deficits compared to typically developing controls [79].

Motor skill deficits appear to persist into adulthood [74, 77]. Adults with FASD display poorer motor function compared to typically developed individuals, especially in balance, motor control, and hand-eye coordination [1].

History and Future Directions

The study of neuropsychological effects of prenatal alcohol exposure has evolved over nearly 50 years. Initial reports documented global abnormalities such as overall IQ scores. Subsequent studies honed in on specific tasks and domains and documented a multitude of difficulties experienced by individuals living with an FASD. Neuroimaging allowed a different level of examination and revealed changes in the brain that may underlie everyday difficulties. What is needed now is a reversal of sorts. No longer do we need to focus on specific deficits in FASD. Rather, we need to focus on how to effectively detect both weaknesses and strengths and use the information gathered to more accurately identify and diagnose those with an FASD. With the prevalence of FASD as high as it is [81] and the accuracy of detection as low as it is [4], we need to increase the number of clinicians trained to accurately detect FASD. Similarly, we need to move away from the stigmatizing treatment of those living with an FASD and their families and instead focus on the creation and implementation of effective tools for identification and treatment. Identifying strengths will serve this goal, creating more optimism and understanding around the disorder and opening more opportunities for strength-base interventions [3].

Acknowledgements The authors thank the families who graciously participate in our studies. The authors have no financial or other conflicts of interest. Preparation of this chapter was funded by a grant from the National Institute on Alcohol Abuse and Alcoholism (NIAAA): U01 AA014834. Additional support was provided by grant T32 AA013525 from NIAAA and grant R25 GM058906 from the National Institutes of Health (NIH).

Glossary

Affective prosody Nonlinguistic aspect of language that conveys emotions and attitudes during discourse [67]

Auditory attention The ability to attend to relevant auditory stimuli and filter out irrelevant auditory stimuli

Fluency The ability to produce multiple responses, in either verbal or nonverbal domains, within time constraints [1]

Memory encoding Learning or the process by which memories are transferred from short-term to long-term storage

Perseveration The continuation or repetition of an activity without the appropriate stimulus [82]

Response inhibition The ability to suppress irrelevant stimuli or behavioral impulses to facilitate efficient, goal-directed behavior [47]

Set-shifting The ability to switch from one conceptual category to another [2]

Spatial attention The ability to attend to the relative location of one's self and/or objects in space

Spatial processing The sensing and integration of information pertaining to a location in space [83]

Visual attention The ability to attend to relevant visual stimuli and filter out irrelevant visual stimuli

Visual-spatial memory Memory for the relative locations and orientation of objects in space

Working memory The process by which information can be held and manipulated in the mind for a short period of time [48]

References

1. Mattson SN, Bernes GA, Doyle LR. Fetal alcohol spectrum disorders: a review of the neurobehavioral deficits associated with prenatal alcohol exposure. Alcohol Clin Exp Res. 2019;43(6):1046–62.
2. Mattson SN, Crocker N, Nguyen TT. Fetal alcohol spectrum disorders: neuropsychological and behavioral features. Neuropsychol Rev. 2011;21(2):81–101.

3. Skorka K, McBryde C, Copley J, Meredith PJ, Reid N. Experiences of children with fetal alcohol spectrum disorder and their families: a critical review. Alcohol Clin Exp Res. 2020;44(6):1175–88.

4. Chasnoff IJ, Wells AM, King L. Misdiagnosis and missed diagnoses in foster and adopted children with prenatal alcohol exposure. Pediatrics. 2015;135(2):264–70.

5. Weyrauch D, Schwartz M, Hart B, Klug MG, Burd L. Comorbid mental disorders in fetal alcohol spectrum disorders: a systematic review. J Dev Behav Pediatr. 2017;38(4):283–91.

6. Mattson SN, Riley EP, Gramling L, Delis DC, Jones KL. Neuropsychological comparison of alcohol-exposed children with or without physical features of fetal alcohol syndrome. Neuropsychology. 1998;12(1):146–53.

7. Mattson SN, Riley EP, Gramling L, Delis DC, Jones KL. Heavy prenatal alcohol exposure with or without physical features of fetal alcohol syndrome leads to IQ deficits. J Pediatr. 1997;131(5):718–21.

8. Sampson PD, Streissguth AP, Bookstein FL, Barr HM. On categorizations in analyses of alcohol teratogenesis. Environ Health Perspect. 2000;108(Suppl 3):421–8.

9. Raldiris TL, Bowers TG, Towsey C. Comparisons of intelligence and behavior in children with fetal alcohol spectrum disorder and ADHD. J Atten Disord. 2018;22(10):959–70.

10. Williams JF, Smith VC, Abuse C. Fetal alcohol spectrum disorders. Pediatrics. 2015;136(5):e1395–406.

11. Popova S, Lange S, Poznyak V, Chudley AE, Shield KD, Reynolds JN, et al. Population-based prevalence of fetal alcohol spectrum disorder in Canada. BMC Public Health. 2019;19(1):845.

12. Mattson SN, Riley EP. A review of the neurobehavioral deficits in children with fetal alcohol syndrome or prenatal exposure to alcohol. Alcohol Clin Exp Res. 1998;22(2):279–94.

13. Ferreira VKL, Cruz MS. Intelligence and fetal alcohol spectrum disorders: a review. J Popul Ther Clin Pharmacol. 2017;24(3):e1–e18.

14. Ervalahti N, Korkman M, Fagerlund A, Autti-Rämö I, Loimu L, Hoyme HE. Relationship between dysmorphic features and general cognitive function in children with fetal alcohol spectrum disorders. Am J Med Genet A. 2007;143A(24):2916–23.

15. Wozniak JR, Mueller BA, Mattson SN, Coles CD, Kable JA, Jones KL, et al. Functional connectivity abnormalities and associated cognitive deficits in fetal alcohol spectrum disorders (FASD). Brain Imaging Behav. 2017;11(5):1432–45.

16. Price AD. The impact of traumatic childhood experiences on cognitive and behavioural functioning in children with foetal alcohol spectrum disorders. Salford: University of Salford; 2019.

17. Streissguth AP, Bookstein FL, Barr HM, Sampson PD, O'Malley K, Young JK. Risk factors for adverse life outcomes in fetal alcohol syndrome and fetal alcohol effects. J Dev Behav Pediatr. 2004;25(4):228–38.

18. McLachlan K, Flannigan K, Temple V, Unsworth K, Cook JL. Difficulties in daily living experienced by adolescents, transition-aged youth, and adults with fetal alcohol spectrum disorder. Alcohol Clin Exp Res. 2020;44(8):1609–24.

19. Ali S, Kerns KA, Mulligan BP, Olson HC, Astley SJ. An investigation of intra-individual variability in children with fetal alcohol spectrum disorder (FASD). Child Neuropsychol. 2018;24(5):617–37.

20. Burton CL, Strauss E, Hultsch DF, Hunter MA. The relationship between everyday problem solving and inconsistency in reaction time in older adults. Neuropsychol Dev Cogn B Aging Neuropsychol Cogn. 2009;16(5):607–32.

21. Kodituwakku PW. Neurocognitive profile in children with fetal alcohol spectrum disorders. Dev Disabil Res Rev. 2009;15(3):218–24.

22. Louth EL, Bignell W, Taylor CL, Bailey CD. Developmental ethanol exposure leads to long-term deficits in attention and its underlying prefrontal circuitry. eNeuro. 2016;3(5):2016.

23. Mattson SN, Calarco KE, Lang AR. Focused and shifting attention in children with heavy prenatal alcohol exposure. Neuropsychology. 2006;20(3):361–9.

24. Coles CD, Platzman KA, Lynch ME, Freides D. Auditory and visual sustained attention in adolescents prenatally exposed to alcohol. Alcohol Clin Exp Res. 2002;26(2):263–71.

25. Li Z, Ma X, Peltier S, Hu X, Coles CD, Lynch ME. Occipital-temporal reduction and sustained visual attention deficit in prenatal alcohol exposed adults. Brain Imaging Behav. 2008;2(1):39–48.
26. Connor PD, Streissguth AP, Sampson PD, Bookstein FL, Barr HM. Individual differences in auditory and visual attention among fetal alcohol-affected adults. Alcohol Clin Exp Res. 1999;23(8):1395–402.
27. Vaurio L, Riley EP, Mattson SN. Neuropsychological comparison of children with heavy prenatal alcohol exposure and an IQ-matched comparison group. J Int Neuropsychol Soc. 2011;17(3):463–73.
28. Coles CD, Platzman KA, Raskind-Hood CL, Brown RT, Falek A, Smith IE. A comparison of children affected by prenatal alcohol exposure and attention deficit, hyperactivity disorder. Alcohol Clin Exp Res. 1997;21(1):150–61.
29. Moore EM, Riley EP. What happens when children with fetal alcohol spectrum disorders become adults? Curr Dev Disord Rep. 2015;2(3):219–27.
30. Anderson P. Assessment and development of executive function (EF) during childhood. Child Neuropsychol. 2002;8(2):71–82.
31. Malloy PF, Richardson ED. Assessment of frontal lobe functions. J Neuropsychiatry Clin Neurosci. 1994;6(4):399–410.
32. Mattson SN, Goodman AM, Caine C, Delis DC, Riley EP. Executive functioning in children with heavy prenatal alcohol exposure. Alcohol Clin Exp Res. 1999;23(11):1808–15.
33. Nguyen TT, Glass L, Coles CD, Kable JA, May PA, Kalberg WO, et al. The clinical utility and specificity of parent report of executive function among children with prenatal alcohol exposure. J Int Neuropsychol Soc. 2014;20(7):704–16.
34. Khoury JE, Milligan K. Comparing executive functioning in children and adolescents with fetal alcohol spectrum disorders and ADHD: a meta-analysis. J Atten Disord. 2019;23(14):1801–15.
35. Kingdon D, Cardoso C, McGrath JJ. Research review: executive function deficits in fetal alcohol spectrum disorders and attention-deficit/hyperactivity disorder—a meta-analysis. J Child Psychol Psychiatry. 2016;57(2):116–31.
36. Connor PD, Sampson PD, Bookstein FL, Barr HM, Streissguth AP. Direct and indirect effects of prenatal alcohol damage on executive function. Dev Neuropsychol. 2000;18(3):331–54.
37. Kerns KA, Don A, Mateer CA, Streissguth AP. Cognitive deficits in nonretarded adults with fetal alcohol syndrome. J Learn Disabil. 1997;30(6):685–93.
38. Malisza KL, Allman AA, Shiloff D, Jakobson L, Longstaffe S, Chudley AE. Evaluation of spatial working memory function in children and adults with fetal alcohol spectrum disorders: a functional magnetic resonance imaging study. Pediatr Res. 2005;58(6):1150–7.
39. Aragón AS, Kalberg WO, Buckley D, Barela-Scott LM, Tabachnick BG, May PA. Neuropsychological study of FASD in a sample of American Indian children: processing simple versus complex information. Alcohol Clin Exp Res. 2008;32(12):2136–48.
40. Olson HC, Feldman JJ, Streissguth AP, Sampson PD, Bookstein FL. Neuropsychological deficits in adolescents with fetal alcohol syndrome: clinical findings. Alcohol Clin Exp Res. 1998;22(9):1998–2012.
41. Rasmussen C, McAuley R, Andrew G. Parental ratings of children with fetal alcohol spectrum disorder on the behavior rating inventory of executive function (BRIEF). J FAS Int. 2007;5(e2):1–8.
42. Bernes GA, Villodas M, Coles CD, Kable JA, May PA, Kalberg WO, et al. Validity and reliability of executive function measures in children with heavy prenatal alcohol exposure: correspondence between multiple raters and laboratory measures. Alcohol Clin Exp Res. 2021;45(3):596–607.
43. Rangmar J, Sandberg AD, Aronson M, Fahlke C. Cognitive and executive functions, social cognition and sense of coherence in adults with fetal alcohol syndrome. Nord J Psychiatry. 2015;69(6):472–8.

44. McGee CL, Schonfeld AM, Roebuck-Spencer TM, Riley EP, Mattson SN. Children with heavy prenatal alcohol exposure demonstrate deficits on multiple measures of concept formation. Alcohol Clin Exp Res. 2008;32(8):1388–97.
45. Schonfeld AM, Mattson SN, Lang AR, Delis DC, Riley EP. Verbal and nonverbal fluency in children with heavy prenatal alcohol exposure. J Stud Alcohol. 2001;62(2):239–46.
46. Rasmussen C, Bisanz J. Executive functioning in children with fetal alcohol spectrum disorders: profiles and age-related differences. Child Neuropsychol. 2009;15(3):201–15.
47. Fryer SL, Tapert SF, Mattson SN, Paulus MP, Spadoni AD, Riley EP. Prenatal alcohol exposure affects frontal-striatal BOLD response during inhibitory control. Alcohol Clin Exp Res. 2007;31(8):1415–24.
48. Baddeley A. Working memory: looking back and looking forward. Nat Rev Neurosci. 2003;4(10):829–39.
49. Burden MJ, Jacobson SW, Sokol RJ, Jacobson JL. Effects of prenatal alcohol exposure on attention and working memory at 7.5 years of age. Alcohol Clin Exp Res. 2005;29(3):443–52.
50. Gautam P, Nuñez SC, Narr KL, Mattson SN, May PA, Adnams CM, et al. Developmental trajectories for visuo-spatial attention are altered by prenatal alcohol exposure: a longitudinal FMRI study. Cereb Cortex. 2015;25(12):4761–71.
51. O'Hare ED, Lu LH, Houston SM, Bookheimer SY, Mattson SN, O'Connor MJ, et al. Altered frontal-parietal functioning during verbal working memory in children and adolescents with heavy prenatal alcohol exposure. Hum Brain Mapp. 2009;30(10):3200–8.
52. Moore EM, Glass L, Infante MA, Coles CD, Kable JA, Jones KL, et al. Cross-sectional analysis of spatial working memory development in children with histories of heavy prenatal alcohol exposure. Alcohol Clin Exp Res. 2021;45(1):215–23.
53. Mattson SN, Riley EP, Delis DC, Stern C, Jones KL. Verbal learning and memory in children with fetal alcohol syndrome. Alcohol Clin Exp Res. 1996;20(5):810–6.
54. Mattson SN, Roebuck TM. Acquisition and retention of verbal and nonverbal information in children with heavy prenatal alcohol exposure. Alcohol Clin Exp Res. 2002;26(6):875–82.
55. Willford JA, Richardson GA, Leech SL, Day NL. Verbal and visuospatial learning and memory function in children with moderate prenatal alcohol exposure. Alcohol Clin Exp Res. 2004;28(3):497–507.
56. Lewis CE, Thomas KG, Dodge NC, Molteno CD, Meintjes EM, Jacobson JL, et al. Verbal learning and memory impairment in children with fetal alcohol spectrum disorders. Alcohol Clin Exp Res. 2015;39(4):724–32.
57. Uecker A, Nadel L. Spatial locations gone awry: object and spatial memory deficits in children with fetal alcohol syndrome. Neuropsychologia. 1996;34(3):209–23.
58. Willoughby KA, Sheard ED, Nash K, Rovet J. Effects of prenatal alcohol exposure on hippocampal volume, verbal learning, and verbal and spatial recall in late childhood. J Int Neuropsychol Soc. 2008;14(6):1022–33.
59. Fryer SL, Mattson SN, Jernigan TL, Archibald SL, Jones KL, Riley EP. Caudate volume predicts neurocognitive performance in youth with heavy prenatal alcohol exposure. Alcohol Clin Exp Res. 2012;36(11):1932–41.
60. Coles CD, Lynch ME, Kable JA, Johnson KC, Goldstein FC. Verbal and nonverbal memory in adults prenatally exposed to alcohol. Alcohol Clin Exp Res. 2010;34(5):897–906.
61. Poth LD, Mattson SN. Profiles of language and communication abilities in adolescents with fetal alcohol spectrum disorders. J Int Neuropsychol Soc. 2022;2022:789.
62. Greene T, Ernhart CB, Martier S, Sokol R, Ager J. Prenatal alcohol exposure and language development. Alcohol Clin Exp Res. 1990;14(6):937–45.
63. Church MW, Eldis F, Blakley BW, Bawle EV. Hearing, language, speech, vestibular, and dentofacial disorders in fetal alcohol syndrome. Alcohol Clin Exp Res. 1997;21(2):227–37.
64. McLaughlin SA, Thorne JC, Jirikowic T, Waddington T, Lee AKC, Astley Hemingway SJ. Listening difficulties in children with fetal alcohol spectrum disorders: more than a problem of audibility. J Speech Lang Hear Res. 2019;62(5):1532–48.

65. Church MW, Gerkin KP. Hearing disorders in children with fetal alcohol syndrome: findings from case reports. Pediatrics. 1988;82(2):147–54.
66. Thorne JC, Coggins TE, Carmichael Olson H, Astley SJ. Exploring the utility of narrative analysis in diagnostic decision making: picture-bound reference, elaboration, and fetal alcohol spectrum disorders. J Speech Lang Hear Res. 2007;50(2):459–74.
67. Monnot M, Lovallo WR, Nixon SJ, Ross E. Neurological basis of deficits in affective prosody comprehension among alcoholics and fetal alcohol-exposed adults. J Neuropsychiatry Clin Neurosci. 2002;14(3):321–8.
68. Mattson SN, Gramling L, Riley EP, Delis DC, Jones KL. Global—local processing in children prenatally exposed to alcohol. Child Neuropsychol. 1996;2(3):165–75.
69. Kaemingk KL, Halverson PT. Spatial memory following prenatal alcohol exposure: more than a material specific memory deficit. Child Neuropsychol. 2000;6(2):115–28.
70. Doney R, Lucas BR, Jones T, Howat P, Sauer K, Elliott EJ. Fine motor skills in children with prenatal alcohol exposure or fetal alcohol spectrum disorder. J Dev Behav Pediatr. 2014;35(9):598–609.
71. Crocker N, Riley EP, Mattson SN. Visual-spatial abilities relate to mathematics achievement in children with heavy prenatal alcohol exposure. Neuropsychology. 2015;29(1):108–16.
72. Flannigan K, Pei J, Rasmussen C, Potts S, O'Riordan T. A unique response to offenders with fetal alcohol spectrum disorder: perceptions of the Alexis FASD Justice Program. Can J Criminol Crim Justice. 2018;60(1):1–33.
73. Goldschmidt L, Richardson GA, Stoffer DS, Geva D, Day NL. Prenatal alcohol exposure and academic achievement at age six: a nonlinear fit. Alcohol Clin Exp Res. 1996;20(4):763–70.
74. Lucas BR, Doney R, Latimer J, Watkins RE, Tsang TW, Hawkes G, et al. Impairment of motor skills in children with fetal alcohol spectrum disorders in remote Australia: the Lililwan project. Drug Alcohol Rev. 2016;35(6):719–27.
75. Simmons RW, Thomas JD, Levy SS, Riley EP. Motor response selection in children with fetal alcohol spectrum disorders. Neurotoxicol Teratol. 2006;28(2):278–85.
76. Nguyen TT, Levy SS, Riley EP, Thomas JD, Simmons RW. Children with heavy prenatal alcohol exposure experience reduced control of isotonic force. Alcohol Clin Exp Res. 2013;37(2):315–24.
77. Kalberg WO, Provost B, Tollison SJ, Tabachnick BG, Robinson LK, Eugene Hoyme H, et al. Comparison of motor delays in young children with fetal alcohol syndrome to those with prenatal alcohol exposure and with no prenatal alcohol exposure. Alcohol Clin Exp Res. 2006;30(12):2037–45.
78. Barr HM, Streissguth AP, Darby BL, Sampson PD. Prenatal exposure to alcohol, caffeine, tobacco, and aspirin: effects on fine and gross motor performance in 4-year-old children. Dev Psychol. 1990;26(3):339.
79. Lucas BR, Latimer J, Pinto RZ, Ferreira ML, Doney R, Lau M, et al. Gross motor deficits in children prenatally exposed to alcohol: a meta-analysis. Pediatrics. 2014;134(1):e192–209.
80. Roebuck TM, Simmons RW, Mattson SN, Riley EP. Prenatal exposure to alcohol affects the ability to maintain postural balance. Alcohol Clin Exp Res. 1998;22(1):252–8.
81. May PA, Chambers CD, Kalberg WO, Zellner J, Feldman H, Buckley D, et al. Prevalence of fetal alcohol spectrum disorders in 4 US communities. JAMA. 2018;319(5):474–82.
82. MacNalty AS. The British medical dictionary. Acad Med. 1963;38(12):1061.
83. Ruocco AC, Irani F. Spatial processing. In: Kreutzer JS, DeLuca J, Caplan B, editors. Encyclopedia of clinical neuropsychology. New York: Springer; 2011. p. 2331–2.

Chapter 12
Physical and Mental Health in FASD

Karen M. Moritz, Lisa K. Akison, Nicole Hayes, and Natasha Reid

Introduction

In addition to the well-documented effects on the developing brain, exposure to prenatal alcohol is known to be associated with a range of co-morbid conditions [1]. Some of these may be evident very early in life, including the facial dysmorphology and heart defects, and can be attributed to the teratogenic effects of alcohol at particular stages of development. However, more recently it has become apparent that prenatal alcohol exposure may be associated with a large range of chronic health conditions that are not readily apparent in childhood but emerge during adolescence and adult life. A recent community survey developed by three adults with FASD examined the health of more than 500 adults with FASD. They concluded that FASD was a "whole-body diagnosis" and that: "…*individuals with FASD have higher frequencies of a wide range of health conditions and develop these earlier than individuals in the general population*" [2]. It is particularly important to establish the links between prenatal alcohol and adult health to allow early intervention measures to be implemented that may prevent or at least delay the onset of secondary health conditions.

The concept that early life exposures may contribute to chronic disease in later life has been extensively examined through studies testing the Developmental

K. M. Moritz (✉) · L. K. Akison
The Child Health Research Centre, The University of Queensland, Brisbane, QLD, Australia

School of Biomedical Sciences, The University of Queensland, Brisbane, QLD, Australia
e-mail: k.moritz@uq.edu.au; l.akison@uq.edu.au

N. Hayes · N. Reid
The Child Health Research Centre, The University of Queensland, Brisbane, QLD, Australia
e-mail: nicole.hayes@mater.uq.edu.au; n.reid1@uq.edu.au

O. A. Abdul-Rahman, C. L. M. Petrenko (eds.), *Fetal Alcohol Spectrum Disorders*,
https://doi.org/10.1007/978-3-031-32386-7_12

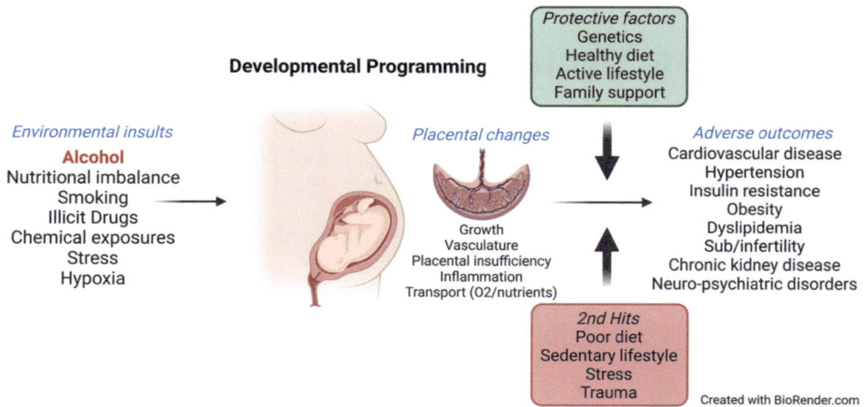

Fig. 12.1 The Developmental Origins of Health and Disease (DOHaD) hypothesis through which prenatal factors influence long-term health

Origins of Health and Disease (DOHaD) hypothesis (for review see Gluckman et al. [3]; Fig. 12.1). This hypothesis put forward by Barker and colleagues in the late 1980s suggests that exposures that occur in early life, particularly during fetal development in the womb, may contribute to altered development of organs and hormonal systems. This may result in babies being born of a low birth weight, with individuals then at increased risk of developing conditions such as high blood pressure, diabetes, cardiovascular disease, and osteoporosis. These alterations in normal development are not considered teratogenic effects (that is, causing birth defects or congenital abnormalities) but rather more subtle changes in growth and homeostatic mechanisms that are likely not immediately obvious at birth.

This chapter will focus on the evidence that prenatal alcohol contributes to physical and mental health outcomes as well as behavioral changes in children and adults. Given in some areas there are relatively few studies examining these outcomes in cohorts, we shall draw on findings from animal models and integrate these with the clinical data. The use of animal models can give insights in the timing and doses of alcohol that may impact health in later life and additionally provide information on the mechanisms involved and potential treatments that may be beneficial. We will also consider the supports and barriers in the health system to obtaining care for the physical and the mental health needs of people affected by prenatal alcohol exposure and finally, the areas where future research could provide beneficial strategies for prevention and intervention.

Early Life Links to Physical and Mental Health Outcomes: The DOHaD Hypothesis

Overview of the DOHaD Hypothesis

The DOHaD hypothesis has predominantly examined how maternal nutrition impacts fetal growth and contributes to long-term health and risk of chronic disease. Focus for many years was on inadequate maternal intake of calories or deficiencies in specific dietary components (e.g., iron, vitamin A). More recently, studies have also examined the impacts of excess dietary intake of calories that contribute to maternal obesity and/or diabetes during pregnancy. Another major factor investigated is the impact of inadequate oxygen supply to the fetus (fetal hypoxia) that can occur due to a poorly functioning placenta, maternal smoking, high altitude or maternal health conditions such as asthma. Finally, the impact of maternal stress, mediated through increased concentrations of hormones such as cortisol, has been examined. All of these exposures during pregnancy have been linked to an increased risk of chronic health conditions in adulthood [3]. The strongest evidence supporting this hypothesis relates to the development of metabolic dysfunction, in particular insulin resistance and type II diabetes, and cardiovascular disease, including coronary heart disease and stroke. It must be noted that outcomes are in part dependent upon the timing and severity of the exposure as well as the sex of the fetus. This "developmentally programmed" predisposition for chronic health conditions may be further exacerbated by factors after birth including poor nutrition (e.g., diets high in sugar, fats, and salt), lack of exercise, stress, and adverse childhood experiences.

The mechanisms contributing to developmental programming include changes in placental function (discussed further below, see Fig. 12.1), altered structural development of organs (leading to suboptimal organ function) and changes in hormone production and regulation. Epigenetic changes (such as DNA methylation or histone modifications) may also be involved. Many organs and hormonal systems have been shown to be affected, with organs such as the kidney shown to be particularly susceptible [4]. The hypothalamic–pituitary–adrenal (HPA) axis has also been shown to be especially susceptible to programming by prenatal events. Given the well-established associations between HPA function and neuropsychiatric disorders as well as metabolic/cardiac function, programming of the fetal HPA may be a common pathway linking early-life events to adult-onset chronic diseases.

Role of the Placenta

An important component of the DOHaD hypothesis is the role played by the placenta. As the placenta supplies all the nutrients and oxygen required by the fetus, maternal conditions that result in poor placental development (placental insufficiency) can contribute to fetal growth restriction. In relation to alcohol, there is evidence that prenatal alcohol exposure during pregnancy can contribute to increased rates of miscarriage and stillbirth, probably via mechanisms involving poor implantation and/or placental function. A recent systematic review and meta-analyses demonstrated that prenatal alcohol consumption caused a reduction in placental weight and increased the likelihood of placental abruption [5]. Detailed analysis of the placenta showed prenatal alcohol consumption caused structural changes in the placenta including alterations in blood vessel development and changes in expression of genes regulating processes such as placental growth and development. Together, these results suggest that in addition to the direct effects of alcohol on the fetus, prenatal alcohol may contribute to reduced placental function and therefore, may cause a degree of placental insufficiency. Recent studies using animal models support this concept. For example, in rats that consumed alcohol around the time of conception, placental development was impaired by the middle of pregnancy and by late pregnancy, expression of genes that regulate glucose and nutrient transfer was altered, likely contributing to the fetal growth restriction [6, 7].

Considerations of Prenatal Alcohol Exposure (PAE) in the Context of DOHaD

PAE has well-documented teratogenic effects, but consideration of the role PAE plays in the context of the DOHaD hypothesis has not historically been considered. More recently, the relationship between prenatal alcohol exposure and the risk of chronic disease has become particularly relevant since more widespread understanding and screening/assessment for FASD over the last 20–30 years has led to increased childhood diagnosis. Many of these individuals first diagnosed in the 1980s and 1990s are now entering their 30–40s and are reporting a range of health problems [2]. In many cases, these health issues are not considered related to the FASD diagnosis or are thought to be side-effects of other medications that an individual with FASD is taking. This can result in concerns being ignored or downplayed by health professionals and may lead to under-reporting of secondary health conditions experienced by people living with FASD.

A major challenge in understanding the contribution of PAE to the development of chronic disease in adulthood is in delineating the effects of the PAE from other exposures during pregnancy (such as maternal smoking/drug use and nutrition) as well as current lifestyle factors (e.g., drug and alcohol use, diet, and exercise). The prevalence of FASD varies with maternal poverty, nutritional deficiencies as well as socio-historical factors, such as the impacts of colonialism on indigenous people. Indeed, it has previously been stated that: *"…fetal alcohol syndrome is not an equal opportunity birth defect"* [8]. Studies examining patterns of maternal alcohol consumption suggest that women from upper socioeconomic status (SES) groups are more likely to drink alcohol during pregnancy but have significantly lower rates of FASD than women in lower SES groups. This suggests the adverse developmental effects of prenatal alcohol exposure may be amplified by factors linked with poverty such as other substance use, nutritional deficiencies, stressful social circumstances, and poor prenatal care [9]. This is also true regarding the influence of postnatal experiences for children with FASD. Previous research has documented that children who are biologically vulnerable as a result of prenatal alcohol exposure are often also exposed to postnatal environmental risks (e.g., poverty, trauma) and therefore are at "double jeopardy" for poor outcomes [10]. Interactions between multiple stressors both during pregnancy and in early postnatal life are well recognized in the DOHaD field and have led to the concept of a "second" or "multiple-hit" hypothesis (see Fig. 12.1 below).

Physical Health Outcomes

Since the first diagnosis of fetal alcohol syndrome (FAS) and the associated diagnoses that make up FASD, there have been numerous case reports and small clinical studies reporting on a wide range of health outcomes. A number of recent systematic reviews have examined the comorbid conditions associated with FASD [1] or have focused on particular physical health outcomes associated with PAE including metabolic disorders and body composition [11], cardiovascular and renal conditions [12], immune function [13], and reproductive health [14] (Table 12.1). These reviews report that clinical evidence is scarce or lacking for many health outcomes, with studies either containing small numbers of participants or only examining young children or adolescents where chronic conditions may not yet have emerged. Further evidence of impacts of PAE on physical health comes from two recent health surveys; one undertaken by caregivers reporting on children/adolescents (average age 12 years, Reid et al. [15]) and the other, a health survey completed by over 500 adults with FASD or related diagnoses (average age 27.5 years, Himmelreich et al. [2]). Both surveys identified a range of disorders in people with FASD occurring at rates significantly higher than the general population and/or with an earlier onset (discussed in more detail below). However, at this time, the strongest evidence for PAE impacting physical health comes from preclinical studies in models where the dose and timing of alcohol exposure can be controlled, and animals can be studied over their entire life. Preclinical studies have also shed light on the biological mechanisms through which alcohol alters developmental processes, as well as enabled intervention strategies to be investigated.

Clinical Studies of Physical Health Outcomes Associated with FASD

Metabolic Outcomes (Including Diabetes and Plasma Hormones/Lipids)

A small number of studies have examined metabolic outcomes in people with FASD. A study of young children (aged 6–7 years) with FAS reported normal glucose but increased fasting insulin concentrations and evidence of glucose intolerance and insulin resistance (see Table 12.1 and the review of Akison et al. [11]). More recent studies have found altered insulin levels in adults with FASD [16] and

Table 12.1 Physical health outcomes in children and adults following PAE and/or a FASD diagnosis

Study cohort	Health domain	Outcome (age)
Children/adults with FAS/ FASD (data derived from systematic reviews)	Metabolic Body composition Cardiovascular Renal Immune	Glucose intolerance/insulin resistance (6–7-year-olds) Altered insulin concentrations (adults) ↓ HDL and elevated triglycerides (adults) ↑ Rates of type II diabetes (adults) ↓ BMI and body fat (children, especially males) ↑ Rates of hypertension (adolescents and young adults) Impaired ability to concentrate urine/altered electrolyte excretion (6-year-olds) ↑ Rates of major/minor infections (all ages)
Children/adults with FAS/ FASD (data from health surveys)[a]	Bone Cardiovascular Immune Other (eye)	Bone and muscle problems (e.g., stiff, painful, swollen joints; lack of flexibility; hypermobility of joints in adults) Heart conditions (e.g., cardiomyopathy in adults) ↑ Rates of infection (especially ear and kidney infections in both children and adults) ↑ Prevalence (and often earlier onset) of autoimmune disorders in adulthood ↑ Rates of dermatitis/eczema and psoriasis (both children and adults) Eye conditions (both children and adults)
Longitudinal birth cohorts[a]	Body composition Renal	↑ BMI and rates of obesity in adolescent girls but not boys ↑ Rates of kidney disease at 30 years of age
Documented PAE but no FAS/ FASD diagnosis[a]	Immune	↑ Risk of infections and sepsis (newborns) ↑ Rates of asthma/dermatitis in some but not all studies (young children)

Data summarized from systematic reviews [11–14] and health surveys [2, 15] or cited in text (e.g., longitudinal birth cohorts). PAE in these cohorts was variable or unrecorded
[a]Includes only outcomes or details not captured in the systematic reviews

increased rates of type II diabetes [17]. One of these studies [17] also found lower levels of the high density lipoprotein (HDL) and elevated triglyceride levels in people with FASD, both of which are associated with an increased risk of cardiovascular problems such as stroke and heart attack. The adult health survey found that rates of type 1 diabetes were 5 times higher in adults with FASD and episodes of hypoglycemia, unrelated to diabetes, occurred in nearly a third of those with FASD compared to rates of less than 1% in the general population [2]. Of note, clinically evident hypothyroidism was present in approximately 5% of those with FASD, a rate more than 180 times that of the general population. In the caregiver survey, elevated rates of thyroid problems were also reported in children and adolescents [15]. Given hypothyroidism is an important metabolic cause of reversible cognitive impairment, alterations in thyroid function warrant further investigation in young people with FASD.

Body Composition (Including Risk of Underweight/Overweight/ Obese and Changes in Bone Health)

Body mass index (BMI), used to detect people who are either underweight or overweight/obese, was found to be lower in children with FASD prior to puberty, particularly in males [18]. Similarly, percentage body fat was also lower in children with FAS/pFAS compared to non-exposed children or those exposed to prenatal alcohol but not displaying signs of FAS [19]. Both health surveys showed increased rates of underweight in those with FASD. Conversely, a more recent study using a large longitudinal cohort of children from the general population found BMI and rates of obesity were increased in adolescent girls exposed to prenatal alcohol exposure [20]. These studies suggest outcomes related to body composition will depend on the level of alcohol exposure but also may change with age. Puberty is likely to be a key time where differences may emerge, and this may involve not only hormonal changes but social changes including alterations to physical activity. With regard to bone health, there is some evidence that PAE may disrupt fetal bone development; however, studies examining bone densitometry are lacking in children with FASD. One recent study found that PAE was associated with increased rates of fractures in childhood [21] although the mechanism contributing to this outcome was unclear. Bone and joint problems were common conditions reported by adults with FASD, with rates of osteoarthritis increased 3.7-fold. In both health surveys, many respondents reported more generalized problems such as chronic joint pain and/or swelling.

Cardiovascular and Renal Outcomes (Including Heart Defects, High Blood Pressure, and Kidney Disease)

With regard to cardiovascular and kidney health following PAE, clinical evidence is limited (for review, see Reid et al. [12]). A recent study has shown that adolescents and young adults with FASD were more likely to be hypertensive after accounting for factors including age, sex, race/ethnicity, medication use, and obesity status [22]. Other outcomes in children with FASD included changes in heart rate and heart rate variability, particularly in response to minor physical challenges [13]. The health surveys showed increased rates of congenital heart defects, including the need for cardiac surgery in early childhood. However, the adult health survey also found increased rates of many other conditions including cardiomyopathy, high blood pressure, and valvular heart disease. Many of these emerged relatively early in life compared to the general population where they are more often considered diseases of middle/old age.

A series of studies has examined renal function in a small cohort of young children with FAS and found they presented with episodes of excess urine production and dehydration likely due to an inability to concentrate urine (see Reid et al. [13]). This may be a contributing factor to the increase rates of urinary incontinence that has been reported by caregivers of children with FASD [15]. In adults with FASD, the rates of diagnosed kidney disease were almost 5 times higher than the general population. Effects of relatively modest amounts of alcohol may also impact renal function; in a longitudinal study of women where PAE was well documented, alcohol consumption during early and late pregnancy was associated with mild to moderate chronic kidney disease in adults at approximately 30 years of age [23].

Immune Function (Including Infections, Allergies, and Asthma)

A recent systematic review identified 12 clinical studies where outcomes focused on allergy and infection in individuals with PAE, although only one study included a group with diagnosed FAS/FASD [12]. In newborns, PAE has been reported to increase the risk for sepsis and infections. In neonates and children, some but not all studies reported an increased risk of dermatitis, skin rashes, and/or eczema. Some studies concluded that PAE may have exacerbated a predisposition to dermatitis or asthma rather than being a causal factor. Children and adolescents with PAE may have increased risk of infection and be hyper-responsive to stress (for review see Reid et al. [15]). Alcohol consumption has also been shown to alter immune function in the mother, which has been linked to adverse neurodevelopment in children [24]. The health surveys provided strong evidence that children and adults with

FASD have a much greater incidence of immune disorders. In children, chronic infections were reported in over 20% of respondents and in adults, rates of infections were up to 200-fold higher than the general population for conditions such as sinusitis, chronic ear infections, and kidney infections. Skin conditions such as eczema/dermatitis and psoriasis were reported at increased rates in children with FASD and this trend continued in adults. Autoimmune diseases, which routinely occur in 5–7% of the general population, were reported in 35% of adults with FASD, with high rates of rheumatoid arthritis and fibromyalgia. Some other less common autoimmune disorders/conditions (e.g., lupus, Crohn's disease, sarcoidosis), were also more prevalent and often developed at a younger age in adults with FASD.

Reproductive Outcomes (Including Onset of Puberty and Fertility)

In one study, adolescent girls who were exposed to high levels of alcohol prenatally had delayed puberty onset (age at first menarche), although other studies have shown no effect (for review see Akison et al. [11]). In boys, there was a tendency for delayed pubertal development and in men, decreased sperm volume and concentration. In both sexes, there was increased salivary testosterone in adolescents with PAE. These outcomes may relate to effects of alcohol on the development of the hypothalamic–pituitary–gonadal (HPG) axis which have been explored in more detail in animal models (see below). Reproductive health problems were not reported in the child health survey but in the adult survey, women with FASD had much higher rates of premature menopause and recurrent miscarriages while men had a higher incidence of undescended testicles.

Other Health Conditions

The systematic review of Popova et al. [1] identified over 400 co-morbid conditions in people with a FASD diagnosis, with many related to the teratogenic effects of alcohol (such as congenital malformations) or those conditions noted above. The health surveys captured a range of other conditions experienced by people living with FASD including eye/vision problems, increased rates of infections, and gastrointestinal problems. The child health survey also reported that children with FASD were likely to have more than one other diagnosed health condition, with over 20% having three or more.

Preclinical Studies of Physical Health Outcomes Associated with PAE

Animal models of PAE have been used to explore the long-term health outcomes that may result from prenatal alcohol exposure (see Akison et al. [11, 14], Reid et al. [12, 13] for review; Table 12.2). Generally, rodents (rat and mice) have been given alcohol at various levels during particular stages of development and the fetus or offspring studied to determine the impacts on organ development and health outcomes. In interpreting animal studies, differences in exposure levels and how animals metabolize alcohol, as well as timing of organ development compared to

Table 12.2 Examples of physical health outcomes in animal models of prenatal alcohol exposure

Dose of alcohol (~BAC if known)	Timing of exposure (human pregnancy trimester equivalent)	Species	Outcome
High dose			
8 g/kg/day via gavage, ~280 mg/dL	Throughout pregnancy (first, second, third trimester)	Guinea pig	↑ Adiposity in adults ↔ Fasting blood glucose
Moderate to high dose			
12.5% (vol:vol) in liquid diet, ~120–240 mg/dL	Periconceptional: 4 days prior to GD4 (first trimester)	Rat	Glucose intolerance and insulin resistance, exacerbated by HFD ↑ Adiposity males most affected
10% Ethanol in saccharin solution	Early-mid gestation until PD10 (first, second, third trimester)	Rat	Precocious puberty onset in males and reduced mating performance/motivation
Moderate dose			
25–30% (vol:vol) in drinking water or ~35% ethanol-derived calories (EDC) in liquid diet	Preconception (4 weeks) and throughout pregnancy (first and second trimester)	Rat	Insulin resistance in juveniles, persisting into adulthood Altered glucose and fatty acid metabolism Delayed puberty onset in females Behavioral signs of feminization in males
1.25–3.75 g/kg via IP injection	Early gestation "binge" (GD7 only) (first trimester)	Mouse	↓ Electrolyte (Ca^{2+}, P^{3-}) excretion in adult males
30% EDC in liquid diet	Early-mid gestation (GD5–11) (first trimester)	Mouse	Delayed puberty onset in females
3 g/kg/day via gavage, ~100–150 mg/dL	Mid-late gestation (GD12–17) (second trimester)	Mouse	↔ Adiposity ↔ Glucose control or metabolic rate ↑ Heart rate but no evidence of hypertension
0.75 g/kg/day IV infusion, ~120 mg/dL	Late gestation (GD95–133) (third trimester)	Sheep	↓ Nephron # in late gestation fetus ↔ Kidney/fetal growth

Table 12.2 (continued)

Dose of alcohol (~BAC if known)	Timing of exposure (human pregnancy trimester equivalent)	Species	Outcome
4 g/kg/day via gavage or 35% EDC in liquid diet, ~100–150 mg/dL	Various timings: throughout, mid-late gestation to birth (first and/or second trimester)	Rat	Some studies found glucose intolerance and insulin resistance but others no change ↑ Estrogen levels, shortened reproductive lifespan and/or delayed puberty onset in females; other studies no reproductive changes Delayed spermatogenesis when PAE in first tri Diuresis and defective renal tubular transport ↑ Water intake ↑ Heart rate Nephrotic syndrome, indicative of kidney damage
Low dose			
10% (vol:vol) in drinking water	Early pregnancy (to GD8) (first trimester)	Mouse	↑ Adiposity in adult males
5–6% (vol:vol) in liquid diet, ~30–50 mg/dL	Throughout pregnancy (first and second trimester)	Rat	↔ Body composition Sex-specific effects on glucose control Structural and functional deficits in cardiovascular system in aged offspring (↑ blood pressure, heart weight, fibrosis)
1 g/kg/day via gavage, ~50 mg/dL	Mid-late gestation (GD13.5–14.5) (second trimester)	Rat	Insulin resistance in adult males only ↔ Plasma lipids ↔ Female puberty onset or fertility ↓ Nephron # in juveniles; sex-specific impairments in glomerular filtration rate and hypertension in adults

Data summarized from systematic reviews [11, 12, 14]) and Nguyen et al. [25] and McReight et al. [26]
GD gestational day, *HFD* high fat diet, *PD* postnatal day

humans, must be carefully considered (Fig. 12.2). Rats are often given very high doses of alcohol, but they metabolize alcohol considerably faster than humans and thus comparable blood alcohol levels may be achieved to a person consuming relatively lower amounts. For example, a dose of 3 g of ethanol per kg body weight in a rat typically results in a peak blood alcohol level of ~100–150 mg/dL, while a similar dose in humans would be equivalent to >18 standard drinks for an average weight woman.

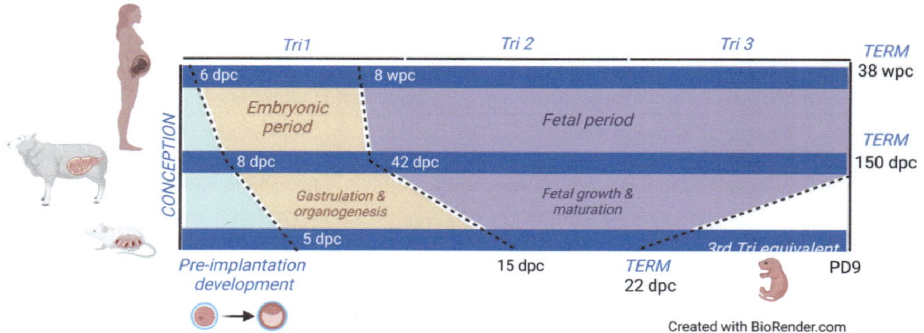

Fig. 12.2 Differences in timing of embryo and fetal development between different species. *dpc* days post conception, *wpc* weeks post conception, "term" refers to the timing of delivery in a normal pregnancy

With respect to timing of development, the processes that occur in the human brain (and other organs, including the kidney and ovary) during the third trimester of pregnancy occur during the first week after birth in the rat (Fig. 12.2). Also, definitions of human disease including "hypertension" and "diabetes" do not apply in animals so instead differences in measurable outcomes are compared to a non-alcohol exposed ("control") group.

Metabolic Outcomes (Including Glucose Intolerance, Insulin Resistance, and Plasma Hormones/Lipids)

Our systematic review identified nearly 30 publications examining metabolic outcomes in animal models [11]. These studies provide strong evidence that PAE at nearly any stage of pregnancy may result in adult rats with elevations in fasting blood glucose and/or insulin compared to non-alcohol exposed animals. These alterations to glucose homeostasis were typically demonstrated by performing a glucose tolerance test or insulin challenge in PAE and control animals. However, in many cases these outcomes only occurred when the dose of alcohol was high, and was often sex-specific, with male offspring appearing to be particularly vulnerable. Metabolic dysfunction was also sometimes only apparent when the PAE was combined with another adverse lifestyle factor, such as a "second hit" of a postnatal high fat diet. These physiological changes occurred together with changes in other hormones, such as leptin, which are known to control hunger. In addition, expression of genes in the liver, fat, and muscle that regulate blood glucose concentrations was affected by PAE. In terms of lipids, low-dose alcohol throughout pregnancy did not affect blood lipids in the offspring but higher doses, including when alcohol was limited to the time around conception, resulted in elevated triglycerides and, in some cases, total cholesterol concentrations.

Body Composition (Including Fat Mass and Bone Density)

Studies where PAE occurred at relatively high levels around conception or throughout pregnancy resulted in male offspring with increased fat mass. This did not occur in female offspring or where alcohol exposure was relatively low (for review see Akison et al. [14]). As many of these studies used dual-energy X-ray absorptiometry, it was also possible to assess bone density and other measures of bone health. In most studies these were unaltered, although PAE has been shown to affect fetal bone development in rats [27].

Cardiovascular and Renal Outcomes (Including Organ Development)

Animal studies have examined heart and cardiovascular outcomes including heart function (measured by echocardiography), blood pressure, heart structure, and cardiovascular responses to various stressors (for review see Reid et al. [12]). A high-dose 2 day "binge" model of PAE resulted in elevated blood pressure in adult offspring, however low-dose alcohol or alcohol around conception either had no effect or slightly decreased blood pressure [28, 29].

One study in sheep found that prenatal alcohol exposure resulted in impaired vasodilation function and increased vascular stiffness in fetuses in late gestation although it is unknown if these changes persist in offspring [30]. A couple of studies have also identified PAE as contributing to left ventricular hypertrophy and impaired cardiac function, such as reduced cardiac output and contractility, as well as markers of cardiac fibrosis (see Reid et al. [12]).

In response to PAE, animal studies have described impaired kidney growth and development. This has resulted in less nephrons (the filtering unit) in the kidney, alterations in renal function (changes in the glomerular filtration rate and urinary responses to challenges such as dehydration), and signs of kidney disease such as renal fibrosis. However, these outcomes were not consistent and depended upon the timing and dose of alcohol. In particular, the early stages of development of the permanent kidney seem especially susceptible. Using in vitro culture of fetal kidneys from the rat, alcohol has been shown to directly impact the rate at which the cells within the kidney could grow and divide. Excitingly, these effects could be prevented by the addition of retinoic acid (a metabolite of vitamin A).

Immune Function (Including Markers of Inflammation and Immune-Related Conditions Such as Arthritis)

In terms of the impact of PAE on the immune system, most preclinical studies have used rat models of PAE (>80%), with moderate high doses over the first and/or second trimester equivalent period of pregnancy (see Reid et al. [13] for review). These studies have examined the effect of PAE on cell-mediated immune responses, particularly splenic or thymic lymphocyte proliferation in response to an immune challenge. Most studies reported that PAE attenuated immune responses to an experimental infection and therefore had an immunosuppressive effect, perhaps explaining the increased rates of infection seen in individuals with PAE in clinical studies. In addition, there was evidence of an attenuated febrile response in response to infection in PAE offspring, which may explain the reduced resistance to infection observed in animals and humans following PAE. Although PAE-induced alterations in immune responses have been reported at all ages, in many instances, the altered immune response was transient, with younger offspring exhibiting alterations that were normalized by adulthood.

Numerous studies have demonstrated changes in cytokine production either in circulating levels or within the brain. In some studies, when challenged with infection, animals exposed to PAE had an attenuated response. In a model of adjuvant-induced arthritis, female offspring exposed to PAE were found to have more severe inflammation and a prolonged course of disease compared to controls [31]. More recently, a study in rats has shown that peripheral inflammation, as measured by circulating and tissue-specific immune cells and cytokines, can show sex-specific changes in response to PAE [32]. Importantly, this study found that immune status was a predictor of glucose intolerance and neurobehavioral dysfunction in adult PAE offspring.

Reproductive Outcomes (Including Onset of Puberty and Fertility)

Animal studies demonstrate numerous impacts of PAE on both the male and female reproductive systems (see Akison et al. [11] for review). This is perhaps not surprising, given the importance of the hypothalamic–pituitary regulation of the gonads and the known impacts of prenatal alcohol on the developing brain. PAE has been shown to alter gonadotropin hormone secretion, activity, and responsiveness in both males and females (see Weinberg et al. [33] for review), and this can result in altered estrogen production from the ovaries in females and testosterone production from the testes in males.

PAE at any stage of pregnancy, but particularly in late gestation, results in an increased age at vaginal opening in female offspring during adolescence, indicative of delayed puberty onset. However, very few other reproductive outcomes have been examined in females. A more recent study has examined ovarian reserve (i.e., primordial follicle numbers in neonates), estrous cyclicity, and pregnancy success in 6-month-old rat offspring and found no effects from a low-dose, acute exposure in late gestation [26].

A greater range of reproductive defects have been reported in male offspring with PAE. At birth, there is often evidence of a reduced anogenital distance compared to controls, suggestive of feminization. There is also evidence for reduced weight of the testes and accessory organs (e.g., prostate and seminal vesicles), reduced testosterone levels, delayed spermatogenesis, and altered mating behavior, resulting in reduced motivation and performance. However, there are inconsistencies in development of these adverse reproductive outcomes, with no clear links to the timing or level of alcohol exposure.

Other Health Outcomes (Including Impacts on the Lung, Gastrointestinal Tract)

Aside from the health outcomes described above, there are also a few studies reporting impacts of PAE on liver and gastrointestinal tract structure and function in offspring (see Akison et al. [14] for review). Aside from the impacts on liver function that manifest in altered regulation of glucose metabolism (described above), PAE has also been shown to increase susceptibility to development of fatty liver disease later in life, particularly in females. In the intestine, PAE has been shown to reduce absorption and transport of nutrients, such as folic acid, and alters the intestinal brush border enzymes of the intestinal villi, which are important for digestion. There is also one study that describes impacts on the structure of the lung in a low-dose, chronic exposure model in the rat [34]. This showed pulmonary fibrosis (i.e., increased collagen deposition) and reduced surfactant proteins, specifically in adult males, in these PAE animals.

Mental Health and Behavioral Outcomes (Including Sleep)

Mental health conditions are recognized as one of the most prevalent comorbidities with FAS or FASD, occurring in up to 70% of adults [1]. This includes psychiatric conditions such as depression, anxiety, and mood disorders as well as behavioral changes including conduct and externalizing disorders and hyperactivity. These conditions and behaviors contribute to challenges with social interactions (for review see Burgess and Moritz [35]; Table 12.3) as well as sleep.

A wide variety of animal models have been used to investigate behavior associated with PAE but extrapolating animal behavior to a defined clinical mental illness

Table 12.3 Mental health and behavioral outcomes associated with PAE

Timing and dose of alcohol	Study cohort	Outcome
Various timing throughout pregnancy	Children/adults with FAS/FASD diagnosis	Behavioral difficulties Externalizing disorders (including hyperactivity) Anxiety and mood disorders Psychiatric illness (including depressive disorders) Conduct and emotional disorders
>5 Drinks on one or occasions during pregnancy	Children with documented PAE but no FASD diagnosis	Externalizing disorders in boys Psychiatric illness Behavioral difficulties Difficult temperament Sleeping problems (infants, <2 years) Conduct disorders Disinhibited behaviors
~1 Drink/day, first trimester of pregnancy	Children and adults with documented PAE FASD diagnosis	Attention disorder (children) Alcohol use disorder (adults at 22 years) Anxiety and depression Conduct disorder Increased emotional and conduct difficulties Hyperactivity and inattention
<2 Drinks per occasion or 1–2 units per week throughout pregnancy	Children with documented PAE but no FASD diagnosis	Depressive symptoms Conduct and emotional symptoms
Various doses and timing throughout pregnancy	Adults with FAS/FASD (health surveys)[a]	↑ Rates of schizophrenia, psychosis, bipolar disorder ↑ Rates of attempted suicide

Adapted from Burgess and Moritz [35] and Himmelreich et al. [2]. Children refers to people under 12 years of age

[a]Includes only outcomes or details not captured above

has limitations. The experimental paradigms used have subjective interpretation and are often inconsistent in the ways they measure and report animal behaviors. Also as noted above, much of the later stages of brain development (the equivalent of the third trimester in humans) occur postnatally in rats and mice. Therefore, results need to be interpreted very carefully. However, animal models have been very useful to explore effects of alcohol on specific areas of brain development and have enabled researchers to investigate potential treatments.

Clinical Studies of Mental Health Outcomes Associated with FASD

Mental Health

Mental health issues are highly prevalent in people with prenatal alcohol exposure and/or FASD. Some of these conditions may present in early childhood. For example, in a small study of children prenatally exposed to alcohol, more than 85% developed a psychiatric illness, with the majority being mood disorders such as major depressive disorder [36]. Other mental health conditions associated with PAE may only become apparent and/or diagnosed during adolescence or adulthood. These most commonly include anxiety and depression. However, the adult health survey found a large range of mental health issues also occurred at much higher rates in individuals with FASD than the general population including panic attacks (17-fold higher), schizophrenia (4–5 times higher), bipolar disorder (sixfold higher), and psychosis (tenfold higher). Alcohol and substance abuse disorders also occurred at higher rates in adults diagnosed with FASD. These serious mental health conditions likely contributed to the survey identifying almost 30% of adults with FASD attempting suicide.

Behaviors (Including Hyperactivity)

Behavioral disorders including conduct disorders, disruptive behaviors, hyperactivity, and impulse control are common in children with a FASD diagnosis (see Table 12.3). However, studies have determined that even occasional or relatively low levels of alcohol during pregnancy may impact behaviors, irrespective of a FAS or FASD diagnosis. For example, a single occasion of binge drinking during the first trimester was associated with childhood emotional and conduct difficulties. A similar outcome was observed in children exposed to a low amount of alcohol (1 drink/day) during pregnancy or even when the exposure was only in the first trimester. The health survey found that almost 80% of adults with FASD also had attention deficit hyperactivity disorder (ADHD) or attention deficit disorder (ADD). Other common issues included personality disorders, oppositional defiant disorder, and obsessive-compulsive disorder, which occurred in people with FASD at 2–4 times the prevalence rates in the general population.

Sleep (Including Circadian Rhythms)

Caregivers of children with FASD commonly report sleeping problems in affected children including difficulty falling and staying asleep, early waking, and an overall reduction in total sleep time compared to non-affected children. A systematic review highlighted that these sleep issues may contribute to sleep deprivation and contribute to the cognitive and behavioral problems characteristic of FASD [37]. Indeed, a study has demonstrated that in families with a school age child with FASD, the sleep problems were associated with increased behavioral issues, increased caregiver anxiety and negative impacts on caregiver and family quality of life [38]. A recent study in children with FASD found more than 90% had disrupted circadian rhythm sleep disorders and insomnia, but during the day, experienced sleepiness as well as hyperactive behaviors [39]. The health survey identified sleep as a major issue for adults living with FASD, suggesting this is not just a problem that occurs in childhood. Difficulties in falling and staying asleep occurred in 50–70% of adults with FASD, who also reported many other sleep-related issues including nightmares, night sweats, and a general feeling of being tired all the time.

Changes in sleep patterns suggest that prenatal alcohol may induce changes in control of circadian rhythms. Circadian rhythms control biological processes including hormone secretion, sleep/wake cycles, body temperature, glucose homeostasis, and immune function that oscillate over a 24-h period. Children with FASD were observed to have increased salivary cortisol levels in the afternoon and at night, thereby implicating changes in the circadian regulation of the hypothalamic–pituitary–adrenal (HPA) axis [40]. Given the importance of sleep for normal circadian rhythms, including hormonal balance, sleep issues likely contribute to many other conditions including high blood pressure, diabetes, and obesity.

Animal Studies of Mental Health Outcomes Associated with PAE

Anxiety and Depressive-Like Outcomes

Animal studies using high doses of alcohol throughout pregnancy provide strong evidence that offspring exposed to prenatal alcohol display a range of altered behaviors. Rats and mice are most commonly used, and offspring exposed to prenatal alcohol display increased anxiety and depression (see Table 12.4). As shown in Fig. 12.2, much of brain development that takes place in the third trimester of a human pregnancy takes place in the first week after birth in rodent species. To examine effects of alcohol during this period, some studies have administered alcohol to the rat throughout pregnancy and then given alcohol directly to the pup for the first 10 days after birth. Outcomes were similar, with offspring showing signs of anxiety and depression. Studies using much lower doses of alcohol throughout

Table 12.4 Examples of mental illness-like and behavioral outcomes in animal models of prenatal alcohol exposure

Dose of alcohol (~BAC if known)	Timing of exposure (human pregnancy trimester equivalent)	Species	Mental illness-like phenotype (age and sex examined)
High dose			
~4 g/kg in liquid diet, ~155–225 mg/dL	All of pregnancy and lactation: GD1-PD10 (first, second, third trimester)	Rat	↑ Anxiety-like behavior ↑ Depressive-like behavior
20% (vol:vol) in liquid diet	"Binge" at GD7 (first trimester)	Rat	↑ Social interaction (males)
Moderate to high dose			
2–4 g/kg in sucralose solution, ~170–250 mg/dL	All of pregnancy (first, second, third trimester)	Guinea pig	↑ Locomotor activity (hyperactivity) ↓ Learning and memory
12.5% (vol:vol) in liquid diet, ~120–240 mg/dL	Periconceptional: 4 days prior to GD4 (first trimester)	Rat	↑ Anxiety (females) ↓ Anxiety (males)
2–4 g/kg in liquid diet (~36% ethanol-derived calories), ~130–190 mg/dL	All of pregnancy (first and second trimester)	Rat	↑ Depressive-like behavior (often males only) ↑ Anxiety-like behavior Hyperactivity Altered social interaction (often ↓ in males, ↑ in females) ↓ Recognition memory (males) ↓ Engaging and responding to playful interactions
Low dose			
5–6% (vol:vol) in liquid diet, ~30–50 mg/dL	All of pregnancy (first and second trimester)	Rat	↑ Anxiety-like behavior No effect on memory and learning ↓ Social interaction (females)

Adapted from Burgess and Moritz [35]
GD gestational day, *PD* postnatal day

pregnancy found evidence of anxiety and depression both in relatively young animals and in aged animals, indicating that the effects persist throughout life. Interestingly, the low dose alcohol throughout pregnancy did not cause significant changes in memory and learning, suggesting impacts on mental health may occur at lower doses of alcohol than other common outcomes related to prenatal alcohol exposure. Alcohol given only around conception (periconceptional exposure) caused changes in measures of anxiety but effects were dependent upon sex; female offspring showed increased levels of anxiety-like behaviors, but male offspring tended to have decreased levels.

Social Interactions and Hyperactivity

Rodent models have explored the effects of prenatal alcohol exposure on social behaviors using a range of different experimental situations. Most often this involves placing an animal exposed to prenatal alcohol in an environment with a control animal (not exposed to alcohol) and observing interactions including non-aggressive (sniffing, licking, playing) and aggressive (fighting, rearing, biting) behaviors as well as avoidance/non-social behaviors. High doses of alcohol throughout pregnancy (first and second trimester equivalent) commonly reduced the social interactions of offspring, including engaging and responding to playful interactions, especially in male offspring. In some studies, hyperactivity in rat and guinea pig offspring was noted together with changes in social behaviors aligning with clinical observations in children with FASD.

Sleep and Circadian Rhythms

In a rat model of prenatal alcohol exposure throughout pregnancy, young offspring, both before and during puberty, spent less total time asleep and more time awake compared to control animals [39]. Similarly, when alcohol was administered postnatally to male rats (days 4–9, third trimester human equivalent) and they were studied as adults, it was found they took longer to enter rapid eye movement (REM) sleep and that the amount of time spent in REM sleep was considerably less [41]. Changes in circadian rhythms such as altered diurnal changes in body temperature and locomotor activity have been observed in rat offspring following prenatal alcohol exposure throughout pregnancy [42]. These outcomes have been associated with changes in the genes that control circadian rhythms ("clock" genes) in the brain [42, 43].

Barriers to Care in Physical and Mental Health Care Systems

While awareness of the impacts of PAE, including acknowledgment of FASD, has been increasing in many countries, individuals with FASD still face substantial barriers to accessing appropriate care for their developmental, physical, and mental health needs. Many of these barriers occur at a system level and stem from a lack of knowledge around FASD, both within the health sector (e.g., general practitioners, speech pathologists, physiotherapists etc.) and across other sectors (including education and the justice system; see Petrenko et al. [44] for review). This lack of knowledge inevitably results in delayed assessment, diagnosis, and appropriate supports being provided. Many parents and caregivers report seeing a large number of health care professionals before FASD is even considered, let alone diagnosed. Along the way, many children will have received an incorrect diagnosis and, in some cases, inappropriate treatment. Even when FASD is suspected, waiting lists to specialist diagnostic services are often extremely long or prohibitively expensive to access.

Once diagnosed, children with FASD may experience challenges qualifying for services, as FASD is not as well recognized as other conditions such as autism spectrum disorder and ADHD. From a health perspective, following diagnosis, the focus is usually then centered on the neurobehavioral aspects of the condition and other aspects of health are often dismissed or considered side-effects of other medications. Additionally, mental health interventions are often not targeted or adjusted to the neurodevelopmental needs of individuals with FASD and are therefore less effective, which can result in frustration and distress for individuals with FASD at not being able to meet the demands of the treatment program.

Individuals with FASD also face barriers due to the multiple systems of care required to meet their physical and mental health support needs (Fig. 12.3). The range of health conditions, comorbidities, and complexities associated with FASD requires the provision of support across a broad array of medical and allied health specialists that tend to be provided "in silos," often with little communication and coordination of care across service providers. Navigating these separates services can be difficult for caregivers, who also report frustration at continually needing to initiate and lead conversations about FASD and the impacts of prenatal alcohol exposure with health providers [46, 47]. This can also be relevant when interacting with other formal support services that are often required, for example, in the education or legal systems.

Stigmatization associated with FASD can also be a significant barrier to care whereby affected individuals and their caregivers may experience external shame in the form of feeling judged or blamed for the challenges associated with the disability. This can lead to a reluctance to seek support and/or disclose prenatal alcohol exposure when accessing services [45, 48].

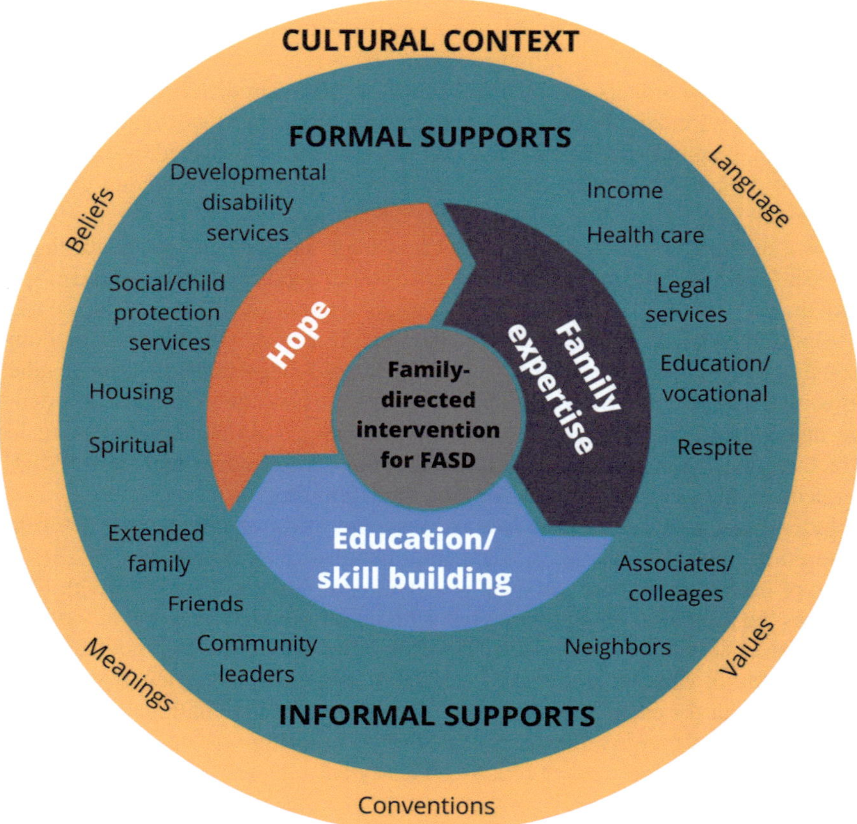

Fig. 12.3 Summary of the formal and informal supports and services that require navigation by caregivers and individuals diagnosed with FASD. (Reproduced with permission from [45])

Historical and Future Trends

Since FAS was first recognized as a condition resulting from prenatal alcohol exposure in the mid 1970s, the emphasis has been on establishing clear criteria for diagnosis as well as focusing on prevention of further alcohol-exposed pregnancies. The initial criteria included the facial features as a key component, but the last 20 years has seen a move to consider the presentation of an individual exposed to prenatal alcohol on a spectrum, with the facial features absent in the majority of cases. Some early studies included a focus on identifying and reporting some of the physical health impacts (e.g., congenital heart defects, the range of physical anomalies).

Although this has continued, overwhelmingly the focus has moved to "proving" the teratogenic effects of alcohol on the developing brain. However, given that alcohol can freely cross the placenta into all cells of the developing fetus, it is surprising that there has been little focus on investigating the impact of prenatal alcohol on development of other fetal organs. With a large number of people who were diagnosed with FAS or FASD as young children now reaching their 30s and 40s, they are experiencing a wide range of conditions not previously considered part of the spectrum.

Recent interest in other aspects of FASD has provided important direction for researchers and the need for education for clinicians and other health professionals in how to provide more effective care for individuals with FASD. The application of a more integrated model of care that brings together professionals across multiple disciplines will ensure the diverse developmental, physical and mental health needs of individuals with FASD are met. Importantly, taking an interprofessional approach provides an opportunity to deliver client-centered, FASD-informed collaborative care for individuals and their families. One example of an integrated and holistic approach that is yet to be widely considered in the care of individuals with FASD is the International Classification of Functioning, Disability and Health (ICF) Framework. The ICF provides an interprofessional, strengths-based, participation and context specific approach to assessing and supporting individuals with FASD. While in the past, there was a need to focus on deficits to evidence the teratogenic effects of alcohol, effective care requires a strength-based approach that incorporates a person's individual strengths and interests and focuses on improving outcomes that are meaningful to individuals with FASD and their families. Interventions and supports that increase participation in school, social, and work activities, for example, are important for improving quality of life and are likely to have long-term flow-on benefits for physical and mental health [45, 49, 50].

Finally, there is increasing recognition that FASD is not necessarily a condition associated with exposure at levels consistent with an alcohol use disorder during pregnancy. Given there are high rates of alcohol consumption in women of reproductive age in most countries around the world, it is perhaps not surprising that there is alcohol exposure during pregnancy [51]. This can partly be explained by the fact that approximately 50% of pregnancies are unplanned, with some women consuming alcohol prior to pregnancy recognition but then stopping or reducing their consumption for the remainder of their pregnancy [52]. However, there is also the misconception that only "strong" alcohol, or alcohol in large quantities is harmful during pregnancy [53].

While abstinence is the only solution to prevent FASD, this is not feasible on a population basis. Therefore, there has been much interest in developing effective intervention strategies to ameliorate the adverse outcomes of PAE. One potential intervention is supplementation with choline, an essential nutrient that contributes to multiple important processes in the body including formation of cell membranes and brain function. Given these roles, the requirement for choline consumption during pregnancy is high but many women fail to consume a diet that provides recommended levels [54]. Additionally, alcohol has been shown to reduce circulating choline levels in both preclinical [5, 7] and clinical studies. There is currently abundant preclinical and clinical evidence to suggest that choline supplementation, either in the mother during pregnancy or of the offspring in early life, can ameliorate some of the brain, growth, and placental deficits from prenatal alcohol exposure [55–58]. However, the integration of this supplement into prenatal care needs to be considered carefully, so that the over-arching message of avoiding alcohol when pregnant or planning a pregnancy is not dismissed.

Conclusions

Broadening the focus on the full range of health issues experienced by people exposed to prenatal alcohol has led to a more inclusive view of a whole-body approach to FASD. Much of the renewed interest in the effects of alcohol on organs other than the brain has emerged due to the insights and experiences of people with FASD. On-going research to fully understand the full range of health problems faced by individuals exposed to prenatal alcohol is important to enable them to access appropriate healthcare throughout their lives and for healthcare professionals to be able to advise of potential prevention or intervention measures.

References

1. Popova S, Lange S, Shield K, Mihic A, Chudley AE, Mukherjee RAS, Bekmuradov D, Rehm J. Comorbidity of fetal alcohol spectrum disorder: a systematic review and meta-analysis. Lancet. 2016;387(10022):978–87.
2. Himmelreich M, Lutke CJ, Travis ET. The lay of the land: fetal alcohol spectrum disorder (FASD) as a whole-body diagnosis. In: Begun AL, Murray MM, editors. The Routledge handbook of social work and addictive behaviors. New York: Routledge; 2020. p. 191–215.
3. Gluckman PD, Hanson MA, Cooper C, Thornburg KL. Effect of in utero and early-life conditions on adult health and disease. N Engl J Med. 2008;359(1):61–73.
4. Dorey ES, Pantaleon M, Weir KA, Moritz KM. Adverse prenatal environment and kidney development: implications for programing of adult disease. Reproduction. 2014;147(6):R189–98.
5. Steane SE, Fielding AM, Kent NL, Andersen I, Browne DJ, Tejo EN, Gardebjer EM, Kalisch-Smith JI, Sullivan MA, Moritz KM, Akison LK. Maternal choline supplementation in a rat model of periconceptional alcohol exposure: impacts on the fetus and placenta. Alcohol Clin Exp Res. 2021a;45(10):2130–46.
6. Gardebjer EM, Cuffe JS, Pantaleon M, Wlodek ME, Moritz KM. Periconceptional alcohol consumption causes fetal growth restriction and increases glycogen accumulation in the late gestation rat placenta. Placenta. 2014;35(1):50–7.
7. Kalisch-Smith JI, Steane SE, Simmons DG, Pantaleon M, Anderson ST, Akison LK, Wlodek ME, Moritz KM. Periconceptional alcohol exposure causes female-specific perturbations to trophoblast differentiation and placental formation in the rat. Development. 2019;146(11):dev172205.
8. Abel EL. An update on incidence of FAS: FAS is not an equal opportunity birth defect. Neurotoxicol Teratol. 1995;17(4):437–43.
9. Skagerstrom J, Chang G, Nilsen P. Predictors of drinking during pregnancy: a systematic review. J Womens Health (Larchmt). 2011;20(6):901–13.
10. Yumoto C, Jacobson SW, Jacobson JL. Fetal substance exposure and cumulative environmental risk in an African American cohort. Child Dev. 2008;79(6):1761–76.

11. Akison LK, Moritz KM, Reid N. Adverse reproductive outcomes associated with fetal alcohol exposure: a systematic review. Reproduction. 2019a;157(4):329–43.
12. Reid N, Akison LK, Hoy W, Moritz KM. Adverse health outcomes associated with fetal alcohol exposure: a systematic review focused on cardio-renal outcomes. J Stud Alcohol Drugs. 2019a;80(5):515–23.
13. Reid N, Moritz KM, Akison LK. Adverse health outcomes associated with fetal alcohol exposure: a systematic review focused on immune-related outcomes. Pediatr Allergy Immunol. 2019b;30(7):698–707.
14. Akison LK, Reid N, Wyllie M, Moritz KM. Adverse health outcomes in offspring associated with fetal alcohol exposure: a systematic review of clinical and preclinical studies with a focus on metabolic and body composition outcomes. Alcohol Clin Exp Res. 2019b;43(7):1324–43.
15. Reid N, Hayes N, Young SB, Akison LK, Moritz KM. Caregiver-reported physical health status of children and young people with fetal alcohol spectrum disorder. J Dev Orig Health Dis. 2021;12(3):420–7.
16. Kable JA, Mehta PK, Coles CD. Alterations in insulin levels in adults with prenatal alcohol exposure. Alcohol Clin Exp Res. 2021;45(3):500–6.
17. Weeks O, Bosse GD, Oderberg IM, Akle S, Houvras Y, Wrighton PJ, LaBella K, Iversen I, Tavakoli S, Adatto I, Schwartz A, Kloosterman D, Tsomides A, Charness ME, Peterson RT, Steinhauser ML, Fazeli PK, Goessling W. Fetal alcohol spectrum disorder predisposes to metabolic abnormalities in adulthood. J Clin Invest. 2020;130(5):2252–69.
18. Amos-Kroohs RM, Fink BA, Smith CJ, Chin L, Van Calcar SC, Wozniak JR, Smith SM. Abnormal eating behaviors are common in children with fetal alcohol spectrum disorder. J Pediatr. 2016;169:194–200.
19. Carter RC, Jacobson JL, Molteno CD, Jiang H, Meintjes EM, Jacobson SW, Duggan C. Effects of heavy prenatal alcohol exposure and iron deficiency anemia on child growth and body composition through age 9 years. Alcohol Clin Exp Res. 2012;36(11):1973–82.
20. Hayes N, Reid N, Akison LK, Moritz KM. The effect of heavy prenatal alcohol exposure on adolescent body mass index and waist-to-height ratio at 12–13 years. Int J Obes. 2021;45(9):2118–25.
21. Parviainen R, Auvinen J, Serlo W, Jarvelin MR, Sinikumpu JJ. Maternal alcohol consumption during pregnancy associates with bone fractures in early childhood. A birth-cohort study of 6718 participants. Bone. 2020;137:115462.
22. Cook JC, Lynch ME, Coles CD. Association analysis: fetal alcohol spectrum disorder and hypertension status in children and adolescents. Alcohol Clin Exp Res. 2019;43(8):1727–33.
23. Das SK, McIntyre HD, Alati R, Al Mamun A. Maternal alcohol consumption during pregnancy and its association with offspring renal function at 30 years: observation from a birth cohort study. Nephrology (Carlton). 2019;24(1):21–7.
24. Bodnar TS, Raineki C, Wertelecki W, Yevtushok L, Plotka L, Zymak-Zakutnya N, Honerkamp-Smith G, Wells A, Rolland M, Woodward TS, Coles CD, Kable JA, Chambers CD, Weinberg J, Collaborative Initiative on Fetal Alcohol Spectrum Disorders (CIFASD). Altered maternal immune networks are associated with adverse child neurodevelopment: impact of alcohol consumption during pregnancy. Brain Behav Immun. 2018;73:205–15.
25. Nguyen TMT, Steane SE, Moritz KM, Akison LK. Prenatal alcohol exposure programmes offspring disease: insulin resistance in adult males in a rat model of acute exposure. J Physiol. 2019;597(23):5619–37.
26. McReight EK, Liew SH, Steane SE, Hutt KJ, Moritz KM, Akison LK. Moderate episodic prenatal alcohol does not impact female offspring fertility in rats. Reproduction. 2020;159(5):615–26.
27. Snow ME, Keiver K. Prenatal ethanol exposure disrupts the histological stages of fetal bone development. Bone. 2007;41(2):181–7.
28. Dorey ES, Walton SL, Kalisch-Smith JI, Paravicini TM, Gardebjer EM, Weir KA, Singh RR, Bielefeldt-Ohmann H, Anderson ST, Wlodek ME, Moritz KM. Periconceptional ethanol expo-

sure induces a sex specific diuresis and increase in AQP2 and AVPR2 in the kidneys of aged rat offspring. Physiol Rep. 2019;7(21):e14273.

29. Walton SL, Tjongue M, Tare M, Kwok E, Probyn M, Parkington HC, Bertram JF, Moritz KM, Denton KM. Chronic low alcohol intake during pregnancy programs sex-specific cardiovascular deficits in rats. Biol Sex Differ. 2019;10(1):21.

30. Parkington HC, Kenna KR, Sozo F, Coleman HA, Bocking A, Brien JF, Harding R, Walker DW, Morley R, Tare M. Maternal alcohol consumption in pregnancy enhances arterial stiffness and alters vasodilator function that varies between vascular beds in fetal sheep. J Physiol. 2014;592(12):2591–603.

31. Zhang X, Lan N, Bach P, Nordstokke D, Yu W, Ellis L, Meadows GG, Weinberg J. Prenatal alcohol exposure alters the course and severity of adjuvant-induced arthritis in female rats. Brain Behav Immun. 2012;26(3):439–50.

32. Bake S, Pinson MR, Pandey S, Chambers JP, Mota R, Fairchild AE, Miranda RC, Sohrabji F. Prenatal alcohol-induced sex differences in immune, metabolic and neurobehavioral outcomes in adult rats. Brain Behav Immun. 2021;98:86–100.

33. Weinberg J, Sliwowska JH, Lan N, Hellemans KG. Prenatal alcohol exposure: foetal programming, the hypothalamic–pituitary–adrenal axis and sex differences in outcome. J Neuroendocrinol. 2008;20(4):470–88.

34. Probyn ME, Cuffe JS, Zanini S, Moritz KM. The effects of low-moderate dose prenatal ethanol exposure on the fetal and postnatal rat lung. J Dev Orig Health Dis. 2013;4(5):358–67.

35. Burgess DJ, Moritz KM. Prenatal alcohol exposure and developmental programming of mental illness. J Dev Orig Health Dis. 2020;11(3):211–21.

36. O'Connor MJ, Shah B, Whaley S, Cronin P, Gunderson B, Graham J. Psychiatric illness in a clinical sample of children with prenatal alcohol exposure. Am J Drug Alcohol Abuse. 2002;28(4):743–54.

37. Inkelis SM, Thomas JD. Sleep in infants and children with prenatal alcohol exposure. Alcohol Clin Exp Res. 2018;42:1390–405.

38. Hayes N, Moritz KM, Reid N. Parent-reported sleep problems in school-aged children with fetal alcohol spectrum disorder: association with child behaviour, caregiver, and family functioning. Sleep Med. 2020;74:307–14.

39. Ipsiroglu OS, Wind K, Hung YA, Berger M, Chan F, Yu W, Stockler S, Weinberg J. Prenatal alcohol exposure and sleep-wake behaviors: exploratory and naturalistic observations in the clinical setting and in an animal model. Sleep Med. 2019;54:101–12.

40. Keiver K, Bertram CP, Orr AP, Clarren S. Salivary cortisol levels are elevated in the afternoon and at bedtime in children with prenatal alcohol exposure. Alcohol. 2015;49(1):79–87.

41. Volgin DV, Kubin L. Reduced sleep and impaired sleep initiation in adult male rats exposed to alcohol during early postnatal period. Behav Brain Res. 2012;234(1):38–42.

42. Guo R, Simasko SM, Jansen HT. Chronic alcohol consumption in rats leads to desynchrony in diurnal rhythms and molecular clocks. Alcohol Clin Exp Res. 2016;40(2):291–300.

43. Chen CP, Kuhn P, Advis JP, Sarkar DK. Prenatal ethanol exposure alters the expression of period genes governing the circadian function of beta-endorphin neurons in the hypothalamus. J Neurochem. 2006;97(4):1026–33.

44. Petrenko CL, Tahir N, Mahoney EC, Chin NP. Prevention of secondary conditions in fetal alcohol spectrum disorders: identification of systems-level barriers. Matern Child Health J. 2014;18(6):1496–505.

45. Reid N, Crawford A, Petrenko C, Kable J, Olson HC. A family-directed approach for supporting individuals with fetal alcohol spectrum disorders. Curr Dev Disord Rep. 2022;9(1):9–18.

46. Anderson T, Mela M, Rotter T, Poole N. A qualitative investigation into barriers and enablers for the development of a clinical pathway for individuals living with FASD and mental disorder/addictions. Can J Commun Ment Health. 2020;48(3):43–60.

47. Doak J, Katsikitis M, Webster H, Wood A. A fetal alcohol spectrum disorder diagnostic service and beyond: outcomes for families. Res Dev Disabil. 2019;93:103428.

48. Roozen S, Stutterheim SE, Bos AER, Kok G, Curfs LMG. Understanding the social stigma of fetal alcohol spectrum disorders: from theory to interventions. Found Sci. 2020;27:753–71. https://doi.org/10.1007/s10699-020-09676-y.
49. Imms C, Granlund M, Wilson PH, Steenbergen B, Rosenbaum PL, Gordon AM. Participation, both a means and an end: a conceptual analysis of processes and outcomes in childhood disability. Dev Med Child Neurol. 2017;59(1):16–25.
50. Olson HC, Sparrow J. A shift in perspective on secondary disabilities in fetal alcohol spectrum disorders. Alcohol Clin Exp Res. 2021;45(5):916–21.
51. Popova S, Lange S, Probst C, Gmel G, Rehm J. Estimation of national, regional, and global prevalence of alcohol use during pregnancy and fetal alcohol syndrome: a systematic review and meta-analysis. Lancet Glob Health. 2017;5(3):e290–9.
52. Muggli E, O'Leary C, Donath S, Orsini F, Forster D, Anderson PJ, Lewis S, Nagle C, Craig JM, Elliott E, Halliday J. Did you ever drink more? A detailed description of pregnant women's drinking patterns. BMC Public Health. 2016;16:683.
53. Popova S, Dozet D, Akhand Laboni S, Brower K, Temple V. Why do women consume alcohol during pregnancy or while breastfeeding? Drug Alcohol Rev. 2021;41:759–77.
54. Zeisel SH. Nutrition in pregnancy: the argument for including a source of choline. Int J Womens Health. 2013;5:193–9.
55. Akison LK, Kuo J, Reid N, Boyd RN, Moritz KM. Effect of choline supplementation on neurological, cognitive, and behavioral outcomes in offspring arising from alcohol exposure during development: a quantitative systematic review of clinical and preclinical studies. Alcohol Clin Exp Res. 2018;42(9):1591–611.
56. Steane SE, Young SL, Clifton VL, Gallo LA, Akison LK, Moritz KM. Prenatal alcohol consumption and placental outcomes: a systematic review and meta-analysis of clinical studies. Am J Obstet Gynecol. 2021b;225(6):607.e601–22.
57. Warton FL, Molteno CD, Warton CMR, Wintermark P, Lindinger NM, Dodge NC, Zollei L, van der Kouwe AJW, Carter RC, Jacobson JL, Jacobson SW, Meintjes EM. Maternal choline supplementation mitigates alcohol exposure effects on neonatal brain volumes. Alcohol Clin Exp Res. 2021;45(9):1762–74.
58. Wozniak JR, Fink BA, Fuglestad AJ, Eckerle JK, Boys CJ, Sandness KE, Radke JP, Miller NC, Lindgren C, Brearley AM, Zeisel SH, Georgieff MK. Four-year follow-up of a randomized controlled trial of choline for neurodevelopment in fetal alcohol spectrum disorder. J Neurodev Disord. 2020;12(1):9.

Chapter 13
FASD-Informed Care and the Future of Intervention

Heather Carmichael Olson, Misty Pruner, Nora Byington, and Tracy Jirikowic

Introduction

About 50 years ago, the full fetal alcohol syndrome (FAS) was recognized in the scientific literature as a condition resulting from prenatal alcohol exposure (PAE) and was soon acknowledged to last lifelong [1–3]. Over the next 25 years, studies revealed that a much wider range of neurodevelopmental conditions were associated with PAE [4, 5]. The overarching term "FASD" to denote "fetal alcohol spectrum disorder(s)" gradually came into use and was formalized in the early 2000s (e.g., [6, 7]). From the beginning of the field, effective treatment for FASD was of interest, although it was daunting to know what to do.

Starting early and building momentum, energetic family support networks emerged to respond to FASD through self-help, peer support, and advocacy in the 1970s and 1980s. Governmental public health and research initiatives also began in

H. C. Olson (✉)
Department of Psychiatry and Behavioral Sciences, University of Washington School of Medicine, Seattle, WA, USA

Center on Child Health, Development and Behavior, Seattle Children's Research Institute, Seattle, WA, USA
e-mail: heather.carmichaelolson@seattlechildrens.org

M. Pruner
Center on Child Health, Development and Behavior, Seattle Children's Research Institute, Seattle, WA, USA
e-mail: mpruner@uw.edu

N. Byington
Masonic Institute for the Developing Brain, University of Minnesota, Minneapolis, MN, USA
e-mail: bying015@umn.edu

T. Jirikowic
Department of Rehabilitation Medicine, University of Washington School of Medicine, Seattle, WA, USA
e-mail: tracyj@uw.edu

© The Author(s), under exclusive license to Springer Nature Switzerland AG 2023
O. A. Abdul-Rahman, C. L. M. Petrenko (eds.), *Fetal Alcohol Spectrum Disorders*,
https://doi.org/10.1007/978-3-031-32386-7_13

the 1970s, appearing gradually over time in a growing number of countries. FASD screening and diagnostic efforts took off in the 1990s, though a constant barrier to diagnosis was the lack of effective treatment [8]. Families and providers continually asked: "Why get a diagnosis when there is nothing to <u>do</u> about it?" Yet, over the years, prevalence studies and advocacy efforts increasingly revealed those living with FASD as a surprisingly large, under-recognized, under-served global clinical population with neurodevelopmental disabilities that deserved (and needed) services over the lifespan (e.g., [9–11]). The high costs of FASD were periodically estimated, such as a 2019 estimate of the lifetime (global) cost of care per diagnosed individual (by age 43) of over $1 million US [12, 13], provoking interest in treatment as a way to reduce these costs.

FASD came to be understood as a set of "brain-based" conditions characterized by wide-ranging, individually variable teratogenic alcohol effects. Along with many correlated prenatal and postnatal risk factors, this meant lifelong neurodevelopmental complexity with additional health and mental health complications. But in the 1990s, US-based data uncovered a stark reality: there were also high rates of a full range of what have been called "secondary conditions" among those living with FASD, especially as they grew older. Current data gathered nearly 20 years later, echoed this unfortunate message. Evidence continued to reveal high rates of adverse life experiences and problems in daily life for those with FASD—even in Canada, a country with more responsive social services [14].

Starting in the 1990s, awareness of this difficult reality galvanized both necessary action and stigma [15]. Pressure for effective treatment and adequate service systems grew. Protective factors were identified, providing direction for treatment. It rapidly became clear that stable, nurturant caregiving, and adequate social and developmental disability services were central protective influences for those with FASD [16]. But what also became clear was the heavy, lifelong burden of FASD on caregivers and families—because there was no organized social safety net for FASD in any country. So, in the late 1990s, it became of vital interest to find and build caregiver and family support, because it was clearly lacking. In the 2000s, interest also turned to finding treatment for young children with PAE, given their high risk for FASD paired with the hope that later problems could be prevented by early intervention (e.g., [17–20]). However, early intervention was also lacking. In the 2000s, periodic calls to action and needs assessments were published (e.g., [21, 22]), a trend that continues to the present time [11, 13], pointing out many gaps in treatment research and services. While FASD was known to be a worldwide problem, in the mid-2000s, the global nature of FASD really began to sharpen into focus and, over time, magnify (e.g., [10]). This meant that the need for treatment services was also worldwide.

While momentum for action was growing, it was fortunate that a foundation of knowledge-based treatment was also being built. Solid basic research and study of animal models highlighted useful treatment directions for human studies (e.g., [23, 24]). As communities slowly began to recognize FASD, clinical wisdom accumulated on intervention for children, youth, and families. Parent support and advocacy networks, and a small group of "champions" in clinical practice and research, spread the word. Shared in newsletters, booklets, and a few books, and later online, this clinical wisdom was derived from the families themselves, interested providers, and specialized FASD diagnostic clinics. Knowledge was based on lived experience and clinical expertise (e.g., [25–29]). Efforts to remediate common areas of impairment among those with FASD emerged as an early treatment direction. At the same time, the range and variability of alcohol's teratogenic neurobehavioral effects were increasingly described by research. This dictated the need for individualized, multi-faceted treatment, because each individual affected by PAE showed a unique, com-plex profile of cognitive-behavioral impairment (e.g., [30, 31]). More holistic efforts to provide family support emerged as another treatment direction. Through advocacy and creativity, family support services aimed to link families to a range of services. This type of treatment responded to the many unmet needs identified for individuals living with FASD (and their families)—and to the lack of available school and com-munity resources and supports tailored to this clinical population (e.g., [26, 32, 33]).

In the mid-2000s, the term "FASD-informed care" was coined by "champions" in clinical care. Efforts began to define it, which have continued to the present time as applied to different types of programs and clinical situations (e.g., [29, 34–37]). Through the 2000s, grassroots efforts to help families have been maintained by dedicated parent support networks, self-advocates, community groups, clinical experts, and some governmental programs. Also, finally, starting in the early 2000s, spurred by coordinated advocacy and governmental action, funding for systematic intervention research began for individuals with FASD, and their families.

Systematic intervention research is vital because it can demonstrate what works. In recent years and in a growing number of countries, treatment efficacy research has become increasingly necessary. This is because of growing societal require-ments for "evidence-based care" or "evidence-based treatments" in physical and mental health. This approach mandates evidence from published studies that meet strict systematic research criteria. These criteria are aimed to ensure treatments are effective (and having these research data is linked to whether or not permission is granted for insurance or governmental funding to pay for treatment). At this point, two decades of findings on intervention for FASD have come from two sources. One source has been a number of "service-to-science" program evaluation studies, sometimes not formally published, which are valuable but do not necessarily con-tribute to defining evidence-based care. Another source has been a relatively small number of controlled quantitative or mixed methods studies of innovative or exist-ing treatments adapted to FASD/PAE, published for peer review, which do help to define evidence-based care.

All this research has been productive. Intriguing treatment ideas have emerged for individuals with PAE or living with FASD across the lifespan, and their families. Ideas have come from around the world. Advances have been made. But at this point the problems are much larger than the solutions found so far.

Progress on FASD intervention is at an important tipping point.

Where are we now? The field has reached good understanding on what defines many of the essential elements of FASD-informed care, presented in this chapter. A complement of interventions has been tested in controlled research, also presented here. This means that, despite limited recognition of FASD and other barriers, systematic research is proceeding and best practices for "evidence-based care" are emerging. A variety of systematic and critical reviewers have carefully analyzed existing data from different angles, with excellent ideas proposed for next research steps, also presented here. The strengths of those living with FASD, and those of their families, and the power of self-advocacy, have come to the fore. Stigma has been recognized as a major barrier to progress on FASD-informed care and providing intervention for those living with FASD. In response, the need to overcome stigma toward FASD has been recognized, no matter how large the task, and ways to do so have been proposed. Pressure to act has grown overwhelming. There are treatment dilemmas to solve and promising treatments to try. Telehealth, app-based, and online treatment methods allow treatment to scale up and be more accessible, and the recent global pandemic has led to new methods, flexible thinking, and global responses. There are decisions to make about strategic directions in FASD intervention, and information is available to make those decisions. All this is discussed here.

It is time to accelerate, shape the future, and move ahead, finding the right interventions to try. The ultimate goal is to change practice in meaningful and sustainable ways to truly help the many families worldwide living with PAE or FASD. The next decade will be exciting and pivotal. The hope is that the treatment response to FASD will now strategically expand more quickly with an increasingly global reach, and that communities and researchers will collaborate and respond on a larger scale.

The Overall Importance of Cultural Perspectives and Lived Experience

There is an important point to make before going further. At this point in history, there is growing awareness of the overall importance of cultural perspectives, and the idea that treatments should be culturally informed. A family's own culture and subculture—and, beyond that, the larger community and cultural context in which an individual with FASD and their family live—must be taken as fully as possible into account to ensure treatment is appropriate and effective. FASD is a global public health problem, so treatments must be created for a wide range of communities and cultures. Yet cultural awareness is simply a first step toward creating culture-centered practices, a process which must be led by individuals and families in the communities themselves.

In conversation with colleagues and inspired by a recent publication [38], it became clear this chapter was written from the standpoint of academics from a western tradition. This meant that careful reflection was needed. FASD is a global public health concern. Therefore, the authors wish to acknowledge the important historical and contextual implications for indigenous, Black, LatinX, Asian—and other diverse communities worldwide from a non-western tradition—for whom there are considerations grounded in cultural context that apply to FASD intervention. The current chapter has taken an inclusive approach by integrating lived experiences data. But the authors recognize that useful learning will come from other cultures and other researchers. The authors also acknowledge a requirement for genuine effort to work alongside our counterparts from diverse communities to be guided to deeper understanding and invite input from all.

This reflection fits well with other themes in this chapter. One of these themes is the importance of gathering lived experience data from groups (cultural, subcultural, community) to inform how treatments are created. Another is working alongside and being led by "stakeholders" (those who have a stake in the treatment) when designing interventions. This reflection also fits with the theme, discussed later, of keeping in mind the fundamental importance of self-determination and basic rights for those living with FASD when collaboratively designing treatments and choosing treatment goals for this important and valued group of individuals and families. Lived experience can illuminate what really matters to the quality of life for those living with FASD. This should be applied to creating interventions. As summarized in a perceptive social media source about FASD, which (among other insights) captures the voices of self-advocates: *"FASD: Nothing about us, without us"* [39].

Goals and Structure of This Chapter

To help direct and accelerate intervention in the field of FASD now and in the future, this chapter first discusses conceptual models, then brings these ideas together with findings from lived experiences research. This is done to define 12 essential elements of FASD-informed care related to intervention. Figure 13.1 captures these essential elements of FASD-informed care as a "visual." The current complement of published intervention studies systematically tested with those with PAE or FASD, from infancy to young adulthood, and their families, are presented in tables and briefly discussed, followed by a short research critique. Promising treatments, chosen from other fields as future research directions, are presented for consideration by readers, as they may help advance the field more quickly. The chapter ends with a discussion of dilemmas and promising directions for work on FASD intervention. The comprehensive reference section provides many resources on the topic of FASD intervention which readers can explore.

If readers are inspired to collaboratively share knowledge—and be led by communities to develop and participate in FASD-informed care, including culture-centered practices—this chapter will have met its most important goals.

Building the Foundation for FASD-Informed Care: Important Theories

FASD-informed care, as it relates to treatment, is built on the foundation of several influential developmental theories, which are important to understand and so are briefly explained here. Based on this solid theoretical foundation, the next section of this chapter presents 12 essential elements of FASD-informed care, that also take into account the "real world" knowledge of those living with FASD. These essential elements of FASD-informed care guide the design and development of useful and effective interventions at multiple levels.

Thinking About Both the Individual and the Family

Scientists have advocated that a *developmental systems model* be applied to understanding how alcohol's teratogenic effects on an individual play out over time, and to developing appropriate interventions (e.g., [18, 40–42]). Among other ideas, as seen in Chap. 2 of this book, this theoretical model suggests that important risk and protective factors be derived from study of typical development (which identifies universal factors), and from population-specific research. In 2009, FASD researcher Olson and her colleagues joined this developmental systems perspective with a *family systems approach,* integrating these two models to allow a focus on both the individual and family in intervention development [26]. Development of family support and positive parenting treatments for families raising those with FASD have been guided, in large part, by this combined model.

Developmental systems thinking suggests that, over time, characteristics of an individual interact back-and-forth with those of caregivers (and those of the larger ecological context, including the family and other larger societal influences, especially as the individual grows older). A developmental systems approach considers the whole lifespan, and how developmental outcomes and influences differ or change in importance at various life stages. Intervention is then designed to reduce disabling individual and environmental risks over the lifespan, while also enhancing protective factors (including strengths of the individual). That means care must be developmentally appropriate, since risk and protective influences change at different life stages. Using this approach, interventions should be designed to alter systems in order to support the life path of an <u>individual</u> with disabilities in a positive direction over time.

According to Olson and her coauthors, developmental systems thinking can be joined with a family systems approach in the field of FASD. This approach suggests that life paths, influences, and outcomes be measured not only at the level of the individual, but at other levels—such as the levels of the caregiver–child relationship and/or the family. Family systems thinking suggests that treatment also be directed toward family members as needed, so as to impact the entire family system. Using a family systems approach, interventions should try to alter family systems (and the impact of formal and informal systems that support families) in order to shape the path of <u>family adaptation</u> in a positive direction over time. Very recent thinking in treatment for FASD is using these ideas as a foundation to create increasingly precise, operational theoretical models that conform to additional elements of FASD-informed care. For instance, there is a very new model of family-directed intervention for FASD that shows how some existing practices match up to this model [38]. Other fields have also recently pursued the idea of joining developmental systems and family systems thinking, such as the field of early intervention [43].

Thinking How to Respond to Secondary Conditions and Mental Health Problems

Many individuals living with FASD or PAE have strong protective factors and personal strengths. Resilience, "grit," and a growth mindset (a belief that talents can be developed through hard work, good strategies, and input from others) are important characteristics shown by many of individuals with FASD or PAE [44]. It is vital to keep all these strengths in mind in thinking about treatment, as they are powerful influences on development.

But research data do show that individuals living with the biological risk presented by FASD or PAE also often have past or present experiences of psychosocial disruption, such as multiple home placements or living with parental substance abuse. Research so far suggests they may often contend with difficult relationships or problems with service systems and, as a group, show an elevated rate of trauma experiences (such as abuse or neglect, victimization, or even violence). They also face possible other biological risk factors of prenatal exposures and family history of mental health and learning problems. As a result, they may encounter these secondary conditions (real-world difficulties that might better be thought of as "secondary impacts"), such as school disruption or difficulties with independent living. They may also experience co-occurring mental health conditions (psychopathology) [45–47].

The *field of developmental psychopathology* is an approach that was born of out developmental systems thinking—but went further to help understand how psychopathology develops over the lifespan. Insights from this theoretical model are needed to build the foundation for FASD-informed care in treatment because so many with FASD face mental health challenges and trauma, and this model also lays a good foundation in other ways. For instance, the field of developmental psychology suggests that interventions focus on improving relationships and provides many insights into how treatment can be trauma-informed to reduce the impact of maltreatment on development.

Among other ideas, this model suggests that early appearing problems, such as the neurocognitive, self-regulation, and adaptive function difficulties that come from the teratogenic effects of alcohol, have a cascade of effects on development (and the capacity to form healthy relationships). Because these effects start early, over time they spread across many levels of function and have a major impact. Practically speaking, this means it is vital to provide comprehensive, intensive early intervention to head off the cascade of effects. That means that not only does treatment for FASD or PAE need to be ongoing, but it also needs to be flexible and collaborative, occurring in interdisciplinary teams and across multiple systems (such as in health care, school, social services, and more). This is because the cascade of effects often leads to problems that multiply and grow more troublesome as an individual matures over the lifespan and encounters new demands and roles in life. In other words, the field of developmental psychopathology holds that to act early and provide the right ingredients for healthy development from the start, produces better outcomes than trying to fix problems later.

A central (and complex) idea in this model is that development can be thought of as occurring in "pathways" toward mental health problems (psychopathology). To best create treatments, the model states that these atypical pathways should be studied and described. This means it is important to figure out what are the different processes that underlie different pathways that lead, over time, to the same problematic outcomes. For instance, it is now thought that conduct disorders can develop along one pathway characterized by problems in impulse control. Alternatively, they can develop along a different pathway characterized by limited prosocial emotions [48]. Practically speaking, to be effective, the pathway an individual is on has to be identified—and then the treatment tailored to the appropriate pathway. In this example, one pathway would require treatment to reduce someone's impulsivity, while the other would require treatment that teaches someone empathy. This idea of tailored treatment needs to be applied along with taking a neurodevelopmental viewpoint for those living with FASD, when mental health problems are being treated. This requires real insight on the part of the provider, who cannot simply use the treatment "usually" applied for a particular set of symptoms. They need to try to understand both the mechanism underlying the symptoms (such as conduct problems) _and_ the unique cognitive-behavioral profile of the individual with FASD.

Thinking About Remediating Specific Areas of Impairment

The models discussed so far do not explain how to intervene to remediate specific areas of impairment that often occur because of the damage alcohol can do to the brain and central nervous system. Yet targeting individual-level impairments is so important it is actually one of the 12 essential elements of FASD-informed care. In 2010, FASD researcher Kodituwakku proposed a model of how to do this [31]. His model takes what is called a *neuroconstructivist view*. This view assumes that reciprocal interactions between neural activity and the brain's hardware gradually form (construct) neural connections, within and between regions of the central nervous system. This is a dynamic and interactive view of how development occurs. It is very true to developmental neuroscience.

Practically speaking, Kodituwakku describes behavioral interventions as a series of "guided experiences" for the child, typically led by an adult. Behavioral interventions, such as doing attention training or mindfulness practice, are designed to produce neural activation. In neural activation, a neuron (nerve cell) is activated by other neurons to which it is connected—and that neuron then stimulates other connected neurons to be activated. If effective, neural activation leads to plasticity of neural structures, which leads to substantial changes in experience. All this, in turn, leads to changes in brain structures, leading to progressive formation of neural circuitry supporting a specific skill. Research shows that there are certain skills that are more powerful predictors of long-term developmental outcomes, such as "executive attention" and "self-regulation." Because of this, Kodituwakku further hypothesizes that interventions targeting executive attention and self-regulation may produce outcome effects that are more generalizable than do interventions that try to enhance specific skills (such as literacy training).

Kodituwakku goes on to emphasize that a successful intervention should have a theoretical foundation. In other words, there should be both an underlying <u>logic model</u> and <u>theory of change</u> that aim to account for how the components (variables) of an intervention are related to each other, the processes involved, and how all this operates to create intervention effects. This actually also fits with insights from the field of developmental psychopathology. True to the idea that treatments should have an underlying logic model and theory of change, more recent researchers have sought increasingly specific theoretical models in order to more precisely understand and/or effectively treat common areas of deficit seen among individuals living with PAE or FASD, such as self-regulation [49] and executive attention [50].

From a practical perspective, based on this neuroconstructivist view, Kodituwakku suggests helpful treatment guidelines that may improve the outcomes of interventions designed for individuals living with the teratogenic effects of PAE and other associated risk factors. These guidelines are presented later in this chapter as part of the discussion of the essential elements of FASD-informed care.

Thinking About Self-Determination and Quality of Life

FASD is a lifelong challenge to health and well-being, recently described as a "whole body" diagnosis [51]. It might be further thought of as a "whole body, whole life" issue. An up-to-date definition of FASD-informed care must take this into account. The *life course health development framework* is a very wide-ranging synthesis of ideas, developed over the past few decades, that incorporates rapidly developing evidence on the biological, physical, social, and cultural contributors to the development of health and disease [52, 53]. While many ideas from this model fit well with those from theories already discussed, this framework adds to the foundation of FASD-informed care. Some key ideas are discussed here.

The life course health development framework prioritizes the goal of attaining a better state of health for <u>all</u> people, for both the short term and long term. Therefore, the goal is lifelong wellness and health equity for all groups. As part of FASD-informed care, this means building a useful "social scaffolding" (changed societal thinking and coordinated, effective systems of care) which can lift those with PAE or FASD toward well-being and health equity with other groups. This framework points the field of FASD toward state-of-the-art thinking from the field of intellectual and developmental disabilities (IDD) and basically suggests that a key measure of treatment outcome is "quality of life" (QOL). Recent ideas in IDD include a focus on self-advocacy and the application of strengths-based approaches to supporting individuals with IDD over the lifespan [54]. Current trends emphasize the goal of improving QOL as a way to drive service delivery for persons with IDD [55]. Current treatments are designed to result in outcomes in line with basic human rights and, importantly, the need for self-determination [56].

Practically speaking, using this framework mandates a shift in perspective in the field of FASD. Treatment design should shift from a primary focus on reducing secondary impacts or psychopathology, especially for older individuals, toward adding a focus on improving QOL, adaptive function and self-determination—and on emphasizing real participation in life activities [15, 57]. Treatments should take into account the actual circumstances (context) in which an individual and their family live, including their socioeconomic and cultural context. Treatments should take realistic, observable steps to improve and adapt the environment, and intervention should include specific, individualized actions to make a positive difference in the actual daily lives of those with FASD [57]. Treatments should aim toward practical outcomes that support full and meaningful life participation. This approach honors basic human rights. Further, a focus on self-determination suggests that treatment researchers be led by, and learn from, the lived experiences and self-advocacy of persons with FASD, and those who care for them. That means asking what outcomes <u>they</u> regard as important, and then designing supports to achieve <u>those</u> outcomes. This shift in perspective and in treatment research is accord with the view that (to the extent possible) individuals with FASD should be causal agents in their own lives [15, 54–56].

Defining 12 Essential Elements of FASD-Informed Care for Intervention with Individuals and Families

The theoretical models discussed above lay the foundation for defining the 12 essential elements of FASD-informed care as they relate to treatment. The next section brings life to these theories by informing them with evidence drawn from systematic study of the lived experiences of those affected by PAE or FASD, and their families. This research comes from qualitative research using data such as direct interviews and focus groups.

Recognizing FASD: An Important First Step

Before discussing the essential elements of FASD-informed care related to treatment and looking at Fig. 13.1, it is important to bring up a central insight from lived experiences research: *FASD is not fully understood or recognized* [58, 59]. While data documenting this fact are US-based, this appears to be true across most societies (e.g., [60]). This is deeply concerning. Without recognition, there can be no FASD-informed care. Lack of recognition means no diagnosis or qualification for services. Lack of recognition automatically limits resource availability and the opportunity for intervention. Without adequate recognition of FASD, no social safety net will be built. That means there will be none of the vital "social scaffolding" that can raise the health of those affected by PAE or living with FASD, and those who care for them. This group cannot achieve health equity, even compared to other neurodiverse groups (such as those with autism). In her definition of FASD-informed care for programs working with women with FASD (and their families), researcher Rutman notes that "having an awareness of FASD" is the starting point [35].

To recognize FASD means moving through a multiple-step process of education, identification and diagnosis that must be put in place in many communities and societies. Yet even now, in the 2020s and in countries that have paid attention to FASD, successful identification remains incomplete [11]. Fortunately, though, progress on identification is being made and, with determination, will continue. If we can continue to take these steps, we can offer access to intervention for the many who are in need.

Twelve Essential Elements of FASD-Informed Care for Intervention with Individuals and Families

Integrating theoretical models with insights gleaned from lived experience research yields the 12 essential elements of FASD-informed care as they relate to intervention, with specific examples provided in each section. Figure 13.1 presents these essential elements in a circular figure.

Briefly put, this model of FASD-informed care can be used to guide intervention at three different levels. The essential elements of FASD-informed care can guide care at the level of: (1) Person-centered planning (for the care of individuals with FASD); (2) Development of treatments for those living with FASD and/or their families (to ensure treatments have all relevant elements to meet the definition of FASD-informed care; and (3) Analysis of the overall complement of FASD interventions (to identify what treatments are still needed to fully offer FASD-informed care to this clinical population) [152].

Discussion starts at the top and inside of the figure, moves clockwise, and ends with a review of the elements presented around the edge of the circle.

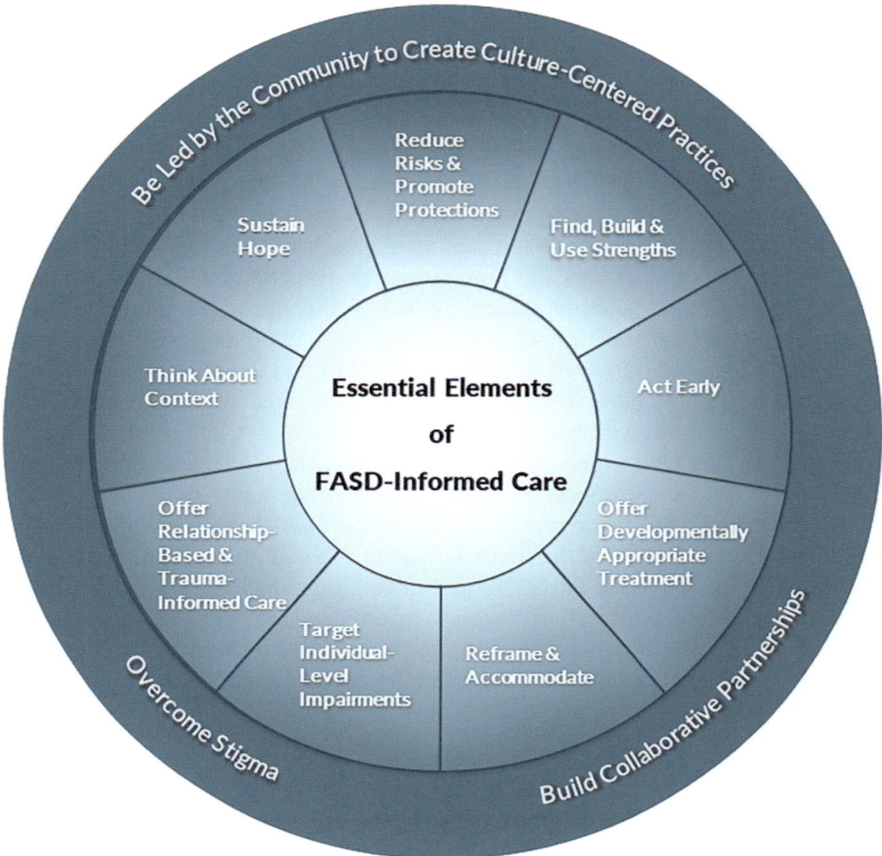

Fig. 13.1 Essential elements of FASD-informed care

Reduce Risks and Promote Protections

Starting at the top and inside of Fig. 13.1 is the element of "Reduce Risks and Promote Protections." After identifying that an individual is affected by PAE, which is a risk factor, theoretical models suggest it is essential to identify other important risk and protective factors for an individual and a family. This is necessary in order to carry out treatment that is FASD-informed. Knowing these factors allows treatment to be designed so individual, family, and environmental risks can be reduced—and protective factors enhanced. The presence of PAE can be a signal to look for associated prenatal and postnatal risk factors, such as other prenatal exposures, or psychosocial risks such as multiple placements, or child maltreatment. However, evidence should be gathered rather than assumptions made. For instance, just because there was drinking during pregnancy does not mean that the family environment was disrupted during pregnancy, or that there is currently a troubled parent–child relationship.

Recent qualitative research on lived experiences has provided detail on treatment-related risk and protective factors regarding caregivers in this clinical population across the lifespan. Caregivers of children with PAE aged birth to 3 years expressed feelings of stress, exhaustion, and being overwhelmed, all parenting risk factors and potential causes of poor outcomes. These parents found value in the protective influence of social-emotional support groups, where they could speak freely without judgment to other parents going through a similar journey [61]. For caregivers with older children with FASD, recent survey data revealed increased rates of concern about caregiver QOL as individuals with FASD mature [62]. These data show that caregivers become the child's advocate and work tirelessly to create adaptations to make day-to-day life more manageable [63]. This can come at a cost of the caregiver's own well-being [59]. Lived experiences data show that needs and priorities vary by family structure, differing among biological, adoptive, and foster caregivers (e.g., [61]). For example, one study found that adoptive parents of adults living with FASD experienced moderate levels of perceived stress. Investigators concluded the risk of stress could be reduced by the protective influence of providing resources in areas specially flagged by these parents (e.g., help in transition into adult housing, support in managing finances for adult children) [64].

Find, Build, and Use Strengths

Moving clockwise around the inside of Fig. 13.1, theoretical models and lived experiences research both emphasize the importance of strengths-based treatment as part of FASD-informed care. In the past, however, treatment for those with FASD was largely deficit-focused. Yet there were earlier data that showed many children with FASD take pride in doing activities independently, are engaged with their families, and are willing to receive (and even seek) help [26]. New strengths data for children with PAE or FASD reveal character strengths such as high social motivation and positive effort/persistence, individual talents, positive mood states/personality—as well as positive influences on the family [65]. Recent evidence emphasizes the intrinsic strengths of those with FASD as older transition-aged youth and adults. These include character strengths such as strong self-awareness [66]. Also, no matter what the family structure, caregivers, and families of those living with FASD also have many strengths, find positive adaptations, have good basic parenting skills, and work to provide protective influences for their child and themselves [19, 26, 59, 63, 67–69].

Data such as these generate promising ideas for strengths-based treatments. Three examples are provided here, based on references cited above. First, birth mother support and mentoring networks can build social support, a factor identified as a strength among women who achieve positive recovery outcomes, using natural support as a treatment mechanism. Second, since many caregivers of individuals with FASD have good basic parenting skills, the focus in parent training can be on strengthening specialized parenting practices (such as learning positive behavior support techniques for school-aged children, or the strategies of monitoring/continency management and supporting autonomy skills for adolescents). Parent training can also focus on sustaining hope through caregivers realizing the "special benefits" of raising a child with FASD. Third, since self-awareness of one's own strengths and challenges is essential to success as an independent adult and is a strength in those with FASD, young adults can be helped toward an understanding of their FASD diagnosis and profile of strengths and challenges. In a collaboration, they can be helped to see what accommodations help them learn and function at their best— and as the key to (and reason for) services.

Act Early

All theoretical models discussed above strongly support the importance of early intervention in FASD-informed care. The capacity of the brain to learn from experience is greatest during the first 3 years of life [70]. The neuroconstructivist view highlights that early intervention has the potential to take advantage of the plasticity of the developing brain to improve at least some of the neurological impairment resulting from alcohol's teratogenic effects, improving brain "hardware" in order to lay a better foundation for later learning. It is notable that the early environmental experiences of children with PAE or FASD are often less than optimal, making early intervention also important to counter psychosocial risk [71]. Lived experiences data have started to detail what caregivers and providers believe should be the content of early intervention for children with PAE or FASD [61, 72].

One important goal of early intervention is to prevent later emergence of troubling secondary impacts and co-occurring mental health conditions. Lived experiences data gathered from caregivers of young children with PAE found that support for child social-emotional needs was apparently lacking in early intervention, even though caregivers did describe their children as receiving support for needs in other domains [61]. Also, the social-emotional well-being of caregivers did not seem to be a primary focus during these first years, as parents stated they lacked support for real-life stressors, problems of living, and respite care. Caregivers said they valued providers who offered reflective developmental guidance, who helped manage expectations for the future, and who connected them with peer support groups. The field of developmental psychopathology, which explains how mental health struggles develop, notes that the early years have a cascading effect on later development. All this means that an important part of FASD-informed care, if PAE and developmental problems can be identified when children are young, is comprehensive, sufficiently intensive, sustained, interdisciplinary early intervention—that takes a neurodevelopmental viewpoint. These early intervention services should fully support child development, caregiver needs, and the caregiver–child relationship.

Offer Developmentally Appropriate Treatment

Developmentally appropriate treatment, directed toward positive outcomes and adaptation, is recommended as part of FASD-informed care by all theoretical models discussed earlier. First, this means working to improve developmental outcomes, for the individual and the family, that typically matter at a particular life stage, such as improving security of attachment in infancy. This also means thinking about treatment that focuses on the developmental influences important at that life stage, such as offering treatment in infancy to increase caregiver sensitivity and responsiveness to a baby. Second, developmentally appropriate treatment means changing treatment goals over time. When children are young, treatment goals are for preventive intervention, to head off problems that might occur, and prevent a cascade of effects that multiply over time. As children grow through the school years and into adolescence, treatment goals center more on remediating deficits and supporting adaptive function. In the past, when individuals with FASD or PAE reached later adolescence and beyond, with needs growing more complex, treatment goals have shifted to more to a responsive approach of mitigating risk and reducing harm [45]. But in adolescence and emerging adulthood, treatment goals should also support the development of agency, autonomy, and self-efficacy. As lived experience research reveals, treatment in the older years should expand and reorient to also address successful accomplishment of the developmentally appropriate goals of increased self-determination and adult QOL.

Third, offering developmentally appropriate care also means coming up with (and applying) treatments aimed at remediating specific impairments arising from PAE at the time that makes the best developmental sense. This may be during critical or sensitive periods when developmental plasticity is heightened. One example is training what the neuroconstructivist view highlighted as the very important skill of "executive attention" at the right time in a "sensitive period." An example of this is the GoFAR metacognitive intervention (discussed later; see also Table 13.7), which is offered starting at age 5 years (just at the time that developmental capacity is just emerging). Fourth, true to the insights of the field of developmental psychopathology, offering developmentally appropriate care can mean customizing treatment to subgroups that are following different developmental pathways toward mental health problems so that treatment can succeed. This truly important (but complex idea) is considered more in the "Discussion" section.

Fifth and finally, to offer developmentally appropriate treatment also means providing intervention across the lifespan. Treatment can lead to improvement, even among older individuals, and this chapter discusses some treatments designed for adolescence and beyond. Because of the dynamic interplay of development, change is always possible. In some ways, change may become easier in the later years (as people mature, recognize they need assistance, and both self-advocate and accept help). In other ways, change may become harder when people are older, as brain plasticity lessens and individuals move down an increasingly fixed life path.

Reframe and Accommodate: Take a Neurodevelopmental Viewpoint

As both theoretical models and lived experiences research make clear, a central, essential part of FASD-informed care is to change perspective. For caregivers and providers, this means to take a "neurodevelopmental viewpoint." This important idea, which arises from understanding FASD is a "brain-based" condition, has been part of the collective clinical wisdom in the field of FASD for decades [18, 19, 27, 28, 31], and woven into some evidence-based treatments (e.g., [73–76]). As FASD researcher Olson has written, taking a neurodevelopmental viewpoint can make it easier to see when certain types of intervention are not appropriate, or how to adapt treatment approaches (and change expectations) to increase intervention effectiveness.

A central element of FASD-informed care (and treatment) is that a neurodevelopmental viewpoint allows caregivers, families, and providers to go through a process of "reframing," as a treatment mechanism. As it is defined here, to "reframe" means to view the challenges of learning, behavior, and daily function of the individual living with FASD as, at least in part, "brain-based." This requires knowing about that particular individual's cognitive-behavioral profile. For parenting or family support interventions, as FASD researcher Olson has written, reframing helps caregivers (and family members) gain a more positive "cognitive appraisal," or view of the individual impacted by PAE or living with FASD, and view of their relationship with that individual. A more positive view can help jumpstart improvements in motivation to change, a sense of parenting efficacy, and use of the most appropriate caregiving methods (positive behavior support) as a first line of treatment [19]. For interventions directed to the individual, an ability to reframe helps define what skills to build in treatment (and what guided experiences to suggest from the neuroconstructivist view) [31]. An ability to reframe prompts creation of tailored "accommodations" in treatment to modify the individual's context. Coming up with ways to accommodate improves how well the environment fits with an individual living with FASD so as to maximize adaptive function, self-determination, and QOL. Modifications of the environment can be extended to home, respite, childcare, school, job, recreation, therapy, and other settings [57]. Learning to take a neurodevelopmental viewpoint, and making efforts to reframe and accommodate, and then changing parenting practices, can help move both the individual and family down a more positive life path [77]. This is evidenced by several interventions (all derived from the standard Families Moving Forward (FMF) Program) that use this logic model and theory of change [19, 73, 78, 79].

Target Individual-Level Impairments

PAE brings wide-ranging neurobehavioral deficits that show up as cognitive-behavioral profiles that vary from one individual to another. With this in mind, in the neuroconstructivist view, FASD researcher Kodituwakku offers a useful set of guidelines for FASD-informed care to maximize treatment outcomes designed for children with PAE or FASD. Kodituwakku's original paper deserves to be read for more detail about these guidelines [31].

The first of Kodituwakku's guidelines is to *"pay heed to the child's overall cognitive-behavioral profile when designing an intervention program for [the child]."* Interestingly, lived experience data echoes the importance of FASD diagnosis, and the positive impact and utility of a feedback session about the diagnosis (and functional profile) for families and school staff, to help appropriately reframe [80]. Diagnosis and feedback can provide useful access to intervention recommendations—and an assessment can generate valuable feedback and linkages even without a definitive FASD diagnosis [81]. The lived experience literature also finds that older individuals with FASD often do not understand their diagnosis as a disability, making feedback to the individual themselves an important treatment [82]. Another important guideline from Kodituwakku is to *"provide enriched input in a guided fashion,"* which builds on a vast animal and human literature showing that enriched environmental input (such as learning opportunities, or chances for the right kind of physical activity) enhances cognitive functioning. Kodituwakku goes on to explain and provide an additional guideline to show how input might be guided to enhance impact on neural structures and child development by staying just within the child's optimal learning zone.

Another guideline from Kodituwakku is to *"provide training in attention and self-regulation early."* Indeed, both self-regulation and attention are developmental capacities that unfold at different biological and cognitive levels, building on each other and gradually integrating together, from the start of life on. In treatment that is FASD-informed, these capacities should receive special support early on, as the neuroconstructivist model suggests improvement in these areas is most likely to generalize to other areas of cognitive and behavioral function. Real-world experience supports the importance of training to remediate impairments in these areas. For instance, impairment in behavior regulation is literally part of the definition used to describe conditions on the fetal alcohol spectrum in DSM-5, the diagnostic manual used by mental health providers [83]. Finally, Kodituwakku suggests that treatments *"combine evidence-based behavioral and pharmacological intervention, unless clinically contra-indicated.*" The idea of using evidence-based treatments is key and will be discussed further later in this chapter. However, despite the frequent real-world use of medications for individuals with PAE or FASD, there is still quite limited guidance for pharmacological care in the field of FASD (see recent systematic reviews [84, 85] and a suggested treatment algorithm based on expert opinion [86]). Note that psychopharmacology treatments are outside the scope of this chapter. Importantly, behavioral and family support interventions are, at least in pediatric populations, nearly always recommended as the optimal first line of treatment.

Offer Relationship-Based and Trauma-Informed Care

The field of developmental psychopathology makes clear that healthy and secure early parent–child relationships are important to a positive life path, and that child maltreatment and trauma are significant risk factors in the onset of psychopathology. Descriptive research has highlighted the high rate of other prenatal and postnatal risks experienced by children with the biological risk factors signaled by PAE or FASD. They often have histories of early life stress and psychosocial disruption and sometimes have experienced maltreatment such as child abuse or neglect (e.g., [46, 87, 88]). It seems clear that young children living in families with the risks of parental substance use and/or psychosocial stressors can especially benefit from relationship-based early interventions. Such treatments are informed by attachment theory and aim to improve both family well-being and child developmental outcomes. They provide preventive intervention. Relationship-based interventions are designed to enhance the quality of parent–child interactions by supporting exchanges that are warm, sensitive, responsive, and adaptive to the young child's needs (e.g., [89, 90]). Improved exchanges can promote emotional security and social competence in the child and, for the caregiver, lead to an increased sense of parenting competence and reduced child-related stress.

Trauma-informed treatment, when relevant, is crucial for this clinical population, as made clear by the field of developmental psychopathology. Indeed, some studies have shown that children with FASD <u>and</u> maltreatment have less positive outcomes than children experiencing trauma who did not have the biological risk factor of PAE [91]. Even the risk of neurodevelopmental impairment may be greater for those who have both trauma and PAE (though this is not entirely clear) [88], suggesting that more intensive remediation of individual-level impairments may be required for those with trauma.

Trauma-informed treatment can be woven directly into treatment following the essential elements of FASD-informed care, as is done in many of the relationship-based interventions listed in Tables 13.1, 13.2, and 13.3, or the positive parenting programs listed in Tables 13.4, 13.5 and 13.6. This kind of care can also be offered an adjunct service that focuses on direct treatment of trauma. Research on responses to child maltreatment recommends various approaches depending on severity, ranging from intensive family preservation services to caregiver education on strategies to counteract lasting harm. There are also flexible and time-tested child-directed approaches such as teaching relaxation and desensitization skills, training concrete skills such as the "rules of touching," or providing therapeutic education using social stories or bibliotherapy [19]. One well-established, evidence-based intervention approach is called Trauma-Focused Cognitive Behavioral Therapy (TF-CBT) [92]. This approach has been adapted to extend to younger children and their families, a process that appears feasible and for which there are published clinical considerations [93]. TF-CBT is stated to be appropriate for children and youth aged 3–18 years. It is notable that TF-CBT may have to be adapted using a neurodevelopmental viewpoint to be appropriate for those living with FASD or PAE, and their families. This is because core techniques used in TF-CBT (such as "cognitive coping" and "trauma narration and processing"), and other aspects of TF-CBT, may not function as expected for individuals with neurodevelopmental differences.

Think About Context

The theoretical models discussed earlier all emphasize the importance of considering the individual with FASD in context, and lived experiences data help in understanding how to "think about context." This brings wide-ranging implications for FASD-informed care, grouped here into three topics.

First, thinking about context as the individual's "ecology," this means the focus should not just be on supporting and treating the individual living with FASD. Instead, *FASD-informed care should also focus on providing treatment and consultation at increasingly broader levels of the child's ecological context,* such as at the levels of the caregiver, family, daycare and school, coaches and mentors, therapists, service systems, community, and culture. Lived experience research, for example, finds real difficulties for those with FASD in the school setting. A caregiver report study acknowledged there were ongoing child behavior and social problems at school, but also pointed out difficulties in the mainstream schooling context such as a lack of attitude shift from school staff after an FASD diagnosis was given [80]. FASD-informed treatment must also try to impact important levels of the child's "ecology." For instance, parenting intervention for caregivers raising children with PAE/FASD likely needs to go beyond coaching the caregiver on new parenting practices to include additional components—such as modules on school advocacy for caregivers, and targeted consultation directly offered to school staff and other providers, as is done in the positive parenting intervention called the Families Moving Forward Program.

Second, thinking about context in a different way, this means that *interventions that are FASD-informed may often focus on strategies to change the context (changing caregiver behavior, household routines, environmental structure),* rather than focusing on remediating specific impairments through training the individual showing effects of PAE. For example, FASD researchers Olson and Montague note that putting into place "accommodations" (or "antecedent-based behavior strategies," as termed in a positive behavior support approach) may be a more efficient and effective way to achieve more positive behaviors for someone living with FASD, compared to the technique of applying consequences to correct misbehavior. Very recent qualitative data from caregivers found that "accommodations" were perceived as generally effective parenting strategies for children diagnosed with an FASD. Study findings revealed that parents of children with FASD who used fewer accommodations reported less success with their behavior management plans. In fact, those parents who reported a specific target behavior was "still a problem" used an average of 1.50 accommodations—compared to those who said a target behavior was "no longer a problem" (who used an average of 3.54 accommodations) (research colleague and predoctoral trainee, University of Rochester, Kautz-Turnbull C, written communication, 2021, 22nd October and 2022, 26th July).

Third, additional insights about context come from an analysis of lived experiences data and, theoretically, from the life course health development framework. FASD researcher Skorka and her colleagues suggest *context should be taken into account in defining successful intervention outcomes for FASD-informed care, and an individual's strengths should also be assessed* [57]. These researchers point out that real-world environments need assessment to see what treatment strategies will meaningfully help an individual with FASD have the most adaptive outcome. For instance, it is not really a successful intervention outcome if a child with disabilities simply has <u>access</u> to soccer (yet constantly sits on the bench watching others play). But it is a potentially successful outcome if the child <u>participates</u> in soccer (and actually has a satisfying and active role in the game). Taking the ideas of these researchers further, context is important in defining what treatment outcomes <u>actually</u> lead to improved QOL in the real world. This is especially important as individuals with FASD grow older. This is because in adolescence and adulthood, QOL becomes harder to achieve as individuals move out into the world—and are expected to be more independent and operate in more environments day-to-day. This means that <u>all</u> the environments in which someone living with FASD needs to function, such as their job or living situation, <u>and</u> the client's strengths, require person-centered assessment to understand what treatment outcomes will really matter to that particular person in their own daily life. Thinking about context means that "person-centered planning" is important.

Sustain Hope

In 1997, some of the earliest and far-seeing thoughts about FASD-informed care were written by pioneering researcher Streissguth, who stated: "Hope and a good grasp of reality are two important characteristics of good [FASD] advocates" [28] (p. 180). In 2009, caregivers of children with FASD and behavior problems reported that one top unmet important family need was to "have help in remaining hopeful about my child's future" [26]. To build and sustain hope with families, providers must reflect on their own comfort level regarding FASD and obtain the support they need to act in a positive, realistic, non-judgmental way. FASD researcher Reid, writing with a group of experienced intervention researchers in the field, has described promoting hope as a key aspect of what they termed "family-directed intervention" in FASD, noting that hope predicts well-being. None of the theoretical models discussed above, that lay the foundation for FASD-informed care, explicitly discuss hope—even though lived experiences data and clinical wisdom in the field have so clearly highlighted this central element. To remedy this important theoretical gap, Reid led the integration of hope theory into a proposed description of FASD-informed care for families. Among other important points, Reid and her colleagues write that hope theory posits "there must be pathways for support in order for families to be hopeful about the future" [38] (p. 4). Indeed, some relationship-based, positive parenting and family support treatments designed for this clinical population have already been deliberately designed or adapted to increase caregiver attitudes related to hope (e.g., [32, 73, 78, 79, 94–97]).

Discussion now moves to the "overarching essential elements" around the edge of Fig. 13.1.

Overcome Stigma

Moving to the outside edge of Fig. 13.1 on the left, an important, overarching essential element of FASD-informed care is to "Overcome Stigma." It might seem jarring to move from the element of "Sustain Hope," to discussing the need to overcome stigma. Yet, as the very insightful FASD researcher Streissguth made clear, those who care and advocate for individuals living with FASD are not only hopeful, but are also realistic [28]. Lived experiences research reveals the stark reality that FASD is stigmatized. This means that FASD-informed treatment is limited, or even blocked, by the pressures of stigma. Early lived experiences research uncovered the heavy burden of stigma experienced by biological parents [98]. More recent data has revealed the many complexities of stigma, with layers ranging from self-stigma to stigma by association. The effects of stigma are wide-ranging, affecting not only the individuals with FASD and biological parents, but also their adoptive and foster parents, siblings—and reverberating further, even to providers [99, 100]. But recent theory and lived experience line up to emphasize the need to strive for health equity and design treatment that is in line with basic human rights [52–56]. That means that to provide intervention to much-deserving individuals with FASD and their families, an overarching essential element of FASD-informed care is to overcome stigma—first recognizing that it exists, and then tackling it—no matter how large the task. To sustain hope, it is necessary to overcome stigma so that advocacy can succeed, and doors can be opened to identification, diagnosis, service eligibility, and intervention.

In this cause, there has been a call for change toward dignity-promoting language regarding FASD [99, 101]. There has also been a call for a shift in perspective in the field of FASD—away from its historical "deficits" focus, and away from its single-minded focus on heading off risk factors and adverse outcomes. Instead, it has been suggested that the field of FASD should move toward: (1) an emphasis on self-advocacy; (2) the application of strengths-based approaches; and (3) a focus on improving measurable indicators of a more positive quality of life and adaptive function. It has also been suggested that this shift in focus can be a catalyst for equitable care that respects the rights of persons with FASD. Further, this shift in thinking may help providers understand why FASD diagnosis is needed—and act as a stimulus for meaningful intervention ideas that make a positive difference in the actual daily lives of those with FASD [15]. In itself, this shift in perspective may, in part, address the pervasive stigma that has impeded progress in the field of FASD [15, 100, 102]. But there is also a clear need for organized, widespread stigma reduction programs specific to FASD [99, 100]. Characteristics of effective FASD stigma reduction programs have been described, with more effective FASD reduction strategies going beyond simple education on PAE and FASD. The best route to decreasing stigma is by contact [103]. This includes meeting people with FASD, hearing them talk, hearing their stories. This helps others to understand the condition better. In a 2017 pre-conference collaborative discussion meeting, many ideas were shared for overcoming stigma. Among these were creating and sharing stories of success and thriving (rather than detriment, weakness or failure), talking about strengths and surviving, and developing continuous opportunities for conversation. Also mentioned was working in partnerships with individuals living with FASD and birth mothers. The idea was that providers and researchers could start to talk <u>with</u> (rather than talk for), and listen with intent to, those who actually live with FASD day-to-day [99, 100, 103].

Build Collaborative Partnerships

Moving down the outside edge of Fig. 13.1, on the right, is another important element of FASD-informed care as it relates to intervention. The field of developmental psychopathology makes clear that effective treatment needs to occur across multiple systems and be flexible and collaborative. Echoing this, the life course health development framework suggests building social scaffolding that includes coordinated and effective systems of care in the interest of health equity. This framework adds that, as much as possible, individuals with FASD should be causal agents in their own lives. Building collaborative partnerships, a continuum of care *and support* between professionals, families (and other support persons), and individuals living with FASD, is a much needed, overarching element of FASD-informed care.

Lived experiences data highlight the many unmet family needs that occur when living with FASD and emphasize that the caregiving process (while rewarding) is highly stressful for all families over the life course [26, 59, 61, 64]. In the field of FASD, lived experiences data (and clinical wisdom) suggest that one important treatment mechanism in FASD-informed care is providing caregiver support. Caregiver support can reduce stress as parents contend with worry about the future and try to come to a realistic understanding of their child's behavior (e.g., [26, 61, 104]). In a recent dissertation that begins to shed light on treatment mechanisms, for example, researcher Kapasi has examined the role that resources and support for families play in caregivers' belief that self-regulation in adolescents with FASD can change for the better. It appears that support is one mechanism sustaining hope and promoting a growth mindset that can help with family functioning and reduce adverse outcomes [44]. Research from the field of developmental disabilities suggests that parents and families with the right kind of support do better later on [105]. Peer and informal parent support and assistance with advocacy, either through parent groups or one-on-one, informal relationships with other parents who have gone through the same situation, is one essential type of support. There are other types of support that are important, including social and emotional support, and therapeutic support.

Researcher Rutman offers more insights about support, building on the work of FASD clinical expert Dubovsky and others. She makes clear that FASD-informed programming recognizes the critical role that healthy family and support people play in the lives of adults with FASD. More fundamentally, she notes that *interdependent living* should be seen as a more accurate and positive reality for all people in society [35].

Research points out that externalizing behaviors and social difficulties/maladjustment are the two most prevalent real-world childhood challenges for families raising those with FASD or PAE, though cognitive difficulties are also mentioned [106]. The positive parenting literature, which guides treatment for families raising children with these difficulties, increasingly emphasizes the importance of close collaboration between therapist and caregivers in supportive, motivating, knowledgeable treatment, in a stance that empowers both family members and providers. This stance was used in early positive parenting and parenting support, education, and advocacy interventions tested with families raising those with FASD (e.g., [32, 73]). It is also a key aspect of what has recently been termed "family-directed intervention" by a group of experienced FASD intervention researchers [38].

Be Led by the Community to Create Culture-Centered Practices

The final element, at the top edge of Fig. 13.1, is vital. Several theoretical models discussed earlier, clinical wisdom, and lived experience data, all indicate that it is important to add creating culture-centered practices as an overarching element of FASD-informed care. The family's own subculture and community—and, beyond that, the larger cultural context in which the individual with FASD and family live— must be taken as fully as possible into account to ensure treatment is appropriate and effective. FASD is a global public health issue, so treatments must be created for a wide range of cultures. This means it is vital to understand the importance of cultural beliefs, values, conventions, and childrearing customs, as part of designing and carrying out interventions for the many different individuals living with FASD and their families all over the world (e.g., [38, 107–110]).

But this element of FASD-informed care is best stated as to "Be Led by the Community to Creating Culture-Centered Practices." The community also includes self-advocates. The idea is to ask community members what is getting in the way of quality of life (and what practices can really help make a difference)—and to ask those who may be offered treatment whether it is actually needed. Even the word "intervention" is not appropriate to some cultures, such as in Aboriginal Australia where it has acquired a negative meaning and raises issues of historical trauma. If treatment is needed, input from the community can lead decisions on what treatment goals and outcomes should be, what treatment should look like, and what are possible mechanisms for how treatment may work. This fits with the fundamental importance of valuing self-determination and basic human rights for those living with FASD.

Cultural and community context change what resources are needed, and what language and interpersonal approaches are used. But taking community and culture into account does not just mean offering community-specific resources. It does not simply mean using interpreters to translate the intervention that is provided or offering treatment in the primary language of the participants. It does not mean simply being culturally sensitive to interpersonal style. These are all important, but are not sufficient to creating culture-centered practices. Taking culture into account requires the participation of cultural navigators and community leaders in designing and implementing treatment that reflects the texture of the community and culture. Taking culture into account requires gathering lived experience data from groups (cultural, subcultural, community, self-advocates) to inform how treatments are created, and working alongside and being led by "stakeholders" (those who have a stake in the treatment) when designing interventions.

Current Peer-Reviewed Intervention Research with Samples of Those Living with PAE/FASD

As discussed so far in this chapter, the field has progressed over 50 years, and essential elements of FASD-informed care have been defined as they relate to treatment. Calls to action to advance services for FASD have been heard. Since the early 2000s, peer-reviewed intervention research with samples specifically identified with PAE or FASD has gradually grown. This body of research is presented here. Treatments discussed in this chapter focus on parent-child or family wellness and support, and/or on building skills for individuals living with FASD. Presented in Tables 13.1, 13.2, 13.3, 13.4, 13.5, 13.6, 13.7, 13.8, 13.9, 13.10, 13.11, 13.12, 13.13, and 13.14, studies are arranged from infancy through adulthood. In this section, existing research will be briefly discussed, and ideas for next research steps discussed. *At this point in time, the authors strongly believe that intervention research in the field of FASD could be strategically expanded, enhanced, and accelerated.*

Table 13.1 PUBLISHED relationship-based and multicomponent early interventions (birth to 5 years)

Intervention name	Description	Participants studied in key references	Key outcomes
Breaking the Cycle (BTC) [154, 155]	A comprehensive and relationship-focused program that includes early childhood intervention, addiction counseling, various parenting programs and other health and social supports[a,b].	Pregnant and early parenting mothers who are using alcohol or other substances, and their children, ages birth-3 years	Pre- to posttreatment improvements in child developmental outcomes, maternal mental health and relationship capacity, as well as decreased maternal substance use [154]. No group differences in child developmental outcomes [155].
Circle of Security (COS) [94]	An attachment-focused intervention designed to increase caregiver observation skills, sensitivity and responsiveness, and self-reflection. Involving a series of activities and repeated videotaped interactions with child-caregiver dyads, a therapist serves as a secure base and safe haven for the caregiver to explore new and unfamiliar feelings and behaviors[a,b].	Children with prenatal alcohol exposure (PAE) or fetal alcohol spectrum disorders (FASD), ages 2–5 years, and their caregivers	Pre- to posttreatment reductions in child behavioral challenges and increased capacity of children to communicate their needs to their caregiver. Improved ability of caregivers to attend to their child's cues and reduced caregiver stress.
Home-U-Go Safely (HUGS) program [156]	A home-based nursing intervention that monitors infant health and growth, provides parents with developmental information and emotional support, and teaches the use of a Snugli to promote close contact time between parent and child[a].	Children with prenatal drug and alcohol exposure, ages 1 week–18 months, and their caregivers	Improvements in child internalizing and externalizing behaviors (based on parent report) relative to comparison group. A trend toward reduced parent stress.

(continued)

Table 13.1 (continued)

Intervention name	Description	Participants studied in key references	Key outcomes
Neurosequential Model of Therapeutics (NMT) [74]	A relationship and developmentally based intervention focused on improving the attachment relationship, symptoms of post-traumatic stress, and building caregiver self-reflection and mindfulness skills. Children and caregivers received child parent psychotherapy (CPP) and caregivers also received mindful parenting education (MPE)[c].	Maltreated children with FASD, ages 10–53 months, and their caregivers	Pre- to posttreatment improvements in child developmental functioning and regulatory capacity. Reductions in caregiver stress.
Strategies for Enhancing Early Developmental Success (SEEDS) [157]	A multicomponent intervention designed to promote school readiness by engaging caregivers to build their child's self-regulatory capacities through the development of collaborative parent–child, teacher–child, and parent–teacher relationships as a foundation for school readiness[a,d].	Children with PAE and early trauma, ages 3–5 years, and their caregivers	Pre- to posttreatment improvements in classroom behavior and caregiver interactions and care in two of three cases. Mixed results in one case.

Note: There is one additional published FASD early intervention referenced in the California Evidence-Based Clearinghouse (cebc4cw.org): the Safe Babies Court Team (SBCT) Project [153]. This is a community engagement and systems-change initiative focused on reducing trauma and improving how courts, child welfare, and child-serving organizations work together to support infants and toddlers in, or at risk of entering, the child welfare system, including but not limited to children with PAE. This intervention does not fit into the category of interventions covered in this table, but has been deemed by CEBC an effective practice useful for very young children with FASD or PAE

[a] Home

[b] Community

[c] Clinic

[d] Classroom

Table 13.2 IN DEVELOPMENT relationship-based and multicomponent early interventions (birth to 5 years)

Intervention name	Description	Participants studied in key references	Key outcomes
Families Moving Forward (FMF) Bridges Jirikowic et al. (in development)	Derived from the standard FMF Program (see Table 13.4), FMF Bridges is an intervention for infants/toddlers with PAE or FASD, birth to 3 years of age. FMF Bridges targets the developmental and relational needs of infants/toddlers with PAE and their caregivers. It is intended to enhance existing EI practices while retaining multiple core features of the standard FMF Program[a,b].	Children with PAE, ages birth to 3, and their primary caregiver	To be determined, study in design phase.
Relationship-Based Early Intervention (RB-EI) Kalberg et al. (under review)	A relationship-based, developmental enhancement to promote emotional security and social competence for children with PAE (ages birth to 3). Using the Heart Start Model, caregiver/child dyads work toward secure and positive interactions by being in a calm and alert regulatory state, by understanding the importance of close proximity and by sharing a specific focus[a].	Children with PAE, ages 9–36 months, and their mothers	Pre- to posttreatment improvements in caregiver involvement and responsivity, and also in children's living environments for both groups. Increases in positive interactions between child and caregiver, reflecting an increased quality of relationship. The greatest benefits were seen for the highest risk children.

[a] Home
[b] Early intervention centers

Table 13.3 FUTURE DIRECTIONS relationship-based and multicomponent early interventions (birth to 5 years)

Intervention name	Description	Participants studied in key references	Key outcomes
Attachment Biobehavioral Catch-up (ABC) [159, 160]	An attachment-focused intervention designed to help children develop regulatory capacities by helping caregivers learn: (1) to provide an environment that promotes regulatory development; (2) to re-interpret a child's alienating behaviors; and (3) to override their own issues that interfere with providing nurturing care[a].	Children in foster care, ages 1–39 months, and their caregivers	Children in the ABC group (and the comparison group who had never been in foster care) showed lower initial levels of cortisol (i.e., enhanced ability to regulate physiology) relative to those in the control intervention [160]. Children of parents in ABC group showed less avoidance after distressful episodes compared to in the comparison group [159].
Attachment Vitamins (AV) [161]	A trauma-informed, psychoeducational group intervention designed to address and repair the impact of chronic stress and trauma on the family unit. AV focuses on increasing: (1) trauma-informed parenting knowledge of emotional development and child individual differences; (2) emotional attunement; (3) mindfulness related to positive parent–child interactions; (4) executive functioning; and (5) reflective functioning[a].	Caregivers of children who are coping with toxic stress and trauma, ages birth to 5 years	Pre- to posttreatment increases in parenting sense of competence, emotional regulation, and warmth toward the child. An observed decrease in parenting stress was not significant.

Table 13.3 (continued)

Intervention name	Description	Participants studied in key references	Key outcomes
Child-Parent Psychotherapy (CPP) [162, 163]	CPP is designed to support and strengthen the caregiver–child relationship as a way to restore and protect the child's mental health. Essential components of CPP focus on safety, affect regulation, reciprocity in relationships, the traumatic event and continuity of daily living. CPP also focuses on contextual factors such as culture, socioeconomic and immigration related stressors[a–c].	Children, ages birth to 5 years, who have experienced a trauma, and their caregivers	Children in CPP group showed significantly more improvements than those in comparison group. Reductions in child post-traumatic stress disorder (PTSD) symptoms and behavior problems. Reductions in mother's avoidant symptoms, general distress, and PTSD symptoms. At 6 month follow-up: reduction in problem behaviors compared to control group.
Early Start Denver Model (ESDM) [74, 162]	ESDM is a comprehensive early behavioral intervention. ESDM promotes developmental and social communication skills in young children with ASD. ESDM integrates applied behavior analysis with relationship-based and developmental approaches and is delivered by therapists and parents[a].	Children with Autism Spectrum Disorder (ASD), ages 18–30 months	Children who received ESDM showed significantly more improvements in IQ, adaptive behavior (communication, motor and daily living skills), and diagnostic status than those in the comparison group.
Nurse-Family Partnership [164]	A community health program aimed at reducing maternal and child mortality and promoting healthier pregnancies and child health outcomes in first-time low-income mothers and their children. Home visiting nurses promoted improvements in prenatal health behaviors and sensitive and responsive caregiving, helped build supportive relationships with family and friends, and linked mothers with needed services in the community[a].	Pregnant and early parenting women with at least two risk factors (i.e., unmarried, less than 12 years of education, unemployed), and their first-born child	A substantial program of research has shown overall improvements in birth outcomes, child abuse and neglect, injuries, and compromised parental life course (i.e., fewer subsequent pregnancies, greater workforce participation, reduced dependence on public assistance).

(continued)

Table 13.3 (continued)

Intervention name	Description	Participants studied in key references	Key outcomes
Promoting First Relationships (PFR) [165]	Strength-based and attachment-based intervention that uses reflective consultation strategies and video feedback to focus on the deeper emotional feelings and needs underlying difficulties in the parent-child relationship[a].	Maltreated children in foster care, ages 10–24 months, and their caregivers	Observational ratings of caregiver sensitivity and attitudes improved more among dyads in the PFR condition relative to the comparison group.

Note: Treatment Foster Care Oregon is also available for preschoolers (previously termed Multidimensional Treatment Foster Care for Preschoolers [158]) (see Tables 13.13 and 13.14, which describes the adolescent version of this treatment)

[a] Home

[b] Community

[c] Clinic

Table 13.4 PUBLISHED parenting interventions

Intervention name	Description	Participants studied in key references	Key outcomes
(a) Positive parenting interventions			
Families Moving Forward (FMF) Program [73]	A caregiver-focused intervention that combines skill-building in positive behavior support with motivational interviewing and cognitive-behavioral treatment approaches to change key caregiving attitudes and behaviors. Can be customized. Caregivers are provided support, education on FASD and advocacy, coaching on skills and attitudes, and connection to community linkages. Targeted school and provider consultation are also offered[a–c].	Children with FASD, ages 4–12 years, and their caregivers	Relative to the comparison group, caregivers receiving the intervention reported improvements in sense of parenting self-efficacy and family needs met, self-care and FASD/advocacy knowledge, and, immediately posttreatment, reported their children showed less problematic disruptive behavior.

Table 13.4 (continued)

Intervention name	Description	Participants studied in key references	Key outcomes
Families on Track Integrated Preventative Intervention [78, 110]	A multicomponent intervention designed to improve family functioning and reduce challenges later in life. Incorporates the FMF Program, a positive parenting intervention, with the Promoting Alternative Thinking Strategies (PATHS) curriculum, a weekly child-skills group that aims to prevent behavior problems by promoting social competence[a].	Children with FASD, ages 4–8 years, and their caregivers	Relative to the comparison group, the intervention was associated with improvements in caregiver knowledge, attitudes, targeted parenting practices, support, and self-care. Improved child regulation and self-esteem were also shown.
Parents Under Pressure (PuP) Program—adapted version [166]	A multi-component intervention designed to improve children's self-regulatory skills by focusing on improving the parent–child relationship and incorporating mindfulness techniques for both parents and children. Using an individualized approach, caregivers are provided psychoeducation about FASD and school consultation, in addition to strategies for enhancing child self-regulatory skills[a].	Children with FASD, ages 9–12, and their caregivers	For participants who completed the program, recruitment and intervention procedures were found to be feasible/acceptable and improvements in child's level of psychosocial distress, and quality of parent–child relationship were reported.
(b) Parent management training			
Parent-Child Interaction Therapy (PCIT) [73]	A behavioral parent training program designed to enhance parent–child relationships, increase appropriate child social skills, reduce inappropriate child behaviors, and institute a positive discipline program. Parents and children receive live, coached practice of behavioral parenting skills. This was a group adaptation of PCIT[a,b].	Children with FASD, ages 3–7 years, and their caregivers	Study compared two interventions: (1) Group adaptation of PCIT; (2) Parent-only Parent Support and Management Program (PSM) based on other effective behavioral programs. The PSM group offered psychoeducation and discussion/problem-solving about FASD and behavioral principles. Approximately half of each group completed treatment, not known if final data include non-completers. Improvements over time in child behavior problems and caregiving stress were seen for both PCIT and PSM groups, with no group differences.

(continued)

Table 13.4 (continued)

Intervention name	Description	Participants studied in key references	Key outcomes
(c) Parenting support, education, advocacy programs			
Coaching Families (CF) [32]	A program designed to educate families about FASD, provide access to community supports and teach advocacy skills to families and caregivers of children with FASD. The CF mentor and caregiver work together to establish high priority needs and goals for the program[a,d].	Caregivers of a child with FASD, ages 1–23 years	Pre- to posttreatment reductions in all areas of family needs, with the exception of mental health issues. An increase in goal achievement was also shown.
Key Worker and Parent Support Program [33]	Family-centered program that provides support, education and intervention services links caregivers to community services and support groups. It also provides consultation to other professionals to ensure a coordinated and effective approach to FASD management[a,b,d].	Families of children and youth with FASD, ages birth to 19 years	Pre- to posttreatment improvements in welfare outcomes among families as reported by caregivers. Positive caregiver perceptions of program were also shown.
Parent-Child Assistance Program (PCAP) [167]	A 3-year home visitation intervention designed to promote substance use recovery, reduce associated challenges and improve child outcomes. Program goals were that individualized and paraprofessional advocates linked mothers to community services such as health care, parenting classes, and therapeutic childcare[a].	Pregnant or postpartum women, reporting alcohol or drug use during pregnancy	Pre- to posttreatment improvements included alcohol/drug treatment completion, abstinence from alcohol/drugs; subsequent pregnancies with PAE. Increased maternal employment and linkages with services. More permanent child custody placements.
Parent Training Program [168]	The parent-focused component of the MILE (math interactive learning experience) intervention [169, 170] was delivered via a workshop or web-based format to compare effectiveness[a,b,e].	Caregivers of children with FASD, ages 3–10 years	Both workshop and web-based groups showed improvement in their knowledge of behavioral regulation principles, FAS and advocacy. Improvements in child behavior for workshop group only.

[a] Home
[b] Clinic
[c] Telehealth
[d] Community
[e] Web-based

Table 13.5 IN DEVELOPMENT parenting interventions and parenting support, education, and advocacy programs

Intervention name	Description	Participants studied in key references	Key outcomes
FMF Connect Mobile Health Intervention [97, 171]	Derived from the clinician-delivered standard FMF Program, the goal of this mHealth app is to provide information and tools directly to caregivers of children with PAE or FASD to help manage their children's condition. Unique features include a family forum for peer support, an in-app dashboard and video library[a].	Caregivers of children with PAE or FASD, ages 3–12 years	Beta-testing showed the FMF Connect intervention appears acceptable and feasible for caregivers of children with FASD, with results guiding additional app refinement prior to feasibility trial and large-scale randomized control trial testing.
Strongest Families FASD [172, 173]	A caregiver-focused, internet-based intervention that is designed to reduce challenging behavior of children with FASD, as well as parental distress. One new parenting skill is introduced each week via the online application and is supplemented by a weekly telephone coaching session to reinforce the skill, answer questions and provide support[b,c].	Caregivers of children with FASD, ages 4–12 years	Not yet available.
Triple P Positive Parenting Program (adapted for a remote community in Western Australia) [107]	Small group positive parenting intervention aimed at improving caregiver confidence and capacity to manage complex child behaviors. Learning strategies include discussion, visual teaching aids, modeling and role play, delivered by specially trained parent coaches. Using community-based participation research methods, this program was adapted to be culturally sensitive, as well as trauma-informed[d,e].	Caregivers of school-age children with complex needs (i.e., complex language environment, very remote community, historical and current trauma, social disadvantage)	Not yet available.

(continued)

Table 13.5 (continued)

Intervention name	Description	Participants studied in key references	Key outcomes
Tuning Into Kids (TIK) [174–176]	A parent-focused group intervention designed to improve emotion regulation skills and reduce behavior problems of children with FASD. Using an emotion coaching approach, parents learn and practice effective ways of responding to their children's emotions and behaviors[e,f].	Caregivers of children with FASD, ages 4–12 years	Not yet available.

[a] Mobile Health app (for smartphone, tablet, or computer)
[b] Internet
[c] Phone coaching
[d] Home
[e] Community
[f] Clinic

Table 13.6 FUTURE DIRECTIONS parenting interventions and parenting support, education, and advocacy programs

Intervention name	Description	Participants studied in key references	Key outcomes
Family Check-Up Model [177, 178]	Prevention program designed for families at high psychosocial risk. Combines motivational interviewing techniques and promotes parent use of positive behavior support in visits at strategic developmental timepoints. Provides links to parenting support services. Delivered by specially trained parent consultants in a variety of settings[a,b].	Mother-child dyads; children ages 2–4 years, at high risk and involved in the Women, Infants, and Children (WIC) Nutrition Program	Reductions in child behavior problems, and increases in caregiver involvement and direct observations of positive behavior support practices relative to comparison group.

Table 13.6 (continued)

Intervention name	Description	Participants studied in key references	Key outcomes
Research Units in Behavioral Intervention (RUBI) [179]	A parent-mediated intervention designed to decrease challenging behaviors in children with ASD. RUBI is delivered individually by trained therapists. Focused on identifying the function of a behavior, preventing disruptive behaviors from happening, promoting positive behaviors, and responding to challenging behaviors[a,c].	Parents of children with ASD and disruptive behaviors, ages 3–7 years	Reductions in parent-reported disruptive and noncompliant behavior were superior for the RUBI group compared with parent education group. Overall improvement rating by blinded clinician was greater for RUBI group.
Stepping Stones Triple P [180] Note: The Triple P Program has recently been adapted for use with children with FASD in a proposed protocol using the Stepping Stones curriculum, though findings are not yet published [107, 181, 182]	A positive parenting program, developed specifically for families of children with disabilities, aims to reduce problem behavior. Parents learn descriptive praise and planned-ignoring strategies, and how to encourage child communication. Uses a group format for teaching parenting strategies and individual sessions for observation, practice and feedback[a,c].	Parents of children with ASD, ages 2–9 years	Reduction in parent-reported child behavior problems and dysfunctional parenting styles (i.e., less reactive, less verbose) relative to the comparison group.

[a] Home
[b] Community
[c] Clinic

Readers should note that although an effort was made to survey the literature as widely as possible, tables in this chapter could not be fully comprehensive. These tables are meant <u>only</u> to inform readers of the range of intervention literature available and are not presented as, or meant to be, a systematic review. In particular, Table 13.1 could include only a sampling of early interventions, given that many treatment studies have been done with "polysubstance-exposed" or "at-risk" young children. In many studies, prenatal alcohol exposure (PAE) is often not clearly specified (or not documented, even though it is likely present). Non-peer-reviewed

Table 13.7 PUBLISHED child-focused skill-building interventions: self-regulation, social skills and communication, and behavioral outcomes (2–12 years)

Intervention name	Description	Participants studied in key references	Key outcomes
(a) Self-regulation			
Alert Program for Self-Regulation [183, 184]	An individualized intervention designed to improve self-regulation and executive function using sensory integration and cognitive strategies. Children engage in activities that focus on emotion sensitization and recognition, behavioral regulation, and social problem-solving[a].	Children with FASD, ages 8–12 years	Improvements in parent-rated child behavior and emotional regulation relative to comparison group [183]. Positive changes observed in brain regions critical for self-regulation among children in the Alert group relative to those in comparison group.
Cognitive Control Therapy (CCT) [122]	A progressive skill-building intervention that is designed to enhance a child's ability to understand their own learning style and learning challenges. Using a metacognitive approach, CCT teaches children self-regulation and self-observation strategies[b].	Children with FASD, ages 8–9 years	Improvements in teacher-rated behaviors of children (i.e., classroom behavior, academic achievement, writing and communication skills). Qualitative improvements in children's self-efficacy, motivation, cooperation, self-confidence, and emotionality.
GoFAR [75, 76]	A computerized intervention designed to improve adaptive functioning and disruptive behavior. GoFAR uses a metacognitive approach (FAR: Focus/Plan, Act, Reflect) to address hurried and impulsive problem-solving. Involves parent training on child behavioral regulation, and behavior analog therapy where parent and child implement the learning strategy[a].	Children with FASD, ages 5–10, and their caregivers	Children in the GoFAR intervention showed greater improvements in disruptive behaviors relative to comparison groups [75]. Children, whose computerized instruction was delivered consistent with parent training, showed greater self-regulation improvements than those receiving incongruent instruction [76].

Table 13.7 (continued)

Intervention name	Description	Participants studied in key references	Key outcomes
Parents and Children Together (PACT), aka Neurocognitive Habilitation Therapy [73, 185]	A group-based intervention that integrates components of the Alert Program to improve executive function skills including memory, cause and effect reasoning, sequencing, planning, and problem-solving[a].	Foster/ adopted children with PAE, ages 6–12 years, and their caregivers	Children in the PACT group demonstrated significant improvement in executive functioning skills relative to comparison group [73]. Improved parent-reported executive functioning and emotional problem-solving skills seen relative to comparison group [185].
Self-Management Intervention [186]	An individualized intervention designed to improve behavior. Informed by a functional behavior assessment, child was explicitly taught self-monitoring strategies and received contingent reinforcement[c].	Child with FASD, 11 years	Pre- to posttreatment improvements in behavior and independence with task completion.

Note: See also Table 13.4a–c. Many parenting interventions focus, in part, on improving child behavioral outcomes. Some positive parenting interventions, such as Families on Track and Parents Under Pressure, also focus on improving child self-regulation or decreasing psychosocial distress

(b) Social skills and communication

Intervention name	Description	Participants studied in key references	Key outcomes
Children's Friendship Training (CFT) [187, 188]	A multicomponent intervention that focuses on developing friendship skills through didactic instruction, modeling, rehearsal and parent coaching. Includes parent-assisted activities to promote generalization of skills outside of intervention sessions[a].	Children 6–12 years with FASD, and their caregivers	Children in the CFT group showed improved knowledge of appropriate social behaviors, improved self-concept and improvements in parent-reported social skills relative to the comparison group.
Kid's Club [189]	A multicomponent, group-based intervention designed to improve social skills by accommodating the sensory needs of children with FASD and providing structure and consistency[d].	Children with FASD, ages 7–12 years, and their caregivers	Pre- to posttreatment improvements in parent-reported, child social skills.

(continued)

Table 13.7 (continued)

Intervention name	Description	Participants studied in key references	Key outcomes
Social Communication Intervention [190]	An intervention designed to address social communication difficulties. Involved group role play of social scripts, a checklist with guidance for resolving social situations, and clinician modeling of socially appropriate responses[a].	Child with FASD, age 9	Increased use of language and generation of socially appropriate strategies for more effective management of social situations.
Theater-based Intervention [191]	A theater-based arts intervention designed to facilitate social communication and engagement in a group setting. Activities focused on collaboration, self-awareness/awareness of others and the environment, relaxation, listening, and curiosity and imagination[b].	Children with FASD, ages 9–14 years	Pre- to posttreatment improvements in child self-esteem, social skills, and emotional awareness as perceived by various stakeholders.
(c) Behavioral outcomes			
Good Behavior Game [192]	A group-based intervention designed to improve challenging behaviors. Involved therapist-delivered praise, corrective feedback, and positive reinforcement[b].	Child with FAS, age 4	Pre- to posttreatment reductions in disruptive behaviors.
Verbal Behavior Intervention [193]	An ABA intervention designed to improve adaptive skills and functional communication with 1:1 instruction. Intervention was informed by an assessment of child strengths and challenges[a].	Child with FASD, age 3 years, 10 months	Pre- to posttreatment improvements across all domains of functional communication, increase in verbal intellectual skills, improved adaptive functioning and emotional/behavioral functioning (per caregiver report).

Note: There are no known interventions IN DEVELOPMENT or with research underway for child-focused skill-building focused on child self-regulation, social skills and social communication, or behavior that are not already discussed in other tables

[a] Clinic

[b] Classroom/school

[c] Home

[d] Community

Table 13.8 FUTURE DIRECTIONS child-focused skill-building interventions—self-regulation, social skills and communication, and behavioral outcomes (2–12 years)

Intervention name	Description	Participants studied in key references	Key outcomes
Incredible Years Dinosaur School [194]	A classroom or group-based program designed to promote children's social competence, emotional self-regulation, and school behavior. Trained teachers promoted social skills and conflict management strategies through the use of puppets, homework activities, picture cue cards and games[a]. Note: The evidence-based IY Dinosaur School curriculum is available for children aged 4–8 years [195].	Students, in kindergarten and first grade, participating in a Head Start program	Students receiving the Dinosaur School curriculum showed more social competence and emotional self-regulation, as well as fewer conduct problems, than those in the comparison group.
Mindful Yoga Programs [196, 197]	Two yoga interventions designed to promote children's behavioral and attention regulation. Included physical postures, breathing techniques, meditation, and relaxation. Delivered by a certified yoga instructor or classroom teacher. Music, books, props and/or videos incorporated into yoga sessions[a].	Preschool students, ages 3–5 years, participating in a Head Start program	Increases in children's behavioral and attention regulation relative to comparison group [197]. Gains on a behavioral task of self-regulation and declines in teacher-rated submissive venting and total behavior problems relative to comparison group [196].
Promoting Alternative Thinking Strategies (PATHS) Program [198]	A universal classroom intervention designed to improve children's social competence and reduce problem behavior[a]. Note: The evidence-based PATHS curriculum is available through Grade 5 (for children through age 10–11 years) [199]. Note: PATHS has been used as part of the preventative, multicomponent Families on Track Program; see Table 13.4a.	Students in a Head Start program, ages 3–4 years	Children in the PATHS group had higher emotion knowledge skills and were rated as more socially competent and less socially withdrawn than the comparison group.
Tools of the Mind (Tools) [200]	A preschool curriculum designed to promote self-regulation skills, within the context of early literacy and math skills, and with a focus on play. The tools curriculum guides teachers' daily practices to help children develop and use tools to facilitate learning[a].	Preschool students, ages 3–4, from a low-income urban school district	The Tools curriculum was found to improve classroom quality and children's executive function skills relative to the comparison group.

(continued)

Table 13.8 (continued)

Intervention name	Description	Participants studied in key references	Key outcomes
Mindfulness techniques [201] Note: This is presented as an example of a category of techniques to explore, with a reminder that a larger treatment plan is important. See interpretation of findings in righthand column.	A mindfulness exercise requiring children to perform small physical movements (e.g., "close your eyes," "put your hands on your belly"). This was a 5 min, 40 sec task designed for children played on an Apple iPad that could be considered as a child version of a "body scan," as it required children to focus their breath and attention on different parts of their body[b]. This was a feasibility study, and more research is needed.	Children with FASD, ages 6–10	Children with FASD were effectively able to follow mindfulness task instructions. Baseline respiratory sinus arrhythmia (RSA: physiological measure related to behavioral regulation) increased after the mindfulness task. Findings are interpreted to suggest: (1) when planning treatment, assessments of the caregiving environment should be included to guide interventions; and (2) if children are living in stressful environments, it is important that any mindfulness-based strategies be provided in conjunction with approaches targeting the broader family environment.

Note: Results of a recent series of meta-analyses aimed to assess all available evidence regarding the efficacy of different behavioral interventions promoting children's executive function skills (working memory, inhibitory control, and cognitive flexibility) in one study to allow for comparison. Long-term effects were assessed via a meta-analysis examining follow-up data. Highlights for non-typically developing children were: (1) EF skills can be trained; (2) effects may not be sustained though more research is needed; (3) interventions offering new strategies of self-regulation, such as mindfulness, biofeedback-enhanced relaxation, and specific strategy interventions were found effective with a generally large average effect; and (4) explicit practice was only effective with a much smaller effect size. Authors concluded different interventions were useful for typically and non-typically developing children [138]

Based on these findings, to enhance executive function outcomes, possible treatment recommendations are: (1) EEG or EMG biofeedback-induced relaxation training; (2) the "Unstuck and On Target" or Alert Program curriculum or other specific strategy learning interventions; and (3) mindfulness meditation in everyday routines. Working these into a child's enjoyable and meaningful daily routine, and a cost/benefit analysis for families, are important additional ideas

[a] Classroom/school

[b] Clinic

program evaluation studies are not included, even though many have been done in the field of FASD. Intervention studies that are in-process or in the design phase <u>are</u> included, though some may not be known. Psychopharmacological and nutritional supplementation treatment studies are not included, though brief mention is made of these important intervention research directions in the Discussion. School-based studies are generally not included. Most published studies have been subjected to

Table 13.9 PUBLISHED child-and adolescent-focused skill-building interventions: toward varied other outcomes (3–16 years)

Intervention name	Description	Participants studied in key references	Key outcomes
(a) Attention and memory skills (see also note on Table 13.8)			
Dino Island/ Caribbean Quest [202] (in beta version, called Cognitive Carnival) [203, 204]	A computerized intervention program designed to strengthen attention and working memory skills using a series of game-like tasks. While being individually coached, in the final game five increasingly demanding cognitive tasks are presented as a motivating "serious" (designed for training and skill development) computer game. The final intervention includes metacognitive strategies provided by trained assistants to help generalization[a].	Children with FASD, ages 8–16 years (Cognitive Carnival: beta version); Children with FASD or autism, ages 6–13 years (Caribbean Quest: final version)	Using the beta version (Cognitive Carnival), children acquired 26 different metacognitive strategies which helped to improve performance during gameplay from pre- to posttreatment. Spontaneous strategy use increased over the course of the intervention [203, 204]. The final version (Caribbean Quest) was delivered within a school setting by educational assistants (EAs). This game-based process specific intervention was feasible, with improved working memory and attention performance, and improved reading fluency suggesting generalization to classroom performance. Preliminary results support use as part of an overall treatment plan [202].
Computerized Progressive Attention Training (CPAT) [205]	A computerized training program involving four sets of tasks that activate sustained attention, selective attention, orienting of attention, and executive attention. Task demands are advanced hierarchically based on a child's improvements in speed and accuracy[a].	Children with FASD, ages 6–15 years	Pre- to posttreatment improvements in sustained and selective attention, spatial working memory, math, and reading fluency.

(continued)

Table 13.9 (continued)

Intervention name	Description	Participants studied in key references	Key outcomes
Transcranial Direct-Current Stimulation (tDCS) and Cognitive Training (CT) [50]	An intervention combining CT (i.e., repeated practice of working memory, attention control and processing speed tasks) with tDCS, a non-invasive method of delivering low intensity electrical current to the brain[b].	Children with FASD, ages 9–16 years	Intervention was feasible and well tolerated in the tDCS group. Nominal improvement in attention compared to control group. Correlation between improvement in attention scores and decrease in parent-reported attention deficits in the tDCS group.
(b) Academic achievement			
Copy, Cover, and Compare Procedure in Spelling [206]	A self-managed proofreading drill and practice program involving a visual prompt and written cues (i.e., copy, cover, and compare) to improve the accuracy of written work (i.e., detect errors, correct spelling)[a].	Child with FASD, 7 years	Pre- to posttreatment increase in frequency of correct words spelled and reduction over time in frequency of spelling errors.
Literacy and Language Training (LLT) [207, 208]	Cognitive intervention focused on the development of phonological awareness and acquisition of early literacy skills. Used multi-sensory stimulation strategies[a].	Children with FASD, ages 9–10 years	Relative to comparison groups, the LLC group showed improvements in specific tests of language and literacy, but no significant gains in general scholastic assessments.
Math Interactive Learning Experience (MILE) [115, 169, 170]	A multi-component intervention, using a metacognitive approach (i.e., focus & plan, act, and reflect) to improve math ability and behavior. Children received individualized 1:1 math tutoring, while caregivers were trained on how to support math learning and behavior regulation at home[a–c].	Children with PAE or FASD, ages 3–10 years, and their caregivers	Greater gains in math performance for the MILE groups. Treatment gains were shown at 6-month follow-up.
Rehearsal training [209]	Rehearsal training designed to improve working memory for numbers[b].	Children with FASD, ages 4–11 years	Intervention group showed improvement in recalling numbers and increased use of rehearsal strategies relative to comparison group.

Table 13.9 (continued)

Intervention name	Description	Participants studied in key references	Key outcomes
(c) Adaptive function skills			
Fire and Street Safety Skills Training [210, 211]	A virtual reality game training designed to teach home fire or street safety skills in small incremental steps, while restricting incorrect or dangerous movements[a,b,d].	Children with FASD, ages 4–10 years	Pre- to posttreatment increase in knowledge of fire safety skills and generalization to real-world simulation 1 week later.
(d) Sensory-motor skills and physical activity			
FAST club: A physical activity (PA) intervention [212, 213]	An individualized, strength-based physical activity program developed to improve executive function. Intervention administered in a group setting (school gym)[a].	Children with FASD, ages 6–14 years	The PA intervention did not influence the stress response (i.e., no change in cortisol levels) in children with FASD [212]. Improvements in executive function skills post-intervention relative to comparison group were maintained at 3 month follow-up [213].
Sensorimotor Training to Affect Balance, Engagement, and Learning (STABEL) [214, 215]	A virtual reality intervention designed to improve sensory control of balance and motor performance. Tasks involved goal-directed movement demands, active problem-solving and adaptation to changes in the sensory environment in the context of the computer game[b,d].	Children with FASD, ages 8–15 years	Children who received the intervention showed greater improvements in balance (including overall ability and reaction to sensory conditions during standing and motor performance) relative to the comparison group.

Note: There are no known interventions IN DEVELOPMENT or with research underway for child and adolescent-focused skill-building that are not presented in other tables. See Chap. 16 on Education and Developmental Disabilities Systems for information on academic strategies and interventions

[a] Classroom/school

[b] Clinic

[c] Community

[d] Home

Table 13.10 FUTURE DIRECTIONS child and adolescent-focused skill-building interventions—toward varied other outcomes (3–16 years)—sleep, physical activity, and adaptive function outcomes

Intervention name	Description	Participants studied in key references	Key outcomes
Cognitive Orientation to Occupational Performance (CO-OP) [218]	A task-specific, cognitive-based, problem-solving intervention that guides individuals to independently discover and develop cognitive strategies to perform targeted tasks of everyday living such as dressing, grooming, writing, bicycling[a,b].	Children, 8–12 years, with developmental coordination disorder (DCD), and children with DCD and co-occurring attention deficit hyperactivity disorder (ADHD)	Improvements in self-perceived functional motor performance and movement quality were seen in both groups. Functional motor improvements were maintained at 3 months follow-up. Children with DCD only showed skill transfer to other motor skills.
Sleep Health in Preschoolers (SHIP) [219]	A family-centered and personalized intervention to address behavioral sleep problems (bedtime resistance, frequent night wakings, insufficient sleep duration) in young children. Provides parents with the knowledge, motivation and skills for setting and achieving goals, adapting to setbacks, problem-solving and improving their child's sleep[a].	Parents of preschool-age children with behavioral sleep problems	Not yet available.
Sleep Intervention for Kids and Parents (SKIP) [220]	A web-based, shared management intervention that emphasizes goal setting, action planning, and self-monitoring to improve sleep. Engages both children and parents to work together to select and later appraise sleep improvement activities. Includes education on the importance of bedtime routine, an optimal sleep environment, and sleep hygiene. Also incorporated elements of cognitive therapy for insomnia: relaxation techniques and stimulus control[c].	Children, ages 6–11 years, with asthma and behavioral sleep disturbances and their parents	Pre- to posttreatment improvements in child and parent sleep outcomes including wake after sleep onset, sleep efficiency, and bedtime range. SKIP was feasible and acceptable.

Table 13.10   (continued)

Intervention name	Description	Participants studied in key references	Key outcomes
Sports Therapy for Attention, Cognitions and Sociality [221]	A sports-activity intervention designed to improve attention, social competency, and cognitive functions in children with ADHD. Children participated in a 90-min athletic activity twice a week including both aerobic (e.g., shuttle runs, jump rope) and goal-directed exercises[b]. Note: This is presented as a practical, meaningful example of a category of physical activity techniques to explore, but is not necessarily the "best" choice of an intervention. There are many aspects of physical activity interventions to consider. These include: (1) cognitively engaging, aerobic, etc.; (2) chronic (higher-intensity or vigorous) vs not; (3) differences when physical activity is a meaningful part of a child's life vs. not; (4) and more.	Children with attention deficit hyperactivity disorder (ADHD), ages 7–9 years	Children in the sports-activity group showed greater improvements in attention, cognitive functions (i.e., flexibility, impulsivity) and speed, and social competence relative to the comparison group.

Note: Results of a recent series of meta-analyses aimed to assess all available evidence regarding the efficacy of different behavioral interventions promoting children's executive function skills (working memory, inhibitory control, and cognitive flexibility) in one study to allow for comparison. Long-term effects were assessed via a meta-analysis examining follow-up data. Physical activity was examined. Results were imprecise, but indicated a significant, moderate effect for non-typically developing children with need for research on the physiological mechanisms underlying the impact of physical activity. In study of children with ADHD, physical activity is suggested as an adjunct treatment, and among those with ADHD or ASD more vigorous (chronic) physical activity does appear to increase some aspects of executive function and gross (but not fine) motor skills [138, 216, 217]

[a] Home and phone support

[b] Clinic

[c] Online support

Table 13.11 PUBLISHED adolescent, transition-aged youth, and adult interventions

Intervention name	Description	Participants studied in key references	Key outcomes
(a) Adolescent interventions			
Adapted Alert Program for Adolescents with FASD [222]	Designed to teach adolescents to monitor, maintain, and regulate their alert levels (high, low, just right). Sensory-based strategies were explored as a way to change alert levels in different contexts. The program was modified to ensure ecological validity in Canada and with the FASD population[a].	Youth with FASD, ages 11–17 years	Adolescents used both sensory and non-sensory strategies to regulate and they reported an increase in use of self-regulation strategies from pre- to posttreatment.
Project Step Up—Adolescent Group [223]	A multicomponent intervention designed to reduce alcohol consumption and alcohol-related negative outcomes. Included education, modeling, coaching, behavioral rehearsal, and performance feedback strategies. Caregiver groups were educated on the effects of PAE on the brain and how to handle associated parenting challenges[a].	Youth with FASD, ages 13–18 years, and their caregivers	Decrease in self-reported alcohol risk and in alcohol-related negative behaviors in light/moderate drinkers relative to the comparison group. Intervention found to be acceptable and helpful for both adolescents and caregivers.
Saturday Cognitive Habilitation Program [224]	A community intervention program designed to improve youth's ability to plan, organize, shift, and evaluate problem-solving strategies. Adapted from the MILE intervention[b].	Youth with FASD, ages 10–14 years	Pre- to posttreatment gains on measures of nonverbal reasoning, reading comprehension, or mathematics reasoning for 4/5 participants.
The Brain Unit [225]	A universal school-based program that combined mental health literacy and dialectical behavioral therapy (DBT) skills to improve students' self-concept, coping skills, and social support. Program was delivered by teachers, who were provided with core instructional goals, but could flexibly adapt instructional methods for their students (i.e., bibliotherapy, role play, videos, class meetings, visual scripts, or social stories)[c].	Youth with FASD and other developmental disabilities, in grades 3–12, and their peers without disabilities	Large effect sizes for intervention schools on all measures of self-concept, coping, and social support. Strong fidelity to the program reported by teachers.

Table 13.11 (continued)

Intervention name	Description	Participants studied in key references	Key outcomes
(b) Transition-aged youth and adult interventions			
Mind, Body, and Spirit program (MBS) [226]	Designed to develop and strengthen the ability of adult male offenders to transition from a correctional facility to the community prior to release. The MBS program focused on improving communication, interpersonal skills, personal strengths, and physical health using an activity-based format[d].	Incarcerated adult men with FASD, ages 19–50 years	Participant-reported improvements in anger and stress management, self-esteem, and coping skills over the course of the intervention. Increased self-awareness and insight into patterns of behavior and improved relationships with family and children.
Parent-Child Assistance Program (PCAP) adapted [167]	A paraprofessional home visitation and advocacy intervention aimed at decreasing the risk for future alcohol- or drug-exposed births. Case managers assist clients in accessing treatment, family planning needs, and connect patients with support groups and help secure stable housing[e].	Women with FASD or suspected FASD, ages 14–36 years	Pre- to posttreatment reductions in alcohol and drug use, as well as increased use of contraceptives, medical and mental health care services, and stable housing.
Step by Step Program [227]	A community-based intervention designed to reduce the risk of breakdown in families, strengthen life and parenting skills, and increase success and independence within families. Mentors support parents on a 1:1 basis to access supports related to housing, addiction treatment, finances and parenting[b].	Parents with FASD or suspected PAE, ages 19–47 years	Reduction in severity of needs specific to each parent (i.e., experience of abuse, social problems, housing and transportation, and community resources) and gains made toward achieving individual goals over the course of the intervention.

[a] Clinic
[b] Community
[c] Classroom/school
[d] Correctional facility
[e] Home

Table 13.12 IN DEVELOPMENT adolescent, transition-aged youth, and adult interventions

Intervention name	Description	Participants studied in key references	Key outcomes
Aware Program Parker et al. (findings in preparation)	An interactive, web-based program designed to teach mindfulness skills to adolescents with FASD to improve their self-regulatory abilities and decision-making skills. Parents are provided with online resources, including a guide describing the topics and skills that will be taught to teens, to support their teen's use of the Aware Program[a].	Adolescents with FASD	Pre- to posttreatment improvements in emotion regulation abilities and executive functioning. Adolescents successfully used the program and were engaged with the online program activities. Adolescents and parents provided positive satisfaction ratings.
My Health Coach app Petrenko and Tapparello (funded, grant underway)	A mobile health application that provides adults with FASD evidence-based education about their condition and tools to promote their own self-management and health advocacy goals. This app is being designed in partnership with adults with FASD.	Population to be determined	Not yet available.
Self-Regulation Intervention adapted from the Alert Program Rasmussen, Pei and Oberlander (in preparation)	The Alert Program, adapted for adolescents with FASD, was designed to improve a range of self-regulatory functions including cognitive, behavioral and physiological measures (sleep and cortisol regulation)[b].	Adolescents with FASD	Not yet available.

[a] Home
[b] Clinic

Table 13.13 FUTURE DIRECTIONS adolescent, transition-aged youth, and adult interventions

Intervention name	Description	Participants studied in key references	Key outcomes
Attachment, Regulation, and Competency (ARC) Program [228]	A multicomponent intervention framework designed to build developmental competencies, stabilize internal distress, and strengthen security of the care-giving system. Core components include establishing routines and rituals, increasing caregiver affect management, improving caregiver-child attunement, and increasing use of positive praise and reinforcement[a–c].	Children/ adolescents with complex trauma, ages 2–21 years, and parents	Pre- and posttreatment reductions in child behavior problems (internalizing, externalizing and total problems). Improvements in symptoms of PTSD and child/adolescent needs and strengths.
Cognitive Therapy for Insomnia (CBTI) for Adolescents [229]	Based on CBTI for adults, this protocol was adapted for the treatment of adolescents with insomnia. It consists of psychoeducation, sleep hygiene, restriction of time in bed, stimulus control, cognitive therapy, and relaxation techniques[c].	Adolescents with insomnia, ages 12–19 years	Both CBTI groups (group therapy and guided internet therapy) showed clinically significant improvements on sleep efficiency, sleep onset latency, wake after sleep onset, and total sleep time relative to comparison group.
Supporting Teens' Autonomy Daily, aka Supporting Teens' Academic Needs Daily (STAND) [230]	A multicomponent intervention delivered in the style of motivational interviewing to enhance family engagement in therapy. STAND targets identified academically important executive function skills for adolescents (i.e., organization, time management, and planning (OTP skills)) and parent-based behavior management practices (i.e., monitoring and contingency management)[c].	Children/ adolescents with ADHD, ages 11–15 years, and their parents	Children receiving the STAND intervention showed greater improvements in OTP skills, homework behavior, parent-teen contracting, implementation of home privileges, and parenting stress relative to comparison group.

(continued)

Table 13.13 (continued)

Intervention name	Description	Participants studied in key references	Key outcomes
Trauma Affect Regulation: Guide for Education and Therapy (TARGET) [215]	TARGET is a strengths-based, trauma-focused psychotherapy designed to regulate intense emotions, manage intrusive trauma memories, and promote self-efficacy. TARGET teaches skills using a seven-step sequence, the FREEDOM steps (focus, recognize, emotions, evaluate, define, option, make a contribution), to help individuals learn to process and manage trauma-related reactions to stressful situations[c,d].	Adolescents with full/partial PTSD, involved in delinquency, ages 13–17 years	TARGET showed a reduced severity of PTSD symptoms and gains on outcomes of depression, anxiety and, post-traumatic cognitions
Treatment Foster Care Oregon-Adolescents (TFCO-A) [231] Note: Previously referred to as "Multidimensional Foster Care"	TFCO-A is a model of foster care treatment. TFCO-A aims to create opportunities for youths to successfully live with families rather than in groups or institutional settings, and to simultaneously prepare their parents (or other long-term placement) to provide them with effective parenting. Four key treatment elements are: (1) a consistent reinforcing environment with mentoring and encouragement to develop academic and positive living skills; (2) daily structure with clear expectations and limits and well-specified consequences; (3) close supervision; and (4) helping youth avoid deviant peer associations while providing support for establishing prosocial peer relationships[a,c,d].	Youth with severe emotional and behavioral disorders and/or severe delinquency, ages 12–18 years Note: There are also versions for preschoolers (which has been tested) and for children (which has not been tested separately).	TFCO-A has received the highest rating of "1" (well-supported by research evidence) on the California Evidence-Based Clearinghouse for a wide variety of child welfare-related outcomes (e.g., reduced disruptive behavior, reduced placement disruption).

Note: Cognitive behavioral therapy (CBT), and approaches built on CBT such as trauma-informed CBT (TF-CBT), are often used with those living with FASD. CBT techniques, adapted appropriately for neurodevelopmental differences, may be helpful. These techniques can certainly help *caregivers* raising children and youth with FASD or PAE. But assisting the individuals living with FASD may often require specialized or multicomponent approaches for troubling symptoms (e.g., insomnia), difficult life tasks (e.g., academic success), more complicated presentations (e.g., complex developmental trauma), or major and chronic difficulties (e.g., delinquency). Presented in this Future Directions table are evidence-based, effective treatments that respond to these significant challenges

[a] Home

[b] Community

[c] Clinic

[d] Classroom/school

Table 13.14 FUTURE DIRECTIONS adolescent and transition-aged youth, and adult interventions—well-known mental health approaches beyond CBT to be studied with targeted FASD sub-populations

Intervention name	Description	Participants studied in highly selected key references	Key outcomes
Dialectical Behavioral Therapy (DBT) [232]	A multicomponent cognitive-behavioral intensive intervention that targets treatment engagement and the reduction of self-harm and suicide attempts. DBT focuses on teaching skills for enhancing emotion regulation, distress tolerance, and building a life worth living. Core components include individual psychotherapy, multifamily group skills training, youth and parent telephone coaching, and weekly therapist team consultation[a].	Adolescents who are highly suicidal, ages 12–18 years	Participants in the DBT group showed a reduction in suicide attempts and self-harm relative to the comparison group.
Functional Family Therapy (FFT) Model [233]	A systems-oriented, behaviorally based model of family therapy designed to reduce youth referral problems (i.e., delinquency, oppositional behaviors, violence, substance use), and improve prosocial behaviors by enhancing support and communication within the family[a–c].	Adolescent offenders, ages 11–17 years, and their families	Adolescents in the FFT group showed a reduction in youth behavioral problems, including felony and violent crime recidivism (when therapist adherence to the FFT model was high).
Multisystemic Therapy (MST) [234]	An intensive family-based intervention designed to reduce adolescent antisocial behavior (i.e., criminal activity, substance use, conduct problems) and improve their functioning across family, peer, school and community contexts. Family strengths (i.e., love for the adolescent, social support) are used to overcome barriers (i.e., caregiver substance use, stress, hopelessness) to caregiver effectiveness[b–d].	Adolescents with juvenile justice involvement, ages 12–17 years, and their caregivers	Youth who received MST showed a reduction in recidivism and improved youth functioning in the home, at school and in the community relative to the comparison group.

Note: DBT, FFT, and MST are effective therapies with large research literatures. These therapies are for use with adolescents and transition-aged youth who show very significant, chronic mental health, and lifestyle difficulties. Such problems can include suicide attempts, conduct disorders, and/or juvenile justice involvement. DBT has also been successfully used with adults, for prevention of problems with youth, and for target symptoms beyond suicide and self-harm. FFT and MST both focus on the entire family system, and so also include treatment for adults. MST also involves

Table 13.14 (continued)

working with other systems with which a youth interacts, such as peers, school and community systems. These three therapy approaches, which likely would require adaptation for use with those living with FASD or PAE, seem quite promising for those with serious secondary impacts

[a] Clinic

[b] Home

[c] Community

[d] Classroom/school

critical or systematic review elsewhere, so quality assessment is often available in other publications and is not presented here. Intervention studies included are listed with short descriptions and 1–2 key references, participants of interest (those with PAE/FASD), and delivery settings. Findings of key references are briefly discussed, *focusing on outcomes that have shown change.* For the purposes of these tables, only selected studies from larger research programs could be included. This means that only one of a series of studies may be presented, and readers are encouraged to further explore and find the full age range and types of participants to which these treatments can apply—and all outcomes which have been studied. A few notes are included.

To help catalyze intervention research, also listed in certain tables are the authors' recommendations of highly selected, wide-ranging existing treatments from other fields that address concerns common in FASD/PAE, with references and descriptions. Readers are encouraged to use these selected references to prompt further independent exploration of promising treatment ideas. These "future directions" treatments are theoretically sound and typically have a robust, or at least developing, evidence base. Among the promising options to be explored, some school-based treatments are included. This is because school-based mental health interventions (and enhancements to early intervention and other settings where children are already present) are cost-effective options for service provision. The authors believe these existing interventions are worth consideration for study with the clinical population of those with FASD or PAE, though these programs will likely need some adaptation taking a neurodevelopmental viewpoint. It is crucial to remember that all promising treatments should be informed by lived experiences data drawn from those living with FASD or PAE. True to the essential elements of FASD-informed care, adaptation should be led by the community to create culture-centered practices. Even the fact of whether treatment is needed should be led by the community and the input of self-advocates.

Relationship-Based and Multicomponent Early Interventions (Birth to 5 Years)

Tables 13.1 and 13.2 include a range of approaches to relationship-based and multicomponent early interventions that have been specifically tested with samples of children aged birth to 5 years with PAE or FASD, and their caregivers. These tables should be considered a sampling of available interventions. There are many treatment studies that have been done with young children with polysubstance or drug exposure (where PAE is not a specific focus), or with "at-risk" young children (who may have PAE). These many other studies are not included here, but there is an in-depth synthesis article that reviews a large portion of this work [111].

Certainly, much more research remains to be done specifically with children with PAE or FASD, using bigger samples and a wider range of treatments. Many of these are pilot trials or are still in development. Fortunately, though, these treatments fit with most essential elements of FASD-informed care. For instance, all are designed to "act early" based on similar theories of change, and all reduce risks and promote protections. All share an aim to improve the caregiver–child relationship and are inherently trauma-informed. All offer developmentally appropriate treatment in that they promote mutual regulation between parent and child, or the way in which parents and children interact together and stay in a calm and responsive state—and build child self-regulation (a common area of impairment for children born with PAE).

One intervention, shown in Table 13.1, the Circle of Security, is an existing evidence-based treatment for caregivers used in this trial on an individualized basis. With adaptation, it was found to be efficacious for caregivers and children with PAE or FASD in a small study. Another, shown in Table 13.1, the SEEDS Program, is a novel multicomponent treatment, developed especially for young children with PAE and early trauma. The SEEDS Program aimed to provide comprehensive and inter-disciplinary early intervention, promoting a spirit of collaboration between parent and teacher, with outcomes yet to be fully discussed.

To truly provide FASD-informed care, early interventions should include educating caregivers to reframe and accommodate (and thus take a neurodevelopmental viewpoint). As shown in Table 13.1, this is something Zarneger and colleagues clearly aim to do with their novel model, already published as a pilot study. This model integrates two evidence-based treatment approaches (Child-Parent Psychotherapy and Mindful Parenting Education). As shown in Table 13.2, one promising novel "early intervention (EI) enhancement" in development, called FMF Bridges, aims to do this by including a caregiver curriculum based on the existing, scientifically validated Families Moving Forward (FMF) Program. This curriculum educates caregivers of children aged birth to 3 years on the neurodevelopmental viewpoint as it applies to young children. FMF Bridges integrates developmentally appropriate material from the FMF Program with elements of an existing, well-studied evidence-based relationship-based intervention. Note that EI enhancements are integrated into settings already attended by young children with

PAE, such as birth-to-three centers, intensive outpatient substance abuse treatment settings for parents, or home visitation programs.

Traditional early interventions typically aim toward building child self-regulation, but may not always try to target <u>other</u> individual-level impairments. However, the approach of Zarnegar and colleagues appears to customize skill-building to each individual child. This is an approach the neuroconstructivist view would suggest. Interestingly, the SEEDS multicomponent early intervention (with findings published so far as a case study series) appears to train a wider range of skills (such as precursors of executive function and other aspects of learning readiness).

Table 13.3 shows some very promising evidence-based, relationship-based interventions or multicomponent early intervention programs not yet studied with samples with known PAE or FASD. The full range of these treatments, often known as "infant and early childhood mental health interventions," is discussed in more detail by Olson and Montague [19]. For the current chapter, the authors recommend several interventions that might strategically be tested next as future directions. These are designed for a variety of family structures, are developmentally appropriate and trauma-informed, and most target the parent–child relationship as a way to support child self-regulation. Many take place through home visiting or bringing families into clinics. Among these are the Attachment, Biobehavioral Catch-Up (ABC) Model (originally designed for foster parents), Promoting First Relationships (originally designed for high-risk parents), The Nurse-Family Partnership (originally designed for pregnant and early-parenting persons with risk factors), and others.

It is crucial to remember that all these promising treatments may need adaptation and should be informed by lived experiences data. Adaptation should be led by the community in which they are deployed to create culture-centered practices. As will be repeated throughout this chapter, even the fact of whether treatment is needed should be led by the community. This is even true of early interventions, which tend to target goals that are "universal" to all cultures, such as improving the quality of parent-child attachment or enhancing cognitive stimulation. Yet exactly <u>how</u> to go about improving the security of attachment between parent and child, or <u>how</u> to offer ways to help children improve their developmental potential, differs around the world. Measuring whether these early interventions are effective must be done in ways that are meaningful to those to whom treatment is provided.

All this means that early interventions should be examined across a variety of cultures using samples with PAE or FASD, adapting as needed, and ascertaining when novel treatments must be developed. Fortunately, this is starting to happen. For example, now being published is a study on an effort to provide a new, relationship-based early intervention enhancement in two rural communities in a South African context for children with PAE and their caregivers (see Table 13.2). This treatment encourages caregiver-child dyads to attain a calm and alert regulatory state as a precursor to secure and positive engagement. This treatment adds value to natural settings children already attend. Benefits were seen for all children, with the greatest benefits for the highest-risk children (research colleague and investigator, University of New Mexico, Kalberg W, 2021, written communication, 22nd October).

Parenting and Family Support Interventions

Tables 13.4a–c and 13.5 include a robust set of what can be grouped into: (1) positive parenting interventions; (2) parent management training; and (3) parenting support, education and advocacy programs. Tested so far are treatments that are typically offered in-person (at home or in the clinic), with at least one known now to be offered via telehealth. Online treatments are now being developed. Several of these treatments, such as Coaching Families and the Key Worker Program, have been sustainably implemented for 10–20 years in several communities in Canada. Programs fit with almost all essential elements of FASD-informed care. For instance, these programs find, build, and use strengths, aim to overcome stigma, build collaborative partnerships, offer developmentally appropriate care, think about context (intervene at different levels of a youth's ecology), sustain hope, and more. With the possible exception of parent management training (Table 13.4b), all reframe and accommodate (take a neurodevelopmental viewpoint). Positive parenting interventions also attempt to target a range of individual-level impairments.

Positive parenting interventions in Table 13.4a are aimed toward families raising children in the preschool and elementary school years and include explicit use of a positive behavior support approach (drawn from the developmental disabilities literature) [112]. For these interventions, initial efficacy studies have been done, with at least some translational research. Some are novel treatments, such as the Families Moving Forward (FMF) Program, which has also been used with good feasibility in gradually growing real-world practice since 2010, including most recently through telehealth. The FMF Program offers parent training and advocacy education specialized for families raising children with PAE or FASD and behavior problems, with additional important elements such as a focus on child joys and rewards, caregiver self-care, and planning for the future with hope. Positive parenting interventions, which teach caregiving methods to deal with challenging behavior, have also been combined with child-focused skills-building in multicomponent approaches, such as the Families on Track Program, Parents Under Pressure Program, or the MILE Program (MILE components are listed in both Tables 13.4 (parent training program); and Table 13.9 (child skills-building component, discussed later).

Presented in Table 13.4c, the wide range of parenting support, education, and advocacy approaches are used with families raising an individual with PAE or FASD, with the broadest age range for any program from birth to young adulthood. These approaches offer specialized parenting education and typically also customized family support/case management that offers caregiver support and education and emphasizes connecting families with needed services. One program of interest offering education is the workshop or web-based parent training program that accompanied the MILE learning readiness/self-regulation program. Parent support programs range from the Key Worker and Parent Support Program and Coaching Families, which serve all families raising an individual with PAE, to the more targeted Parent-Child Assistance Program (PCAP). PCAP serves pregnant and parenting persons (birth mothers) at very high risk for chemical dependency and has spread widely to community practice in multiple states and countries.

Listed in Table 13.5, in efficacy studies now underway, are several parenting interventions that have moved beyond telehealth, to administration online in order to increase accessibility and scalability. One is a web-based parent training program based on an existing model for children with neurodevelopmental disorders, that includes supportive phone-based coaching, called Strongest Families FASD. Another is a mobile Health application ("mHealth app") called FMF Connect. This app takes content and treatment principles from the FMF Program and adds unique features such as an in-app Family Forum (moderated parent support group) and more. FMF Connect allows the intervention to be self-administered or coached. Also undergoing ongoing study of efficacy is a caregiver-focused intervention with a relationship-focused stance, using techniques of emotion coaching (which predict positive child outcomes), called Tuning into Kids.

To fully provide FASD-informed care as a positive parenting or family support intervention, further thought is needed about overcoming stigma, thinking about context, and being led by the community to create culture-centered practices. Specifically, outcomes should be measurably defined in terms of what is necessary to improve QOL for children, parents, and families. Measures should be meaningful and consider the influence of context (participation and environmental factors) on daily functioning. The logic model and theory of change underlying each intervention need to be defined and described and should be clear and precise. In addition, given the wide cultural variation of parenting practices, outcomes, logic models, and theories of change need consideration across a range of cultures. Interventions should be adapted to different cultures as needed, but novel treatments should also be developed when required.

Positive parenting interventions are especially suited to families raising children with PAE or FASD. There are several promising existing interventions with a developing evidence base that have features that complement the three positive parenting programs already tested with this clinical population. Listed in Table 13.6 are the Family Check-Up Model (designed to be offered as part of integrated primary care), the program known as Research Units in Behavioral Intervention (RUBI; delivers basic positive parenting skills and designed for children with autism, but might be adaptable), and the Stepping Stones Triple P Program (which can be used with groups).

In addition, there are a range of evidence-based parent management training methods available based on social learning theory, including those primarily developed for young children at risk for (or with) disruptive behavior disorders or ADHD, or focused on promoting school readiness. These tend to focus more on consequences for misbehavior and rewards for desirable behavior and may or may not fit well with samples with the neurodevelopmental problems seen in FASD. While the scientific literature for social learning theory-based parent training is very robust, of this category of treatments only Parent-Child Interaction Therapy (PCIT) has been studied explicitly with samples with PAE or FASD, with mixed evidence for efficacy. Recent reviews of the behavioral parent training literature continue to support that these are well-established, efficacious approaches for children with ADHD, who have symptoms similar to those of children living with FASD or PAE. The data are especially strong in the school years, but there are data showing these approaches work in the preschool years and, with the addition of other components, to a lesser extent in adolescence [113]. Therefore, it remains of interest to see if the "usual" treatments work for families raising children with PAE or FASD. It is also of interest to explore whether they can work with appropriate adaptation. Notably, the broad evidence base for these programs has not yet included secondary analysis to see if there is differential efficacy for children with PAE or FASD. This seems like an important omission in that literature. For more information, see discussion of both positive parenting and social learning theory-based approaches in Olson and Montague [19].

Child-Focused Skill-Building Interventions: Self-Regulation, Social Skills and Communication, and Behavioral Outcomes

Table 13.7a–c presents a range of skill-building, child-focused interventions aimed toward improving social and friendship skills, social communication, self-regulation, and behavioral outcomes (not including parent training). These are primarily aimed at remediating these areas of deficit among children in the preschool and elementary school years (about 2–12 years). Both descriptive neurobehavioral research and lived experiences data make clear that impairment in these domains creates daily life challenges, increased caregiving stress, and reduced family and child QOL. As a consequence, this has been an area of more intensive research activity, including programmatic research on some interventions with replication studies, and at least initial real-world translational research. Of course, more research is needed, and many of the samples have been small (or case studies using single subject design). All these treatments conform with at least some essential elements of FASD-informed care in that they take a neurodevelopmental viewpoint, target individual-level impairments, are developmentally appropriate, and take context into account.

True to guidelines of the neuroconstructivist view, self-regulation has been a significant intervention research topic (Table 13.7a). Early on, efforts were made to have children observe their own learning style using Cognitive Control Therapy and, more recently, using contingency reinforcement, with a goal of improving self-regulation. A newer, robust metacognitive approach to improve child self-regulation was designed as a computerized intervention (delivered along with trained parent assistance) called GoFAR (FAR: Focus/Plan, Act, Reflect). It is notable that GoFAR was actually a *multicomponent* program because the child skills-building component was combined with parent training on behavioral regulation and behavior analog therapy where the parent and child together implemented the learning strategy. A program designed by occupational therapists, called the Alert Program for Self-Regulation, has been successfully used in both an individualized and group format, and adapted in several ways, with both neurobiological (brain function) and behavior outcomes assessed. Multiple studies have been done on the Alert Program by several research labs. As shown in Table 13.7b, treatment to improve child social skills has been investigated most robustly in a series of studies by one lab on Children's Friendship Training (CFT) with promising efficacy data. It is notable, in a small study, that CFT was apparently more effective when coupled with a specific type of medication therapy compared to other groups [114]. There have also been several small exploratory studies of innovative treatments for group social skills improvement or individual social communication support for children with FASD. Most studies focusing on child behavior are actually included in Table 13.4a–c, as parent training programs often target reductions in child disruptive behavior. However, included in Table 13.7c are two case studies of children with FASD whose behavior (and functional communication) improved with classic applied behavior analysis techniques used as treatment.

Note that no "in-process" treatments of child-focused skill-building interventions aimed toward self-regulation, social skills and communication, and behavioral outcomes were identified for this chapter, so there is no corresponding table. However, this literature survey could not be fully comprehensive, so it is possible that some research underway was missed.

There are many other promising ideas for treatment of self-regulation, and of social skills and communication, for children with PAE and FASD. The authors recommend finding existing programs to treat these areas of common individual-level impairment that have an evidence base, and then adapting as needed taking a neurodevelopmental viewpoint. Listed in Table 13.8 are a wide-ranging set of programs with a convincing (or at least developing) evidence base. Thinking about the outcome of self-regulation, the preschool curriculum called "Tools of the Mind" is literally designed to promote self-regulation in a play-based learning format. Further, Mindful Yoga Programs are treatments that include physical activity, breathing, meditation, and relaxation to improve both self-regulation (and executive attention). Addressing the outcome of social skills, the Incredible Years Dinosaur School and Promoting Alternative Thinking Strategies (PATHS) Program are two child group programs (often delivered in the classroom, but which can also be delivered in community or clinic settings), which have a strong evidence base and concrete materials that could easily be adapted for children with PAE or FASD. In fact, PATHS has been combined with the FMF Program as a multicomponent intervention in the Families on Track intervention listed in Table 13.4 [78, 79].

Beyond just trying these promising treatments, intervention research in the area of child skill-building in self-regulation, social skills and communication and behavior should continue to assess both behavioral and neurobiological outcomes, following the lead of research with the Alert Program. Additional interventions focusing on increasing executive function skills are a particularly important area to consider, especially because they can enhance everyday function and overall quality of life. Also, considering guidance of the field of developmental psychopathology, to really make a difference in the cascade of developmental effects, intervention should be as intensive as possible in the early years. This makes more intensive multicomponent treatments, such as GoFAR, and treatments such as Tools of the Mind, which immerse a child fully in a preschool curriculum focused on self-regulation, more attractive intervention options. While these may be more costly in short term, they may ultimately prove more worthwhile in long term. It may also be vital to start self-regulation treatment even earlier, using relationship-based and multicomponent early interventions in the first years of life (as presented in Tables 13.1 and 13.2). These can help very young children with more basic levels of physiological, attentional, and emotional regulation, literally laying a better neurological foundation for attaining success in achieving developmentally more advanced levels of self-regulation (i.e., behavioral and executive regulation) [49]. It is also likely that child skill-building treatments in this area should sometimes be coupled with carefully individualized medication treatment, as suggested by Kodituwakku, to enhance treatment effectiveness [31].

As discussed earlier, those living with FASD or PAE often experience psychosocial risk factors, such as maltreatment or other adverse childhood experiences. Child-focused skill-building interventions aimed to improve problems in self-regulation, social skills, and behavior may be responding to symptoms that have emerged not only because of PAE—but because of these risk factors. Interventions in this area are likely to be especially important and respond to the essential element of FASD-informed care to "offer treatment that is trauma-informed."

Of course, to fully provide FASD-informed care in child skill-building interventions, further thought is needed about context and culture, especially when the target domains are social skills and social communication. For instance, there are thought-provoking questions as to whether "neurotypical" social skills are what should be taught to individuals who are neurodiverse (such as those with FASD). Also, social skills and social communication differ widely from culture to culture, so what is taught in treatment must also differ. Treatment goals, and even the fact of whether treatment is needed, should be led by the community and the input of self-advocacy.

Child and Adolescent-Focused Skill-Building Interventions: Toward Varied Other Outcomes

Table 13.9a–d presents skill-building child and adolescent-focused interventions aimed toward remediating additional areas of deficit identified in descriptive neurobehavioral research with the clinical population of those at high-risk because of PAE, or those living with FASD. These are aimed at youth from preschool through adolescence (3–16 years). Some are computerized and one is built on a virtual reality platform. Included are metacognitive interventions (such as attention and memory training), treatments designed to improve academic achievement, one adaptive function intervention (safety skills training), and sensory-focused and physical activity interventions. Also included are very new, innovative multicomponent interventions, such as the combination of transcranial direct-current stimulation and cognitive training. Of course, more research remains to be done.

These skill-building treatments are targeted toward children and youth in the preschool through early high school years (about 3–16 years). Treatments are proliferating because there are many domains in which this clinical population shows individual-level impairments, and this is a good age range for remediation. Several of these interventions have been studied in randomized control trials. Most thoroughly investigated (in the US) has been the Math Interactive Learning Experience (MILE) program. MILE is actually a multicomponent intervention, focused on developing math skills while accommodating and remediating underlying problems with neurocognition. In the primary trial of MILE, children aged 3–10 years received individualized 1:1 math tutoring using a metacognitive approach, while caregivers were trained on how to support their child's math learning and behavior regulation at home. This has been successfully replicated (in Canada) using child tutoring only, extended to include children with PAE only (rather than only those with FASD), and offered in natural settings like school or home, with a broader study design [115].

This set of treatments fits with some essential elements of FASD-informed care. Most centrally, all offer developmentally appropriate care, reframe and accommodate (take a neurodevelopmental viewpoint), and target individual-level impairments. Some find, build, and use strengths. What is now needed is to further incorporate a strengths-based view in design and deployment of these treatments. For instance, the typically high social motivation and desire for the attention seen among individuals with FASD (a clear strength) might be used to enhance learning, such as ensuring that treatments include adult assistance (and, importantly, mobilize the individual's attention as a reward). This was done, for example, in the MILE program. It is also vital to gather lived experience data to ensure that treatment goals are informed by the actual context in which children and adolescents with PAE or FASD function, and whether what is being worked on in treatment will help them during actual school participation and meaningfully raise their QOL. For instance, it is possible that children in the MILE treatment saw the value of getting better at math (and doing better at school). But they may not always have understood the value of outcomes targeted in some other interventions, and how that would make their daily life better. Also, like treatments listed in Tables 13.7a–c and 13.8, if there are hypothesized neurological changes resulting from the interventions in Tables 13.9a–d and 13.10, neurobiological outcomes should be assessed. This is clearly possible for attention and memory, academic achievement, or physical activity interventions, especially if these treatments are delivered sufficiently early in life—and would also be possible for sleep interventions, if they were tested.

Also important will be to adapt, or develop, interventions for these varied outcomes that fit different cultures, led by the community and self-advocates in creating culture-centered practices. This is a vital theme for every treatment section in this chapter.

There is an important point to make about adaptive function interventions, since Table 13.9c lists only one treatment study that has apparently done in this area. This is very surprising, since adaptive function is a broad domain and impairment in this area is very common among those living with FASD and affected by PAE. In truth, there are many, many treatments relevant to adaptive function. Why? First, adaptive function impairment is a fundamental criterion of the current proposed DSM-5 definition of "neurobehavioral disorder associated with prenatal alcohol exposure" (ND-PAE). In the diagnosis of ND-PAE, briefly put, adaptive function difficulties can occur as evidence of significant impairment in two or more domains, including: communication (past or present); social skills or social communication; daily living skills; or motor skills (past or present) [83]. This means that social skills and social communication treatments listed in Tables 13.7 and 13.8 are also relevant to adaptive function. Second, so are physical activity interventions in Tables 13.9d and 13.10. Third, treatments that impact behavior problems (which, in turn, lower adaptive function), listed in Tables 13.4c, 13.5, 13.6 and 13.7a–c, 13.8, are also relevant to the area of adaptive function.

Note that no "in-process" treatments of child-focused skill-building interventions aimed toward varied other outcomes were identified for this chapter, so there is no table that presents these in this chapter. However, this literature survey could not be fully comprehensive, so it is possible that some research underway was missed.

As listed in Table 13.10, there are several interventions with a developing evidence base the authors believe might be useful for future research with the population of those with PAE or FASD, and there are certainly many more than are mentioned here. Metacognitive interventions have already received considerable investigation and should continue to do so. Drawn from literatures on ADHD and neurodevelopmental disorders, the authors have identified the most important intervention domains for future research as: (1) sleep; (2) physical activity; and (3) adaptive function. Given clear evidence of sleep difficulties among individuals with PAE and its profound impact on the parent–child relationship and family QOL [116, 117], two sleep-related treatments are recommended (one for preschoolers and one for children in the school years). Because of the known efficacy of physical activity for improving attention and executive function, one physical activity intervention is suggested, simply as an example. The note at the top of Table 13.10 provides additional evidence from the broader literature on physical activity intervention to guide further research in this area. Finally, an interesting method for guiding individuals to independently discover strategies for how to perform daily living tasks, and improve adaptive function, is recommended as a promising research direction to pursue.

Interventions for Adolescence, Transition-Aged Youth, and Adulthood

Table 13.11a, b lists published treatments tested with adolescent, transition-aged youth (TAY; age 15–26 years) and/or adults with PAE or FASD. This area of study is only just emerging, with remarkable research gaps and opportunities. For this broad age range, holistic management or community interventions has also been tested, as listed in Table 13.4. Other tested treatments listed in Table 13.11a, b aim to build self-regulation, coping or other skills or to prevent secondary impacts and mental health conditions, or build knowledge and skills to reduce specific adverse conditions (such as alcohol misuse). Treatments listed in Table 13.11a, b conform to most of the essential elements of FASD-informed care, but considerable work needs to be done to improve the quality and range of treatments. Importantly, in these life phases, needs are highly individualized and person-centered planning is needed. At these later stages of life, it is important to also adhere to the essential element of FASD-informed care and "build collaborative partnerships" to create support.

Some interventions studied so far have been described as aimed at mitigating or reducing harm [45]. This is reasonable as, by this age, a surprising number of individuals with PAE or FASD may be experiencing a range of secondary impacts, such as difficulties in independent living, a disheartening fact documented first in 1996 and shown again in 2020 [14, 118]. Among those with typical development, the life stages of adolescence and TAY are vulnerable times for the onset of psychopathology, and this is also true for those living with FASD. For adolescents with FASD, there is generally increased risky behavior (including suicide) [119], and adults show increased rates of mental health difficulties [120]. Recent survey data has documented a wide range of concerning negative health outcomes for transition-aged youth and adults with FASD [51]. While health consequences associated with PAE in adult humans are not known, animal research suggests that humans may be more vulnerable to chronic diseases such as hypertension, diabetes, immune dysfunction, and cancer [121, 122].

But portraying these later developmental stages for those living with FASD only as a set of adverse life experiences is an incomplete, misleading and even detrimental picture. Only recently have lived experience data, and the efforts of self-advocates begun to document the many strengths and protective factors among older individuals living with FASD, and their families. For example, recent evidence emphasizes the intrinsic strengths of those with FASD, including older transition-aged youth and adults, such as strong self-awareness, receptiveness to support, capacity for human connection, perseverance through challenges, and hope for the future [66].

During adolescence and the time of transition-aged youth (TAY), relationships with caregivers and other adults are in flux. Adolescents/TAY are in search of an independent identity and more intimate interpersonal and romantic relationships. For these life stages, interventions must more fully take context into account, and squarely aim toward improvement in a sense of agency, self-determination, and QOL as outcomes. Finding, building, and using strengths in treatment are necessary and should be further emphasized. For instance, one intervention approach could be to teach the skills of self-advocacy, and teach awareness of the FASD diagnosis and one's individual profile of skill deficits and (especially) strengths. Interventions aimed at the phases of adolescence/TAY must involve a broader social context than the family, and so might include mentoring by a trusted adult, peer-to-peer interventions, and/or new ways for parents to be involved in assisting treatment. Interventions might also train caregivers on skills of "autonomy supportive parenting" [123, 124].

These life phases also require increased mental health support that is concrete, experiential, and adapted to the developmental level of the individual. Further, influences now pivotal in typical development at this time in cultural history, such as social media, mobile health apps, and online information, can be leveraged to provide FASD intervention in these later life phases.

These intervention ideas are also applicable to young adulthood, including the notion of "autonomy supportive parenting"—but as it applies to navigating young adult life tasks for someone whose functional level may not be the same as their chronological age. It is important to note that recent life experiences data have shown different rates of certain secondary impacts for adults living with FASD vs adolescents or youth [14]. This means that, in young and perhaps middle adulthood, there are different or additional intervention needs. Therefore, treatment must support outcomes relevant to young adulthood, such as successful independent living, effective management of health conditions, post-secondary education, employment, and creation of adaptive life partnerships. Focusing on these outcomes, developmentally appropriate to adulthood, supports the basic human right of self-determination, promotes agency, allows life participation (rather than just access), and ultimately raises <u>adult</u> QOL.

Table 13.12 lists several interventions with research underway. One feasible web-based mindfulness intervention with promising efficacy, the Aware Program, apparently improved indicators of self-regulation and executive function for adolescents and youth with FASD. Two other projects underway are an adaptation of the Alert Program for adolescents, and an interesting adult-directed FASD intervention now in development. The latter project is a mobile health app, called My Health Coach. True to the essential element of FASD-informed care to "be led by the community to create culture-centered practices," this app is being designed with concrete input from self-advocates who themselves are living with FASD. This app is designed to help young adults with FASD act as their own self-managers to achieve their own customized health and life goals.

As listed in Tables 13.13 and 13.14, there are many "promising" interventions with a developing or solid evidence base the authors believe might be useful to try with adolescents, TAY or adults living with FASD. In Table 13.13, highly selected intervention domains include (1) adolescent autonomy development paired with autonomy supportive parenting; (2) sleep; and (3) trauma/affect regulation. Offering developmentally appropriate treatment for the stages of adolescence and TAY centers around helping parents assist their offspring to attain the pivotal outcomes of autonomy and psychological well-being, which appear to be important across cultures as they are important to self-determination. Promising interventions applicable across this wide age range (and across cultures) have also been chosen given clear evidence of sleep difficulties among those living with FASD, and the frequent co-occurrence of trauma in this clinical population.

Beyond these promising treatment directions, the authors also note that many older individuals living with FASD are served in the mental health system for co-occurring mental health conditions, and sometimes contend with serious issues such as suicide. In these systems, providers will typically use well-known evidence-based practices, such as functional family therapy or dialectical behavior therapy. As shown in Table 13.14, a fruitful area of future research will be to examine, with samples of individuals living with FASD, whether these evidence-based practices show the expected treatment effects. If not, it will be important to determine what treatment adaptations are needed, or whether other mental health practices are more effective.

Of course, to fully provide FASD-informed care for older individuals living with FASD, and those who care for them, especially careful thought is needed about context and culture. For instance, a cultural framework is mandatory in consideration of diagnosis and treatment of mental health concerns. Cultural roles, values, and resources shape the roles and life paths of adolescents, transition-aged youth and adults, whether they are of a typical or atypical course. Treatment goals, and even the fact of whether treatment is needed, should be led by the community and the input of self-advocacy.

Critical and Systematic Reviews: A Brief Summary of Scientific Critique of FASD Intervention Research

As intervention data have accumulated in the field of FASD, critical and systematic reviews of research evidence have periodically been published. Such reviews help to shape, stimulate, and improve the field. Early reviews noted the small amount of intervention research and commented about limitations of the evidence as a whole, or suggested improvements for early research on behavioral and family support interventions. Later reviews reported encouragement by the slowly increasing breadth of evidence and examined treatment research from different angles. The very brief summary provided here will give an overview of these reviews [8, 45, 71, 110, 125–129]. Also included are a few key implications drawn from this information by the authors. (This summary does not include reviews of medication or basic science interventions.)

One consistent and repeated theme in critical and systematic reviews has been the gaps in research aimed at treatment for those with PAE or FASD in infancy/toddlerhood, and in adolescence and beyond. But now, as evident from Tables 13.1 and 13.2, and 13.11 and 13.12, these research gaps are slowly being remedied. Reviewers have also noted that many intervention studies have focused on samples drawn from clinic settings. In addition, reviewers have pointed out that epidemiological studies to establish prevalence in the general population, and in settings without many services (such as rural or remote areas, or areas without diagnostic clinics), are lacking, so the full scope and pattern of the problem of FASD are not known. All this means that treatment findings so far might not apply to the full range of individuals with FASD—such as those with milder central nervous system impairment or those not connected to services. It is certain that there are individuals with milder effects. It is quite likely that those not connected to services have different needs than those with access to community resources. An implication is that treatment may ultimately have to be set up as a "tiered" [34] or "stepped" system of care, from less intensive through more intensive care, with a wide range of resources, that can then serve everyone within communities.

Over time, reviewers have rated the quality of intervention research in several ways, finding multiple strengths in study design and outcome measurement. But clear methodological weaknesses have also been noted, even though there has been slow improvement in study methodology as the field has matured. Limitations have included small sample sizes, and design flaws such as the potential for selection bias and issues raised by lack of blinding of examiners and families, poor description of randomization, and limited choice of treatment targets and outcome measures. Reviewers have noted a restricted focus on immediate posttreatment outcomes (with less attention to examining sustained effects), and lack of attention to factors that moderate treatment outcome—or to factors that promote or maintain gains. To refine interventions, reviewers have suggested examining mechanisms of change, identifying active treatment ingredients, and examining the impact of modifiable parameters (such as treatment length) that affect feasibility and cost. They have also suggested looking at treatment "responders" and "non-responders," and trying to understand the reasons for why some respond and some do not. Further, reviewers have recommended exploring whether effects generalize to other settings or other outcomes, and building a more robust evidence base for treatments aimed at this clinical population by carrying out programmatic research. Reviewers have also recommended carrying out translational research to examine whether treatments work in the community.

Thinking About a Transdiagnostic Approach

Because alcohol is a teratogen, it has wide-ranging and individually variable effects. Despite years of high-quality research, a neurobehavioral "phenotype" (characteristic pattern that typifies a disorder) has not been fully described, though progress has been made. Some have questioned whether FASD is a discernable disorder separable from other conditions (e.g., [130]). At present, it is still considered a "proposed condition in need of study" (under the term "neurobehavioral disorder associated with PAE," or "ND-PAE") in the current DSM-5 manual of mental health conditions [83]. All this means it is difficult to "see" the central characteristics of FASD. It also means this clinical population has symptoms that overlap with others (such as those whom ADHD researchers categorize as having "complex ADHD").

Discussion of these issues is ongoing, important, and complicated.

All this raises several challenging questions for treatment. First, is treatment specialized for this population necessary or practical? Also, many times, PAE is not known because providers do not ask, stigma prevents birth parents from revealing PAE, or a child is adopted or in foster care and there is no way to know. So, there is a second puzzling question: is the application of specialized treatment even <u>possible</u> much of the time, since PAE is often unknown?

Because children and families need to be served, clinicians have moved forward, quite often, without answers to these two questions. Instead, clinicians have taken a "transdiagnostic" approach, or have applied other diagnoses and treated those instead. Essentially, clinicians have applied treatments for youth from other clinical populations who share symptoms with those seen in the clinical population. "Transdiagnostic" means that the same treatment logic and procedures can be applied beyond a particular diagnosis. This may have been done because PAE was unknown, or FASD was unrecognized—or, perhaps, PAE was known, but FASD could not be reliably diagnosed. This has allowed clinical work to go forward, but clinicians have not been able to take advantage of the developing evidence on FASD treatment.

The authors of this chapter have taken the stance that evidence-based treatment for individuals living with FASD, and their families, is important, practical and necessary. But even from this perspective, thinking about a transdiagnostic approach can still be very helpful. Several useful research ideas are discussed here.

Reflecting on a transdiagnostic approach suggests important research directions. Of course, research on FASD diagnostic systems is needed to reliably and validly discern the condition. But in the area of treatment research, a major need is to test existing evidence-based treatments (EBTs) for youth with similar symptoms, and their families, with those living with PAE or FASD. Clinicians are using these treatments, so it is important to see if they work or not. It does seem likely that these treatments need adaptation to become part of the complement of useful FASD interventions. Such testing has already been done with interventions such as the Alert Program, which was designed for youth with various diagnoses that include symptoms of self-regulation impairment. The Alert Program has needed adaptation, as have many of the existing EBTs tested so far.

Interestingly, the flip side of thinking of a transdiagnostic approach is the possibility that some innovative, specialized treatments specifically developed for those with FASD or PAE may be useful for youth from <u>other</u> clinical populations who share the symptoms that are the focus of those treatments. In other words, it is possible that some treatments developed for FASD may be able to be applied in a broader, "transdiagnostic" manner. One possible example is the Families Moving Forward (FMF) Program, which is composed of a number of "modules" which can be customized for families. The FMF Program was specifically developed for those with FASD or PAE and challenging behavior. But this program may actually be very appropriate for certain overlapping, complex, and very diverse clinical subpopulations of individuals with neurodevelopmental differences from other or multiple causes coupled with problematic behavior. These might include those diagnosed with complex ADHD arising from a variety of causes, or those with *suspected* PAE and documented prenatal polydrug exposure. One future research direction is that the FMF Program, though specially developed for those with PAE, could be tested for efficacy with these groups and might be found to have broader applicability.

Discussion

Progress on intervention for those living with FASD and PAE, and those who care for them, is at a tipping point. Interest in effective treatment has never been higher. Recognition of FASD is still a major stumbling block. But there are a growing number of providers and policymakers, and especially families, who know about the condition of FASD—and are concerned about the risks presented by alcohol's teratogenic effects from the prenatal period on.

As shown in Fig. 13.1, the essential elements of FASD-informed care related to treatment have been defined, based on solid theoretical foundations. It is validating that other researchers have named some similar principles for children with polysubstance exposure [111] and for women with FASD and their families [35, 111]. Especially validating is discussion of the guiding concept of "thriving" in the field of FASD. Researchers Petrenko and Kautz-Turnbull propose ways to move science forward to promote thriving when living with FASD, using what they term the *"From Surviving to Thriving"* model. This model illustrates a proposed paradigm shift from deficit-based to strengths-based research and intervention in order to recognize strengths and improve quality of life for people with FASD [131]. The elements of FASD-informed care outlined in the current chapter fit well with their model—and align well with the powerful concept of "thriving" with FASD.

As laid out in this chapter's tables, there is a small but expanding body of treatment literature specifically tested with samples with PAE or FASD, which matches up well with the essential elements of FASD-informed care. But there are many gaps in the complement of treatments that are available. We do need to create an adequate set of effective interventions across the lifespan, and we need to build evidence to define a solid standard of best practices. To help families, we also need to move rapidly to implement these evidence-based practices with fidelity in a sustainable manner in community settings. It is fortunate that very recent calls for grant applications have begun to solicit treatment studies in the field of FASD.

But what is <u>really</u> required in the field is a strategic plan for progress on FASD intervention with funding to support this plan. The field faces a set of tasks. Each task presents a set of dilemmas (some quite complex), which must be solved. This Discussion section lays out many of those tasks and their underlying dilemmas and proposes solutions framed as action steps.

Enhance FASD Recognition

<u>Dilemma</u>: In most countries, FASD is not well-recognized. The public, providers of all types, and most service systems still lack sufficient awareness of FASD. Providers fail to screen because they do not ask about PAE, or do not ask in an adequate manner. That means they do not refer for diagnosis. All may be halted by stigma. Treatment that is FASD-informed cannot even be delivered. If FASD is not

recognized, families, agencies, and service systems (and funders) do not see the full scope of the public health problem, and community uptake of treatments is minimal, even when treatments have been shown to be efficacious. What does this mean for a strategic plan for progress on intervention for those living with FASD, and those who care for them?

Solutions: Community education about the effects of PAE and FASD must continue. Professional education about screening must increase, including how to sensitively ask about PAE (and, importantly, the need to systematically document PAE data to make it available). This is needed across many systems (obstetrics, primary health care of all types, mental health, child welfare, education, justice, and more). In addition, funders and treatment researchers must divert some of their energies toward effective stigma reduction. Guidance exists on how to proceed. Recently, stigma about FASD and alcohol use during pregnancy have been described as pervasive and multilayered [99, 100]. Ideas for effective programs for stigma reduction have been identified and should be tested (e.g., [103]). As an essential element of FASD-informed care, the effort to "overcome stigma" must be woven into family support and education treatments, relationship-based interventions, all types of parenting interventions—in fact, into all treatments for this clinical population.

Provide Basic "Evidence-Informed" Care

Dilemma: Despite the fact that many efficacious treatments have been developed for individuals and families (see Tables 13.1, 13.2, 13.4, 13.5, 13.7, 13.9, 13.11, and 13.12), there is still limited community availability of these treatments. Treatment is simply not very accessible. Few providers have been trained across disciplines, and most geographic locations do not have adequate services. Systems of FASD-informed care are under development, but do not exist in most countries. Funding for appropriate treatment is limited or unavailable. Evidence-based best practices are not fully known, as there are major gaps in what is known about treatment. What should be done?

Solutions: At the very least, providers and systems could follow the consensus advice of experts that is already available. If *"evidence-based"* care is not yet fully available, providers and systems could at least provide *"evidence-informed"* care appropriate for FASD. How can this be done?

Scientifically accurate, clinically useful provider education about PAE and FASD could be required across multiple disciplines. PAE screening programs that refer for diagnosis could be initiated or, if they exist, enhanced. At a minimum, providers and systems could adopt a neurodevelopmental viewpoint to modify their usual practices. This means incorporating the essential elements of "reframe and accommodate" into treatment as usual, which helps providers (and their clients) see problems differently and act accordingly. This should be combined with the essential element of "offering relationship-based and trauma-informed care," given the high frequency of adverse childhood experiences among those with PAE or living with FASD.

Some resources for training providers on evidence-informed care in FASD are already available. Developed through expert consensus, the Treatment Improvement Protocol #58 on Addressing FASD (TIP #58), created by SAMHSA in the US, provides clinically relevant, evidence-informed guidance on FASD-informed care, at least for mental health and substance abuse treatment settings [36]. Evidence-informed care can also be raised to a higher level of sophistication through the use of formal training curricula for providers. One effective method for this is through models of learning and guided practice, such as the ECHO model. This type of provider education increases workforce capacity to provide evidence-informed (or even evidence-based) care and is now beginning in the field of FASD treatment [132].

Evidence-informed care can also be made accessible to families by offering it directly to the public. As research has taught more about intervention for those living with FASD, there have been many evidence-informed educational efforts. Some are very high quality. These have not necessarily been evaluated, but often have anecdotal evidence or final reports that document their usefulness. For example, Triumph Today, an evidence-informed parenting education program, is now in a video-based format offered freely online via YouTube through the Ohio Guidestone website [133]. As another example, the US Centers for Disease Control and Prevention offers training and education opportunities (i.e., videos, podcasts, links to training), materials, and multimedia (i.e., infographics, fact sheets, brochures, posters) [134].

Offer Person-Centered Planning

Dilemma: As a teratogen, prenatal alcohol exposure has wide-ranging and individually variable effects. A neurobehavioral "phenotype" (characteristic pattern that typifies a disorder) has not been fully described. What methods can be used to efficiently offer intervention for those living with FASD, without disparities, to this widely variable clinical population? At least in certain cultures?

Solutions: Person-centered planning is recommended, as it is in the field of intellectual and developmental disabilities (IDD)—and efficient methods are needed to carry out person-centered planning and make sure it is the standard of care in the field of FASD. Person-centered planning is thought to apply across the lifespan, from the early years through the end of life, and is integral to the very definition of FASD-informed care.

Person-centered planning fits with all theoretical models discussed earlier and is often the story told in the lived experiences data from the field of FASD. Person-centered planning is a method that fits well with the essential elements of FASD-informed care presented in this chapter. FASD researcher Rutman, writing about programs for women with FASD, makes "person-centered accommodations" one of her core principles of FASD-informed care for adults [35]. In this chapter, person-centered planning is seen as an approach in which the person is placed at the center of the services, and individualized services (including accommodations) are developed collaboratively and in partnership between professionals, families, and the individual living with FASD. The focus is on the person and what they can do, not on their condition or disability. This fits with other essential elements of FASD-informed care, such as "thinking about context," and "being strengths-based." It also fits with emphasizing self-determination and self-advocacy. This person-centered planning process would likely differ a great deal by culture.

Explore Existing Evidence-Based Treatments

Dilemma: Practically speaking, providers are using unmodified, existing evidence-based treatments (EBTs) all the time to respond to symptoms among those with PAE or FASD. This is because PAE is often unknown (or no one has asked), FASD is unrecognized, or providers know about FASD but are not yet offering FASD-informed care. With good reason, clinicians often ask: Why can't I just use the interventions I already have available to me?

<u>Solutions</u>: The fundamental assumption that EBTs do not work for this clinical population needs critical examination using controlled research. This can be done through intervention studies that include groups with FASD or PAE <u>and</u> appropriate comparison groups. This can also be done through secondary data analysis of interventions for youth with similar symptoms (such as ADHD), if treatment researchers in those fields adequately assess PAE.

It is essential to know if existing interventions work with the clinical population of those with PAE or FASD. This is especially true in mental health settings, where a range of EBTs are employed. Flannigan and her colleagues have written that commonly used mental health treatments, such as cognitive behavioral therapy (CBT), or therapies for especially serious symptoms [such as functional family therapy (FFT), dialectical behavior therapy (DBT), or multisystemic therapy (MST)], really need research because they are so broadly applied to those living with FASD [45]. There is also need to further explore the efficacy of the "third wave" mental health treatments that are increasingly in use, such as mindfulness-based approaches or strategies such as acceptance and commitment therapy (ACT).

Understand What Treatment Adaptations Are Needed
for Existing EBTs (and Should Be Built into Novel Treatments)

Dilemma: Over the years, clinical wisdom and caregiver report has led to the fundamental assumption that existing EBTs do not work well for those with PAE or FASD. This has led to the further idea that EBTs must be adapted. At times, this assumption has motivated development of interesting novel treatments to add to the complement of existing EBTs. The assumptions that existing EBTs do not work as efficiently or effectively for those living with FASD or PAE (or do not work at all) are convincing, but so far only based on lived experience. What should be done?

Solutions: Research on the efficacy of existing, non-adapted EBTs with groups living with FASD or PAE is needed, as there is no real source of data to confirm the hypothesis that non-adapted EBTs do not work. But continued systematic research is also needed on what adaptations are needed for existing EBTs, and on the efficacy of novel treatments. This is because adapted and novel treatments may sometimes be needed, because assumptions drawn from lived experience could well be true for some types of intervention (and for different cultural contexts).

For example, family support or positive parenting programs for those living with FASD do basically look different from those in other fields. They necessarily include new types of parent support, as they sometimes require creation of innovative community resources and often involve specialized, thorough education and assistance on advocacy. This is because societal service systems have not yet been built for FASD, eligibility criteria often exclude those with FASD, and stigma must be overcome. As another example, given that FASD is a global health problem, family support programs look very different when developed for English-speaking Western populations living in mixed urban/suburban/rural locations vs. multilingual Indigenous communities living in remote locations.

In addition, this assumption could be true in some cases because individuals with FASD or PAE may travel a range of developmental pathways to problem outcomes that look similar to those of other children (but really aren't). These pathways may be quite complicated given alcohol's wide-ranging, individually variable effects. For example, taking a neurodevelopmental viewpoint, some individuals in this clinical population may show conduct problems because of *impulsivity* arising from PAE, while others show conduct disorders due to *delays in emotional understanding* related to their clinical condition [135]. That would mean some individuals with FASD truly might not respond to "usual" treatments—but not so much due to the simple fact that individuals have the diagnosis of FASD. Instead, the reasons may be much harder to figure out. Why? Because individuals within this group are following variable, diverse developmental pathways influenced by different innate characteristics (that only partly come from the impact of PAE on the brain). In neuroscience, this is termed the "heterogeneity problem" [136]. The usual treatments do not always work because, from individual to individual, the symptoms occur for different reasons than expected, or because PAE results in variable symptoms, and so these individuals require different treatments.

A few researchers have provided practical guidance for how to adapt treatments using a neurodevelopmental viewpoint (how to "reframe and accommodate"). For example, FASD researchers Olson and Montague [19], in a useful resource, offer examples of suggested adaptations for EBTs that can be generally applied, which are described and added to here. First, *services should be offered over a longer period of time,* perhaps with more sessions and/or repetition as needed. Second, *slower intervention progress should be expected,* given the need for considerable review and practice, and caregiver assistance to help children consolidate learning. Third, for individuals with PAE or FASD, *sensory sensitivities and behavior regulation problems should be accommodated in treatment,* which can be done in many ways. Fourth, *treatment procedures and goals should be adapted to the functional level and different cognitive-behavioral profiles of the treated individuals, including strengths.* (For example, use visual prompts if visual processing is a strength, limit verbal input if verbal processing is a challenge, and rely on experiential methods such as roleplay or real-world practice. Also try to focus on improved adaptive behavior in every intervention.) Finally, no matter what the intervention, *individual and caregiver emotional support should be built in.* This is important so everyone can tolerate slow progress, deal with high stress and personal distress, and improve their sense of competence.

Build the Evidence-Base and Address Treatment Gaps (Which Points to Future Research Directions)

Dilemma: There is a developing evidence base of controlled research, as laid out in the tables in this chapter. Clinicians should learn about this evidence base, and use it when they can. But systematic and critical reviewers have noted many gaps in the treatment research. Simply put, research has not yet produced an adequate complement of interventions for those living with FASD or PAE, and their families, and there is certainly not a complete set of evidence-based best practices. What are fruitful future research directions?

Solutions:

Intervention for different developmental phases: Given its importance from so many theoretical perspectives, early intervention with samples with clearly diagnosed FASD or adequately assessed PAE has not received enough attention, and should be an area of intense research interest, with larger samples. Recently, researchers found that a wide range of early interventions were generally effective in reducing ADHD symptoms and enhancing working memory, a promising finding [137]. Enhancing services that can be integrated into existing early intervention settings are of special interest, because they are cost-effective and can reach larger numbers of children. For the preschool years, there are also multiple skill-building interventions that take advantage of neuronal plasticity and sensitive periods in development that have been (or could be) tested to move the field forward.

Clearly, treatments for transition-aged youth and older individuals living with FASD are sorely needed. Beyond this, however, geriatric care for those living with FASD must become a focus. It is now being revealed that this population may face more (and perhaps earlier) significant bodily health conditions as they age [121], and recent data show they continue to contend with challenging mental health issues [120]. In Tables 13.1, 13.2, 13.3, 13.4, 13.5, 13.6, 13.7, 13.8, 13.9, 13.10, 13.11, 13.12, 13.13, and 13.14, and earlier in this chapter, the authors have discussed what might fill treatment gaps at different developmental phases.

Remediation of individual-level impairment: For individuals with PAE or FASD, important research directions continue to emphasize intensively enhancing self-regulation and executive function skills across the age range. Examples of promising treatments and ideas are given in Table 13.8. For instance, a series of meta-analyses suggested that promising interventions for non-typically developing populations included the categories of strategy learning (such as the Alert Program or a curriculum called "Unstuck and On Target") and biofeedback-enhanced relaxation training [138]. Remediation of sleep deficits appears vital, and physical activity interventions appear important at least as an adjunct treatment. These physiological interventions can have multiple benefits. Academic interventions are discussed elsewhere in this book. As can be seen in the tables, authors of the current chapter could find no "in process" intervention studies for outcomes for a wide variety of child-focused skills. While this could simply be that these studies are underway and not yet published, it seems vital to expand research to remediate individual-level impairment so treatments are available for person-centered planning.

One especially interesting intervention, presented as a promising direction in Table 13.10, is the Cognitive Orientation to Occupation Performance (CO-OP). This is a task-specific, cognitively-based, problem-solving intervention that guides individuals to independently discover and develop cognitive strategies to perform specific everyday tasks of living. While this may require adaptation for different levels of intellectual function, and careful strategy learning approaches, the CO-OP approach could potentially be used as a treatment to increase adaptive function for specific outcomes that are meaningful for a youth living with FASD or PAE.

Multicomponent interventions: Another important research direction is toward use of multicomponent interventions bringing together treatments that, each on their own, are promising. Together, these can leverage even more positive outcomes— and the "whole may be greater than a sum of the parts." However, multicomponent interventions often become more complicated, less feasible and flexible, and more costly. Sometimes a multicomponent intervention means combining parent-directed and child-directed treatment. But it can also mean bringing together different types of treatments—such as combining direct consultation to parents with consultation with community providers, or applying several types of treatment to the child, youth, or adult. It can even mean providing a preschool curriculum (such as Tools of the Mind), modular treatments (such as STAND), or a longer term, multilayered treatment, such as Treatment Foster Care Oregon (TFCO, which has many components and versions for preschoolers, children, and adolescents; see Tables 13.13 and 13.14), which can be very complicated but effective. Multicomponent interventions have been tested with efficacy in the field of FASD, such as the MILE program or Families on Track, yielding sustained treatment effects or a broader range of impact on child outcomes. Multicomponent treatments may be especially important for lasting neurobiological change, for more complex problems (such as serious trauma, foster care, or delinquency), and for older individuals living with FASD.

Also bringing together multiple components is the innovative idea of integrating child-directed neurobiological and metacognitive strategies. A prime example is new, feasible FASD intervention research combining transcranial direct-current stimulation and working memory training (see Table 13.9). Applying this integration technique to other metacognitive strategies, especially those thought to have more generalizable effects across neurocognitive domains (such as attention training), may be an intriguing direction to explore.

Tiers of care: FASD researcher Olson [34] has proposed the idea of three "treatment tiers" as a solution, which can be helpful in identifying what treatments are most needed to fill gaps in the continuum of care, and what could be a major focus of the effort to create best practices [34]. The notion is that the complement of FASD interventions can be organized into types and levels of treatment on a practical basis. The *first tier* involves a range of preventive interventions, preventing or reducing early harm from PAE, even though some of these interventions may involve more cost. Examples include brief intervention to reduce or stop alcohol use (and therefore prenatal impact) among pregnant persons showing social or binge drinking during a current pregnancy, intensive early intervention, or lower-cost enhancements offered to very young children with PAE involved in existing early intervention services. The *second tier* includes less resource-intensive interventions useful when alcohol-related problems have already made themselves known, but are less functionally impairing. For example, these might be group interventions for particular symptoms, such as controlled social skills training or self-regulation training for groups of children. As other examples, these might include a 1–2 session therapeutic feedback with a transition-aged youth or adult with FASD to offer them self-awareness of their own cognitive-behavioral profile, self-administered app-based interventions, web-based parent education, or networks of natural parent support. The *third tier* includes more resource-intensive interventions for individual or family problems that are more functionally impairing. For example, these might be group or individualized positive parenting interventions, individualized school-based child tutoring to improve math and meta-cognition, or intensive case management support for women who themselves have FASD or who show serious chemical dependency and associated psychosocial risks.

Outcome measurement at the level of neurobiology: When appropriate, FASD intervention research should examine brain–behavior relationships, going beyond outcome measurement through interview, questionnaires, or observations of change in behavior. The central concern about alcohol is that it is a neurobehavioral teratogen and, ingested during pregnancy, can damage central nervous system (CNS) development. More than this, PAE is often associated with serious psychosocial risks (such as trauma) which can also negatively impact CNS development and function. For treatments that may improve underlying neurobiology, it seems vital to examine the impact of treatment on CNS structure and function through neuroimaging methods and neurochemistry. If a treatment can improve underlying neurobiology, it is even more possible that developmental trajectories made atypical by PAE and associated risk factors can be normalized.

Potential experimental treatments derived from basic research: Although not a topic for this chapter, it is worth mentioning promising treatment directions arising as potential experimental treatments derived from basic research. Categories include blocking alcohol's teratogenic effects, enhancing neuroprotective factors, and providing nutritional supplementation. An earlier, seminal overview of these ideas by Idrus and Thomas is available to readers [23]. There are many intriguing updates of these ideas, with the focus still primarily on basic research. For example, a recent paper discusses possibilities derived from research in animal models examining the impact of antioxidant treatments on adverse outcomes of PAE resulting from the presumed mechanism of oxidative stress [139]. But it is research on choline, a nutritional supplement first identified as promising in animal models and then in careful human study, that has really moved forward as an FASD intervention. Choline has been identified as a substance that may be effective in reducing the impact of PAE when administered during pregnancy, which may possibly even be effective during some periods of postnatal development. One set of studies on choline by FASD researcher Wozniak and his team tells an interesting story. An initial, randomized, double-blind placebo-controlled pilot study of choline vs. placebo was carried out with children with FASD, finding choline safe and well tolerated. Additional studies were carried out, with mixed findings on choline effectiveness. Then participants from the first two trials were examined at a 4-year follow-up. When this sample of 31 children with FASD were seen at an average of 8.6 years of age, there were group differences. Compared to 16 children who had received a placebo, the 15 who had been given choline as young children had better scores across a number of domains. These included nonverbal intelligence, visual-spatial skills, working memory, and verbal memory ability, and they showed fewer behavioral symptoms of ADHD [140, 141].

Psychopharmacology is also not a topic for this chapter. However, given Kodituwakku's guideline regarding the need for appropriate pharmacologic intervention to accompany the behavioral treatments [31] discussed in this chapter, one point is important here. Psychopharmacology is an area strikingly in need of systematic treatment research. There are two recent systematic reviews of medication use in FASD [84, 85] that reveal how much research needs to be done, with a strong recommendation for doing clinical trials. At present, there exist no empirically based guidelines for treatment of children in this clinical population. There is only a recent treatment algorithm, based on expert opinion, designed to treat the complex symptoms of this clinical population. But this algorithm needs validation. The stated aims of this algorithm are to reduce polypharmacy and result in functional improvements. But the authors acknowledge multiple limitations presented by the absence of specific experiments that inform diagnostic symptom clusters, and the lack of clinical trials that support the efficacy of selected medications [86].

Create Scalable Treatments

Dilemma: Prevalence data show that FASD is a remarkably common problem, and, as the process of FASD identification accelerates, that means a great many families to serve. Treatments tested so far have been efficacious. But they have not been especially scalable or cost-effective. Some require labor-intensive home visiting, and some have multiple components hard to offer in real-world settings because of the need for lengthy training or materials that are hard to use. Many have been studied outside natural community environments. Further, interventions for those with PAE or FASD actually developed in "grass roots" clinical service settings have rarely been fully evaluated. What should be done?

<u>Solutions</u>: Treatment looks different in the transformed digital age. Some individual and family-level treatments can readily be translated to a less expensive, more flexible telehealth delivery modality, as has been done for the FMF Program. Some existing tested treatments are suitable for (or designed for) online delivery, or for mobile health (mHealth) application formats, or are being developed (see Tables 13.5 and 13.9). Online and mHealth app treatments can be self-administered or supported by text-based coaching or phone- or video-based clinician assistance.

For increased efficiency, interventions can be offered in natural environments where individuals already gather, such as schools (e.g., MILE [115], Alert Program [142, 143]), early intervention settings (FMF Bridges [95, 96]), or prisons (see Table 13.11). Online networks are also efficient and potentially very cost-effective interventions that are also strengths-based. These have been used in the community but not necessarily evaluated, yet could be examined in well-designed studies. Ideas include birth mother support networks or transition-aged youth/young adult self-advocacy social media networks.

Treatments developed in actual clinical service settings should be evaluated. This is important so their efficacy can be fully documented, with data to show whether or not they are effective. Finally, "active ingredients," or components of treatments that are found to work well, should be identified, treatments streamlined, and then these more efficient treatments scaled up.

Build a Robust Evidence Base and Set of Best Practices Through Research and Use of Implementation Science

<u>*Dilemma*</u>: *Beyond just developing an adequate complement of interventions, it is also necessary to build a robust evidence base for the most promising treatments. It is then necessary to define a set of best practices. How can this be done?*

<u>Solutions</u>: The solution here requires programmatic research. To do this, independent research groups validate a treatment's efficacy used with fidelity (delivered according to actual treatment model). Studies are also conducted to show that a treatment is effective when actually used in the community, in what is called translational research. This programmatic research generates the evidence that, if sufficient, can allow a practice to be deemed an "evidence-based treatment" or EBT. In the US and in some countries, there are "evidence-based registries" that rate treatments according to the quality and amount of evidence available, such as the California Evidence-Based Clearinghouse [144]. Funding that allows treatments to be delivered to youth and families, such as insurance or Medicaid funding in the US,

is increasingly dependent upon how robust is the evidence base for a treatment. It is difficult to build this evidence base, especially for novel or innovative treatments (even when they are needed for a population with new characteristics). This is because treatment research is lengthy, labor-intensive, and (therefore) costly. But with a good evidence base, "best practices" emerge. Ultimately, according to systematic and critical reviewers, best practices (and concomitant policy change to encourage use of best practices) are what is really needed to make intervention for those living with FASD and PAE a reality.

In building treatments, studies need to aim for a scientific understanding of how and why, and for whom and when, problems arise and treatments work. In fact, the conceptual models used to define the essential elements of FASD-informed care emphasize that it is vital to understand the underlying logic model and theory of change of each intervention. With that understanding, treatments can be streamlined down to their active ingredients so the least amount of resources can be used when they are moved into the community. The solution here is also programmatic research.

It is also vital to ensure that treatments are moved out into the community—and, once used in real-world settings, are used as intended. Implementation science offers solutions. This is the scientific study of methods and strategies that help the uptake of evidence-based practice and research into regular use by providers and policy makers. The field of implementation science tries to close the gap between what we know and what we do by finding and addressing the barriers that slow or stop the uptake of proven evidence-based interventions [145]. This usually involves the input of all key stakeholders in an important process of collaboration. In the field of FASD, it is imperative to systematically examine how best to disseminate, implement, and sustain treatments with fidelity, so they are actually delivered as designed, over time—and thus most likely to yield expected outcomes in community settings. Among other important questions, examining a treatment using implementation science techniques means studying barriers to and facilitators of treatment at all different levels—or using special research designs that more quickly provide information on real-world effectiveness than do the usual study-after-study approaches to programmatic treatment research. The typical time for "bench-to-bedside" intervention research is 20 years. For the field of FASD, this needs to speed up.

Of course, there are also cultural considerations given the fact that FASD is a global health problem, discussed in the next section. Cultural considerations make it even more of a challenge to speed up the intervention research process.

Be Led by the Community to Create Culture-Centered Practices

<u>Dilemma</u>: The 12 essential elements of FASD-informed care may have a relatively "universal" definition that applies across societies and cultures. But, to be effective, specific treatments developed, tested, and implemented must either fit well with the culture and context in which they are deployed—or be appropriately adapted. How

can culture-centered practices be created in a process that involves being led by the community?

Solutions: Interventions not only need to be developed, tested, disseminated, and implemented. But they also must adapted (or created anew) for different cultural contexts, and then disseminated and implemented in these diverse contexts. As FASD researchers Petrenko and Alto have written, each cultural context presents unique elements—and barriers to the implementation process. These researchers note that it is crucial to keep building the complement of published interventions, and to publish all results (even those that are nonsignificant) as well as writing up less rigorously designed community trials. This allows those developing interventions for FASD to be aware of all intervention options. They raise the need for research on cultural barriers to addressing FASD, from awareness to treatment. Further, they advocate for partnerships that extend across countries, and sharing of expertise and experience as widely as possible across local, national, and international levels [110]. Fortunately, international research collaborations do exist, such as that of the Collaborative Initiative on Fetal Alcohol Spectrum Disorders (CIFASD), funded in the US by the NIAAA, but these have only recently moved to a strategic focus on treatment [146].

But how can culture-centered practices be created in a process that involves being led by the community? This is an essential element of FASD-informed care. It is important to conduct community-engaged research, which involves collaborative inquiry with a diversity of stakeholders. This aligns research and service goals with community priorities. Community members should be involved as leaders and co-creators of culturally relevant FASD-informed care and treatment. When needed, developing treatment that is culture-centered means gathering lived experience information that can be used to adapt treatments or even create novel interventions. This is a deeply important, complex process that takes time, sensitivity, and respect for the culture and the people. Here, the process is best illustrated in examples.

One team of Australian researchers collected information from caregivers in individual interviews, and another from community members and providers through a workshop. Information-gathering was via an Australian First Nations conversational process of "yarning," or telling and sharing stories and information, which is both a process and an exchange. In one study, by talking directly with caregivers, researchers learned more about cultural patterns in responses to diagnostic processes for neurodevelopmental impairments and FASD among both Aboriginal and non-Aboriginal caregivers. This could allow needed cultural and contextual adaptation of the diagnostic process [147, 148], which would take time and many additional steps.

Also from Australia is an example of strong community leadership and community-research partnership in creating culture-centered practices: the Marulu Strategy. This was an overall community response developed to respond to FASD and early life stress in a set of almost solely Indigenous remote communities in Western Australia [109]. FASD (and early life stress) prevalence studies in this area had been requested by and conducted alongside, and in collaboration with, those living in the communities. Community leaders had further requested that these prevalence studies be strategically followed, in community partnership, by intervention efforts (and studies) to respond to problems identified by prevalence efforts and to follow the children over time. True to the Marulu Strategy, treatment steps were taken after the prevalence studies were completed. The steps taken were to adapt existing evidence-based interventions to the cultural context, which is a truly challenging process. Among these efforts was the school-based adaptation of the evidence-based Alert Program in these remote Aboriginal Australian communities (e.g., [142, 143]). Another effort was a modification of the Triple P parent training program, which was simultaneously adapted both for FASD and for use in these Aboriginal Australia remote communities to become Jandu Yani U ("For All Families") [107]. The Marulu Strategy has been implemented over a number of years.

Build a Successful Continuum of FASD-Informed Care

<u>Dilemma</u>: There is usually no organized continuum of care for those living with FASD, and their families. When useful services do exist, a major critique has been lack of coordination and continuity of services from one developmental phase to another across the lifespan, without methods for clear transitions (e.g., [58, 61]). For example, researcher Pruner and her colleagues, who gathered lived experiences data from caregivers of children with PAE aged birth to 3 in the US, found that parents did not feel adequately prepared for systems transitions, such as into the school system [61]. Successfully making transitions is also a problem when individuals with FASD are older and expected to be independent and coordinate across multiple types of systems, as there are simply few (or no) methods set up to support change and transition for those who cannot navigate without support. Beyond this, supporting transitions is a particular problem for youth with FASD in complex systems, such as foster care. What are solutions to building a successful continuum of care?

<u>Solutions</u>: Providers need help in building a successful continuum of care for those living with FASD, and their families. Earlier sections of this chapter have discussed what programs have been tested, how research can be done to fill treatment gaps, how to organize treatment into tiers so families can be referred in an organized manner, how to create evidence-informed and evidence-based care, and how to be led by the community to create culture-centered practices.

But families need help in using the care systems that are built. Across different societies, individuals with FASD and their families need organized procedures that route them from one system to another. They need help with transitions. This is important when individuals living with FASD move from one developmental phase to another, when families move to a new geographic location, when eligibility criteria change, and more.

So far, there have been different efforts to solve the problem of building a continuum of FASD-informed care and moving through transitions. At the "grass roots" level, some holistic FASD case management-type interventions, such as the key worker program or Coaching Families program, have been built to solve this problem. Using person-centered planning, these programs place a major focus on helping families establish linkages and navigate systems, to build individual care systems and improve system coordination. This fits well with the essential element of FASD-informed care of "building collaborative partnerships." These programs have been in place in a few Canadian provinces for several decades with good success.

Some agencies, communities, and state systems are trying to build organized care networks for FASD at higher administrative levels in different types of systems. For example, one US state public health system is attempting to strategically build an FASD system of care focused on mental health in a multi-year process. This is a statewide effort, based in community mental health agencies, to provide: (1) mental health provider education on FASD; (2) screening for youth at risk because of PAE who also have behavioral and/or developmental issues; and (3) treatment for youth at risk with either evidence-informed or evidence-based mental health services that are both FASD-informed and trauma-informed (i.e., the Michigan State Department of Public Health FASD State Initiative [149]). Ideally, formal program evaluation would be conducted for any of these efforts to see if outcome change takes place. Governments are also working on transformational policy to create FASD-informed care, such as a strategic policy effort in South Africa [150].

FASD researcher Pei and colleagues have written that the societal response to FASD, at least in Canada, is moving toward a more integrated model. This includes a cohesive process of: (1) early screening, referral, and support for pregnant and postpartum persons; (2) early identification; (3) inclusion of neurological impairment and secondary social and environmental dysfunction with diagnostic criteria; and (4) multilevel and multisystem care and support throughout the lifespan for individuals living with FASD [151]. This Canadian response is a model solution for other countries.

Conclusions

FASD is a global public health problem. Despite progress in community education and prevention efforts, drinking during pregnancy still occurs nearly everywhere. This means every society must face the challenges raised by FASD. Bringing FASD-informed care to communities using culture-centered practices is imperative around the world and will need country-specific health care policy to support it. A vital part of FASD-informed care is to have an adequate complement of treatments that are effective in real-world settings, that can serve to create "best practices." The challenge before us all is to strategically and swiftly move forward in a planful way, and create, test, disseminate, and implement treatments in the real world that raise health, well-being, and quality of life for the courageous individuals living with FASD and PAE, and those who care for them.

Acknowledgments Dr. Carmichael Olson acknowledges the generous, far-seeing, and ongoing support of the Bernard FASD Family Trust. The support of the Trust has truly made possible this work and expanded new research on the Families Moving Forward Program. Also acknowledged with gratitude is the long-term, continuing support of research and clinical services for fetal alcohol spectrum disorders (FASD) by the Center on Child Health, Development and Behavior of the Seattle Children's Research Institute, the Institute on Human Development and Disability, and the Washington State Fetal Alcohol Syndrome Diagnostic and Prevention Network (FAS DPN) based at the University of Washington. Finally, Dr. Carmichael Olson recognizes the pioneering and lasting support of the field of FASD by the Division of Child and Adolescent Psychiatry and Department of Psychiatry and Behavioral Sciences of the University of Washington School of Medicine.

Dr. Carmichael Olson also wishes to acknowledge the deeply valuable input on cultural perspectives integrated throughout the chapter from conversations with a research colleague from the Department of Psychological Medicine, Faculty of Medical and Health Sciences, University of Auckland, NZ (Crawford A 2022, oral communication, 13th and 22nd February).

Dr. Pruner wishes to acknowledge the valuable support of Seattle Children's Research Institute for her postdoctoral fellowship during which she worked on this chapter. Ms. Byington recognizes with appreciation the support of fellow clinicians/researchers who continue to move the field forward and expand the interventions available to this population. Dr. Jirikowic acknowledges the ongoing and meaningful support of the Department of Rehabilitation Medicine in the University of Washington School of Medicine as well as that of the Washington State FAS DPN.

The authors note that Dr. Carmichael Olson is a developer of the Families Moving Forward (FMF) Program, and participant in derivative works. Drs. Pruner and Jirikowic are developers of the in-process FMF Bridges intervention. This could influence discussion of these interventions as they are used as examples. However, the authors have made every effort to be objective in their review throughout this chapter.

The authors wish to thank, with gratitude, the careful, attentive, scholarly manuscript support of Marilyn Haas, MPH, Clinical Research Coordinator II, and Stacy Riffle, RN, Clinical Research Coordinator II, of the Seattle Children's Research Institute.

Finally, the authors dedicate this chapter to the inspiring and resilient individuals living with FASD, and those who care for them with such dedication and determination.

References

1. Jones KL, Smith DW, Ulleland CN, Streissguth P. Pattern of malformation in offspring of chronic alcoholic mothers. Lancet. 1973;1(7815):1267–71.
2. Lemoine P, Harousseau H, Borteyru JP, Menuet JC. Children of alcoholic parents—observed anomalies: discussion of 127 cases. Ouest Med. 1968;8:476–82.
3. Jones KL, Smith DW. Recognition of the fetal alcohol syndrome in early infancy. Lancet. 1973;302(7836):999–1001.
4. Smith DW. Fetal alcohol syndrome and fetal alcohol effects. Neurobehav Toxicol Teratol. 1981;3(2):127.
5. Institute of Medicine (IOM). In: Stratton K, Howe C, Battaglia FC, editors. Fetal alcohol syndrome: Diagnosis, epidemiology, prevention, and treatment. Washington, DC: The National Academies Press; 1996.
6. Streissguth AP, O'Malley K. Neuropsychiatric implications and long-term consequences of fetal alcohol spectrum disorders. Semin Clin Neuropsychiatry. 2000;5(3):177–90.

7. Warren K, Floyd L, Calhoun F. Consensus statement on FASD. Washington, DC: National Organization on Fetal Alcohol Syndrome; 2004.

8. Peadon E, Rhys-Jones B, Bower C, Elliott EJ. Systematic review of interventions for children with fetal alcohol spectrum disorders. BMC Pediatr. 2009;9:35.

9. May PA, Chambers CD, Kalberg WO, Zellner J, Feldman H, Buckley D, et al. Prevalence of fetal alcohol spectrum disorders in 4 U.S. communities. JAMA. 2018;319(5):474–82.

10. Lange S, Probst C, Gmel G, Rehm J, Burd L, Popova S. Global prevalence of fetal alcohol spectrum disorder among children and youth: a systematic review and meta-analysis. JAMA Pediatr. 2017;171(10):948–56.

11. Popova S, Dozet D, Burd L. Fetal alcohol spectrum disorder: can we change the future? Alcohol Clin Exp Res. 2020;44(4):815–9.

12. Ryan DM, Bonnett DM, Gass CB. Sobering thoughts: town hall meetings on fetal alcohol spectrum disorders. Am J Public Health. 2006;96(12):2098–101.

13. Burd L, Popova S. Fetal alcohol spectrum disorders: fixing our aim to aim for the fix. Int J Environ Res Public Health. 2019;16(20)

14. McLachlan K, Flannigan K, Temple V, Unsworth K, Cook JL. Difficulties in daily living experienced by adolescents, transition-aged youth, and adults with fetal alcohol spectrum disorder. Alcohol Clin Exp Res. 2020;44(8):1609–24.

15. Olson HC, Sparrow J. A shift in perspective on secondary disabilities in fetal alcohol spectrum disorders. Alcohol Clin Exp Res. 2021;45(5):916–21.

16. Streissguth AP, Bookstein FL, Barr HM, Sampson PD, O'Malley K, Young JK. Risk factors for adverse life outcomes in fetal alcohol syndrome and fetal alcohol effects. J Dev Behav Pediatr. 2004;25(4):228–38.

17. Kodituwakku PW, Kodituwakku EL. From research to practice: an integrative framework for the development of interventions for children with fetal alcohol spectrum disorders. Neuropsychol Rev. 2011;21(2):204–23.

18. Olson HC, Jirikowic T, Kartin D, Astley S. Responding to the challenge of early intervention for fetal alcohol spectrum disorders. Infant Young Child. 2007;20(2):172–89.

19. Olson HC, Montague RA. An innovative look at early intervention for children affected by prenatal alcohol exposure. In: Adubato SA, Cohen DE, editors. Prenatal alcohol use and fetal alcohol spectrum disorders: diagnosis, assessment and new directions in research and multi-modal treatment. Benthan Science Publisher; 2011; p. 64–107.

20. Streissguth A. Offspring effects of prenatal alcohol exposure from birth to 25 years: the Seattle prospective longitudinal study. J Clin Psychol Med Settings. 2007;14:81–101.

21. Olson H, Ohlemiller M, O'Conner M, Brown C, Morris C, Damus K. A call to action: advancing essential services and research on fetal alcohol spectrum disorders—a report of the national task force on fetal alcohol syndrome and fetal alcohol effect. National Task Force on Fetal Alcohol Syndrome and Fetal Alcohol Effect. 2009; March.

22. Burd LJ. Interventions in FASD: we must do better. Child Care Health Dev. 2007;33(4):398–400.

23. Idrus NM, Thomas JD. Fetal alcohol spectrum disorders: experimental treatments and strategies for intervention. Alcohol Res Health. 2011;34(1):76–85.

24. Murawski NJ, Moore EM, Thomas JD, Riley EP. Advances in diagnosis and treatment of fetal alcohol spectrum disorders: from animal models to human studies. Alcohol Res. 2015;37(1):97–108.

25. Jirikowic T, Gelo J, Astley S. Children and youth with fetal alcohol spectrum disorders: summary of intervention recommendations after clinical diagnosis. Intellect Dev Disabil. 2010;48(5):330–44.

26. Olson HC, Oti R, Gelo J, Beck S. "Family matters": fetal alcohol spectrum disorders and the family. Dev Disabil Res Rev. 2009;15(3):235–49.

27. Malbin D. Fetal alcohol spectrum disorders: trying differently rather than harder. 1st ed. Salem, OR: Oregon Department of Human Services; 2002.

28. Streissguth A. Fetal alcohol syndrome: a guide for families and communities. Baltimore, MD: Paul H. Brookes Publishing Company; 1997.
29. Dubovsky D. Caring for individuals with FASD: what you need to know; what you need to do. CHNET Webinar Presentation; 2014.
30. Mattson SN, Bernes GA, Doyle LR. Fetal alcohol spectrum disorders: a review of the neurobehavioral deficits associated with prenatal alcohol exposure. Alcohol Clin Exp Res. 2019;43(6):1046–62.
31. Kodituwakku PW. A neurodevelopmental framework for the development of interventions for children with fetal alcohol spectrum disorders. Alcohol. 2010;44(7–8):717–28.
32. Leenaars LS, Denys K, Henneveld D, Rasmussen C. The impact of fetal alcohol spectrum disorders on families: evaluation of a family intervention program. Community Ment Health J. 2012;48(4):431–5.
33. Rutman D, Hubberstey C, Hume S. British Columbia's key worker and parent support program: evaluation highlights and implications for practice and policy. In: Riley E, Clarren S, Weinberg J, Jonsson E, editors. Fetal alcohol spectrum disorder: management and policy perspectives of FASD. Wiley-Blackwell; 2011. p. 297–316.
34. Olson HC. Advancing recognition of fetal alcohol spectrum disorders: the proposed DSM-5 diagnosis of "neurobehavioral disorder associated with prenatal alcohol exposure (ND-PAE)". Curr Dev Disord Rep. 2015;2(3):187–98.
35. Rutman D. Article commentary: becoming FASD informed: strengthening practice and programs working with women with FASD. Subst Abuse. 2016;10s1
36. Substance Abuse and Mental Health Service Administration (SAMHSA). Addressing fetal alcohol spectrum disorders (FASD). Rockville, MD: SAMHSA; 2014.
37. Malbin D. Fetal alcohol spectrum disorders: trying differently rather than harder. 2nd ed. Portland, OR: FASCETS; 2011.
38. Reid N, Crawford A, Petrenko C, Kable J, Olson HC. A family directed approach for supporting individuals with fetal alcohol spectrum disorders. Curr Dev Disord Rep. 2022;9:9–18.
39. FASD Changemakers. Nothing about us without us. 2018 [cited 2022 Aug 22]. Available from: https://oursacredbreath.com/2018/09/01/fasd-nothing-about-us-without-us//.
40. Guralnick MJ. A developmental systems model for early intervention. Infant Young Child. 2001;14(2):1–18.
41. Rasmussen C, Andrew G, Zwaigenbaum L, Tough S. Neurobehavioural outcomes of children with fetal alcohol spectrum disorders: a Canadian perspective. Paediatr Child Health. 2008;13(3):185–91.
42. O'Connor MJ, Sigman M, Kasari C. Interactional model for the association among maternal alcohol use, mother-infant interaction, and infant cognitive development. Infant Behav Dev. 1993;16(2):177–92.
43. Guralnick M, Bruder M. Early intervention. In: Matson J, editor. Handbook of intellectual disabilities: integrating theory, research, and practice, Autism and child psychopathology series. Cham: Springer; 2019. p. 717–41.
44. Kapasi A. Achievement motivation and intervention impacts in adolescents with fetal alcohol spectrum disorder. University of Alberta; 2020.
45. Flannigan K, Coons-Harding KD, Anderson T, Wolfson L, Campbell A, Mela M, et al. A systematic review of interventions to improve mental health and substance use outcomes for individuals with prenatal alcohol exposure and fetal alcohol spectrum disorder. Alcohol Clin Exp Res. 2020;44(12):2401–30.
46. Flannigan K, Kapasi A, Pei J, Murdoch I, Andrew G, Rasmussen C. Characterizing adverse childhood experiences among children and adolescents with prenatal alcohol exposure and fetal alcohol spectrum disorder. Child Abuse Negl. 2021;112:104888.
47. Temple VK, Cook JL, Unsworth K, Rajani H, Mela M. Mental health and affect regulation impairment in fetal alcohol spectrum disorder (FASD): results from the Canadian National FASD database. Alcohol Alcohol. 2019;54(5):545–50.

48. Frick PJ, Kemp EC. Conduct disorders and empathy development. Annu Rev Clin Psychol. 2021;17:391–416.
49. Reid N, Petrenko CLM. Applying a developmental framework to the self-regulatory difficulties of young children with prenatal alcohol exposure: a review. Alcohol Clin Exp Res. 2018;42(6):987–1005.
50. Boroda E, Krueger AM, Bansal P, Schumacher MJ, Roy AV, Boys CJ, et al. A randomized controlled trial of transcranial direct-current stimulation and cognitive training in children with fetal alcohol spectrum disorder. Brain Stimul. 2020;13(4):1059–68.
51. Himmelreich M, Lutke C, Hargrove E. The lay of the land: fetal alcohol spectrum disorder (FASD) as a whole-body diagnosis. In: Begun AL, Murray MM, editors. The Routledge handbook of social work and addictive behaviors. 1st ed. London: Routledge; 2020. p. 662.
52. Halfon N, Hochstein M. Life course health development: an integrated framework for developing health, policy, and research. Milbank Q. 2002;80(3):433–79.
53. Halfon N, Larson K, Lu M, Tullis E, Russ S. Lifecourse health development: past, present and future. Matern Child Health J. 2014;18(2):344–65.
54. Wehmeyer ML. Self-determination in adolescents and adults with intellectual and developmental disabilities. Curr Opin Psychiatry. 2020;33(2):81–5.
55. Wehmeyer ML. The importance of self-determination to the quality of life of people with intellectual disability: a perspective. Int J Environ Res Public Health. 2020;17(19):7121.
56. Gómez LE, Monsalve A, Morán ML, Alcedo MÁ, Lombardi M, Schalock RL. Measurable indicators of CRPD for people with intellectual and developmental disabilities within the quality of life framework. Int J Environ Res Public Health. 2020;17(14):5123.
57. Skorka K, McBryde C, Copley J, Meredith PJ, Reid N. Experiences of children with fetal alcohol spectrum disorder and their families: a critical review. Alcohol Clin Exp Res. 2020;44(6):1175–88.
58. Petrenko CL, Tahir N, Mahoney EC, Chin NP. Prevention of secondary conditions in fetal alcohol spectrum disorders: identification of systems-level barriers. Matern Child Health J. 2014;18(6):1496–505.
59. Petrenko CLM, Alto ME, Hart AR, Freeze SM, Cole LL. "I'm doing my part, I just need help from the community": intervention implications of foster and adoptive parents' experiences raising children and young adults with FASD. J Fam Nurs. 2019;25(2):314–47.
60. Elliot E. International overview: the challenges in addressing fetal alcohol spectrum disorders. In: Carpenter B, Blackburn C, Egerton J, editors. Fetal alcohol spectrum disorders: interdisciplinary perspectives. New York: Routledge; 2013. p. 14–26.
61. Pruner M, Jirikowic T, Yorkston KM, Olson HC. The best possible start: a qualitative study on the experiences of parents of young children with or at risk for fetal alcohol spectrum disorders. Res Dev Disabil. 2020;97:103558.
62. Bobbitt SA, Baugh LA, Andrew GH, Cook JL, Green CR, Pei JR, et al. Caregiver needs and stress in caring for individuals with fetal alcohol spectrum disorder. Res Dev Disabil. 2016;55:100–13.
63. Coons K, Watson S, Schinkec R, Yantzid N. Adaptation in families raising children with fetal alcohol spectrum disorder. Part I: what has helped. J Intell Dev Disabil. 2016;41:150–65.
64. Pepper J, Watson S, Coons-Harding K. "Well where's he supposed to live?"—experiences of adoptive parents of emerging adult children with FASD in Ontario. J Dev Disabil. 2019;24(1).
65. Kautz-Turnbull C, Adams T, Petrenko C. The strengths and positive influences of children with fetal alcohol spectrum disorders. Am J Intellect Dev Disabil. 2022;127(5):355–68.
66. Flannigan K, Wrath A, Ritter C, McLachlan K, Harding KD, Campbell A, et al. Balancing the story of fetal alcohol spectrum disorder: a narrative review of the literature on strengths. Alcohol Clin Exp Res. 2021;45(12):2448–64.
67. Brown JD, Sigvaldason N, Bednar LM. Motives for fostering children with alcohol-related disabilities. J Child Family Stud. 2007;16(2):197–208.

68. Astley SJ. Fetal alcohol syndrome (FAS) primary prevention through FAS diagnosis: II. A comprehensive profile of 80 birth mothers of children with FAS. Alcohol Alcohol. 2000;35(5):509–19.
69. Kapasi A, Brown J. Strengths of caregivers raising a child with foetal alcohol spectrum disorder. Child Fam Soc Work. 2017;22(2):721–30.
70. Shonkoff JP, Garner AS, Siegel BS, Dobbins MI, Earls MF, Garner AS, et al. The lifelong effects of early childhood adversity and toxic stress. Pediatrics. 2012;129(1):e232–e46.
71. Reid N, Dawe S, Shelton D, Harnett P, Warner J, Armstrong E, et al. Systematic review of fetal alcohol spectrum disorder interventions across the life span. Alcohol Clin Exp Res. 2015;39(12):2283–95.
72. Pruner ML. Toward earlier identification and strengths-based intervention for infants and toddlers with prenatal alcohol exposure: evidence from the Washington State Fetal Alcohol Syndrome Diagnostic & Prevention Network clinical database. Doctoral dissertation. University of Washington; 2021.
73. Bertrand J, Interventions for Children with Fetal Alcohol Spectrum Disorders Research Consortium. Interventions for children with fetal alcohol spectrum disorders (FASDs): overview of findings for five innovative research projects. Res Dev Disabil. 2009;30(5):986–1006.
74. Zarnegar Z, Hambrick EP, Perry BD, Azen SP, Peterson C. Clinical improvements in adopted children with fetal alcohol spectrum disorders through neurodevelopmentally informed clinical intervention: a pilot study. Clin Child Psychol Psychiatry. 2016;21(4):551–67.
75. Coles CD, Kable JA, Taddeo E, Strickland DC. A metacognitive strategy for reducing disruptive behavior in children with fetal alcohol spectrum disorders: GoFAR pilot. Alcohol Clin Exp Res. 2015;39(11):2224–33.
76. Kable JA, Taddeo E, Strickland D, Coles CD. Improving FASD children's self-regulation: piloting phase 1 of the GoFAR intervention. Child Fam Behav Ther. 2016;38(2):124–41.
77. Petrenko CLM, Pandolfino ME, Roddenbery R. The association between parental attributions of misbehavior and parenting practices in caregivers raising children with prenatal alcohol exposure: a mixed-methods study. Res Dev Disabil. 2016;59:255–67.
78. Petrenko CLM, Demeusy EM, Alto ME. Six-month follow-up of the families on track intervention pilot trial for children with fetal alcohol spectrum disorders and their families. Alcohol Clin Exp Res. 2019;43(10):2242–54.
79. Petrenko CLM, Pandolfino ME, Robinson LK. Findings from the families on track intervention pilot trial for children with fetal alcohol spectrum disorders and their families. Alcohol Clin Exp Res. 2017;41(7):1340–51.
80. Doak J, Katsikitis M, Webster H, Wood A. A fetal alcohol spectrum disorder diagnostic service and beyond: outcomes for families. Res Dev Disabil. 2019;93:103428.
81. Pei J, Baugh L, Andrew G, Rasmussen C. Intervention recommendations and subsequent access to services following clinical assessment for fetal alcohol spectrum disorders. Res Dev Disabil. 2017;60:176–86.
82. Burnside L, Fuchs D. Bound by the clock: the experiences of youth with FASD transitioning to adulthood from child welfare care. First Peoples Child Fam Rev. 2013;8(1):40–61.
83. American Psychiatric Association (APA). American psychiatric association: diagnostic and statistic manual of mental disorders. 5th ed. Arlington, VA: American Pscyhiatric Association; 2013.
84. Mela M, Okpalauwaekwe U, Anderson T, Eng J, Nomani S, Ahmed A, et al. The utility of psychotropic drugs on patients with fetal alcohol spectrum disorder (FASD): a systematic review. Psychiatr Clin Psychopharmacol. 2018;28(4):436–45.
85. Ritfeld GJ, Kable JA, Holton JE, Coles CD. Psychopharmacological treatments in children with fetal alcohol spectrum disorders: a review. Child Psychiatry Hum Dev. 2021;53:268.
86. Mela M, Hanlon-Dearman A, Ahmed AG, Rich SD, Densmore R, Reid D, et al. Treatment algorithm for the use of psychopharmacological agents in individuals prenatally exposed to alcohol and/or with diagnosis of fetal alcohol spectrum disorder (FASD). J Popul Ther Clin Pharmacol. 2020;27(3):e1–e13.

87. Kambeitz C, Klug MG, Greenmyer J, Popova S, Burd L. Association of adverse childhood experiences and neurodevelopmental disorders in people with fetal alcohol spectrum disorders (FASD) and non-FASD controls. BMC Pediatr. 2019;19(1):498.

88. Price A, Cook PA, Norgate S, Mukherjee R. Prenatal alcohol exposure and traumatic childhood experiences: a systematic review. Neurosci Biobehav Rev. 2017;80:89–98.

89. Spieker SJ, Oxford ML, Kelly JF, Nelson EM, Fleming CB. Promoting first relationships. Child Maltreat. 2012;17(4):271–86.

90. Powell B, Cooper G, Hoffman K, Marvin B. The circle of security intervention: enhancing attachment in early parent-child relationships. New York: The Guilford Press; 2014.

91. Henry J, Sloane M, Black-Pond C. Neurobiology and neurodevelopmental impact of childhood traumatic stress and prenatal alcohol exposure. Lang Speech Hear Serv Sch. 2007;38(2):99–108.

92. Cohen J, Mannarino A, Deblinger E. Treating trauma and traumatic grief in children and adolescents. 2nd ed. The Guilford Press; 2017. 126 p.

93. Pollio E, Deblinger E. Trauma-focused cognitive behavioural therapy for young children: clinical considerations. Eur J Psychotraumatol. 2017;8(Suppl. 7):1433929.

94. Hanlon-Dearman A, Malik S, Wellwood J, Johnston K, Gammon H, Andrew KN, et al. A descriptive study of a community-based home-visiting program with preschool children prenatally exposed to alcohol. J Popul Ther Clin Pharmacol. 2017;24(2):e61–71.

95. Jirikowic T. Sensory interventions in early years of childhood. In: Proceedings of the University of Washington 43rd annual Duncan seminar, Seattle, WA; 25 Mar 2022.

96. Jirikowic T, Pruner M. Sensory processing interventions to support behavior regulation and participation for children with FASD and related pre-and postnatal risks. In: Proceedings of the Maine Occupational Therapy Association (MeOTA) conference, 5 Mar 2022. Portland, ME: University of Southern Maine; 2022.

97. Petrenko CL, Parr J, Kautz C, Tapparello C, Olson HC. A mobile health intervention for fetal alcohol spectrum disorders (Families Moving Forward Connect): development and qualitative evaluation of design and functionalities. JMIR Mhealth Uhealth. 2020;8(4):e14721.

98. Salmon J. Fetal alcohol spectrum disorder: New Zealand birth mothers' experiences. Can J Clin Pharmacol. 2008;15(2):e191–213.

99. Let's talk: Stigma and stereotypes-where do we begin. In: Choate PW, Lutke J, Hiemstra K, Stanghetta P, editors. The 7th international conference on fetal alcohol spectrum disorder research, results, and relevance, 1 Mar 2017, Vancouver, BC, Canada. The University of British Columbia (UBC): UBC Interprofessional Continuing Education; 2018. Available from: https://www.interprofessional.ubc.ca/files/2018/06/FASD2017_Stigma_and_Stereotypes_Summary.pdf.

100. Roozen S, Stutterheim SE, Bos AER, Kok G, Curfs LMG. Understanding the social stigma of fetal alcohol spectrum disorders: from theory to interventions. Found Sci. 2020;27:753.

101. Canada Northwest FASD Partnership Ministers. Language guide: promoting dignity for those impacted by FASD. In: Looking after each other: a dignity promotion project; 2017.

102. Choate P, Badry D. Stigma as a dominant discourse in fetal alcohol spectrum disorder. Adv Dual Diagn. 2018;12 https://doi.org/10.1108/ADD-05-2018-0005.

103. Corrigan PW, Lara JL, Shah BB, Mitchell KT, Simmes D, Jones KL. The public stigma of birth mothers of children with fetal alcohol spectrum disorders. Alcohol Clin Exp Res. 2017;41(6):1166–73.

104. Malbin D. Fetal alcohol spectrum disorders: trying differently rather than harder. 3rd ed. Portland, OR: Tectrice Inc.; 2017.

105. Bailey DB Jr. Introduction: family adaptation to intellectual and developmental disabilities. Ment Retard Dev Disabil Res Rev. 2007;13(4):291–2.

106. Green CR, Roane J, Hewitt A, Muhajarine N, Mushquash C, Sourander A, et al. Frequent behavioural challenges in children with fetal alcohol spectrum disorder: a needs-based assessment reported by caregivers and clinicians. J Popul Ther Clin Pharmacol. 2014;21(3):e405–20.

107. Andersson E, McIlduff C, Turner K, Thomas S, Davies J, Elliott EJ, et al. Jandu yani u 'for all families' Triple P-Positive Parenting Program in remote Australian aboriginal communities: a study protocol for a community intervention trial. BMJ Open. 2019;9(10):e032559.
108. Crawford A, Te Nahu LTH, Peterson ER, McGinn V, Robertshaw K, Tippett L. Cognitive and social/emotional influences on adaptive functioning in children with FASD: clinical and cultural considerations. Child Neuropsychol. 2020;26(8):1112–44.
109. Fitzpatrick JP, Oscar J, Carter M, Elliott EJ, Latimer J, Wright E, et al. The Marulu strategy 2008-2012: overcoming fetal alcohol spectrum disorder (FASD) in the Fitzroy Valley. Aust N Z J Public Health. 2017;41(5):467–73.
110. Petrenko CL, Alto ME. Interventions in fetal alcohol spectrum disorders: an international perspective. Eur J Med Genet. 2017;60(1):79–91.
111. Marcellus L, Badry D. Infants, children, and youth in foster care with prenatal substance exposure: a synthesis of two scoping reviews. Int J Dev Disabil. 2021;69:265.
112. Hieneman M, Childs K, Sergay J. Parenting with positive behavior support: a practical guide to resolving your child's difficult behavior. Baltimore, MD: Brookes Publishing Company; 2006. 192 p.
113. Evans SW, Owens JS, Wymbs BT, Ray AR. Evidence-based psychosocial treatments for children and adolescents with attention deficit/hyperactivity disorder. J Clin Child Adolesc Psychol. 2018;47(2):157–98.
114. Frankel F, Paley B, Marquardt R, O'Connor M. Stimulants, neuroleptics, and children's friendship training for children with fetal alcohol spectrum disorders. J Child Adolesc Psychopharmacol. 2006;16(6):777–89.
115. Kully-Martens K, Pei J, Kable J, Coles CD, Andrew G, Rasmussen C. Mathematics intervention for children with fetal alcohol spectrum disorder: a replication and extension of the math interactive learning experience (MILE) program. Res Dev Disabil. 2018;78:55–65.
116. Inkelis SM, Thomas JD. Sleep in infants and children with prenatal alcohol exposure. Alcohol Clin Exp Res. 2018;42(8):1390–405.
117. Kamara D, Beauchaine TP. A review of sleep disturbances among infants and children with neurodevelopmental disorders. Rev J Autism Dev Disord. 2020;7(3):278–94.
118. Streissguth A, Barr H, Kogan J, Bookstein F. Understanding the occurrence of secondary disabilities in clients with fetal alcohol syndrome (FAS) and fetal alcohol effects (FAE): final report to the Centers for Disease Control and Prevention (CDC), Aug 1996. Report No.: Tech. Rep. No. 96-06. Seattle, WA: University of Washington Fetal Alcohol & Drug Unit; 1996.
119. O'Connor MJ, Portnoff LC, Lebsack-Coleman M, Dipple KM. Suicide risk in adolescents with fetal alcohol spectrum disorders. Birth Defects Res. 2019;111(12):822–8.
120. Coles CD, Grant TM, Kable JA, Stoner SA, Perez A. Prenatal alcohol exposure and mental health at midlife: a preliminary report on two longitudinal cohorts. Alcohol Clin Exp Res. 2022;46:232.
121. Moore EM, Riley EP. What happens when children with fetal alcohol spectrum disorders become adults? Curr Dev Disord Rep. 2015;2(3):219–27.
122. Riley EP, Mattson SN, Li TK, Jacobson SW, Coles CD, Kodituwakku PW, et al. Neurobehavioral consequences of prenatal alcohol exposure: an international perspective. Alcohol Clin Exp Res. 2003;27(2):362–73.
123. Joussemet M, Landry R, Koestner R. A self-determination theory perspective on parenting. Can Psychol. 2008;49:194–200.
124. Grolnick W, Levitt M, Caruso A. Adolescent autonomy in context: facilitative parenting in different cultures, domains, and settings. In: Soenens B, Vansteenkiste M, Petegem S, editors. Autonomy in adolescent development: towards conceptual clarity. London: Psychology Press; 2017. p. 240.
125. Ordenewitz LK, Weinmann T, Schluter JA, Moder JE, Jung J, Kerber K, et al. Evidence-based interventions for children and adolescents with fetal alcohol spectrum disorders—a systematic review. Eur J Paediatr Neurol. 2021;33:50–60.

126. Premji S, Benzies K, Serrett K, Hayden KA. Research-based interventions for children and youth with a fetal alcohol spectrum disorder: revealing the gap. Child Care Health Dev. 2007;33(4):389–97.
127. Chandrasena AN, Mukherjee RAS, Turk J. Fetal alcohol spectrum disorders: an overview of interventions for affected individuals. Child Adolesc Mental Health. 2009;14(4):162–7.
128. Paley B, O'Connor MJ. Intervention for individuals with fetal alcohol spectrum disorders: treatment approaches and case management. Dev Disabil Res Rev. 2009;15(3):258–67.
129. Paley B, O'Connor MJ. Behavioral interventions for children and adolescents with fetal alcohol spectrum disorders. Alcohol Res Health. 2011;34(1):64–75.
130. Lange S, Shield K, Rehm J, Anagnostou E, Popova S. Fetal alcohol spectrum disorder: neurodevelopmentally and behaviorally indistinguishable from other neurodevelopmental disorders. BMC Psychiatry. 2019;19(1):322.
131. Petrenko CLM, Kautz-Turnbull C. From surviving to thriving: a new conceptual model to advance interventions to support people with FASD across the lifespan. Int Rev Res Dev Disabil. 2021;61:39–75.
132. Petrenko C, Tapparello C. Leveraging technology to increase quality of life for FASD across the lifespan. National Institute on Alcohol Abuse and Alcoholism: University of Rochester; 2022.
133. OhioGuidestone. Triumph today series. Available from: YouTube.
134. Centers for Disease Control and Prevention. FASDs: materials and multimedia: U.S. National Center on Birth Defects and Developmental Disabilities, Centers for Disease Control and Prevention [updated 2021 May 21, cited 2022 Aug 20]. Available from: https://www.cdc.gov/ncbddd/fasd/materials.html.
135. Petrenko CLM, Pandolfino ME, Quamma J, Olson HC. Emotional understanding in school-aged children with fetal alcohol spectrum disorders: a promising target for intervention. J Popul Ther Clin Pharmacol. 2017;24(2):e21–31.
136. Feczko E, Miranda-Dominguez O, Marr M, Graham AM, Nigg JT, Fair DA. The heterogeneity problem: approaches to identify psychiatric subtypes. Trends Cogn Sci. 2019;23(7):584–601.
137. Shephard E, Zuccolo PF, Idrees I, Godoy PBG, Salomone E, Ferrante C, et al. Systematic review and meta-analysis: the science of early-life precursors and interventions for attention-deficit/hyperactivity disorder. J Am Acad Child Adolesc Psychiatry. 2022;61(2):187–226.
138. Takacs ZK, Kassai R. The efficacy of different interventions to foster children's executive function skills: a series of meta-analyses. Psychol Bull. 2019;145(7):653–97.
139. Zhang Y, Wang H, Li Y, Peng Y. A review of interventions against fetal alcohol spectrum disorder targeting oxidative stress. Int J Dev Neurosci. 2018;71:140–5.
140. Wozniak JR, Fink BA, Fuglestad AJ, Eckerle JK, Boys CJ, Sandness KE, et al. Four-year follow-up of a randomized controlled trial of choline for neurodevelopment in fetal alcohol spectrum disorder. J Neurodev Disord. 2020;12(1):9.
141. Wozniak JR, Fuglestad AJ, Eckerle JK, Fink BA, Hoecker HL, Boys CJ, et al. Choline supplementation in children with fetal alcohol spectrum disorders: a randomized, double-blind, placebo-controlled trial. Am J Clin Nutr. 2015;102(5):1113–25.
142. Wagner B, Latimer J, Adams E, Carmichael Olson H, Symons M, Mazzucchelli TG, et al. School-based intervention to address self-regulation and executive functioning in children attending primary schools in remote Australian aboriginal communities. PLoS One. 2020;15(6):e0234895.
143. Wagner B, Olson HC, Symons M, Mazzucchelli TG, Jirikowic T, Latimer J, et al. Improving self-regulation and executive functioning skills in primary school children in a remote Australian aboriginal community: a pilot study of the alert program®. Aust J Educ. 2019;63(1):98–115.
144. The California Evidence-Based Clearinghouse for Child Welfare. [cited February 15, 2022]. Available from: https://www.cebc4cw.org/.
145. Practical implementation science: moving evidence into action. 1st ed. Springer Publishing Company; 2022. 300 p.

146. Collaborative Initiative on Fetal Alcohol Spectrum Disorders (CIFASD). [cited 2022 Aug 22]. Available from: https://cifasd.org/.

147. Hamilton SL, Maslen S, Watkins R, Conigrave K, Freeman J, O'Donnell M, et al. 'That thing in his head': aboriginal and non-aboriginal Australian caregiver responses to neurodevelopmental disability diagnoses. Sociol Health Illn. 2020;42(7):1581–96.

148. Reid N, Hawkins E, Liu W, Page M, Webster H, Katsikitis M, et al. Yarning about fetal alcohol spectrum disorder: outcomes of a community-based workshop. Res Dev Disabil. 2021;108:103810.

149. Fitzpatrick K. Building an FASD system of care within Michigan's community mental health system. In: 8th International conference on fetal alcohol spectrum disorder, Mar 2019. Vancouver: The University of British Columbia; 2019.

150. Adebiyi BO, Mukumbang FC, Beytell A-M. A guideline for the prevention and management of fetal alcohol spectrum disorder in South Africa. BMC Health Serv Res. 2019;19(1):809.

151. Pei J, Tremblay M, McNeil A, Poole N, McFarlane A. Neuropsychological aspects of prevention and intervention for FASD in Canada. J Pediatr Neuropsychol. 2017;3:25–37.

152. Olson HC, Pruner M, Byington N, Jirikowic T, Kuhn M. Supporting quality of life for individuals and families: a model of FASD-informed care and the future of intervention for fetal alcohol spectrum disorders. In: 6th European conference on fetal alcohol spectrum disorder, Sept 2022. Arendal, Norway.

153. The Safe Babies Court Team (TM): The California Evidence-Based Clearinghouse (CEBC). Available from: https://www.cebc4cw.org/program/safe-babies-court-teams-project/.

154. Koren G. Breaking the cycle (BTC)-20 years of breaking records in managing addicted mothers and their young children. J Popul Ther Clin Pharmacol. 2014;21(3):e505–7.

155. Yazdani P, Motz M, Koren G. Estimating the neurocognitive effects of an early intervention program for children with prenatal alcohol exposure. Can J Clin Pharmacol. 2009;16(3):e453–9.

156. Belcher HME, Butz AM, Wallace P, Hoon AH, Reinhardt E, Reeves SA, et al. Spectrum of early intervention services for children with intrauterine drug exposure. Infant Young Child. 2005;18(1):2–15.

157. Hajal NJ, Paley B, Delja JR, Gorospe CM, Mogil C. Promoting family school-readiness for child-welfare involved preschoolers and their caregivers: case examples. Child Youth Serv Rev. 2019;96:181–93.

158. Gilliam K, Fisher P. Multidimensional treatment foster care for preschoolers: a program for maltreated children in the child welfare system. In: Timmer S, Urquiza A, editors. Evidence-based approaches for the treatment of maltreated children. Child maltreatment, vol. 3. Dordrecht: Springer; 2014. p. 145–62.

159. Dozier M, Lindhiem O, Lewis E, Bick J, Bernard K, Peloso E. Effects of a foster parent training program on young children's attachment behaviors: preliminary evidence from a randomized clinical trial. Child Adolesc Social Work J. 2009;26(4):321–32.

160. Dozier M, Peloso E, Lewis E, Laurenceau JP, Levine S. Effects of an attachment-based intervention on the cortisol production of infants and toddlers in foster care. Dev Psychopathol. 2008;20(3):845–59.

161. Waters SF, Hulette A, Davis M, Bernstein R, Lieberman A. Evidence for Attachment Vitamins: a trauma-informed universal prevention programme for parents of young children. Early Child Dev Care. 2020;190(7):1109–14.

162. Lieberman AF, Ghosh Ippen C, Van Horn P. Child-parent psychotherapy: 6-month follow-up of a randomized controlled trial. J Am Acad Child Adolesc Psychiatry. 2006;45(8):913–8.

163. Lieberman AF, Van Horn P, Ippen CG. Toward evidence-based treatment: child-parent psychotherapy with preschoolers exposed to marital violence. J Am Acad Child Adolesc Psychiatry. 2005;44(12):1241–8.

164. Olds DL. The nurse-family partnership: an evidence-based preventive intervention. Infant Ment Health J. 2006;27(1):5–25.

165. Spieker SJ, Oxford ML, Kelly JF, Nelson EM, Fleming CB. Promoting first relationships: randomized trial of a relationship-based intervention for toddlers in child welfare. Child Maltreat. 2012;17(4):271–86.

166. Reid N, Dawe S, Harnett P, Shelton D, Hutton L, O'Callaghan F. Feasibility study of a family-focused intervention to improve outcomes for children with FASD. Res Dev Disabil. 2017;67:34–46.

167. Grant TM, Ernst CC, Streissguth A, Stark K. Preventing alcohol and drug exposed births in Washington State: intervention findings from three parent-child assistance program sites. Am J Drug Alcohol Abuse. 2005;31(3):471–90.

168. Kable JA, Coles CD, Strickland D, Taddeo E. Comparing the effectiveness of on-line versus in-person caregiver education and training for behavioral regulation in families of children with FASD. Int J Ment Health Addict. 2012;10(6):791–803.

169. Coles CD, Kable JA, Taddeo E. Math performance and behavior problems in children affected by prenatal alcohol exposure: intervention and follow-up. J Dev Behav Pediatr. 2009;30(1):7–15.

170. Kable JA, Coles CD, Taddeo E. Socio-cognitive habilitation using the math interactive learning experience program for alcohol-affected children. Alcohol Clin Exp Res. 2007;31(8):1425–34.

171. Petrenko CLM, Kautz-Turnbull CC, Roth AR, Parr JE, Tapparello C, Demir U, et al. Initial feasibility of the "Families Moving Forward Connect" mobile health intervention for caregivers of children with fetal alcohol spectrum disorders: mixed method evaluation within a systematic user-centered design approach. JMIR Format Res. 2021;5(12)

172. Hundert AS, Huguet A, Green CR, Hewitt AJ, Mushquash CJ, Muhajarine N, et al. Usability testing of guided internet-based parent training for challenging behavior in children with fetal alcohol spectrum disorder (strongest families FASD). J Popul Ther Clin Pharmacol. 2016;23(1):e60–76.

173. Turner K, Reynolds JN, McGrath P, Lingley-Pottie P, Huguet A, Hewitt A, et al. Guided internet-based parent training for challenging behavior in children with fetal alcohol spectrum disorder (strongest families FASD): study protocol for a randomized controlled trial. JMIR Res Protoc. 2015;4(4):e112.

174. Havighurst S, Harley A. Tuning in to kids: emotionally intelligent parenting program manual. Melbourne: University of Melbourne; 2007.

175. Havighurst S, Harley A. Tuning in to kids: emotionally intelligent parenting program manual. Melbourne: University of Melbourne; 2010.

176. Havighurst SS, Wilson KR, Harley AE, Kehoe C, Efron D, Prior MR. "Tuning in to kids": reducing young children's behavior problems using an emotion coaching parenting program. Child Psychiatry Hum Dev. 2013;44(2):247–64.

177. Dishion TJ, Shaw D, Connell A, Gardner F, Weaver C, Wilson M. The family check-up with high-risk indigent families: preventing problem behavior by increasing parents' positive behavior support in early childhood. Child Dev. 2008;79(5):1395–414.

178. Gill AM, Hyde LW, Shaw DS, Dishion TJ, Wilson MN. The family check-up in early childhood: a case study of intervention process and change. J Clin Child Adolesc Psychol. 2008;37(4):893–904.

179. Bearss K, Johnson C, Smith T, Lecavalier L, Swiezy N, Aman M, et al. Effect of parent training vs parent education on behavioral problems in children with autism spectrum disorder: a randomized clinical trial. JAMA. 2015;313(15):1524–33.

180. Whittingham K, Sofronoff K, Sheffield J, Sanders MR. Stepping Stones Triple P: an RCT of a parenting program with parents of a child diagnosed with an autism spectrum disorder. J Abnorm Child Psychol. 2009;37(4):469–80.

181. Bezzina LA. Corrigendum. J Intellect Disabil Res. 2017;61(12):1196.

182. Bezzina LA, Rice LJ, Howlin P, Tonge BJ, Einfeld SL. Syndrome specific modules to enhance the Stepping Stones Triple P public health intervention. J Intellect Disabil Res. 2017;61(9):836–42.

183. Nash K, Stevens S, Greenbaum R, Weiner J, Koren G, Rovet J. Improving executive functioning in children with fetal alcohol spectrum disorders. Child Neuropsychol. 2015;21(2):191–209.

184. Soh DW, Skocic J, Nash K, Stevens S, Turner GR, Rovet J. Self-regulation therapy increases frontal gray matter in children with fetal alcohol spectrum disorder: evaluation by voxel-based morphometry. Front Hum Neurosci. 2015;9:108.

185. Wells AM, Chasnoff IJ, Schmidt CA, Telford E, Schwartz LD. Neurocognitive habilitation therapy for children with fetal alcohol spectrum disorders: an adaptation of the alert program(R). Am J Occup Ther. 2012;66(1):24–34.

186. Griffin MM, Copeland SR. Effects of a self-management intervention to improve behaviors of a child with fetal alcohol spectrum disorder. Educ Train Autism Dev Disabil. 2018;53(4):405–14.

187. O'Connor MJ, Frankel F, Paley B, Schonfeld AM, Carpenter E, Laugeson EA, et al. A controlled social skills training for children with fetal alcohol spectrum disorders. J Consult Clin Psychol. 2006;74(4):639–48.

188. O'Connor MJ, Laugeson EA, Mogil C, Lowe E, Welch-Torres K, Keil V, et al. Translation of an evidence-based social skills intervention for children with prenatal alcohol exposure in a community mental health setting. Alcohol Clin Exp Res. 2012;36(1):141–52.

189. Sparks-Keeney T, Jirikowic T, Deitz J. The Kid's Club: a friendship group for school-age children with fetal alcohol spectrum disorders. Dev Disabil Special Interest Sect. 2011;34(2):1–4.

190. Timler GR, Olswang LB, Coggins TE. "Do I know what I need to do?" A social communication intervention for children with complex clinical profiles. Lang Speech Hear Serv Sch. 2005;36(1):73–85.

191. Keightley M, Agnihotri S, Subramaniapillai S, Gray J, Keresztesi J, Colantonio A, et al. Investigating a theatre-based intervention for indigenous youth with fetal alcohol spectrum disorder: exploration d'une intervention basee sur le theatre aupres de jeunes autochtones atteints du syndrome d'alcoolisme foetal. Can J Occup Ther. 2018;85(2):128–36.

192. Wiskow KM, Ruiz-Olivares R, Matter AL, Donaldson JM. Evaluation of the good behavior game with a child with fetal alcohol syndrome in a small-group context. Behav Interv. 2018;33(2):150–9.

193. Connolly SC, Millians M, Peterman R, Shillingsburg MA. The clinical application of applied behavior analysis in a child with partial fetal alcohol syndrome: a case study. Clin Case Stud. 2016;15(3):225–42.

194. Webster-Stratton C, Jamila Reid M, Stoolmiller M. Preventing conduct problems and improving school readiness: evaluation of the incredible years teacher and child training programs in high-risk schools. J Child Psychol Psychiatry. 2008;49(5):471–88.

195. The Incredible Years. Small group dinosaur curriculum. 2013. Available from: https://incredibleyears.com/programs/child/dinosaur-curriculum/.

196. Rashedi RN, Rowe SE, Thompson RA, Solari EJ, Schonert-Reichl KA. A yoga intervention for young children: self-regulation and emotion regulation. J Child Fam Stud. 2021;30:1–14.

197. Razza RA, Linsner RU, Bergen-Cico D, Carlson E, Reid S. The feasibility and effectiveness of mindful yoga for preschoolers exposed to high levels of trauma. J Child Fam Stud. 2020;29(1):82–93.

198. Domitrovich CE, Cortes RC, Greenberg MT. Improving young children's social and emotional competence: a randomized trial of the preschool "PATHS" curriculum. J Prim Prev. 2007;28(2):67–91.

199. Greenberg M, Kusche C. Building social and emotional competence: the PATHS curriculum. In: Jimerson S, editor. Handbook of school violence and school safety. Mahwah, NJ: Lawrence Erlbaum Associates; 2006. p. 395–412.

200. Barnett WS, Jung K, Yarosz DJ, Thomas J, Hornbeck A, Stechuk R, et al. Educational effects of the tools of the mind curriculum: a randomized trial. Early Child Res Q. 2008;23(3):299–313.

201. Reid N, Harnett P, O'Callaghan F, Shelton D, Wyllie M, Dawe S. Physiological self-regulation and mindfulness in children with a diagnosis of fetal alcohol spectrum disorder. Dev Neurorehabil. 2019;22(4):228–33.

202. Kerns KA, Macoun S, MacSween J, Pei J, Hutchison M. Attention and working memory training: a feasibility study in children with neurodevelopmental disorders. Appl Neuropsychol Child. 2017;6(2):120–37.

203. Bartle D, Rossoff S, Whittaker D, Gooch B, Kerns K, MacSween J. Cognitive games as therapy for children with FAS. Los Angeles, CA: Association for Computing Machinery; 2010.

204. Makela ML, Pei JR, Kerns KA, MacSween JV, Kapasi A, Rasmussen C. Teaching children with fetal alcohol spectrum disorder to use metacognitive strategies. J Spec Educ. 2019;53(2):119–28.

205. Kerns KA, Macsween J, Vander Wekken S, Gruppuso V. Investigating the efficacy of an attention training programme in children with foetal alcohol spectrum disorder. Dev Neurorehabil. 2010;13(6):413–22.

206. Gryiec M, Grandy S, McLaughlin TF. The effects of the copy, cover, and compare procedure in spelling with an elementary student with fetal alcohol syndrome. J Precis Teaching Celerat. 2004;20(1):2–8.

207. Adnams CM, Sorour P, Kalberg WO, Kodituwakku P, Perold MD, Kotze A, et al. Language and literacy outcomes from a pilot intervention study for children with fetal alcohol spectrum disorders in South Africa. Alcohol. 2007;41(6):403–14.

208. Stromland K, Mattson S, Adnams C, Autti-Ramo I, Riley E, Warren K. Fetal alcohol spectrum disorders: an international perspective. Alcohol Clin Exp Res. 2005;29(6):1121–6.

209. Loomes C, Rasmussen C, Pei J, Manji S, Andrew G. The effect of rehearsal training on working memory span of children with fetal alcohol spectrum disorder. Res Dev Disabil. 2008;29(2):113–24.

210. Coles CD, Strickland DC, Padgett L, Bellmoff L. Games that "work": using computer games to teach alcohol-affected children about fire and street safety. Res Dev Disabil. 2007;28(5):518–30.

211. Padgett LS, Strickland D, Coles CD. Case study: using a virtual reality computer game to teach fire safety skills to children diagnosed with fetal alcohol syndrome. J Pediatr Psychol. 2006;31(1):65–70.

212. Keiver K, Bertram CP, Orr AP, Clarren S. Salivary cortisol levels are elevated in the afternoon and at bedtime in children with prenatal alcohol exposure. Alcohol. 2015;49(1):79–87.

213. Pritchard Orr AB, Keiver K, Bertram CP, Clarren S. FAST Club: the impact of a physical activity intervention on executive function in children with fetal alcohol spectrum disorder. Adapt Phys Act Q. 2018;35(4):403–23.

214. Jirikowic T, Westcott McCoy S, Price R, Ciol MA, Hsu LY, Kartin D. Virtual sensorimotor training for balance: pilot study results for children with fetal alcohol spectrum disorders. Pediatr Phys Ther. 2016;28(4):460–8.

215. McCoy SW, Jirikowic T, Price R, Ciol MA, Hsu LY, Dellon B, et al. Virtual sensorimotor balance training for children with fetal alcohol spectrum disorders: feasibility study. Phys Ther. 2015;95(11):1569–81.

216. Welsch L, Alliott O, Kelly P, Fawkner S, Booth J, Niven A. The effect of physical activity interventions on executive functions in children with ADHD: a systematic review and meta-analysis. Ment Health Phys Act. 2021;20:100379.

217. Zhang M, Liu Z, Ma H, Smith DM. Chronic physical activity for attention deficit hyperactivity disorder and/or autism spectrum disorder in children: a meta-analysis of randomized controlled trials. Front Behav Neurosci. 2020;14 https://doi.org/10.3389/fnbeh.2020.564886.

218. Izadi-Najafabadi S, Gunton C, Dureno Z, Zwicker JG. Effectiveness of cognitive orientation to occupational performance intervention in improving motor skills of children with developmental coordination disorder: a randomized waitlist-control trial. Clin Rehabil. 2022;36(6):776–88.

219. Tinker EC, Garrison MM, Ward TM. Development of the sleep health in preschoolers (SHIP) intervention: integrating a theoretical framework for a family-centered intervention to promote healthy sleep. Fam Syst Health. 2020;38(4):406–17.

220. Sonney JT, Thompson HJ, Landis CA, Pike KC, Chen ML, Garrison MM, et al. Sleep intervention for children with asthma and their parents (SKIP study): a novel web-based shared management pilot study. J Clin Sleep Med. 2020;16(6):925–36.
221. Kang KD, Choi JW, Kang SG, Han DH. Sports therapy for attention, cognitions and sociality. Int J Sports Med. 2011;32(12):953–9.
222. Kapasi A, Pei J, Kryska K, Joly V, Gill K, Thompson-Hodgetts S, et al. Exploring self-regulation strategy use in adolescents with FASD. J Occup Ther Sch Early Interv. 2021;14(2):184–206.
223. O'Connor MJ, Quattlebaum J, Castaneda M, Dipple KM. Alcohol intervention for adolescents with fetal alcohol spectrum disorders: project step up, a treatment development study. Alcohol Clin Exp Res. 2016;40(8):1744–51.
224. Millians MN, Coles CD. Case study: Saturday cognitive habilitation program for children with prenatal alcohol exposure. Psychol Neurosci. 2014;7(2):163–73.
225. Katz J, Knight V, Mercer SH, Skinner SY. Effects of a universal school-based mental health program on the self-concept, coping skills, and perceptions of social support of students with developmental disabilities. J Autism Dev Disord. 2020;50(11):4069–84.
226. Brintnell ES, Sawhney AS, Bailey PG, Nelson M, Pike AD, Wielandt P. Corrections and connection to the community: a diagnostic and service program for incarcerated adult men with FASD. Int J Law Psychiatry. 2019;64:8–17.
227. Denys K, Rasmussen C, Henneveld D. The effectiveness of a community-based intervention for parents with FASD. Community Ment Health J. 2011;47(2):209–19.
228. Barto B, Bartlett JD, Von Ende A, Bodian R, Norona CR, Griffin J, et al. The impact of a statewide trauma-informed child welfare initiative on children's permanency and maltreatment outcomes. Child Abuse Negl. 2018;81:149–60.
229. De Bruin EJ, Bögels SM, Oort FJ, Meijer AM. Efficacy of cognitive behavioral therapy for insomnia in adolescents: a randomized controlled trial with internet therapy, group therapy and a waiting list condition. Sleep. 2015;38(12):1913–26.
230. Sibley MH, Graziano PA, Kuriyan AB, Coxe S, Pelham WE, Rodriguez L, et al. Parent-teen behavior therapy + motivational interviewing for adolescents with ADHD. J Consult Clin Psychol. 2016;84(8):699–712.
231. Åström T, Bergström M, Håkansson K, Jonsson AK, Munthe C, Wirtberg I, et al. Treatment foster care Oregon for delinquent adolescents: a systematic review and meta-analysis. Res Soc Work Pract. 2020;30(4):355–67.
232. McCauley E, Berk MS, Asarnow JR, Adrian M, Cohen J, Korslund K, et al. Efficacy of dialectical behavior therapy for adolescents at high risk for suicide: a randomized clinical trial. JAMA Psychiat. 2018;75(8):777–85.
233. Celinska K, Sung H-E, Kim C, Valdimarsdottir M. An outcome evaluation of functional family therapy for court-involved youth. J Fam Ther. 2019;41(2):251–76.
234. Timmons-Mitchell J, Bender MB, Kishna MA, Mitchell CC. An independent effectiveness trial of multisystemic therapy with juvenile justice youth. J Clin Child Adolesc Psychol. 2006;35(2):227–36.

Heather Carmichael Olson, Ph.D. is a Clinical Professor at the University of Washington School of Medicine, and a faculty member at the Seattle Children's Research Institute and Hospital. As a clinical and developmental psychologist, for over 30 years she has explored the effects of prenatal substance exposure on child and family development in research, teaching, public policy, and direct service to children and families. She has dedicated her career to development, testing and implementation of effective interventions for youth at high risk because of prenatal alcohol exposure and fetal alcohol spectrum disorders (FASD), and the families who care for them.

Misty Pruner, Ph.D., OTR/L is a postdoctoral fellow at the Seattle Children's Research Institute and recent graduate from the University of Washington (UW) Rehabilitation Science PhD program. Inspired by front-line work as a pediatric occupational therapist for over 13 years, her dissertation focused on early identification and strengths-based intervention of infants and toddlers with prenatal alcohol exposure. Dr. Pruner has a special interest in clinical research and program development that promotes nurturing parent–child relationships and optimizes long-term neurodevelopmental outcomes. Dr. Pruner also now works as an Occupational Therapist and LEND Faculty at the UW Institute on Human Development and Disability.

Nora Byington, B.S. after receiving a bachelor's degree in Biomedical Sciences from Colorado State University, embarked on a career in pediatric clinical study coordination. Previously a Clinical Research Coordinator at the Seattle Children's Research Institute studying children's developmental trajectories, she currently holds a position as a Neuroimaging Specialist at the Masonic Institute for the Developing Brain at the University of Minnesota. Her expertise includes neuroimaging, psychometrics, biospecimens, and regulatory affairs. Ms. Byington's primary research interests encompass exploration of typical and atypical neurodevelopmental trajectories and the identification and testing of potential early life interventions.

Tracy Jirikowic, Ph.D., OTR/L, FAOTA is a Professor in the Division of Occupational Therapy at the University of Washington. She has held a clinical appointment with the Washington State Fetal Alcohol Spectrum Disorders Diagnostic and Prevention Network for over 20 years. Her research focuses on children affected by prenatal alcohol and substance exposure and family supports and outcomes. This includes early identification and intervention for young children, assessment and interventions to support sensory processing and sensorimotor development, and community-based supports and interventions that promote inclusion and participation for children and their families.

Chapter 14
Ethical and Social Issues in FASD

Christina Tortorelli, Dorothy Badry, Peter Choate, and Kerryn Bagley

Introduction

Ethical and social challenges, exacerbated by stigma are a salient reality for both pregnant individuals and children, youth, and adults who have either suspected or diagnosed fetal alcohol spectrum disorder (FASD). Stigma is the belief or perception of others. Discrimination is the act of treating someone differently based on one's perception. The Canadian Mental Health Association [1] clarifies the difference, "Stigma is the negative stereotype and discrimination is the behaviour that results from this negative stereotype." Ethical and social issues are at play every day for professionals working in the FASD context. Further, community members, afraid of what they do not understand behave in ways that demonstrate discomfort, misinformation, and/or entrenched ideas about persons with FASD. Judgments and biases create further stigma resulting in further trauma, gaps in service delivery, and increased stress. These experiences can compel caregivers to be ultra-strong advocates in the face of numerous barriers [2, 3].

Critical ethical considerations exist for FASD. The term FASD alone raises alarm bells because it directly implicates mothers as responsible for prenatal alcohol exposure (PAE) and as the cause of their child's lifelong disability. There are no

C. Tortorelli (✉) · P. Choate
Department of Child Studies and Social Work, Mount Royal University, Calgary, AB, Canada
e-mail: ctortorelli@mtroyal.ca; pchoate@mtroyal.ca

D. Badry
Faculty of Social Work, University of Calgary, Calgary, AB, Canada
e-mail: badry@ucalgary.ca

K. Bagley
Department of Community and Allied Health, La Trobe University,
Melbourne, VIC, Australia
e-mail: kbagley@latrobe.edu.au

other disabling conditions that so directly denote a social cause of a disability—alcohol use in pregnancy, that is in principle, considered preventable, but not as preventable as one might think when understood and contextually grounded in the complex lives of biological mothers.

Jones and Smith [4] were one of the earliest to demonstrate a causal link between prenatal alcohol exposure and adverse fetal consequences, it unfortunately also set the stage for stigmatization of behaviors during pregnancy that were previously thought to be harmless. They introduced the term fetal alcohol syndrome. Had FASD been named Lemoine [5] or Jones and Smith [4] Syndrome, would that have made a difference to the long-standing experiences of stigma experienced by biological mothers of children with PAE? In 2014, a paper was published that examined a criminal injury claims case in the UK where financial compensation was sought due to prenatal alcohol exposure. The case was initially rejected, overturned on appeal by a tribunal and subsequently overturned on judicial review based on the consideration that a fetus did not have the status of personhood until actually born [6]. This case highlights the ethical, moral, and legal dilemmas surrounding FASD.

This chapter focuses on the strengths and challenges individuals with FASD and their caregivers experience while interacting with systems that do not understand the uniqueness and complexity of this spectrum of disorders. We challenge those stereotypes as not representative of the vast majority of people with FASD. Next, we contemplate alternate ways of thinking about FASD. The differences made by taking a person-first approach are shared, most importantly from the perspective of those with FASD. As you read this chapter, we ask you to reflect on your assumptions, biases, and perspectives, assess your knowledge of FASD, develop a plan for further professional development, and continuously ask yourself "Are you listening?"

In the FASD Context

People with FASD possess dreams, strengths, and hopes for the future as might any other person. We have seen with a variety of disabilities, that when a strengths and possibilities approach is applied, the person gains momentum that increases their quality of life. The person with FASD is deserving of the same. To shift the perspective of FASD to one of a disability with possibility requires a change in the context of professional, research and academic dialogue which tends toward deficit models [7].

PAE is not new, yet knowledge about FASD often remains limited in health and social services. It has long been known that alcohol use during pregnancy can be harmful. Research has traced the linkage between alcohol use and pregnancy from pre-1700, to the eighteenth and nineteenth centuries and into current times highlighting biblical references in the Book of Judges 13:3–4 admonishing women to refrain from alcohol use during conception and pregnancy. Gin Lane is highlighted in England in the eighteenth to nineteenth centuries suggesting drunkenness was relegated to the lower classes of society. A famous illustration by William Hogarth in 1751 showed the mothers in desperation neglecting their children. It was one of a pair of illustrations intended on showing the impact of the dramatic increase in gin consumption and its impact on society. It is noted that the Temperance Movement and Prohibition was less scientific and more "moralistic" [8]. Tracing the history of alcohol use and pregnancy, the work of Roquette [9] (1957), Lemoine [5] (1968), and Jones and Smith [4] (1973) are highlighted, as is the first recommendation suggesting women limit alcohol use in pregnancy to two drinks a day in a US Food and Drug Administration Drug Bulletin [10] published in 1977 [11].

FASD is often termed the 100% preventable disorder—a message that is highly stigmatizing to women. The message fails to understand the underlying trauma that is common to many of the individuals who consume alcohol in pregnancy [7]. This message is typically linked to FASD being the most common cause of brain-based birth defects. Even though FASD exists across a spectrum and expressions of the disability range from mild through to severe, the public discourse is often focused upon the most severe group. The discourse is dominated by incapacity as opposed to capacity. It has been noted in prevalence research that individuals have milder expressions of FASD are not always picked up. Identifying these individuals would increase prevalence rates [12].

Part of the reason that milder cases go undetected is related to the lower severity of impact. If we only consider cases with more severe expressions of FASD, the perception of the disability becomes skewed. There are many expressions of FASD and it is critical to acknowledge that many individuals have strengths and capacities that often go unrecognized when so much attention is paid to individuals with serious problems [13].

In our view, a strengths and possibilities perspective is in line with the United Nations Convention on the Rights of Persons with Disabilities (UNCRPD) [14] which has been signed by all but 8 members of the United Nations (UN). The most notable exception is the United States. The UN Convention on the Rights of the Child [15] is also applicable. The United States is the only member to not have ratified the convention.

There is a particular issue in Canada in that indigenous peoples, who have been subject to cultural genocide are particularly traumatized and more prone to substance abuse issues [16], but also to over surveillance in research regarding FASD [17]. As a result, indigenous peoples with FASD are overrepresented in the criminal justice, health care, and child protection systems [18, 19]. Other colonized countries such as Australia and New Zealand have similar experiences. As the British Columbia Representative for Children and Youth has shown, it is racism, stigma, and classism that lead to indigenous children most often being assessed for FASD. Although FASD occurs across all spectrums of the population, more advantaged children presenting with similar clinical profiles are assessed for autism spectrum disorder (ASD) or attention deficit hyperactivity disorder (ADHD) [20]. Indeed, given the similarity of symptoms between FASD, ASD, and ADHD, all children presenting for assessment within this cluster should be considered for all three possibilities [21]. However, given the information in Charlesworth [20] race may well be acting as a lens through which to determine which diagnosis to consider. As this report shows, an indigenous child will more likely be screened for FASD.

This same report [20] notes that a failure to understand the nature of the disorder, its expressions, as well as the supports needed leave people with FASD out of disability support networks. For example, in the Canadian province of Alberta, the program, Persons with Developmental Disabilities (PDD) [22] has an IQ cut off of 70. Many people with FASD will score higher than 70 but, due to the disability, they face serious challenges in adaptive skills and daily functioning and are desperately in need of disability services.

Charlesworth [20] emphasizes the blame that continues to be placed on persons with FASD, through which the community views the disorder as preventable and the behaviors of the young person or adult as intentional. As a mostly hidden or invisible disability, assumptions prevail. The poignant words of Mr. Myles Himmelreich, a person with FASD, reinforce these perceptions:

> The general public's lack of FASD knowledge leads to our behaviours being seen as "bad." The lack of support leads to failure. The lack of care leads to low self worth. I often refer to the saying "I'm not the only one" as what individuals with FASD say when they have the opportunity to interact with others with the same diagnosis. It is said when talking about not being the only one to struggle in school or to be misunderstood or to have sensory issues or to struggle with showing correct emotions and much more. In doing this project, I got to see these children and youth saying, "I am smart," "I do try," "I care" [20].

Himmelreich et al. [23] (2020) have shown that FASD is not just a brain disorder as it has often been portrayed. Rather, it is a whole-body disorder in which there are a number of physical manifestations that occur in both higher frequency and in earlier stages of life than would be seen in the general population. FASD impacts physical, sensory, mood, behavioral, and cognitive aspects of a person's life in ways that are seen across the FASD population but in very unique ways in personal expression and throughout the life course of the person. This reinforces the need for disability supports that are based in a full understanding of the disorder.

In the Community Context

> Kathy Mitchell wants to share something with you. She's not proud of it, and it's not a behavior she hopes you'll emulate. It's just the truth: As a teen, Kathy drank alcohol while pregnant with her daughter, Karli. It was a perilous if unwitting mistake that has defined both of their lives [24].

As the above quote shows, mothers are seen as primarily responsible for harming their baby in pregnancy and therefore are shamed and blamed [25]. Kathy Mitchell is now a champion of FASD support and prevention. In the story, the mother tells of her own internalized shame and grief which helps us to see how important the value of the relationship is between the parent and professional Ms. Mitchell's story illustrated how she successfully parented her daughter [24].

The work of Choate et al. [18] (2020) shows that parents with FASD are seen as incapable of parenting their own children. These assumptions are so strong that parents, presumed but not diagnosed with FASD, are seen from this perspective. However, as Fig. 14.1 shows, a mother with an FASD child can be required to maneuver her way through multiple systems, all with demands around assessment, eligibility, oversight, lack of coordination, and conflicting expectations. The processes are very time intensive. Fathers are often absent from this web or are seen as ancillary. An ethical approach would be to offer systemic management support, increase inter-agency cooperation, and reduce the complexity that the mother must encounter and traverse.

There are several elements that contribute to inaccurate community perceptions regarding the cause of FASD. Perhaps one of the most inaccurate views is that there is a conscious choice to expose the fetus to alcohol. This fails to consider the lived realities of mothers who may be trying to navigate inter-personal violence, trauma, and lack of access to community supports [18]. This misperception leads to the way that the community treats the parents of individuals with FASD. Mothers are seen as responsible for the lifelong outcomes their child may have as a result of exposure to alcohol in utero. The only preventative measure that is guaranteed to end FASD is for all females to abstain from any alcohol consumption from the onset of puberty to the completion of menopause. At a minimum this is unfair and at most unattainable causing increasing stigma toward women no matter their relationship to a child with FASD [25, 26].

From the perspective of the community, this removes the more compassionate disability language and places the person with FASD squarely in the category of being a burden to society [27, 28]. Greenmyer et al. [29] reviewed the medical costs associated with a diagnosis of FASD (Canada and the United States) concluding

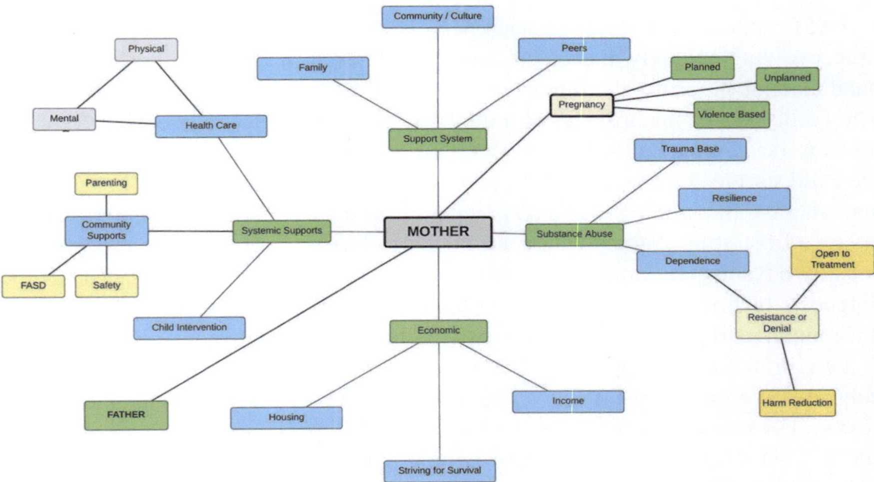

Fig. 14.1 The complexity of managing FASD through multiple systems. In this example, the mother navigates economic, health, mental health, personal, and community supports

that the costs are higher than for other conditions such as autism spectrum disorder. The authors note that "the costs accrued by FASD are the result of both primary exposures to alcohol and adverse developmental outcomes" [29]. When analyzed from a disease burden perspective, then stigma is elevated.

Professional/System Context

Is FASD a disability? This ethical question is raised frequently in relation to FASD. For most childhood disabilities, there is an underlying medical or genetic cause that is outside of the control of the mother. These disabilities are often noted prior to birth or at the time of birth. Disabilities such as Down syndrome or cerebral palsy that are present at birth evolve during childhood requiring multi-system assessment and diagnosis to establish the extent of the disability and identify required interventions. Care and compassion for parents of children with these types of disabilities are strong, with family, community, and medical resources available for support in the developed world.

When considering the impact of a diagnosis of FASD, the Canada FASD Research Network has examined varying definitions of the condition and in a recently published the following definition:

> Fetal Alcohol Spectrum Disorder (FASD) is a diagnostic term used to describe impacts on the brain and body of individuals prenatally exposed to alcohol. FASD is a lifelong disability. Individuals with FASD will experience some degree of challenges in their daily living, and need support with motor skills, physical health, learning, memory, attention, communication, emotional regulation, and social skills to reach their full potential. Each individual with FASD is unique and has areas of both strengths and challenges [30].

FASD appears differently in each person and may be a hidden disability for a time, evolving uniquely in each circumstance. Even if the birth mother reports prenatal alcohol exposure, the impact on the infant is frequently not noted upon birth. The family leaves the hospital with the hope that their child will develop typically meeting developmental milestones within usually anticipated timeframes. Should the child start to show signs of struggling with intellectual function, self-regulation, and adaptive functioning [31] a complex process begins, taking the family/caregivers on a frustrating journey where answers are elusive. For more economically and socially advantaged families, professionals are less likely to explore FASD as the diagnosis of first consideration while families less advantaged are more likely to have inquiries regarding PAE made early on in the investigative process.

Few professionals approach FASD as a spectrum disorder, meaning that they believe you either have FASD or you don't. This is certainly so in the public discourse. For children, youth, and adults with FASD, this complicates their experiences in life as there is one perspective, limiting focus on strengths and adaptability. Moreover, professionals are influenced by their personal stances on alcohol use, substance use disorders, culture, personal experiences, and exposure to accurate information about FASD [3, 32]. Brown [27] discusses the intersection with the justice system and the lack of knowledge that those involved with youth and young adults hold. Barriers to assessment and diagnosis result in limited information coming before the court. Probation, Child Welfare, Lawyers, and the Judiciary have varied levels of accurate knowledge of what it means to have fetal alcohol spectrum disorder and as a result, questions are not asked, planning and sentencing options are not considered nor individualized. Choate et al. [18] reviewed 41 legal cases from across Canada in which the parent's capacity to care for their child long term was in question. In all cases either the parent had a diagnosis of FASD [26] or were suspected to have FASD [7]. The results of the cases overwhelmingly resulted in the state obtaining permanent guardianship of the child. The outcomes in 41 these cases which reinforces the position of Brown and colleagues [27].

The medical model necessary for diagnosis is based on deficits, citing underlying causes from a biological, disease perspective. This model is not a good fit with the social and behavioral challenges of having FASD. A person's identity, based on perceived inadequacies, creates the narrative of being "not enough" [33]. In contrast, the social model of disability recognizes that society is structured in ways that compound the challenges of having FASD and contribute to negative attitudes associated with disability in general. The social model holds society responsible for removing those barriers and shifting the dialogue from challenge to success. It is through the lens of a social model that persons with FASD are treated as respected individuals with strengths and abilities [34].

Of note, there are champions introducing narrative approaches into medical and interdisciplinary conversations [35]. Charon advocates for an "assets-based approach... as opposed to a deficits-based and pathology-replicating paradigm." A blending together of the social model and narrative medicine in the context of FASD would position individuals with FASD as the authors of their own story.

Let's return to the ethical question of whether FASD should be framed as a disability recognizing that it is lifelong and deserving of the requisite support that enhances the person's life. Definitions contained in a publication by the National Academies of Sciences [36] are thought-provoking and provide an alternate way of understanding how FASD could be viewed. Their definition of children's health uses the language of children being able or enabled to succeed by realizing their potential, having their needs satisfied. In contrast, childhood disability [37] is defined as having health-related limitations to successfully interacting with society, still considering the individual's desired level of interaction. Looking at the definition of health—any child with FASD would fall under the definition of health if society provided each child with targeted resources to meet their individual needs and supported them to interact successfully with society. This perspective aligns with the social model of disability and the CanFASD definition which calls attention to the unique strengths and challenges experienced by each child, youth, and adult requiring targeted and lifelong support [38].

We are of the view that the ethical answer is that FASD is a disability deserving supports and services provided to others with developmental disabilities. We are also of the view that the health of the individual with FASD is directly related to the support that they are provided with over their lifetime. This, however, has not been the experience of most individuals and caregivers.

Resources

Concerns of alcohol use and pregnancy spark some of the most contentious ethical debates that exist in modern times. However, it is critical to recognize that prenatal alcohol exposure (PAE) is a point in time over a lifetime that occurs before the birth of the child. It is critical to situate FASD as a lifespan disability that requires supports from birth to adulthood. Once FASD is recognized and diagnosed the need to provide supports and interventions exists. When health professionals recognize that FASD is a concern, it is incumbent upon them to consider effective supports and interventions. The individual who has PAE and has been diagnosed with FASD should have rights and entitlements to disability services to support them over their lifespan. However, things are not that simple. FASD remains a highly stigmatized disability that often goes unrecognized and therefore underserved. Many people go through their whole life without an FASD diagnosis and they struggle. Many become parents and can contribute to the intergenerational cycle of FASD without interventions to support individuals in their challenges with addictions.

FASD is a life span disability, and individuals require supports from early childhood to adulthood including "navigating physical health, mental health, disability, employment, legal, and family services" [39]. It is well known that children and adults impacted by PAE have often had adverse childhood experiences and exposure to trauma. Children and youth with FASD are at high risk of suicidal ideation and attempts as noted in recent Canadian research that also identified higher reported rates of sexual and physical abuse for those with FASD living within the child welfare system in comparison to those in other living situations [40]. FASD is also identified as a transgenerational problem and noted by several researchers as a diagnosis of moral disorder in conceiving and child-bearing women [41, 42] who are subject to "moral policing" [6].

There is a small body of literature on adoptive and foster parents and it is noted in one international study that 15% of children seen through an adoption clinic and below 2 years of age met the diagnostic criteria for FASD [43]. Foster parents caring for children with FASD often receive children who have had severe trauma, have experienced multiple placements and disrupted relationships [44]. Adoptive parents of children with FASD face challenges getting services and often have to actively advocate with child welfare services to provide necessary supports for their children.

Access to Services and Supports

Access typically requires a diagnosis. For those with suspected but not confirmed FASD, this is a gap worth noting. This information gap stems from the stigma and shame of admitting to alcohol consumption during pregnancy. Birth mothers describe deep feelings of regret and responsibility for the challenges their child is facing. As a result, accessing accurate prenatal information is a challenge limiting diagnosis. In addition, government record-keeping for children in the care of child welfare agencies is inconsistent, lacking the detail required for diagnosis. This important, historical information is either not available or it is very difficult to access [45].

Although programs vary across jurisdictions, many governments offer some level of funding and services to support both the child and the caregiver recognizing the challenges of caring for an individual with a disability. Mcdonald and Cooper [46] discuss the status of policy and services across Canada noting that "it is a patchwork of federal and provincial legislation and municipal programs" (p. 185). Work by Finlay [47] responded to recommendations from the UN Committee on the Rights of Persons with Disabilities that Canada addresses the lack of a national process for data collection. National programs are financial in nature such as Canada's Registered Disability Savings Plan (RDSP) and Disability Tax Credit. Provincial and municipal programs are both financial and service delivery focused and may rely on the care-givers to manage the funding and hiring processes. There have been calls for better prevalence data across the globe as well as broader response systems [48].

Globally disability services have specific eligibility criteria that support access to disability services, although they will vary widely across jurisdictions. For example, in Alberta, Canada, the criteria to access the Family Supports for Children with Disabilities (FSCD) require very specific medical documentation that the child has a disability "due to a developmental, physical, sensory, mental or neurological con-dition or impairment, and or a health condition that impacts their daily living activi-ties such as eating, grooming, walking, interacting with others, playing and problem solving" [49]. Generally, most children with an FASD diagnosis will qualify and services can be provided until age 18.

At age 18, the Government of Alberta offers the Persons with Developmental Disabilities (PDD) program to provide services to adults. The transition from FSCD to PDD is a long process that requires extensive planning. The risk exists however that individuals with FASD will not be eligible for these services because the eligi-bility criteria as noted above are based on a person having an IQ below 70 and hav-ing challenges in at least 6 of 24 identified daily living skills as assessed on the Alberta PDD Adaptive Skills Inventory [50]. This criteria unfortunately excludes many individuals with FASD as many have IQs much higher than 70 but have poor adaptive functioning and daily living skills. The situation is complicated further when we add the challenges of FASD and adolescence, involvement with child wel-fare, and the transition to adulthood and the struggles of parents and caregivers to engage with adult services.

Role of the Caregiver in Individualized Planning

Individualized planning based on each child, youth, and adult's needs is a corner-stone of best practice for all disability services, and even more critical for a spec-trum diagnosis where the range of differences in diagnostic and functional profiles is broad. The work of navigating individualized planning and intervention often falls to the primary caregiver. A study by Petrenko and colleagues [49] provides insight into the caregiver experience. Data was collected from interviews and focus groups with 24 foster and adoptive parents who were caring for an individual aged birth—35 years with FASD. Protective factors and stressors are mirror images of one another indicating that with the right resources, stressors decrease allowing the relationships to remain strong within the family/caregiving unit, decreasing stress and increasing success for the individual with FASD. The results (see Fig. 14.2), reflect the need to support the caregiver and the family unit as a whole. Caregiver responsibility to educate various professionals was a strong theme. Increasing the education of professionals in medicine, nursing, justice, child welfare, and disabilities would decrease this burden on caregivers.

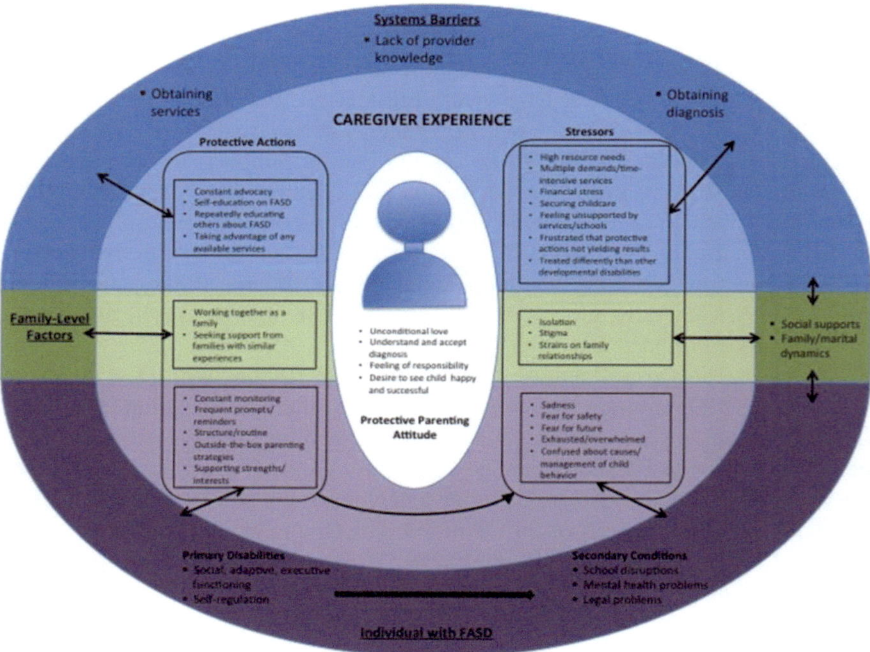

Fig. 14.2 Thematic model. This figure illustrates the transactions between foster and adoptive parents' protective actions and stressors related to raising an individual with FASD across multiple levels of the ecology (individual with FASD, family, and systems). Parents' protective parenting attitude was central to their experience and transcended ecological levels. *FASD* fetal alcohol spectrum disorders. (Reproduced with permission from [51])

Culture and Location Matter

Several studies [52–56] elucidate the challenges of accessing resources in indigenous, rural, and remote communities. The Canada Health Act [57] promises equitable access for all; however, the experience for those living in rural and remote communities is one of disenfranchisement where a one-size-fits-all approach does not work in practice. Research in rural and remote Australia shows similar findings regarding access to services. For indigenous communities, services are limited and not culturally appropriate. Working with indigenous families, Green et al. [52] found that "the lived reality of caring for a child with a disability is not supported or acknowledged by current policy, and this negatively impacted their experience and ability to care for their child." For all these families, the time and frustration spent trying to access a minimal service for their family members far exceed that of what is required by families in or near urban centers.

Obtaining and Maintaining Supports

A review of the Family Support for Children with Disabilities Program by the Government of Alberta in 2018 [58] revealed that parents were concerned about having to advocate for services. There are two main issues that parents have to overcome. The first challenge is to make the case to the caseworker to be approved for services. The second challenge is to demonstrate the need for continued services. The first problem of trying to access resources is attached to obtaining a diagnosis, which, as noted earlier, can be a cumbersome process. The diagnostic process is founded in ruling out other diagnoses that may explain the child's presentation. Investigation is complicated by challenges inherent in locating accurate information about PAE such as clearly documented records that meet diagnostic standards, reluctance of parents to acknowledge PAE as a result of shame and stigma. Given FASD is a life-long disability, the fiscal challenges of maintaining services become apparent. The assessment of the intervention by caseworkers is most often based on identifying positive change, meeting established goals, and the assumption that without the intervention the gains will be maintained. For an individual with FASD that is not the case and the removal of supports and services results in a decline in the entire family structure. A UK study of caregiver impacts found that "problems faced by parents as a result of not receiving support to modify parenting techniques combine with a perceived lack of recognition of difficulties by professionals to produce an inauspicious situation" [59].

Shifting Perceptions, Understanding, and Taking Action

Up to this point, this chapter has focused on discussing and problematizing key themes that arise in the context of FASD, especially the adversities faced by families, mothers, and children, the challenges of working through complex systems and structures, and the applications and limitations of medical and social framings of disability. The deficit discourse in part, arises from a medicalized approach where FASD is presented as an impairment that has no cure and limited success with therapy approaches, promoting a degree of apathy about diagnosis (i.e., "what's the point of pursuing a diagnosis if there's no therapies to then be applied"). In a study on stigma of birth mothers of children with FASD, Corrigan et al. [60] results of a general population survey, participants reported less positive views of mothers who had a child with FASD as opposed to their views of mothers reporting previous experience of mental illness, substance use, and jail experience. It appears that barriers may not only relate to knowledge gaps, but also to attitudinal ones.

There are, however, some good examples of ways in which these impediments can be overcome. We now turn the discussion toward some of the actions and changes in understanding and perception that may help to counter the ethical and social problems such as stigma and inaction that have been identified. Specifically, this discussion encompasses: changes in professionals' perceptions of FASD; the idea of an FASD practice lens; the value of multidisciplinary approaches; the critical realist model of disability; and the inclusion of the "client voice" as a way of informing professional practice.

One example of how practitioners are helping to shift problematic perceptions of FASD that create stigma is increased discussion around the importance of language and how FASD is framed in clinical and community contexts through the development and distribution of language guides. These language guides make suggestions about respectful language that can be used in clinical reports, conversations about FASD, and presentations. They are also a useful tool when engaging with the media about FASD. For example, the use of the phrase "a person suffering from FASD" suggests that person is unhappy and is unable to lead a productive and meaningful life which fits with a deficit discourse. The alternative suggested "person with FASD or living with FASD" does not make assumptions about the experience or perceptions of the person with FASD allowing room to acknowledge strengths, capabilities, and challenges [59].

Another example of effective perception change stems from the adoption of multidisciplinary team (MDT) approaches to FASD. Usually, MDTs are rationalized as groupings that function because they combine unique practice skills that are more effective together than they would be separately. However, an additional and often under-recognized benefit of MDTs is that the MDT members are by default placed in a position of critical reflectiveness by virtue of seeing their work sitting alongside that of other professionals with very different knowledges. This means that they are often able to perceive and remark upon both the strengths and the gaps or practice assumptions that might pertain to the work of their collaborating colleagues. Working in an MDT modality is deemed as best practice [61] for working with those with FASD and their families. The critical reflections inherent in this best practice can render benefits that may not accrue in non-MDT practice contexts.

These examples describe some of the processes that cumulatively produce an "FASD-informed lens" [62], which is a way of describing the process of going beyond just awareness and knowledge of FASD and into a state of informed critical reflection. A possible criticism of past efforts to equip professionals for working with FASD is that the focus on knowledge acquisition through professional education and training, which while necessary, cannot guarantee the development of an FASD-informed lens.

Other avenues exist for countering identified barriers, starting with the reconceptualization of disability itself. When considering how we respond to FASD, it is important to take account both the social and medical aspects of the disorder. The "critical realist model" of disability [63] provides a model in which, both the social (e.g., stigma) and medical (e.g., impaired executive functioning) are encompassed, and where solutions can be sought. In other words, the critical realist model allows us to consider FASD from a holistic perspective that includes addressing medical issues and developmental concerns of the individual at the same time looking at how those around the person, as well as community, services, and societal barriers may create disability for people with FASD. Another compelling model is the bio-ecological model of human development, advanced by Urie Bronfenbrenner. This model views the child within the context of multiple, intersecting systems [64]. Together, the two models urge us to approach FASD in a manner that is inclusive of as many different aspects of the ecosystem (families, services, professionals, education and justice systems, etc.) as can be aligned. For many people living with FASD, the unexamined values, assumptions, and expectations of the society that surrounds them are equally disabling as the neurological effect caused by the disorder itself.

A final, crucial element of this discussion, and of the FASD ecosystem, is the inclusion of the voices of those living with FASD in decision-making and understanding. Overwhelmingly, research into the experience of parents and carers and people with FASD is that they feel unsupported and un-heard by professionals. This is not a specific criticism of professional practice: the strong deficit discourse associated with FASD makes it hard to advocate for support through strengths-based approaches. And yet, when the strengths and capabilities of people living with FASD are acknowledged, this can transform practice. This is reflected, for example, in the proliferation of biographical writing about FASD, including various texts by people living with the disorder and increasing incorporation of adults with FASD as advocates for support in the media, in social media, in health and social service programs, as well as in research programs outlined below.

Support to Succeed

Contemplating the successes of individuals shifts in the dialogue regarding the life course of persons with FASD. The strengths of individuals with FASD are rarely reported in scientific literature but there are some exceptions [65]. For example, a major research project was conducted by adults living with FASD known as The Lay of the Land survey and published in 2020 [23] in The Routledge Handbook of Social Work and Addiction. This research developed from informal conversations held by adults with FASD among themselves about various health problems they were experiencing. Upon discovering some common ailments, and with support from leading FASD researchers and advocates, the anonymous survey identified 25 core research areas. The questionnaire was developed and disseminated and there were 541 participants. The findings highlight the need for health and social service professionals to pay close attention and listen to the health concerns of children and adults with FASD. Further, they identify the need to offer and fund adult diagnosis as a medical right and pose questions about the impact of high levels of chronic stress and mental health issues on physical health.

To illustrate the point about the meaning of a diagnosis to an adult in Alberta, one of the chapter authors was approached by a student taking an addictions studies diploma in Calgary, Alberta in 2014. He stated: "I am 62 years old and I just got diagnosed with FASD. Finally, my whole life makes sense." The Lay of the Land research reflects the authentic voice of adults who have FASD and this group of committed researchers and their consulting supporters have collectively raised the profile of the health and psychosocial health concerns associated with this disability from an insider perspective.

Other examples of success can be found in books published by authors living with FASD. The Best I Can Be—Living with Fetal Alcohol Syndrome or Effects [66] written by Liz Kulp states on the book cover,

> You cannot see my disability on the outside. I like to make myself look pretty… I am adopted and my mom died so no one will ever know when or how much or how often my mom drank. I just know I have to live with it.

Liz wrote this book with her adoptive mother Jodee and both have committed their lives to supporting success for individuals with FASD through promoting positive messages and public education on the Live Abilities-Create Possibilities website [67].

Another adult with FASD, RJ Formanek, is a well-known public speaker and runs a successful Facebook FASD Support Group called Flying with Broken Wings. RJ is a spokesperson for the Red Shoes Rock [68] campaign and runs a blog filled with realistic and positive information [69].

Myles Himmelreich, quoted earlier, is an adult living with FASD who has dedicated his life to educating and developing knowledge about FASD, offering an insider view of what life is like with this disability. We are deeply honored to consider Myles a friend and colleague and he is one of the most well-known, successful public speakers about FASD. One just has to Google Myle's name to find his many contributions to public education on FASD. Recently, Myles was a key consultant in a recent report on FASD published by the Representative for Children and Youth [20].

The academic community has also been considering the ways in which a strengths perspective can be focal to examining the life course of those with FASD. Peterenko and Kautz-Turnbull [70] have proposed a model that thinks about moving from surviving to thriving. They suggest focusing upon six domains within a person-centered approach: reducing stigma, improving strength-based measures, using strength-based frameworks, community knowledge translation, adapting existing effective models for FASD and improving efforts to reach underserved populations. Flanigan et al. emphasize that more needs to be done to enhance a success orientation which includes seeing the intrinsic strengths of the individual, self-awareness, receptivity to support, the capacity for human connection, perseverance. and possessing hope [71]. A strength-based approach also centers upon different areas of intervention such as aspects of intact functioning [72].

Taking Action

Engage in Critical Thinking

Understanding that societal systems and access to resources may require a diagnosis, there is an inherent tension between the language of health/ability and the disability lens. All professionals that interact with humans in some of their most vulnerable moments are entrusted to make informed and accurate decisions. As professionals, we are tasked with using critical thinking to assess the scope and effectiveness of our practice, take a holistic perspective while engaging children and families to achieve the best outcomes. Critical thinking is a rigorous, self-directed, and self-reflective process requiring the uncovering of assumption and biases. This awareness is critical in the prevention of negative impacts on our assessment, intervention, communication, and outcomes for persons with FASD [73]. The medical model of disability can quickly take us down a path of loss, deficit, and risk.

A balanced, critically informed approach engaging in strength-based assessment and planning that embraces the whole child and their caregivers will result in the achievement of positive outcomes. The development of secondary conditions such as school failure, involvement with the justice system, and substance use is "the result of the complex interplay of factors across the levels of the ecology (individual, family, systems of care, and culture" [74]. This ecological approach aligns with the social model of disability discussed earlier. This is a long-term process, a marathon, for which the sustainability of resources over the lifespan is critical. Professionals have a responsibility to work in coordination with one another, the family, and other service providers. Leadership grounded in critical thinking processes is essential.

There is a critical knowledge base required for all professionals working with individuals with FASD and their caregivers [27, 74, 75]. We propose that taking the initiative to learn about FASD from credible sources, making a commitment to deeply listen to the unique experiences, understanding the nuances of strengths and challenges for each individual, and reflecting on one's own perception and biases will place you at the center of positive change.

Acknowledge the Complexity of FASD

It is important to consider the complexity of FASD and to appreciate the challenges individuals face in accessing disability services. As noted, "FASD is not an established category within developmental disabilities or educational systems in the US." Even if children do qualify, FASD-informed services are often locally unavailable [76]. Further, the need exists to recognize FASD as a complex disability, partly because it falls between the cracks of disability, child welfare, and social service systems with no one clear path to support services. It is noted that effective support requires seeing the "whole person in context" and this population is vulnerable, experiences social isolation, has behavioral and safety concerns, struggle with adaptive functioning and family living skills [65].

A Jurisdictional Example of Engagement

Understanding FASD as a disability in and of itself presents an ethical quandary. In the province of Alberta, Canada it is estimated that about 36,000 individuals live with FASD. The FASD Cross Ministry Committee was established in 2007 is responsible for the development and oversight of the coordinate cross ministry response, ensuring that a continuum of services and supports are delivered that are meaningful, evidence based and accessible [76]. Thank and Jonsson (2009) [77] noted while FASD is costly, the Alberta FASD Service Networks were cost-efficient to government through their provision of intervention services in a number of sectors including women's health, child welfare, employment, justice, and education. It is important to note the economic costs on an annual basis is as high as 143 million (CAD), thus warranting investment in an FASD prevention strategy [77]. All allied health and social service ministries sit at this table and meet monthly. Alberta has demonstrated a model of excellence through supporting FASD diagnostic clinics and access to online training on FASD in partnership with the Canada FASD Research Network. The focus of these efforts, The Prevention Conversation Initiative [78] is targeted toward specific professionals including educators/school teachers, justice, and legal professions and those working in women's health. Overall, it is critical to highlight that this an Alberta wide, comprehensive approach to support individuals and families no matter whether they live in urban, rural, or remote communities. It is inclusive of Metis and First Nations Communities. The work that is uniquely done in Alberta ultimately provides the best care possible to infants, children, youth, and adults and this is thanks to the dedicated commitment of those community members whose family members live with FASD. The notion that it takes a community to raise a child has been well embraced in this model and awareness of FASD continues to make gains.

The need exists for expanding the type, range, and availability of supports to families of children with FASD across helping services [75]. The ethical dilemma presented here is the concern that children who qualify for disability supports within families do not have any guarantee when the biological age of 18 is reached. The need for disability supports in FASD across the lifespan exists, and serious consideration to lifelong support with seamless transitions to adulthood services is critical to consider. Young adults with FASD who transition out of the child welfare system and are no longer eligible for supports are highly vulnerable and at risk of poverty, homelessness, victimization, and engagement with the criminal justice system.

Advocacy for Change

FASD is not well accepted in the mainstream disability world. It is therefore a challenge to get a diagnosis, to find programs that effectively support individuals with FASD, to provide FASD informed care, and to obtain grants to conduct research. Research on FASD is among the most highly scrutinized by ethics boards and yet this research is essential in developing knowledge and best practice. Organizations such as the Canada FASD Research Network have served to advance the research agenda on FASD with dedicated, funded research in the areas of prevention, diagnosis, justice, child welfare, and intervention [79]. One core example supporting ethical practice is the FASD Policy Alert on Children's Rights in the Criminal Justice System [80]. A dedicated research network on FASD has the capacity to continue to promote research, knowledge, and education on FASD and to highlight critical information about the distinct needs of children, youth, and adults with FASD, recognizing the greater risk of this population for adverse outcomes. Children with FASD represent a substantial part of the child welfare population yet training on FASD and alcohol and other drug disorders are notably absent in workforce training [81].

No matter your role, we challenge you to engage in social justice advocacy. Invite others into the dialogue and solution building conversations. Place those most impacted by FASD at the center of the conversation by including them in the conversation. Step back and invite those with lived experience to lead the discussion. Resist the status quo by challenging systems to adapt to new ways of thinking. Acknowledge the disability, its' lifelong impact, call out bias, decrease stigma, engage in research opportunities, be innovative, loudly and boldly share success stories. When you listen, and act intentionally with integrity you make a difference.

References

1. Canadian Mental Health Association. Ontario: CMHA Ontario;2021. Stigma and Discrimination. 2021. https://ontario.cmha.ca/documents/stigma-and-discrimination/. Accessed 24 July 2021.
2. Aspler J, Bogossian A, Racine E. "It's ignorant stereotypes": key stakeholder perspectives on stereotypes associated with fetal alcohol spectrum disorder, alcohol, and pregnancy. J Intellect Dev Disabil. 2021;47:1–12. https://doi.org/10.3109/13668250.2020.1865649.
3. Bagley K, Badry D. How personal perspectives shape health professionals' perceptions of fetal alcohol spectrum disorder and risk. Int J Environ Res Public Health. 2019;16(11):1936. https://doi.org/10.3390/ijerph16111936.
4. Jones KL, Smith DW. Recognition of the fetal alcohol syndrome in early infancy. Lancet. 1973;302(7836):999–1001.
5. Lemoine P, Harousseau H, Borteyru JP, Menuet JC. Children of alcoholic parents—observed anomalies: discussion of 127 cases. Ther Drug Monitor. 2003;25(2):132–6.
6. Larcher V, Brierley J. Fetal alcohol syndrome (FAS) and fetal alcohol spectrum disorder (FASD)—diagnosis and moral policing; an ethical dilemma for paediatricians. Arch Dis childhood. 2014;99(11):969–70.
7. Choate P, Badry D. Stigma as a dominant discourse in fetal alcohol spectrum disorder. Adv Dual Diagn. 2019;12(1/2):36–52. https://doi.org/10.1108/ADD-05-2018-0005.
8. Bown JM, Bland R, Jonsson E, Greenshaw AJ. A brief history of awareness of the link between alcohol and fetal alcohol spectrum disorder. Can J Psychiatry. 2019;64(3):164–8.
9. Rouquette J. Influence sur la toxicomanie alcoolique parentale sur le développement physique et psychique des jeunes enfants. 1957. (Doctoral dissertation).
10. Food and Drug Administration (FDA). Food and Drug Administration (FDA) Fetal alcohol syndrome. FDA Drug Bull. 1977;7(4):18.
11. Warren KR. A review of the history of attitudes toward drinking in pregnancy. Alcohol Clin Exp Res. 2015;39(7):1110–7. https://doi.org/10.1111/acer.12757.
12. Popova S, Lange S, Poznyak V, Chudley AE, Shield KD, Reynolds JN, Murray M, Rehm J. Population-based prevalence of fetal alcohol spectrum disorder in Canada. BMC Public Health. 2019;28(19):845. https://doi.org/10.1186/s12889-019-7213-3.
13. Frances A. Saving normal: an insider's revolt against out-of-control psychiatric diagnosis, DSM-5, big pharma, and the medicalization of ordinary life. 1st ed. Cambridge: Cambridge University Press; 2013.
14. United Nations Convention on the Rights of Persons with Disabilities. New York, NY. 2007. https://treaties.un.org/doc/Publication/CTC/Ch_IV_15.pdf.
15. United Nations Convention on the Rights of the Child. New York, NY. 1989. https://www.ohchr.org/en/professionalinterest/pages/crc.aspx.
16. Truth and Reconciliation Commission of Canada. Truth and Reconciliation Commission of Canada interim report. Winnipeg: Truth and Reconciliation Commission of Canada; 2012.
17. Salmon A. Aboriginal mothering, FASD prevention and the contestations of neoliberal citizenship. Crit Public Health. 2011;12(2):171–3. https://doi.org/10.1080/09581596.2010.530643.
18. Choate P, Tortorelli C, Aalen D, Beck J, McCarthy J, Moreno C, Santhuru O. Parents with fetal alcohol spectrum disorder within Canada' Child Protection Trials. Can Fam Law Q. 2020;39:283–307.
19. Bell M, Glowatski K, Pitawanakwat R, Stewart M. FASD and the TRC Call to Action 34.4: a consideration of evaluation methods. Ottawa: Adjust Consulting Ltd; 2019. https://www.justice.gc.ca/eng/rp-pr/jr/fasd-etcaf/fasd-etcaf.pdf
20. Charlesworth J. Excluded: increasing understanding, support and inclusion for children with FASD and their families. Victoria: FASD; 2021. https://rcybc.ca/wp-content/uploads/2021/06/RCY-FASD_Report_FINAL_REVISED_21-JUNE-2021_Web.pdf

21. Lange S, Shield K, Rehm J, Anagnostou E, Popova S. Fetal alcohol spectrum disorder: neuro-developmentally and behaviorally indistinguishable from other neurodevelopmental disorders. BMC Psychiatry. 2019;19:322. https://doi.org/10.1186/s12888-019-2289-y.
22. Alberta PDD–Eligibility. Government of Alberta. 2021. https://www.alberta.ca/pdd-eligibility.aspx.
23. Himmelreich M, Lutke CJ, Hargrove ET. The lay of the land: Fetal Alcohol Spectrum Disorder (FASD) as a whole-body diagnosis. In: Begun AL, Murray MM, editors. The Routledge handbook of social work and addictive behaviors. New York: Routledge; 2020.
24. Fleming AF. This mother drank while pregnant. Here's what her daughter is like at 43. The Washington Post. https://www.washingtonpost.com/national/health-science/this-mother-drank-while-pregnant-heres-what-her-daughters-like-at-43/2016/01/15/32ff5238-9a08-11e5-b499-76cbec161973_story.html. Accessed 18 Jan 2016.
25. Abadir AM, Ickowicz A. Fetal alcohol spectrum disorder: reconsidering blame. Can Med Assoc J. 2016;188(3):171. https://doi.org/10.1503/cmaj.151425.
26. Zizzo N, Racine E. Ethical challenges in FASD prevention: scientific uncertainty, stigma, and respect for women's autonomy. Can J Public Health. 2017;108(4):e414–7. https://doi.org/10.17269/CJPH.108.6048.
27. Brown NN, Burd L, Grant T, Edwards W, Adler R, Streissguth A. Prenatal alcohol exposure: an assessment strategy for the legal context. Int J Law Psychiatry. 2015;42:144–8. https://doi.org/10.1016/j.ijlp.2015.08.019.
28. Shankar I. Risky bodies: allocation of risk and responsibility within Fetal Alcohol Spectrum Disorder (FASD) prevention campaigns. Can J Disabil Stud. 2016;5(2):152. https://doi.org/10.15353/cjds.v5i2.276.
29. Greenmyer JR, Popova S, Klug MG, Burd L. Fetal alcohol spectrum disorder: a systematic review of the cost of and savings from prevention in the United States and Canada. Addiction (Abingdon, England). 2020;115(3):409–17. https://doi.org/10.1111/add.14841.
30. Harding K, Flannigan K, McFarlane A. Policy action paper: toward a standard definition of fetal alcohol spectrum disorder in Canada. Policy. 2019.
31. American Psychiatric Association. Diagnostic and statistical manual of mental disorder. 5th ed. Washington, DC: American Psychiatric Association; 2013. https://doi.org/10.1176/appi.books.9780890425596.
32. Cameron M. This is common factors. Clin Soc Work J. 2014;42(2):151–60. https://doi.org/10.1007/s10615-013-0467-9.
33. Byrne L, Happell B, Reid-Searl K. Lived experience practitioners and the medical model: world's colliding? J Ment Health (Abingdon, England). 2016;25(3):217–23. https://doi.org/10.3109/09638237.2015.1101428.
34. Hughes R. The social model of disability. Br J Healthc Assist. 2010;4(10):508–11. https://doi.org/10.12968/bjha.2010.4.10.79078.
35. Charon R, DasGupta S, Hermann N, Irvine C, Marcus ER, Colsn ER, Spencer D, Spiegel M, Charon R. The principles and practice of narrative medicine. Oxford: Oxford University Press; 2017.
36. National Academies of Sciences, Engineering and Medicine. Opportunities for improving programs and services for children with disabilities. Washington, DC: The National Academies Press; 2018. https://doi.org/10.17226/25028.
37. Halfon N, Houtrow A, Larson K, Newacheck P. The changing landscape of disability in childhood. Future Child. 2012;22(1):13–42. https://doi.org/10.1353/foc.2012.0004.
38. Harding K, Flannigan K, McFarlane A. Policy action paper: toward a standard definition of Fetal Alcohol Spectrum Disorder in Canada. Canada Fetal Alcohol Spectrum Disorder Research Network; 2019.
39. Loock C, Elliott E, Cox LF, et al. Alcohol spectrum disorder. In: The Routledge handbook of social work and addictive behaviors. New York: Routledge; 2020.

40. Burns J, Badry DE, Harding KD, Roberts N, Unsworth K, Cook JL. Comparing outcomes of children and youth with fetal alcohol spectrum disorder (FASD) in the child welfare system to those in other living situations in Canada: results from the Canadian National FASD Database. Child Care Health Dev. 2021;47(1):77–84.

41. O'Malley KD. The knotted cord: transgenerational alcohol related neurodevelopmental disorder (ARND). Hauppauge: Nova Science Publishers; 2014.

42. Armstrong EM. Conceiving risk, bearing responsibility: fetal alcohol syndrome and the diagnosis of moral disorder. Baltimore: JHU Press; 2003.

43. Tenenbaum A, Mandel A, Dor T, Sapir A, Sapir-Bodnaro O, Hertz P, Wexler ID. Fetal alcohol spectrum disorder among pre-adopted and foster children. BMC Pediatr. 2020;20(1):1–6.

44. Fuchs D, Burnside L, Marchenski S, Mudry A. Children with FASD-related disabilities receiving services from child welfare agencies in Manitoba. Int J Ment Health Addict. 2010;8(2):232–44. https://doi.org/10.1007/s11469-009-9258-5.

45. Freeman J, Condon C, Hamilton S, Mutch RC, Bower C, Watkins RE. Challenges in accurately assessing prenatal alcohol exposure in a study of fetal alcohol spectrum disorder in a Youth Detention Center. Alcohol Clin Exp Res. 2019;43(2):309–16. https://doi.org/10.1111/acer.13926.

46. MacDonald JE, Cooper SN. (dis)Ability policy: a tangled web of complexity. In: Harding R, Jeyapal D, editors. Canadian social policy for social workers. Oxford: Oxford University Press; 2018.

47. Finlay B, Dunn S, Zwicker JD. Navigating government disability programs across Canada. Can Public Policy. 2020;46(4):474–91. https://doi.org/10.3138/cpp.2019-071.

48. Jonsson E, Salmon A, Warraen KR. The international charter on prevention of FASD. Lancet. 2014;2(3):e135–7. https://doi.org/10.1016/S2214-109X(13)70173-6.

49. Alberta Family Supports for Children with Disabilities. https://www.alberta.ca/fscd-eligibility.aspx#jumplinks-1. Accessed 30 July 2021.

50. Government of Alberta. PDD Adaptive Skills Inventory. http://www.humanservices.alberta.ca/pdd-online/documents/pdd-adaptive-skills-inventory.pdf. Accessed 1 Aug 2021.

51. Petrenko CLM, Alto ME, Hart AR, Freeze SM, Cole LL. "I'm doing my part, I just need help from the community": intervention implications of foster and adoptive parents' experiences raising children and young adults with FASD. J Fam Nurs. 2019;25(2):314–47. https://doi.org/10.1177/1074840719847185.

52. Green A, Abbott P, Delaney P, Patradoon-Ho P, Delaney J, Davidson PM, DiGiacomo M. Navigating the journey of aboriginal childhood disability: a qualitative study of carers' interface with services. BMC Health Serv Res. 2016;16(1):680. https://doi.org/10.1186/s12913-016-1926-0.

53. DiGiacomo M, Green A, Delaney P, Delaney J, Patradoon-Ho P, Davidson PM, Abbott P. Experiences and needs of carers of aboriginal children with a disability: a qualitative study. BMC Fam Pract. 2017;18(1):96. https://doi.org/10.1186/s12875-017-0668-3.

54. Sage R, Ward B, Myers A, Ravesloot C. Transitory and enduring disability among urban and rural people. J Rural Health. 2019;35(4):460–70. https://doi.org/10.1111/jrh.12338.

55. Johnson E, Lincoln M, Cumming S. Principles of disability support in rural and remote Australia: lessons from parents and carers. Health Soc Care Commun. 2020;28(6):2208–17. https://doi.org/10.1111/hsc.13033.

56. Vilches SL, Pighini MJ, Stewart M, Goelman H. Documenting the urbanistic policy bias in rural early childhood services: toward a functional definition of rurality: urbanistic policy bias. Can Geogr. 2017;61(3):375–88. https://doi.org/10.1111/cag.12359.

57. Government of Canada. The Canada Health Act. 2020. https://www.canada.ca/en/health-canada/services/health-care-system/canada-health-care-system-medicare/canada-health-act.html. Accessed 26 July 2021.

58. Government of Alberta. WHAT WE HEARD: feedback from parents, families and advocates in the Family Support for Children with Disabilities (FSCD) program. GOA. 2018. https://open.alberta.ca/publications/9781460141342.

59. Mukherjee R, Wray E, Commers M, Hollins S, Curfs L. The impact of raising a child with FASD upon carers: findings from a mixed methodology study in the UK. Adopt Foster. 2013;37(1):43–56. https://doi.org/10.1177/0308575913477331.
60. Corrigan PW, Lara JL, Shah BB, Mitchell KT, Simmes D, Jones KL. The public stigma of birth mothers of children with fetal alcohol spectrum disorders. Alcohol Clin Exp Res. 2017;41:1166–73. https://doi.org/10.1111/acer.13381.
61. Masotti P, Longstaffe S, Gammon H, Isbister J, Maxwell B, Hanlon-Dearman A. Integrating care for individuals with FASD: results from a multi-stakeholder symposium. BMC Health Serv Res. 2015;15(1):457. https://doi.org/10.1186/s12913-015-1113-8.
62. Gibbs A, Bagley K, Badry D, Gollner V. Foetal alcohol spectrum disorder: effective helping responses from social workers. Int Soc Work. 2020;63(4):496–509. https://doi.org/10.1177/0020872818804032.
63. Shakespeare R. Disability rights and wrongs revisited. 2nd ed. Florence: Taylor and Francis; 2013.
64. Urie B. The ecology of human development: experiments by nature and design. Cambridge: Harvard University Press; 1981.
65. Skorka K, McBryde C, Copley J, Meredith PJ, Reid N. Experiences of children with fetal alcohol spectrum disorder and their families: a critical review. Alcohol Clin Exp Res. 2020;44(6):1175–88.
66. Kulp L, Kulp J. The best I can be: living with fetal alcohol syndrome/effects. Brooklyn Park: Better Endings New Beginnings; 2009.
67. Live Abilities-Create Possibilities Website. http://www.betterendings.org/services.html.
68. Red Shoes Rock Facebook Group. https://www.facebook.com/RedShoesRock/.
69. Red Shoes Rock Blog. https://redshoesrock.com/blog/.
70. Petrenko CL, Kautz-Turnbull C. From surviving to thriving: a new conceptual model to advance interventions to support people with FASD across the lifespan. In: International review of research in developmental disabilities, vol. 61. New York: Academic Press; 2021. p. 39–75. https://doi.org/10.1016/bs.irrdd.2021.07.002.
71. Flannigan K, Wrath A, Ritter C, McLachlan K, Harding KD, Campbell A, Reid D, Pei J. Balancing the story of fetal alcohol spectrum disorder: a narrative review of the literature on strengths. Alcohol Clin Exp Res. 2021;45(12):2448–64. https://doi.org/10.1111/acer.14733.
72. Kully-Martens K, McNeil A, Pei J, Rasmussen C. Toward a strengths-based cognitive profile of children with fetal alcohol spectrum disorders: implications for intervention. Curr Dev Disord Rep. 2022;9:53–62. https://doi.org/10.1007/s40474-022-00245-5.
73. The Foundation for Critical Thinking. Our concept and definition of critical thinking. California. 2019. https://criticalthinking.org/pages/our-conception-of-critical-thinking/411.
74. Pedruzzi RA, Hamilton O, Hodgson HHA, Connor E, Johnson E, Fitzpatrick J. Navigating complexity to support justice-involved youth with FASD and other neurodevelopmental disabilities: needs and challenges of a regional workforce. Health Justice. 2021;9(1):8. https://doi.org/10.1186/s40352-021-00132-y.
75. Petrenko CL, Tahir N, Mahoney EC, Chin NP. Prevention of secondary conditions in fetal alcohol spectrum disorders: identification of systems-level barriers. Matern Child Health J. 2014;18(6):1496–505.
76. Alberta FASD Cross Ministry Committee. https://www.alberta.ca/fasd-in-alberta.aspx#jumplinks-2. Accessed 27 July 2021.
77. Thanh NX, Jonsson E. Costs of fetal alcohol spectrum disorder in Alberta, Canada. J Popul Ther Clin Pharmacol. 2009;16(1):e80–90.
78. Government of Alberta. The Prevention Conversation. 2021. https://preventionconversation.org.
79. Badry D, Coons-Harding KD, Cook J, Bocking A. Finding answers, improving outcomes: a case study of the Canada fetal alcohol spectrum disorder research network. Adv Dual Diagn. 2019;12(1/2):53–61.

80. FASD Policy Alert. Children's rights in the child justice system: FASD and General Comment 24. 2021. https://canfasd.ca/issue-papers-alerts/#alerts. Accessed 30 July 2021.
81. Badry D, Choate P. Fetal alcohol spectrum disorder: a disability in need of social work education, knowledge and practice. Soc Work Soc Sci Rev. 2014;17(3):20–32.

Chapter 15
FASD and Child Welfare

Dorothy Badry (iD), **Ana Hanlon Dearman** (iD), **Peter Choate** (iD),
Lenora Marcellus (iD), **Christina Tortorelli** (iD), **and Robyn Williams** (iD)

Introduction

Fetal alcohol spectrum disorders (FASD) is a disability that requires lifespan support. The primary response to FASD emerged in North America and was particularly influenced by the Jones and Smith publication in 1973, which identified disabilities caused by alcohol exposure [1]. The life course model posited has relevance to FASD and will be integrated in this chapter [2]. The life course of a person with FASD needs to include the prenatal period, infancy, childhood, adolescence, and adulthood, and each stage comes with unique developmental tasks. Child welfare can become involved at any of these stages including adolescence and adulthood when individuals with FASD become parents. It is critical to recognize that child protection concerns exist at all stages, but it is often in early life that child

D. Badry (✉)
Faculty of Social Work, University of Calgary, Calgary, AB, Canada
e-mail: badry@ucalgary.ca

A. H. Dearman
Max Rady College of Medicine, Pediatrics and Child Health, University of Manitoba, Winnipeg, MB, Canada
e-mail: ahdearman@rccinc.ca

P. Choate · C. Tortorelli
Child Studies and Social Work, Mount Royal University, Calgary, AB, Canada
e-mail: pchoate@mtroyal.ca; christinatortorelli@mtroyal.ca

L. Marcellus
School of Nursing, University of Victoria, Victoria, BC, Canada
e-mail: lenoram@uvic.ca

R. Williams
Curtin Medical School, Faculty of Health Sciences, Perth, WA, Australia
e-mail: robyn.williams@curtin.edu.au

© The Author(s), under exclusive license to Springer Nature Switzerland AG 2023
O. A. Abdul-Rahman, C. L. M. Petrenko (eds.), *Fetal Alcohol Spectrum Disorders*,
https://doi.org/10.1007/978-3-031-32386-7_15

welfare becomes involved due to the challenges associated with parenting and alcohol and substance use disorders.

The UN Convention on the Rights of the Child is described as a human rights treaty for children that recognizes all children have rights to develop and grow, and the consideration of the best interest of the child is at the forefront [3]. The Convention on the Rights of Persons with Disabilities was adopted by the United Nations in 2006 and enacted in 2008 [4]. The child welfare system is focused on the rights of children to be safe in their families and communities. Children with disabilities and FASD in particular often face multiple adversities including historical trauma in the family, social isolation, and stigma. It is critical to note that FASD is not well recognized globally as a childhood disability. Internationally, most children involved in child welfare are unlikely to be screened and assessed for FASD, having limited access to supports that could help improve their quality of life [5]. The intersection of FASD and child welfare is critical, and the need to recognize FASD in frontline child welfare practice is essential for both prevention and intervention.

The role of child welfare at its core foundation is to assure the survival, security, and development of children and families. Child protection issues such as failure to meet the care and developmental needs of children, neglect, and abuse are primary reasons for removal from parental care. Women with substance use disorders often have traumatic histories and mental health problems that can contribute to the removal of children from their care and intergenerational transmission of maltreatment. Given these experiences and often punitive policies, many families are fearful of the child welfare system [6]. However, it has been noted that recognition of FASD in an infant or child offers a crucial opportunity for intervention for both mother and child. Programs such as PCAP (Parent Child Assistance Program) have made substantial contributions in supporting mothers and children involved in child welfare, including reduced alcohol use in pregnancy [7, 8].

Children with FASD are overrepresented yet underrecognized in the child welfare population. Misconceptions of FASD and stigma have played a pivotal role in the lack of FASD diagnosis. The adequate provision of services in childhood, adolescence, and adulthood globally is problematic. FASD may go unrecognized in a child for many years and often the disability is not picked up until children enter the school system or when unexplained behavioral challenges become problematic [9]. Adequate screening and documentation of prenatal alcohol exposure are needed across all systems of care, including child welfare, to effectively identify people with FASD and support children and families. When children have behavior problems, there is a tendency to blame the parents instead of localizing the disabilities associated with FASD. Parents of children with FASD experience high levels of stress, more so than those of children with other developmental disabilities [10]. Creating sound interventions for children and youth with FASD is essential.

Stigma is a major contributor to FASD going unrecognized and underserved. Public stigma of FASD is pervasive across the globe [11, 12]. Stigma contributes to shaming and blaming of women and discrimination of people with FASD. It also creates internalized self-stigma and feelings of low self-worth. Often, we know very little about the lived experiences of children with FASD who end up in the child welfare system and grow up in care. Parents who use alcohol during pregnancy often face life adversities and the use of alcohol is not done with an intent to cause harm to the developing fetus, but rather is a function of interpersonal challenges they are experiencing [7, 8]. For example, Myles Himmelreich who lives with FASD is a well-known public speaker who grew up in the child welfare system and speaks to the effects of this stigma. Myles provides training on FASD, is a father and an advocate for many living with this disability and takes the position that harmful messages about alcohol use and pregnancy can contribute to stigmatizing the person who lives with FASD. In a recent report, Myles stated the following:

> FASD is caused when there is alcohol intake during the pregnancy. This can happen for a number of reasons but please know statements like "FASD is 100% preventable" just leads to more shame and blame. Statements like "The child's mother should have cared enough to not drink" lead to stigma for the mother and child. My mother drank; I have FASD. This is what I HAVE—not who I AM. This is what the children and youth in this report HAVE—not who they ARE [13].

The voice of Myles informs us that it is critical to recognize that the disability of the person who lives with FASD was formulated by pre-birth experiences and often difficult circumstances of families where alcohol use leads to FASD. The identity of the person living with FASD is shaped by many influences, and individuals with FASD are their own persons who want to live and experience life on their own terms. In Myles's case, his experience of growing up in the child welfare system has become a critical tool he has utilized in sharing knowledge about FASD as a successful public speaker, despite having many early disadvantages to overcome.

The stigma and lack of empathy experienced by families with FASD are accompanied by a pervasive lack of understanding about the effects of FASD across systems of care, including child welfare [11]. Families where FASD is a concern often come to the attention of child welfare due to concerns such as poverty, risky behavior of their child, mental health concerns, substance abuse, and issues of neglect [14]. Case workers receive little, if any, training on FASD, and child welfare systems are rarely set up to effectively screen and intervene with this population [15]. Running parallel are the universal voices from foster carers/kinship families raising children with FASD who are experiencing a lack of support, respite, and training. Increasingly, advocacy and access to FASD diagnosis occur when adolescents with FASD involved in the child welfare system become enmeshed within the criminal justice system [5]. This could be addressed and even prevented with adequate screening and supports earlier in their time in care.

Epidemiology of PAE and FASD in Child Welfare and Related Settings

In 2021, almost 50 years after the initial publication on fetal alcohol syndrome, FASD continues to be a leading cause of developmental disability globally [see Chap. 1]. Recent research has identified that limited knowledge exists overall about children with prenatal alcohol exposure in the child welfare system despite the significant role that alcohol has in parental involvement with the child welfare system

[16]. Data collected on 547 children and youth in the US who had been adopted or were in the foster care system concluded that 156 children met the criteria for FASD diagnosis and 125 (80%) had not been diagnosed as having prenatal alcohol exposure [9]. Globally, the themes of undiagnosed and unrecognized FASD have emerged over the past decade across child protection, criminal justice, and health sectors, and this identifies a significant gap in knowledge about FASD amongst professionals [9, 11]. The issue of FASD prevalence is taken up by Popova in Chap. 1 and highlights the global concern of FASD as a critical public health problem of particular concern to children and families. It was identified that there is a 6.0% prevalence rate of children with FASD in the child welfare system and children in the child welfare system are at risk for FASD [17, 18]. While the estimated global prevalence of FASD among special subpopulations, which includes children in care, is identified as 7.7 per 1000, epidemiological research has identified that in the United States the prevalence rate is noted to be 32 times higher in special subpopulations such as children in child welfare care in contrast to the general population [17]. Globally, the overall estimated prevalence of FASD in special subpopulations is considered to be 10–40 times higher than the general population [17] which raises credible concerns about the need to engage in supports for prevention.

Child Welfare Policies Toward PAE and FASD

There are many reasons why individuals may use alcohol prenatally and substance use is a leading reason for parental involvement in the child welfare system [16]. The use of alcohol during pregnancy relates to the same social determinants that influence alcohol use more generally. Many of these reasons include being unaware of their pregnancy, not understanding how alcohol may affect an unborn child, partner or peer pressure, mental health and addictions, and trauma that may include intimate partner violence or victimization. It has been shown that individuals who give birth to children later diagnosed with FASD have higher rates of inadequate prenatal care and experience significant social disparity [19]. Importantly, it has also been shown that both low parental empowerment and parental mental health are important reasons why women may use alcohol [20]. Individuals can also receive conflicting information regarding use of alcohol, particularly in small quantities, during pregnancy [21]. The harmful use of alcohol is a serious health problem and vulnerable populations including those in corrections and the child welfare system are 10–40 times at higher risk for FASD than other populations [17].

In North America, prevention programming and child welfare are generally of the view that no alcohol is acceptable in pregnancy with several states in the US taking the position that alcohol use in pregnancy is child abuse [22]. This is not so in Canada as a result of a Supreme Court of Canada decision concluding that a fetus is not a child within the meaning of child protection [23]. The issue of child welfare involvement due to prenatal substance exposure remains a key public health concern [24] as alcohol exposure has particular health risks impacting fetal growth and contributes to low birth weight [24, 25]. Further, lifelong adverse effects can include impacts on emotional, behavioral, developmental, and cognitive functioning. Children with these challenges who do not have the benefit of their disability being recognized by child welfare have limited opportunity to receive beneficial therapeutic interventions [26].

It is reported that 50–80% of child welfare cases include a parent who uses substances and this is a serious concern given the problems associated with parenting and family functioning, birthing parents being most often involved with the child welfare system [27]. The child welfare system tends to see the child as the client and the complexity of parental substance use require a different lens be applied when considering interventions. This research suggests models such as the Parent Child Assistance Program PCAP—a program that provides home visitation and mentoring to women, including supporting women in accessing treatment programs involving their children, can demonstrate positive benefits [13].

A recently published US report, *Prenatal alcohol and other drug exposures in child welfare study,* identified substance use, socioeconomic and racial/ethnic disparities contribute to involvement in the child welfare system. Substance use by marginalized populations was identified as a significant concern in this reporting noting, "A disproportionate number of Black and low-income women are reported to child welfare because of substance use during pregnancy" (p. iv) [26]. Active parental substance use creates conditions for involvement with the child welfare system and contributes to the risk of loss of parental rights in contrast to those not using substances [28, 29]. Many health and social concerns are noted to be key intersections where active substance use is identified in a person's life such as mental health problems, stress, being a single parent, social isolation, historical trauma, childhood sexual abuse, housing insecurity, unemployment, poverty, and experiences of violence and abuse [27]. This research noted that severity of substance abuse was a key factor leading to out of home child placement [27]. In the US, the Child Abuse Prevention and Treatment Act and the Comprehensive Addiction and Recovery Act passed in 2016 compels states to develop policy and practice plans related to the "safe care" with a particular focus on infants and caregivers [24]. Further, the level of intervention in more serious cases is often determined and defined by both the intensity of FASD related behaviors and the social locations of the parents. It is noted in the US that 23 states identify prenatal substance exposure [PSE] as child abuse, thus contributing to criminalization of mothers who use substances [24]. Mandated reporting of positive substance screening remains in place for many health care providers [24], and it was noted that information on substance use is either disclosed through self-report or toxicology testing [25].

When a referral or report is made to child welfare regarding a child with prenatal substance exposure who is deemed to be at risk, investigations are often undertaken to determine risk and assess safety issues. If intervention is required, it can range from the least intrusive approach which is the provision of support services to families in their home, or the most intrusive approach which is child removal [24]. Safety concerns for infants are paramount given their vulnerability and risk, and in a review of national foster care data in the US from the Adoption and Foster

Care Reporting System (AFCARS) it is reported that confirmed prenatal substance exposure is a factor in child removal in almost 35% of cases reported to child welfare [30]. In this research, infants were identified as children under a year and it was noted that for infants removed due to substance use, there were additional leading reasons for removal from parents including neglect, inadequate housing, caregiver inability to cope, physical abuse, parent incarceration, and disability (86% of cases) [30]. For infants where substance use was the primary reason for removal, it was noted that they were more likely to remain in care, even when a goal of reunification with parents or relatives was documented on their case plans [30]. This suggests that active parental substance use is considered to constitute risk, particularly for infants. This unique study of infants removed due to substance use offers insight into the early life trajectory and experiences with the foster care system.

Child Welfare and Families

Biological parents of children with FASD diagnosed in clinical settings often do not raise their children, which is attributable to many cumulative disadvantages [19]. Pivotal research conducted in Seattle profiled the experiences of 80 birth parents and noted that an FASD diagnosis for their child provided an opportunity to provide care and prevention services to individuals who were at risk of further alcohol exposed pregnancies [20]. The researchers noted that within this sample, 95% of individuals had been physically or sexually abused during their lifetime, 96% had 1–10 mental health disorders, and 61% did not complete high school. Although many individuals demonstrated the ability to overcome their alcohol dependence, they experienced many barriers to accessing substance use, mental health, and reproductive health treatment and support. Alcohol use was also noted to be intergenerational, with parents of children with FASD potentially having FASD themselves [20]. Individuals with FASD are likely to have their children at a younger age than individuals without FASD [31], highlighting their own vulnerability in personal relationships. When FASD is not recognized, the risk of intergenerational cycles exists and there is a high risk for ongoing prenatal alcohol exposure in subsequent generations [32]. Adult diagnosis of FASD remains a developing field and access is fragmented and limited [33], yet it is critically important in child welfare involvement to know if parents have FASD [34].

It is known that when an individual gives birth to a child after prenatal alcohol exposure, the likelihood exists for further affected births without intervention [7]. For example, in a 2008 Australian study research reports that among 65% of children with FASD, with almost half reported to have a sibling with FASD [32]. Biological mothers who have substance use disorders often face many challenges, frequently are single parents and are more likely to be reported to child welfare due to their substance use [30, 35] and to have their child taken into care [36]. There is a strong association between active substance use and perceived risks to infants and children by the child welfare system [37]. In one study, single women with mental health issues were identified as more likely to report their substance use during pregnancy than women who were married and it was suggested that clinical screening for these problems can offer a critical point of intervention in prenatal care [38].

Child welfare often plays a critical role in the lives of families of children with FASD for several reasons including active substance use disorders and challenging child behaviors. Children with FASD are at risk of child welfare often due to what is identified as neurobehavioral problems and it is noted that challenging behaviors are often the reason for referral for support and clinical intervention [9].

Parents who have FASD were involved in a Canadian study identified their desires to break the cycle of addiction in future generations and in the voice of one parent:

> When I grew up, my mom and dad used to always drink around me, and I don't want that. I want to break that cycle, and I don't want to live like that. ... I don't want my kids to have to go through that. So I don't really hang around people who drink or do drugs [39].

Parents identified challenges in working with child welfare and being stigmatized due to the "label of FASD client" [39 , p. 357], often feeling misunderstood and judged by workers with limited knowledge about FASD. Parents with FASD face many barriers including a constant fear of losing the custody of their children and feel particularly vulnerable due to poverty and housing insecurity. A major policy and structural barrier for adults with FASD is that they often do not quality for disability supports [39]. The need exists for FASD informed care in responding to the child protection needs of children and families and this is particularly needed when parents themselves have FASD. It is important to recognize that the parent with FASD requires interventions that are strength-based and person-centered so that accommodations can be provided that consider both relationships and safety [40].

The work done by researchers in British Columbia, Canada has outlined a strengths-based intervention model of FASD informed care for parents who have FASD. There are several best practices including: (1) adopting a non-judgmental and non-stigmatizing approach; (2) using respectful person first language that is clear, concrete, and easy to understand; (3) checking in with the person to ensure they are understanding what is being communicated; (4) offering reminders and use of tools such as visual calendars; (5) providing support through coaching, modeling, and hands on support; (5) setting realistic goals and breaking those down into steps that are achievable; (7) ensure service providers involved with the family have FASD training; (8) provide an individualized and flexible approach to the individual; (9) use outreach support and one-to-one work; (10) use a wholistic, wellness based approach in working with the individual; (11) consider the broader needs of the individual as a person and beyond being a parent; (12) involve a healthy support network of family or other support persons; and (13) attend to the physical environment to ensure it is not overwhelming the person [40].

FASD Screening and Recognition Within Child Welfare

FASD is an etiologic diagnosis that describes specific physical and neurobehavioral characteristics resulting from prenatal exposure to alcohol. The diagnostic assessment is intended to provide understanding of this constellation of features in an individual child and recommend early intervention that is informed by the assessment. The interested reader can learn more about available diagnostic systems and process for evaluation in Chaps. 8 and 9 of this book. Points particularly relevant for the child welfare system will be emphasized here.

The diagnostic assessment of FASD generally requires documentation of PAE. However, documentation of prenatal alcohol exposure in the medical record is often lacking [8]. Prenatal visits and delivery are sensitive times for gathering this information which is best gathered in a trusting and non-judgmental environment with opportunity for harm reduction and supportive intervention available. Visits with a healthcare provider who is trauma informed and culturally sensitive as well as FASD informed is critical to gathering this information which then allows for discussion of PAE and early recognition of affected children. However, it is equally important to recognize mothers who may be unwilling to disclose their alcohol use in pregnancy for fear that the child will be apprehended by child welfare. If the mother has other children, she may fear loss of them as well. In addition, if the mother has her own child welfare history, that, along with a disclosure of use in pregnancy, will almost certainly lead to a referral to child welfare.

Alcohol is also often not the only prenatal exposure, with tobacco and other drugs commonly used. In a Canadian study looking at the complexity of prenatal exposures in children, 82% were found to have multiple exposures [41]. This is consistent with data from the CanFASD Dataform which documents nicotine, cannabis, cocaine/crack, and prescription medications as among the most common co-occurring exposures [42]. The need exists to conduct routine screening for prenatal alcohol exposure given the well-known challenges and neurodevelopmental problems faced by individuals with FASD [42]. It is reported that screening for FASD is often inconsistent, and some support exists internationally for in-school screening to identify cases of FASD [43]. Children who come into care are routinely assessed by a primary health care provider and physicians are well positioned to screen for concerns about alcohol use in parents or prenatal alcohol exposure in children [18]. In relation to children with PAE screening can also assess for child maltreatment, academic and social problems, mental health disorders, behavioral problems, communication skills, educational concerns, physical health issues such as sleep, dental problems, nutrition and growth, and facilitate referrals for appropriate professional supports [ah]. The primary health care provider can also facilitate referrals to child welfare if child protection concerns exist and play a key role in supporting children and foster care providers when children are placed in care [18]. As earlier identified, given the strong connection between alcohol use and child welfare involvement, and the concern about child protection issues for children with PAE and FASD, a critical need exists to develop protocols and practices within child welfare to engage in

FASD informed practice. The reason this is essential is that screening, assessment and diagnosis support the best outcomes for children who have FASD as they are often cared for in the child welfare system [18, 31, 42, 44, 45].

It has been identified that inconsistent approaches to screening for PAE and FASD are a concern in the child welfare system. A notable research project is reported by the Children's Aid Society of Toronto that involves the application of a Neurobehavioral Screening Tool (NST) to screen children and youth coming into care [46]. This brief screening tool asks questions related to behaviors, impulsivity, and hyperactivity and completed by the assigned child protection worker (CPW). There were 106 children and youth involved in this research aged 3–15 and of the 18 children suspected to have FASD, 14 received this diagnosis. This collaborative model of care that includes child protection workers from the outset through engaging in neurobehavioral screening demonstrated the benefit of screening for FASD in child welfare cases. This approach was effective, and psychiatric comorbidity was identified for all youth referred for FASD diagnosis. It was also noted that the psychiatric referrals led to medications being started or changed as necessary and psychosocial concerns for youth were identified leading to recommendations about support needs in their living environments. This research showcased the direct benefit of a collaborative screening and assessment model involving child protection workers, pediatricians, and psychiatrists and strongly recommends the engagement of the CPW in screening for FASD for children involved in child welfare care [46].

Following routine screening, children at risk for an FASD diagnosis should be referred for comprehensive evaluation. The presentation of FASD is often complicated by exposure to trauma and social stressors. The differential diagnosis of FASD requires careful consideration of prenatal and postnatal influences on physical, emotional, and cognitive development that may contribute to behavioral assessments and functioning. In recent work characterizing adverse prenatal and postnatal experiences in children, 2/3 of children in a clinical cohort had experienced both prenatal and postnatal adversity [41]. In the same study, over 80% of children had been prenatally exposed to multiple substances. All of these factors warrant balancing and consideration in a diagnostic assessment.

In a study that examined the relationship between prenatal substance exposure, adverse childhood experiences, and mental and behavioral disorders conducted in Finland, it was noted that exposed children had higher prevalence of diagnosed mental and behavioral disorders (55%) in contrast to the controls (26%) [47]. It was also noted that of those exposed that 8% had an FASD diagnosis while 51% had multiple substance exposures including smoking during the pregnancy (75%) in contrast to the controls (19%). A serious concern noted in the out of home care group was that mothers had a death rate of 15% stating that mothers themselves had a behavioral or emotional disorder diagnosis (77%). It was identified that children and youth with behavioral and emotional disorders who had experienced out of home care were also diagnosed with disorders related to psychological development, mood, stress, and sleep. This was attributed to what was identified as "PSE is associated with a high accumulation of ACES and ACEs independently increase the risk of mental and behavioral disorders. The risk was highest among youths with

PSE (prenatal substance exposure), OHC (out of home care) and a high rate of maternal risk factors" (p. 10). This research identifies the critical point that child welfare involvement needs to consider the mother-child dyad in intervention given the risks for both parent and child.

Concerns and Health Issues for Infants and Young Children

In 2014, the Adoption and Foster Care Analysis and Reporting Systems report indicated that over one-third of children coming into care in the US were infants and young children under five, the largest age group of children coming into care. The number of foster care entries attributable to parental drug use increased 147% between 2000 and 2017 primarily due to increased use of illicit substances including opioids [48]. From 2004 to 2016, the incidence of Neonatal Abstinence Syndrome (NAS, also known as NAS, Neonatal Opioid Withdrawal) increased from 1.6 to 8.8 per 1000 hospital births [49].

Infancy and early childhood are critical stages for identifying the risk factors of prenatal alcohol exposure, as the first 3 years of life is the period of time when the most rapid physical and developmental growth takes place. Infants with FASD may present with small for gestational age or low birth weight growth patterns, prematurity, and decreased length and head circumference in some cases [50]. Related infant health issues associated with prenatal exposure to alcohol and other substances include sudden infant death syndrome (SIDS or crib death), infectious diseases (including hepatitis B and C, HIV, methicillin-resistant *Staphylococcus aureus* (MRSA), and syphilis) if mother tested positive for these infections while pregnant, and breathing problems.

In the very early years of life and if the child is living in a supportive environment, evidence of developmental delays may not apparent [51]. As the developmental stage advances toward emerging independence, problem solving, and abstract reasoning, children with FASD begin to demonstrate more challenges. In infancy and early childhood, problems with self-regulation tend to be most notable [52]. This can include negative affect and difficulties in arousal regulation, stress reactivity, impulse control, sensory integration, early attention skills, sleep and more. They may also show difficulties in fine and gross motor function, coordination and balance, and lowered adaptive functions [52].

Infants and toddlers presenting to child protection services, with or without prenatal substance exposure, may have experienced maltreatment as well as disruptions in their relationships with primary caregivers at a point where these relationships are critical for development. Because their healthy development is interrupted by the lack of security and attachment from their primary caregivers, infants and toddlers in foster care are vulnerable to the effects of neglect, maltreatment, and multiple placements, which can have lifelong implications if not addressed [53]. Alternatively, younger children may have entered foster care from the home of substance-using birth parents and may have experienced irregular and inconsistent daily care.

Developmentally appropriate services are needed at every stage of maturation, starting early. A supportive environment during the first 3 years of life can have a positive impact on long-term outcomes of the children. The benefits of providing early intervention, even without a formal FASD diagnosis, are significant with life-long impacts, including increasing the possibilities of them returning to birth families or experiencing a timely adoption process, identifying health and developmental issues early, and providing a caregiving environment that supports the best possible outcomes.

Most interventions and programs available through child welfare for substance-exposed infants and young children are focused on attachment and mental health [54]. Healthy development of an infant is influenced by the interactions between the infant, the caregiver, and the environment. Two factors which are of great importance in caring for substance-exposed infants are attuned caregivers and supportive environments. Researchers have found that parents and caregivers of special needs infants focus so much on the needs of the infants that they neglect their own well-being. Foster parents consistently identify the feeling of being supported as key to their success and satisfaction with fostering. Support for parents and caregivers can include respite services, childcare, and parenting resources. Birth mothers may also be coping with a mental health issue such as postpartum depression.

Diagnosis before the age of six has been identified as a key protective factor for children with FASD [55]. From a neurodevelopmental viewpoint, tailoring or positively reframing parenting practices to address a child's cognitive-behavioral profile can support development and socio-emotional well-being [52].

Concerns and Health Issues for Children, Adolescents, and Adults

Symptoms of FASD in childhood reflect disordered self-regulation, sensory processing, memory dysfunction, and global developmental and adaptive delays. In the preschooler, significant language delays and difficulties with regulation of attention and disorganized behavior increase the impact of developmental delays. Behavioral dysregulation often with aggression is extremely challenging for parents trying typical means of control and correction with limited success managing their child. For the child in care, this can be a reason for failure of placements and multiple caregiving experiences which places the child further at risk for disordered attachment and emotional dysregulation.

School age children with FASD tend to show increasing difficulties as demands increase with maturation. These include cognitive impairments, learning disabilities, attention deficits, memory deficits, language problems, hyperactivity and behavioral dysregulation with sensory stimulation, difficulties with social judgment, and peer relationships [18]. School age children in care who experience instability in care arrangements and/or in schooling fall even further behind academically and struggle find social supports.

Consideration of FASD in adolescent youth may be missed, often having been seen by other providers who have provided mental health diagnoses. These youth may or may not be attending school where their symptoms may have been more easily recognized. Children in care, particularly those with behavioral challenges, often have multiple school placements creating uneven responses to the child's needs across different settings. They may have experienced considerable trauma and loss and may be using substances themselves. Their language difficulties are often overestimated and may be severe. Gaps in thinking can include difficulties with forming associations, predicting, abstract reasoning, cause and effect, and generalization. They may be very literal and miss subtle social cues. Impulsivity and distractibility impact learning and social behaviors. They may experience difficulty weighing and evaluating decisions and may have difficulty judging difficulty, safety, and danger leaving them at heightened risk of exploitation and victimization. As well, youth with FASD growing up in care typically lose many supports when they transition to adulthood [56]. As adolescents and adults, people with FASD increasingly struggle with organization and have difficulty managing time, money, free time, and schedules. They are often described as socially immature.

School age children and adolescents need routine, structure, and consistency across environments, but unfortunately children with FASD often experience trauma, vulnerability, and adversity. Involvement with child welfare is not uncommon in childhood and adolescence. It is critical to recognize that children with FASD have high needs, and supporting caregivers are important to maintain placement stability for children in care [49]. One particular program, Families Moving Forward, offers consultation and support to caregivers of children aged 3–12 who have PAE and provides critical support in parent/caregiver coaching, psychoeducation supports, and skill building with an aim of looking forward [57]. Currently research is being conducted on an app that will provide support to families in an innovative way [58]. This critical program recognizes that FASD informed care is essential in order to meet the needs of children and families living with FASD and supporting caregivers needs to be an integral part of case management in FASD [59].

In the first paper from the Canada FASD National Database examining adverse outcomes for children and youth with FASD in child welfare care ($N = 665$) in contrast to those in other living situations, it was discovered that youth over the age of 12 living in care report significantly higher rates of physical and sexual abuse, and legal problems as an offender [60]. Almost half the participants lived with either their biological parent or relatives (311), while 184 were in foster care, 136 in adoptive care, and 34 living in a group home. This research also signaled concerns about the risk of suicidal ideation in this population (39%), noting this risk was higher for those children with FASD living with their biological family (27.3%) in contrast to those living in care (21.7%) and the remaining (17.8%) in adoptive living situations. This research opens up areas for potential interventions, recognizing that many young people who are living with their families may require additional mental health supports [60].

A mixed methods study exploring the topic of FASD and suicide was undertaken to explore suicidality—those range of behaviors that include suicidal talk and behavior, suicidal ideation, suicide attempts, and death among children and youth in Canada [46]. A secondary analysis from the National FASD Database was undertaken and included records with PAE confirmed, FASD diagnosis confirmed, and suicidality identified on record. The average age of participants was about 17.5 years, and, in the examination of cases, it was noted that suicidality was identified in this population at almost 26%, a much higher rate than the average population in Canada (3–12%). Higher rates of suicidality were greatest for those with trauma and abuse histories (33.1%), for those with legal problems and for those in group home or institutional settings [46, 60]. A concerning finding was that almost 12% of children in the age range of 6–12 also reported suicidality which raises concerns about the urgent need to recognize risks and vulnerabilities for this population in relation to mental health and well-being.

In summary, it is critical that FASD informed case management be utilized in the care of children with FASD. Infants, children, and youth with FASD are a vulnerable population facing lifelong challenges and often come into care in adverse circumstances such as parental substance use [18]. Early intervention is critical wherever possible and young children benefit from stable home environments with structure and routine [49, 55]. Children and youth with FASD often have trauma histories, and clinical support is needed in dealing with these concerns. It has been identified that children with FASD are far more likely to be cared for and live in the child welfare system [57], and caregiver support is essential in child welfare. Children with FASD benefit from highly structured environments at home, in school and in the community. Families raising children with FASD benefit from disability support such as respite and relief and it is critical to support families in times of crisis as we know parents experience higher levels of stress [10]. Children and youth with FASD are a complex population and research on FASD and suicidality underscores the critical need for professional and caregiver training and support in case management [46, 61]. Challenges are significant in the transition to adolescence and adulthood and the need exists to monitor and support mental health challenges.

Life Course Cumulative Disadvantages Associated with FASD

Childhood trauma and adverse childhood experiences are part of the landscape of FASD and child welfare and this needs to be more broadly understood in child intervention. While it is recognized that children are at risk when active substance use is going on in a home, it is critical to appreciate that FASD alone presents a remarkable vulnerability. FASD due to the nature of its condition sets the stage for a lifetime of vulnerability—the effects of prenatal alcohol exposure on the brain and body cause inherent challenges. The individual with FASD from the time they are an infant is situated to be dependent on others and ideally will grow into adulthood with well-established interdependent relationships to help navigate life. However, the dependence of the child and the ability to have their needs met is entirely dependent on the social structure into which they are born and live. That is to say that the family into which the child is born is expected by society to provide care that will support the child's development and growth. It is in this early stage of life that trajectories are established and infants and young children whose needs go unmet will struggle over their lifetime.

The universal theme and the problematic narrative of the lack of awareness of FASD are unacceptable and must be challenged. Children in the child protection system remain at risk of not being screened and assessed for FASD, and as noted earlier, this is critical in supporting the prevention of further cases within the same family. Misconceptions of FASD and stigma around the cause—alcohol use during pregnancy, have played a pivotal role in the lack of FASD diagnosis and the provision of services throughout the world. Despite a growing body of substantial research legitimizing FASD as a neurodevelopmental disability, FASD is still not perceived and understood as a legitimate and accepted developmental disability and this population remains dramatically underserved and poorly understood [54]. This impacts the delivery of effective services aimed at ameliorating the social, emotional, sensory, physical, psychological, and neurological challenges children living with this disability experience.

Child Welfare Practice

Child welfare workers, supervisors, and managers work within a system that is socially constructed to address the safety and well-being of children. Although each worker has completed intensive child welfare training, there is tension between the academic, legislative, and emotional contexts of lived lives. This gray space between objectivity (required by legislation, policy) and subjectivity (preferred by the front-line worker) is the context in which decisions are contemplated and child welfare workers are human beings with individual experiences that inform their judgment and decision-making [62].

Awareness of FASD within child welfare systems is often inconsistent. There are few child welfare authorities who offer required training in disability or training in FASD. These topics are not usually part of the core required training when one enters the child welfare workforce. Given the numbers of children with prenatal exposure coming to the attention of child welfare, it is confounding that education about FASD is lacking [46, 49, 57].

It is often challenging for those working in the child welfare system to figure out the best ways to screen and assess for FASD in children on their caseload. Screening and case management are key roles in child welfare work. Most child welfare systems are also challenged with high turnover rates at the front line, which compounds these challenges. A systematic review of FASD policy and practice in the US child welfare system notes that none of the studies focused on the assessment and referral process or the support provided to foster families or staff training regarding prenatal exposure [45]. It should therefore be no surprise that those with FASD are under-served in primary care provision within the child protection, criminal justice, education, health, and disabilities systems.

When confronted with a complex situation that involves a child with a disability like FASD, the child welfare system struggles to understand the nature of the diagnosis and how to assess the impact of the disability in relation to child protection concerns. The nature of a spectrum disorder requires unique and individualized planning. Accessible community resources are generalist in nature and rarely specialized enough to meet FASD specific needs. The over representation of high incidence of mental health among individuals with FASD is well documented [46, 48]. FASD informed approaches in clinical settings, particularly in child welfare and mental health are imperative in order to do no further harm.

Caring for children and youth with FASD is important work that often requires supports to help families manage due to the high care needs associated with FASD as a disabling condition. One program providing interventions to families earlier identified in this chapter is the Families Moving Forward Program [58]. It is critical to provide therapeutic interventions to families and caregivers as ongoing support is important for children with FASD, whose high needs often go far beyond the capacity of families and caregivers. While providing therapeutic support to the family is important, child welfare casework can also positively impact families by providing services such as respite and relief. Respite and relief are often essential components in maintaining the placement of a child, whether that be with family or relatives, or foster carers. Loss and grief work is also critical to include in responding to FASD in child welfare practice. Loss occurs on so many levels and can include apprehension at birth and the profound experience of loss by the mother at this time. Child apprehension at any time represents a major loss for both the family and the child. There are many losses along the way when developmental milestones are not met, when children experience rejection and exclusion, and when their disability is not understood by those in their environment and accommodations are not made for the disability.

Understanding of the caregiver experience is critical for professionals working to support families raising children with FASD. Most caregivers of children and adults with FASD are not their biological parents, rather they are kinship, foster, or adoptive families and often have limited experience and knowledge about how to care for a child with distinct needs related to PAE [31, 63]. As a result, caregivers are more likely to require detailed information about the child's history, access to caregiver support groups specific to FASD, and community support to balance daily life with disability needs. In an exploration of the adaptability of 84 caregivers across urban and rural Ontario, it was noted that "the ways in which adaptation is achieved may be unique for families of children with FASD, as compared to other intellectual or developmental disabilities" (p. 160) [63].

Kinship families provide care to children with whom they have a familial, cultural, or community connection. Unlike foster care, kinship families do not apply for this role. Instead, they are contacted, often in an emergency situation or on an urgent basis and asked to provide a safe home. Many of the complexities that exist for foster parents exist for kinship families as well and are compounded by family dynamics, additional demands of taking on the responsibility for their relatives' children, a lack of knowledge of systems, and a lack of knowledge of FASD. The kinship family can feel their sense of privacy is challenged by the very nature of having the child welfare system involved in their lives, often unexpectedly. Kinship families may be reluctant to have multiple professionals in their homes while trying to maintain a sense of family autonomy. Family privacy may be incongruent with the high level of support required in caring for children with FASD.

Adoptive families accept the challenges of raising a child with FASD expecting that there will be appropriate support from the health and social systems. Historically however, adoptive families were not provided with background health information about their children, including prenatal alcohol exposure [54]. Adoptive parents have become vocal advocates for individuals with FASD across the life course more so than birth or foster families as they are not as constrained by stigma or child welfare system processes.

For all caregivers, the level of need, support required, and stress are significant factors contributing to a high risk for placement or family breakdown. Expert consultative support for caregivers is hit and miss, and service delivery continues to be fragmented for this population. The provision of adequate support by frontline social workers in child protection to caregivers impacts placement stability which has been directly linked to enhanced positive outcomes [49]. Engaging caregivers in case planning, putting them in the lead to determine the level of support that the family system requires and can withstand is critical for success. Looking outside the family system for additional support through school, community, friends, and family can result in a more balanced case management plan. Continued advocacy for children and youth with FASD is required in child welfare specifically, and children in child protection deserve to benefit from FASD informed care in the interest of social justice.

It is clearly identified that children and youth with FASD often go undetected in child welfare and justice settings [5, 9] and recent research from Western Australia illustrates this point. The Banksia Hill Detention Centre Study included 99 children who were assessed for FASD and a prevalence rate of 36% was found in youth who had a range of neurodevelopmental conditions [64]. Notably, only two of the young people had previously been assessed for FASD diagnosis before incarceration revealing significant gaps in screening and recognition of FASD in child welfare and in the community. These children who are already often involved in the child welfare system often have serious behavioral and social challenges due to a disability that goes largely unrecognized within child welfare services.

Conclusion

Children with FASD involved with child welfare are a high needs and vulnerable population. One aspect of vulnerability is the fact that FASD goes underrecognized and this contributes to risk for the child. It has been noted globally that children with

FASD are a vulnerable population and often excluded from mainstream disability services. Stigma in relation to FASD remains a significant problem. Lack of education and knowledge in child welfare, social services, education, justice, and health professions sectors remain a significant problem.

One of the biggest challenges facing the child welfare system in Canada, the United States, Australia, and other countries is the failure of child welfare and health professionals to recognize FASD among the population. This is particularly concerning when best practice is predicated on early diagnosis and intervention, and children have better outcomes the earlier that intervention begins. Given children with FASD often have trauma histories and adverse childhood experiences, it is critical that screening, assessment, and diagnosis occur in order to provide interventions to support positive developmental trajectories.

There is no universal model of child protection practice for children and youth with FASD and concerted efforts need to be made to establish national and international practice guidelines. We must act to provide FASD informed care predicated on training and consultation regarding the distinct disability needs of this population. Adopting a life course approach is crucial as FASD is a lifespan disability and points of intervention are critical at every developmental stage from infancy to adulthood.

References

1. Jones K, Smith D. Recognition of the fetal alcohol syndrome in early infancy. Lancet. 1973;302(7836):999–1001.
2. Elder G. The life course as developmental theory. Child Dev. 1998;69(1):1–12. https://doi.org/10.1111/j.1467-8624.1998.tb06128.x.
3. Pais MS, Bissell S. Overview and implementation of the UN convention on the rights of the child. Lancet. 2006;367(9511):689–90.
4. Sabatello M. Children with disabilities: a critical appraisal. Int J Childrens Rights. 2013;21(3):464–87.
5. Williams R, Badry D. A decolonising and human rights approach to FASD training, knowledge, and case practice for justice involved youth in correctional contexts. In: Decolonising justice for aboriginal youth with fetal alcohol spectrum disorders, vol. 111. New York: Routledge; 2020.
6. Stone R. Pregnant women and substance use: fear, stigma, and barriers to care. Health Justice. 2015;3:1–15.
7. Grant TM. Preventing FASD: the parent-child assistance program (PCAP) intervention with high-risk mothers. In: Riley E, Clarren S, Weinberg J, Jonsson E, editors. Fetal alcohol spectrum disorder: management and policy perspectives of FASD. Weinheim: Wiley-VCH Verlag; 2010. p. 193–206.
8. Kartin D, et al. Three-year developmental outcomes in children with prenatal alcohol and drug exposure. Pediatr Phys Ther. 2002;14(3):145–53.
9. Chasnoff IJ, Wells AM, King L. Misdiagnosis and missed diagnoses in foster and adopted children with prenatal alcohol exposure. Pediatrics. 2015;135(2):264–70.
10. Paley B, O'Connor MJ, Frankel F, Marquardt R. Predictors of stress in parents of children with fetal alcohol spectrum disorders. J Dev Behav Pediatr. 2006;27(5):396–404.
11. Choate P, Badry D. Stigma as a dominant discourse in fetal alcohol spectrum disorder. Adv Dual Diagn. 2019;12(3):5.

12. Roozen S, Stutterheim SE, Bos AE, Kok G, Curfs LM. Understanding the social stigma of fetal alcohol spectrum disorders: from theory to interventions. Found Sci. 2020;27:753–71.
13. Charlesworth J. Excluded: increasing understanding, support and inclusion for children with FASD and their families. 2021. https://rcybc.ca/wp-content/uploads/2021/04/RCY-FASD_Report-Apr2021_FINAL_highres.pdf. Accessed 27 July 2021.
14. Gibbs A, Bagley K, Badry D, Gollner V. Foetal alcohol spectrum disorder: effective helping responses from social workers. Int Soc Work. 2020;63(4):496–509.
15. Pelech W, Badry D, Daoust G. It takes a team: improving placement stability among children and youth with fetal alcohol spectrum disorder in care in Canada. Child Youth Serv Rev. 2013;35(1):120–7.
16. Richards T, Bertrand J, Newburg-Rinn S, McCann H, Morehouse E, Ingoldsby E. Children prenatally exposed to alcohol and other drugs: what the literature tells us about child welfare information sources, policies, and practices to identify and care for children. J Publ Child Welfare. 2022;16(1):71–94.
17. Popova S, Lange S, Shield K, Burd L, Rehm J. Prevalence of fetal alcohol spectrum disorder among special subpopulations: a systematic review and meta-analysis. Addiction. 2019;114(7):1150–72.
18. Hanlon-Dearman A, Green CR, Andrew G, LeBlanc N, Cook JL. Anticipatory guidance for children and adolescents with fetal alcohol spectrum disorder (FASD): practice points for primary health care providers. J Popul Ther Clin Pharmacol. 2015;22(1):e27–56.
19. Singal D, Brownell M, Wall-Wieler E, Chateau D, Hanlon-Dearman A, Longstaffe S, et al. Prenatal care of women who give birth to children with fetal alcohol spectrum disorder in a universal health care system: a case-control study using linked administrative data. CMAJ Open. 2019;7(1):E63–72.
20. Astley SJ. Profile of the first 1400 patients receiving diagnostic evaluations for fetal alcohol spectrum disorder at the Washington State Fetal Alcohol Syndrome Diagnostic and Prevention Network. Can J Clin Pharmacol. 2010;17(1):e132–64.
21. Bagley K, Badry D. How personal perspectives shape health professionals' perceptions of fetal alcohol spectrum disorder and risk. Int J Environ Res Public Health. 2019;16(11):1936.
22. Hui K, Angelotta C, Fisher CE. Criminalizing substance use in pregnancy: misplaced priorities. Addiction. 2017;112(7):1123.
23. Winnipeg Child and Family Services (Northwest Area) v. G. (D.F.), [1997] 3 S.C.R. 92. https://scc-csc.lexum.com/scc-csc/scc-csc/en/item/1562/index.do. Accessed 31 July 2021.
24. Peddireddy SR, Austin AE, Gottfredson NC. Factors contributing to level and type of child welfare involvement following prenatal substance exposure: a scoping review. Child Abuse Negl. 2022;125:105484.
25. Behnke M, Smith VC, Levy S, Ammerman SD, Gonzalez PK, Ryan SA, Wunsch MD, Papile LA, Baley JE, Carlo WA, Cummings JJ. Prenatal substance abuse: short-and long-term effects on the exposed fetus. Pediatrics. 2013;131(3):e1009–24.
26. Ingoldsby E, Richards T, Usher K, Wang K, Morehouse E, Masters L, Kopiec K. Prenatal alcohol and other drug exposures in child welfare study: final report. Washington, DC: U.S. Department of Health and Human Services; 2021.
27. Osterling KL, Austin MJ. Substance abuse interventions for parents involved in the child welfare system: evidence and implications. J Evid Based Soc Work. 2008;5(1–2):157–89.
28. Grella CE, Hser YI, Huang YC. Mothers in substance abuse treatment: differences in characteristics based on involvement with child welfare services. Child Abuse Negl. 2006;30(1):55–73.
29. Marcenko MO, Kemp SP, Larson NC. Childhood experiences of abuse, later substance use, and parenting outcomes among low-income mothers. Am J Orthopsychiatry. 2000;70(3):316–26.
30. Boyd R. Foster care outcomes and experiences of infants removed due to substance abuse. J Publ Child Welfare. 2019;13(5):529–55.
31. Fuchs DBL, Marchenski S, Mudry A. Children with FASD involved with the Manitoba child welfare system. 2007. www.cecw-cepb.ca/sites/default/files/publications/en/FASD_Final_Report.pdf.

32. Elliott EJ. Fetal alcohol spectrum disorders in Australia—the future is prevention. Public Health Res Pract. 2015;25(2):e2521516.
33. Badry D, Bradshaw C. Assessment and diagnosis of FASD among adults. A national and international systematic review. Ottawa: Public Health Agency of Canada; 2010.
34. Temple VK, Ives J, Lindsay A. Diagnosing FASD in adults: the development and operation of an adult FASD clinic in Ontario, Canada. J Popul Ther Clin Pharmacol. 2015;22(1):e96–e105.
35. Deutsch SA, Donahue J, Parker T, Hossain J, De Jong A. Factors associated with child-welfare involvement among prenatally substance-exposed infants. J Pediatr. 2020;222:35–44.
36. Wall-Wieler E, Roos LL, Brownell M, Nickel NC, Chateau D. Predictors of having a first child taken into care at birth: a population-based retrospective cohort study. Child Abuse Negl. 2018;76:1–9.
37. Hafekost K, Lawrence D, O'Leary C, Bower C, Semmens J, Zubrick SR. Maternal alcohol use disorder and risk of child contact with the justice system in Western Australia: a population cohort record linkage study. Alcohol Clin Exp Res. 2017;41(8):1452–60.
38. Havens JR, Simmons LA, Shannon LM, Hansen WF. Factors associated with substance use during pregnancy: results from a national sample. Drug Alcohol Depend. 2008;99(1):89–95. https://doi.org/10.1016/j.drugalcdep.2008.07.010.
39. Rutman D, Van Bibber M. Parenting with fetal alcohol spectrum disorder. Int J Ment Health Addict. 2010;8(2):351–61.
40. Rutman D. Article commentary: becoming FASD informed: strengthening practice and programs working with women with FASD. Subst Abuse Res Treat. 2016;10:SART-34543.
41. Lebel CA, McMorris CA, Kar P, Ritter C, Andre Q, Tortorelli C, et al. Characterizing adverse prenatal and postnatal experiences in children. Birth Defects Res. 2019;111(12):848–58.
42. Cook J, Unsworth K, Flannigan K. Characterising fetal alcohol spectrum disorder in Canada: a national database protocol study. BMJ Open. 2021;11(9):e046071.
43. May PA, Gossage JP, Kalberg WO, Robinson LK, Buckley D, Manning M, Hoyme HE. Prevalence and epidemiologic characteristics of FASD from various research methods with an emphasis on recent in-school studies. Dev Disabil Res Rev. 2009;15(3):176–92.
44. Lange S, Shield K, Rehm J, Popova S. Prevalence of fetal alcohol spectrum disorders in child care settings: a meta-analysis. Pediatrics. 2013;132(4):e980–95.
45. Petrenko CL, Alto ME, Hart AR, Freeze SM, Cole LL. "I'm doing my part, I just need help from the community": intervention implications of foster and adoptive parents' experiences raising children and young adults with FASD. J Fam Nurs. 2019;25(2):314–47.
46. Burns J, Badry DE, Harding KD, Roberts N, Unsworth K, Cook JL. Comparing outcomes of children and youth with fetal alcohol spectrum disorder (FASD) in the child welfare system to those in other living situations in Canada: results from the Canadian National FASD Database. Child Care Health Dev. 2021;47(1):77–84.
47. Koponen AM, Nissinen NM, Gissler M, Autti-Rämö I, Sarkola T, Kahila H. Prenatal substance exposure, adverse childhood experiences and diagnosed mental and behavioral disorders—a longitudinal register-based matched cohort study in Finland. SSM Popul Health. 2020;11:100625. https://doi.org/10.1016/j.ssmph.2020.100625.
48. Patel M, Agnihotri S, Hawkins C, Levin L, Goodman D, Simpson A. Identifying fetal alcohol spectrum disorder and psychiatric comorbidity for children and youth in care: a community approach to diagnosis and treatment. Child Youth Serv Rev. 2020;108:104606.
49. Meinhofer A, Angleró-Díaz Y. Trends in foster care entry among children removed from their homes because of parental drug use, 2000–2017. JAMA Pediatr. 2019;173(9):881–3.
50. Leech AA, Cooper WO, McNeer E, Scott TA, Patrick SW. Neonatal Abstinence Syndrome in the United States, 2004–2016: an examination of neonatal abstinence syndrome trends and incidence patterns across US census regions in the period 2004–2016. Health Aff. 2020;39(5):764–7.
51. Kalberg WO, May PA, Buckley D, Hasken JM, Marais AS, De Vries MM, Bezuidenhout H, Manning MA, Robinson LK, Adam MP, Hoyme DB. Early-life predictors of fetal alcohol spectrum disorders. Pediatrics. 2019;144(6):e20182141.

52. Andrew G. Diagnosis of FASD: an overview. In: Riley E, Clarren S, Weinberg J, Jonsson E, editors. Fetal alcohol spectrum disorder: management and policy perspectives of FASD. New York: Wiley-Blackwell; 2010. p. 127–48.
53. Olson H, Montague R. Chapter 4. An innovative look at early intervention for children affected by prenatal alcohol exposure. In: Adubato S, Cohen D, editors. Prenatal alcohol use and FASD: diagnosis, assessment and new directions in research and multimodal treatment. Sharjah: Bentham Science Publishers; 2011. p. 64–107.
54. Center on the Developing Child at Harvard University. Applying the science of child development in child welfare systems. 2016. https://www.developingchild.harvard.edu. Accessed 26 July 2021.
55. Marcellus L, Badry D. Infants, children, and youth in foster care with prenatal substance exposure: a synthesis of two scoping reviews. Int J Dev Disabil. 2021;69(2):1945890. https://doi.org/10.1080/20473869.2021.1945890.
56. Streissguth AP, Barr HM, Kogan J, Bookstein FL. Understanding the occurrence of secondary disabilities in clients with fetal alcohol syndrome (FAS) and fetal alcohol effects (FAE): final report. Atlanta: Centers for Disease Control and Prevention (CDC); 1996. p. 96–106.
57. Pelech B, Badry D, Daoust G. It takes a team: improving placement stability among children and youth with fetal alcohol spectrum disorder in care in Canada. Child Youth Serv Rev. 2012;35(1):120–7. https://doi.org/10.1016/j.childyouth.2012.10.011.
58. Petrenko CL, Kautz-Turnbull CC, Roth AR, Parr JE, Tapparello C, Demir U, Olson HC. Initial feasibility of the "families moving forward connect" mobile health intervention for caregivers of children with fetal alcohol spectrum disorders: mixed method evaluation within a systematic user-centered design approach. JMIR Format Res. 2021;5(12):e29687.
59. Petrenko CL, Parr J, Kautz C, Tapparello C, Olson HC. A mobile health intervention for fetal alcohol spectrum disorders (families moving forward connect): development and qualitative evaluation of design and functionalities. JMIR Mhealth Uhealth. 2020;8(4):e14721.
60. Flannigan K, McMorris C, Ewasiuk A, Badry D, Mela M, Ben Gibbard W, Unsworth K, Cook J, Harding KD. Suicidality and associated factors among individuals assessed for fetal alcohol spectrum disorder across the lifespan in Canada: Suicidabilité et facteurs associés chez les personnes évaluées pour les troubles du spectre de l'alcoolisation fœtale de durée de vie au Canada. Can J Psychiatry. 2021;67(5):361–70.
61. Families Moving Forward. http://familiesmovingforwardprogram.com/.
62. Munro E, Hardie J. Why we should stop talking about objectivity and subjectivity in social work. Br J Soc Work. 2019;49(2):411–27.
63. Coons KD, Watson SL, Schinke RJ, Yantzi NM. Adaptation in families raising children with fetal alcohol spectrum disorder. Part I: what has helped. J Intellect Dev Disabil. 2016;41(2):150–65. https://doi.org/10.3109/13668250.2016.1156659.
64. Bower C, Watkins RE, Mutch RC, Marriott R, Freeman J, Kippin NR, Safe B, Pestell C, Cheung CS, Shield H, Tarratt L. Fetal alcohol spectrum disorder and youth justice: a prevalence study among young people sentenced to detention in Western Australia. BMJ Open. 2018;8(2):e019605.

Chapter 16
Educating School-Aged Children with FASD

Molly N. Millians

Introduction

Fetal alcohol spectrum disorders (FASD) is a descriptive term encompassing the range of physical abnormalities and neurobehavioral deficits associated with the effects of prenatal alcohol exposure (PAE) [1–4]. The clinical diagnosis of fetal alcohol syndrome (FAS), partial fetal alcohol syndrome (pFAS), neurodevelopmental disorder associated with prenatal alcohol exposure (ND-PAE), and alcohol-related neurodevelopmental disorder (ARND) is included within the term of FASD [2, 4]. In the United States, approximately 1–5% of school-aged children may be affected by PAE [5]. While the estimated prevalence of children and youth with FASD in other countries is similar to the United States, meta-analysis and review studies have suggested significantly higher prevalence rates in South Africa, Croatia, and estimated for Ireland [6, 7]. The prevalence of FASD among school-aged children may be an underestimation due to differences in study methodologies and diagnostic models [8, 9]. Nevertheless, based upon the estimates, it is probable that most school systems in the United States and other nations educate children and youth with FASD [10, 11].

The effects of PAE include a range cognitive and functional impairments that may be compounded by other in-utero exposures, genetic factors, and pre-and-postnatal environmental stressors that disrupt development and learning [12] Though some individuals with FASD share similar traits, research has not yet identified a consistent cognitive or behavioral phenotype associated with the disorder [1, 13]. Some children and youth affected by PAE have global developmental delays, while others may exhibit specific deficits in one or more cognitive domains that

M. N. Millians (✉)
Department of Child Psychiatry and Behavioral Sciences, Emory University School of
Medicine, Atlanta, GA, USA
e-mail: molly.n.millians@emory.edu

O. A. Abdul-Rahman, C. L. M. Petrenko (eds.), *Fetal Alcohol Spectrum Disorders*,
https://doi.org/10.1007/978-3-031-32386-7_16

interfere with learning [1, 13]. Irrespective of cognitive impairments, some children and youth with FASD have problems with behavior regulation, emotional regulation, and adaptive functioning [14–16]. Also, among individuals with FASD, there is a high rate of reported co-occurring medical conditions [17]. Many affected by PAE have experienced social and environmental challenges, such as multiple caregiving placements, deprivation, or involvement in foster care that may impact learning readiness [12, 18, 19]. The variable presentation of FASD coupled with common adverse experiences place many children and youth at risk for learning and school problems, especially if they do not receive intervention [20, 21]. Though not all school-aged children with FASD exhibit the same cluster of characteristics, it is important for educators to understand the scope and nuances of the disorder and consider PAE as an indicator that the student may require support or interventions to address potential learning and school problems [22].

However, there are barriers obtaining information about FASD that pose challenges to educators to understand and meet the needs of school-aged children affected by PAE. Many children are not screened or evaluated for the effects of prenatal exposures potentially leading to overlooked or misdiagnosis and ineffective treatment planning [23, 24]. This may occur more often among minoritized populations, children living in poverty, or children in foster care because of disparities in access to healthcare and mental health services [23–26]. Negative stereotypes and misperceptions about FASD may hinder collaboration between caregivers, educators, and allied service providers. Because of misperceptions, such as beliefs that children with FASD have severe behavioral problems due to poor parenting, some caregivers may not disclose information about their children's diagnosis out of concern of being judged by teachers or ostracized by classmates' families [27]. Other misinformed beliefs, such as children with FASD are unable to learn because of permanent brain damage, may inadvertently influence some teachers' interactions and effort with students [28]. Access to accurate information is necessary to counter stigma and respond to the needs of school-aged children with FASD [28, 29].

The neurobehavioral deficits associated with FASD fall within the classification of developmental disabilities, defined as a group of life-long conditions related to physical and or neurocognitive impairments that impact language, learning, and behavior [30, 31]. However, studies examining prevalence and outcomes of different conditions classified as developmental disabilities often do not specify FASD as a subset, contributing to the marginalization of the disorder [30, 31]. Furthermore, few studies have surveyed the number of school-aged children with FASD receiving special education services [32]. Currently, in the United States, there is no long-term coordinated surveillance effort to examine the special education services and educational outcomes of students with FASD in public schools [9, 32]. These and other barriers interfere with understanding and disseminating accurate information about FASD to guide educational policy and best practices to offset potential school problems.

Qualitative studies examining experiences of students with FASD, their caregivers and teachers, provide insight into key components to support students with FASD in schools despite existing barriers [33, 34]. From these studies, increasing awareness through training and dissemination of accurate information about the effects from PAE were associated with improved student–teacher interactions and countering misperceptions [35, 36]. Studies showed that collaboration between school personnel, caregivers, allied services providers, and when developmentally appropriate, individuals with FASD, was associated with better interactions with families and support of students at school [37, 38]. In addition, studies have shown that effective individualized interventions following a habilitative approach improved learning, academics, and functioning at home and at school [39, 40].

This chapter provides an overview of the educational needs of school-aged children with FASD. The chapter presents a review of the literature regarding school functioning, educational experiences, and outcomes of school-aged children affected by PAE. Next, the chapter discusses regulations, school-based services, and best practices in public education that apply to school-aged children with FASD in the United States. Lastly, the chapter concludes with a proposal for an integrative approach that focuses on building and applying skills to promote active engagement, learning, and participation at school so that children and youth with FASD can reach their potential.

School Functioning

School functioning refers to the academic, behavioral, and social skills needed to meet the expectations of an educational setting [41]. Efficient school functioning relies on the interplay between multiple cognitive processes and personal characteristics to engage, maintain motivation, and learn in a school setting [42, 43]. These cognitive processes and personal traits are sensitive to biological, genetic, social, and environmental factors [22, 44, 45].

In the general population, intellectual abilities, language, attention, executive functioning, working memory, and visuospatial processing are associated with scores on standardized academic achievement measures of word reading, reading comprehension, written expression, and mathematics [42, 46, 47]. Also, studies of children have shown associations between graphomotor skills and performance on standardized measures of written expression and mathematics [42, 48, 49]. In school-aged children, better developed executive functioning and self-regulation are associated with higher grades and fewer behavioral problems in the classroom [50–52].

Attention, executive functioning, and self-regulation are interlinked constructs that contribute not only to scores on academic achievement tests but also to traits needed to manage the social demands of a school setting [51–54]. In broad terms, executive functioning refers to a set of cognitive processes that includes inhibition, updating working memory, and shifting that interact to complete goal directed behavior [55, 56]. Neural models of executive functioning suggest that these processes are associated with activation of the prefrontal cortex and basal ganglia [55]. According to this definition of executive functioning, inhibition is the ability to suppress dominant, automatic, or proponent responses when completing a task [55]. The definition defines updating working memory as the ability to monitor, add, and delete information as new content is acquired [55]. Lastly, shifting is the ability to switch between task goals and sets of information [53, 55]. These processes work in coordination to support learning and problem-solving tasks that are critical for the school environment.

Self-regulation, defined as the unconscious and conscious control of one's emotions and behaviors across contexts, shares cognitive resources with executive functioning [57, 58]. As children increase in conscious control of their behavior and emotions, they draw upon the cognitive processes related to executive functioning and other domains, such as language to modulate their responses [53, 57]. In school, self-regulation may be observed by students' focusing, staying on task, coping with frustration, self-monitoring, and maintaining self-control across school settings [43, 57]. Specifically, studies have shown that self-control is associated with changes in grades, increased task completion, and use of prosocial behaviors in the classroom [43, 51]. In the long-term, better developed executive functioning and self-regulation are associated with higher educational attainment and decreased risk of later substance abuse and involvement with the judicial system [43, 59].

Along with cognitive processes, individual learning traits such as self-efficacy contribute to school success [33, 43, 60]. Self-efficacy is one's belief in one's ability to understand, learn, and apply skills to achieve a goal [61, 62]. It assists with students' effort, motivation, and persistence to complete challenging tasks or to maintain performance in less-than-optimal learning settings [62]. Research examining effort in students with learning disabilities has shown that those with positive self-perceptions about learning were more likely to use strategies to persevere with challenging learning tasks when compared to students with learning disabilities who hold negative self-perceptions [63]. Other studies have shown positive relationships between self-efficacy and higher grades in school and reaching goals in the workplace [60, 64]. In school-aged children, self-efficacy is sourced through supportive learning environments with appropriate teacher and parent expectations and positive school experiences [43, 62]. Reviews of strength-based literature suggested that many individuals with FASD exhibit personal traits that align with self-efficacy [65].

FASD, Disrupted School Experiences, and Educational Outcomes

Studies of individuals with FASD referred for clinical services and recruited from the community illustrate the risk for school problems and disrupted school experiences, defined as being suspended, expelled, or dropping out of school in this population [20, 66]. A 1996 summary report from a project examining adverse outcomes and protective factors in individuals with FAS or affected by PAE referred for clinical services indicated that approximately 60% of school-aged children and adolescents with PAE reported difficulties having good relationships with their peers and between 55 and 60% reported exhibiting behaviors that disrupted classes [20]. In addition, approximately 60% of the participants with FAS or affected by PAE indicated having been suspended, expelled, or dropped out of school with only 40% of individuals with PAE between the ages of 21 and 51 having graduated high school or completed the high school general equivalency exam (GED) [20]. Studies of participants with FASD recruited from the community reported somewhat better school experiences and outcomes. For example, a 2006 study examining school functioning with participants recruited from the community in an urban area in the southeastern United States found no differences in conduct problems at school in adolescents with PAE when compared to a special education contrast group, and to a control group of adolescents with no or unknown PAE [67]. A more recent study analyzing the records of adolescents, youth, and adults with FASD from the Canadian National FASD Database indicated that 18% reported school disruptions defined as being suspended or expelled from school [66]. The school disruption rate was lower than reported by participants with FASD referred for clinical services. However, for comparison to a general school-aged population within a Canadian school system, the rate of school disruptions for the adolescents with FASD was higher than the average rate of approximately 3% of students reported to be suspended and expelled in schools under the jurisdiction of the Ontario Ministry of Education [68].

Research suggests that individuals with PAE with more complex cognitive, behavioral, and mental health issues of have poorer educational outcomes [66, 69]. One study, examining the effects of PAE on adaptive functioning in young adults with PAE compared to a control group and a special education contrast group of young adults with no or unknown PAE found that 53% of young adults with facial features and cognitive impairments associated with PAE had graduated high school [69]. For the young adults with cognitive impairments but no facial features associated with PAE, 62% completed high school [69]. The study indicated that 66% of the special education contrast and 81% of the control group reported graduating high school [69]. Except for the group of the more severely impacted adolescents with PAE, the graduation rates for the special education contrast group and the control group were similar to the 2015 graduation rates in the United States in which 66% of students receiving special education and about 84% of all students completed high school [70].

A more recent study conducted in Finland examined the impact of childhood adversity, out-of-home placements or being in foster care, as well as behavioral, mental health, and other diagnoses on secondary school completion in youth with and without prenatal exposure [71]. Individuals were excluded from the study if they had intellectual disabilities to match the groups of individuals with and without prenatal exposures. The results indicated that individuals with prenatal exposure to alcohol and drugs without cognitive impairment were less likely to complete secondary school [71]. For those that completed high school in both the non-exposed and prenatally exposed groups, neuropsychological, mental health, and behavioral disorders including psychiatric disorders as well as dual diagnoses were related to a lag or an extended time to complete secondary school [71]. There was no association between the overall score of reported childhood adverse experiences and out-of-home placements to completion of secondary school [71]. The study indicated that regardless of history of prenatal exposures, those who had more behavioral, mental health, and medical diagnoses fared worse than those without the complications transitioning into adulthood [21, 69, 71]. An earlier study out of Sweden reported that all individuals with FASD completed the compulsory years of education as mandated by the Swedish Education Act that prohibits dropping out of school and allocates special education and other services to ensure completion of education [21]. Overall, these studies reflect the variability in presentation of FASD, individuals' intervention needs, access to services, and policies that have long-term implications.

FASD, Cognitive Processes, and School Functioning

Over the years, studies have shown that neurodevelopmental impairments associated with PAE combined with other medical, environmental, and social factors have detrimental impacts on most aspects of school functioning [1, 19]. Some with FASD exhibit global developmental delays with scores on standardized measures of intellectual and adaptive functioning falling more than 2 standard deviations below the mean when compared to the normative sample [1]. Yet, most individuals affected by PAE do not exhibit global developmental delays but have impairments in one or more specific cognitive domains [1].

Imaging and behavioral studies have identified that brain structure and white matter integrity are susceptible to the effects in-utero alcohol exposure influencing processes drawn upon for learning [13, 72–74]. For example, neuroimaging studies have shown associations between alterations in the prefrontal cortex and frontoparietal region and heavy PAE [72, 75]. Atypical development in one or more of these areas would impair executive functions such as inhibition, planning, and shifting [74, 76, 77]. Decreased white matter integrity and connectivity related to PAE is associated with poorer cognitive efficiency [74, 76, 78]. This would impact academics, behavior, and managing the expectations of a school setting.

Behavioral studies have identified impairments with verbal learning and recall in school-aged children with PAE due to inefficient use of strategies for encoding or deficits with word retrieval [79, 80]. The impairments with verbal learning and recall have remained after accounting for influence of intellectual abilities in children with PAE [80]. In addition, research has indicated that children with FASD show poorer performance encoding spatial information needed for place learning when compared to typically developing, non-exposed peers [81, 82]. Problems with visual and spatial coding not only would interfere with academics but also with navigating a school or classroom layouts, organizing, and locating materials, judging social distance, and following classroom routines [83]. Other studies have indicated aspects of attention, working memory, and executive functioning impacting effective communication, spelling, and written language skills [84, 85].

Across age-groups, studies have found differences in brain activation patterns in individuals with PAE compared to nonexposed individuals and others with behavioral diagnosis such as Attention-Deficit Hyperactivity (ADHD) during mental tasks of numerical processing [86, 87]. Specifically, studies have shown that children with FASD showed less activation in areas of the intraparietal sulcus and activated additional regions to support processing numerical information including determining magnitude, judging proximity of numbers, and basic arithmetic when compared to non-exposed controls [87, 88]. Deficits with number processing combined with weakness in visuospatial abilities, executive processes, and working memory associated with the effects from PAE would impact learning mathematics [89, 90].

Clinically, caregivers and teachers often report children with FASD exhibit difficulties with behavior and self-regulation that interfere with school functioning. Many children and adolescents with FASD are reported as having problems with attention and may be described as unfocused, easily distracted during instruction, and frequently making careless errors when completing assignments or test [91]. Based upon the results of parent and teacher behavioral reports of attention problems, many school-aged children affected by PAE often meet the criteria for or have a diagnosis of Attention-Deficit Hyperactivity Disorder (ADHD) [17, 92]. However, a description of attention problems may mask weaknesses in other cognitive processes that impact learning and classroom functioning.

Studies using cognitive measures in addition to traditional parental and teacher behavioral checklists have found differences in attentional profiles in children affected by PAE when compared to non-exposed children with ADHD [93, 94]. In a 2011 article, Mattson, Crocker, and Nguyen succinctly summarized the similarities and differences between FASD and ADHD. They indicated that FASD is associated with lower intellectual abilities, and more impaired selective attention, problem-solving, encoding, verbal fluency, and adaptive behaviors than ADHD [93]. In comparison to ADHD, FASD may be associated with less impaired motor control, focused attention, sustained attention, and retrieval of information [93]. The article indicated that FASD and ADHD share similarities regarding parental and teacher reports of behavioral problems, challenges with social skills, as well as weaknesses with cognitive flexibility and execution of complex motor tasks [93]. The reliance on parent and teacher reports or checklists does not capture the other underlying neurocognitive impairments that may contribute to or appear as attention difficulties in classroom settings in children affected by PAE [94]. Awareness of the differences between FASD and other behavioral disorders would be necessary when assessing observed behavioral difficulties to determine appropriate interventions.

Many children and adolescents with FASD exhibit deficits with aspects of executive functioning that interfere with academic performance, social interactions, and classroom behavior [95, 96]. Specifically, studies have shown that children with FASD show difficulties with shifting between mental sets, incorporating feedback to adjust problem-solving approaches, recognizing that a response may be correct for one problem but not for another, and learning to regulate attentional resources when tasks and time demands increase [2, 4]. Problems with executive functioning in school-aged children with FASD often are greater than expected when compared to overall cognitive abilities and may persist into adulthood [2, 4].

In addition, school-aged children affected by PAE are described as having difficulties with emotional and behavioral regulation, which overlap with executive functioning [1, 16, 58]. Often school aged with FASD are described as being easily overwhelmed and overreact to common environmental stressors [58, 97]. Clinically, parent and teacher reports indicated that school-aged children with FASD exhibit difficulties modulating their arousal level that interferes with transitioning from high-level activities to seated work, sustaining engagement during group instruction, and refraining from impulsively responding in class [98, 99]. Also, problems with executive functioning and self-regulation in school-aged children affected by PAE may be described as showing lack of persistence to complete work, avoidance of tasks, commenting out of turn during class discussions, and exhibiting behaviors that may be bothersome to classmates [100, 101]. There are ways to address weakness with executive functioning and self-regulation and skills influenced by these processes to improve academic performance and classroom behavior [102, 103]. Some examples include teaching cognitive control strategies and metacognitive awareness, providing instruction to improve use of prosocial skills, and effective problem-solving approaches through repeated practice across contexts, and using various levels of difficulty or challenges [103, 104].

Some school-aged children with FASD are reported has having difficulties managing social interactions [95]. Studies have shown that adolescents affected by PAE may have difficulties explaining a situation possibly due to poor encoding of the event or challenges organizing language to express ideas in a logical sequence [84]. Also, problems with organizing and expressing verbal information clearly would interfere with meaningful participation during classroom discussions and when working cooperatively in groups [85, 105]. In the classroom, children with FASD are reported to demonstrate prosocial skills such as initiating and engaging in social exchanges with peers; however, they are described as showing variability in sustaining these interactions [106, 107]. Some children with FASD due to impulsivity may make comments that are unrelated to a topic or inappropriate to the social situation [95]. The unpredictability of interactions of school-aged children with FASD may result in avoidance by classmates [95]. Also, teachers may misinterpret problems with impulsivity as purposeful disruptive classroom behavior [95]. Providing instruction to sustain engagement and awareness of the social setting and interactions may improve classroom behavior.

A recent review article by Lees et al. has a table of examples of the cognitive indicators related to FASD and common presentations in the classroom. Not all individuals with FASD have the same neurobehavioral deficits and learning profile. The variability among the neurobehavioral traits associated with effects from PAE in school-aged children shows the need for comprehensive evaluations to identify the learning strengths and challenges to prevent misinterpretation of observed behaviors and to guide appropriate intervention planning [99, 108].

FASD and Individual Traits

Recent articles examining personal traits through a strength-based model have suggested that many school-aged children affected by PAE have personal characteristics that are associated with successful school functioning [65, 109]. In a 2021 review study, Flannigan et al. proposed that many individuals with FASD have affinities in arts, music, and sports [65]. The findings from the review indicated that many individuals with FASD were described as socially motivated, curious and demonstrated perseverance [65]. These traits are associated with self-efficacy and better school functioning [65]. Other studies have suggested that school-aged children with FASD who are socially motivated are more receptive to learn through interactive exchanges with instructors [65, 109, 110]. Interactive instructional approaches have been effective when habilitating mathematic skills and learning readiness in children with FASD [110, 111]. Additionally, individuals with FASD, who are socially motivated, might benefit from support to establish and maintain positive relationships with peers and adults [107]. Stable connections with responsible adults and positive peer networks are found to be protective factors in childhood and related to better outcomes in adulthood [108, 109].

FASD and Academic Achievement

Studies examining the timing and dosage of in-utero alcohol exposure have been found to impact scores on academic achievement measures of reading, spelling, and arithmetic [67, 90, 112]. In a 1996 study, Goldschmidt et al. examined academic skills in children affected by PAE at 6 years of age [112]. After controlling for intellectual abilities, social factors, and other prenatal substance exposure, heavy intra-uterine alcohol exposure at the second trimester of pregnancy was associated with lower scores on tests of word reading, spelling, and arithmetic. There was a dose–response relationship between in-utero alcohol exposure during the second trimester and arithmetic test scores. A threshold effect of one drink per day during the second trimester was related to lower scores on tests of word reading and spelling [112]. In a follow-up study when the children were 10 years of age, binge drinking during the second trimester was associated with lower reading scores [113]. Contrary to the earlier study, there was no relationship between PAE and scores on the test of arithmetic; however, scores were generally lower than those in reading and spelling [112, 113]. Furthermore, in-utero alcohol exposure during the first and second trimester was related to poorer teacher's ratings of academic performance across subjects reflecting an association of academic underachievement with PAE [113]. Without controlling for factors that might influence academic performance, a study conducted in Australia found that children with heavy PAE during the first trimester of pregnancy were twice as likely not to meet reading benchmarks on a nationally administered, criterion-referenced academic test [114]. Additionally, the study indicated that maternal binge drinking, defined as consumption of five or more drinks in a single sitting, was related to failing to meet academic benchmarks in expressive writing [114]. The findings demonstrated the of binge drinking and heavy PAE on academic functioning. However, there is little information on the impact of light-to-moderate in-utero alcohol exposure and academic achievement [115].

Other studies have examined the impact of PAE on academic achievement by examining maternal biological factors that may be related to the amount of exposure. Interesting outcomes regarding PAE, and academic achievement came out of a population-based study of pairs of mothers and their children from the United Kingdom participating in the Avon Longitudinal Study of Parents and Children. In a 2013 study, researchers examined the effects of PAE on academic performance using a Mendelian randomization based upon the maternal variant in the alcohol-dehydrogenase gene that is considered to predict higher metabolism of alcohol that may result in lower prenatal alcohol exposure [116]. The results showed that moderate levels of alcohol consumption by women with higher incomes during pregnancy were associated with higher scores on cognitive and academic measures when compared to women who reported light drinking. In this study, women who had higher incomes reported moderate drinking during pregnancy when compared to women who reported light drinking. Additionally, better scores on cognitive and academic standardized tests were noted in children whose mother had the gene variant. The authors concluded that the children of mothers with the gene variant had lower exposure during pregnancy [116]. However, the findings reflected the influence of socioeconomic status and maternal education related to better outcomes on cognitive and academic achievement measures, possibly masking the impact of PAE [45, 116]. A later study examining the dosage, timing, duration, and patterns of maternal drinking during pregnancy applying Mendelian randomization showed clear effects of PAE on academic achievement after accounting for socioeconomic status [117]. These studies point out the need to screen school-aged children for the effects of PAE regardless of social and environmental factors to assess their educational needs. The impact of PAE on cognitive and academic functioning crosses socioeconomic status, race, and other demographic factors [116, 117].

Other studies have shown associations between heavy PAE and impaired cognitive processes impacting spelling and word reading. In 2015, Glass et al. examined spelling and word reading skills of children heavily exposed to alcohol in-utero as compared to a non-exposed contrast group [118]. The results indicated that children with heavy PAE had significantly lower scores on measures of word reading and spelling, phonological processing, and working memory when compared to the contrast group. Comparison of cognitive functioning between the two groups indicated that working memory uniquely contributed to spelling in the children with heavy PAE but not to the contrast group after accounting for the variance of phonological processing and speeded naming. Results indicated that working memory had a stronger relationship to performance on measures of word reading and spelling in children with heavy PAE when compared to the nonexposed contrast group. The authors surmised that a wider range of executive functioning problems may interfere with learning in children affected by heavy PAE [118].

In a recent study, researchers investigated structural and functional brain mechanisms that mediated word reading and phonemic decoding tasks in adolescents with PAE and dysmorphia as compared to a group of adolescents with PAE without dysmorphia, and a control group of typically developing adolescents without reported PAE [119]. The findings showed that adolescents with PAE and dysmorphia showed greater activation in the right precentral gyrus during the phonemic decoding task, and rightward lateralization in the inferior longitudinal fasciculus during both tasks. The study controlled for family socioeconomic status, intellectual abilities, other exposures, and diagnosis of ADHD. In the group of adolescents with PAE and no dysmorphia, activation in the left angular gyrus and white matter organization in the left inferior longitudinal fasciculus was associated with better reading skills; however, the association was weaker when compared to the controls [119]. Overall, the study indicated differences in brain structural characteristics and activation impacting sight word reading and phonemic decoding between adolescents affected by PAE with and without dysmorphia [119].

Across age-groups of children affected by PAE, studies have identified deficits in mathematics. In 2011, Rasmussen and Bisanz examined a range of mathematical skills in young children with and without FASD between 4 and 6 years of age. Children with FASD had lower mean scores on quantitative concepts, applied problems, and math reasoning when compared to a control group of children without FASD [120]. The findings indicated that phonological working memory was associated with performance on the mathematical tests for both groups with children with FASD showing significantly lower scores than the control group [120]. It is not clear from the article if there were group differences in intellectual abilities. The reported correlations suggested that children with FASD drew upon more aspects of verbal working memory that are associated with executive functioning when completing different mathematical tasks when compared to the control group [120]. In this study, there was no association between visuospatial abilities and mathematics.

Other studies have examined associations of cognitive processes and mathematics in children affected by PAE. One study conducted in 2015 examined whether attention, working memory, and aspects of visuospatial abilities would be associated with mathematical abilities in children with and without heavy PAE who were 7–12 years of age [89]. The children with heavy PAE had lower global mathematics achievement scores when compared to the non-exposed control group of children [89]. The findings indicated that after accounting for socioeconomic status and intellectual abilities, spatial attention and memory explained the variance in mathematics achievement scores of children with heavy PAE when compared to the non-exposed controls [89].

The deficits in mathematics associated with PAE continue into adolescence. In a 2006 study, adolescents affected by PAE scored significantly lower on measures of mathematical achievement when compared to adolescents who were exposed but had no effects and to a contrast group of adolescents who received special education services [67]. In a later study, researchers examined academic achievement in correlation with brain surface area in children ages 8–16 with heavy prenatal alcohol exposure to a control group of children with no reported prenatal exposure [90]. The results indicated that atypical brain development was associated with lower scores on mathematics in children with heavy prenatal alcohol exposure [90]. Mathematics is a life skill. Deficits in mathematics would hinder budgeting and managing money, interpreting, and following schedules, measuring for cooking, and other daily tasks [16].

Caregivers, Teachers, and Students with FASD Perspectives on School

Qualitative studies have interviewed caregivers, teachers, and students with FASD regarding their perspectives on school. Biological and non-biological caregivers expressed significant levels of stress advocating for services for their children with FASD. Caregivers reported being hesitant to disclose information about their children's diagnosis of FASD out of fear of being judged or shunned by school staff and classmates' families [27, 121]. Also, caregivers expressed frustration about educators' limited knowledge about the learning needs of their children with FASD [121, 122]. Some caregivers who had obtained school-based services reported they were inadequate addressing the needs of their children with FASD [34, 123, 124].

In other studies, teachers reported having little knowledge about the impact of PAE on learning, school functioning, and available resources [29, 35, 125, 126]. Some teachers stated that reports from clinical or diagnostic evaluations were hard to understand because they were written using medical terminology and provided little information that translated into classroom interventions [29, 122]. Many teachers reported being unaware of having students with FASD in their classes [126]. It is likely that teachers were unaware of students' diagnosis of FASD due to caregivers' reluctance to discuss the diagnosis for fear of stigma, poor communication between school staff, or possible oversight of incorporating medical and other diagnostic reports provided to the school into students' records [127].

Teachers have expressed frustration about having the time and the tools to address learning and behavioral challenges of children with FASD in the classroom [125, 126]. A study conducted in South Africa reported that teachers expressed feeling stressed working with children with FASD in the classroom [128]. Many of the teachers had received information about FASD; however, they stated that the training did not provide enough strategies to address the variability in learning and classroom behavior exhibited by children affected by PAE [128]. Other studies examining training for teachers and school staff about the impact of PAE on behavioral and learning showed positive impacts on supporting children with FASD in the classroom [37]. A quasi-experimental study conducted in British Columbia, Canada showed that teachers who received training about FASD adjusted their approaches to address learning and behavior difficulties of children with FASD in their classroom [37]. The findings showed statistically significant improvement in adaptive functioning in children with FASD. Though not statistically significant, possibly due to the small sample size, the research reported a moderate effect of teacher training on student's academic outcomes [37]. The results suggested that teacher training on the impact of PAE tailored for school settings may improve teacher interactions with students who have learning challenges related to FASD.

Few studies have examined students with FASD views on what helps them to feel successful and motivated at school. In a collective case study of eight adolescents with FASD who received special education instruction, parent support and advocacy, and appropriate academic expectations and instruction, as well as had positive peer or social networks contributed to their motivation to do well and graduate high school [33]. In another qualitative study, high school students with FASD receiving special education reported losing motivation when assignments and materials were either too easy or too difficult, and when the students perceived their teachers to show a limited understanding of their learning needs and were disengaged when providing instruction [123]. The interviews with adolescents with FASD indicated that a social network of peers and parent support were critical in maintaining students' persistence and motivation to complete school [29, 127]. In line with the literature on self-efficacy, realistic expectations, supportive caregivers and teachers, and a positive school environment influenced student motivation and self-efficacy leading to better outcomes in adolescents FASD [33, 35]. The findings from the qualitative studies provide a starting point to examine educational practices to improve the outcomes of children and youth affected by PAE.

FASD and Special Education Services

Survey and review studies have examined the prevalence of children and youth affected by PAE receiving special education services in Canada and other countries. However, there is limited information regarding the type and implementation of special education services and other interventions provided in school settings across nations. In a 2019 study, Popova et al. compared the prevalence of FASD among children and youth classified into special subpopulations, including incarcerated, special education, clinical care, state's care, and Aboriginal populations, to the global estimate of 0.77% from the general population [9]. The study estimated that between 7.58 and 8.81% of children and youth with FASD received special education services. The prevalence of FASD was estimated to be 10–40 times higher in the classified subpopulations when compared to the prevalence of FASD within the general population [9]. In an earlier study, researchers conducted a survey between 2011 and 2012 to estimate the number of Canadian children with FASD, ages 5–14, who received special education in public schools and the cost to provide the services [32]. Based upon completed surveys from two Canadian provinces, 6631 children out of 169,000 were identified as having FASD with an estimated cost of services of 53.5 million Canadian dollars [32]. In a subsequent study, other researchers examined the cost of care for individuals with FASD in Canada, Sweden, New Zealand, and the United States [129]. The estimated mean cost per year for special education services, based upon a review of seven studies, was

7177.00 United States dollars per individual with FASD [129]. The authors stated these are rough estimates in part due to FASD being underrecognized or misdiagnosed impacting surveillance [129].

Studies examining adverse outcomes associated with the effects from PAE have included information about participant's educational placement [20, 67]. In the 1996 summary report by Streissguth et al. 40% of the participants with FAS or affected by PAE reported receiving special education services. The report indicated 65% of the participants with FAS or affected by PAE received interventions to address problems with reading and mathematics, with only 30% receiving interventions to improve functional and life skills [20]. It is not clear in the summary if the reported remedial interventions were special education services or provided through other school programs. In a 2006 study of adolescents affected by PAE, approximately 28% of adolescents with facial features and cognitive impairments, and 16% without facial gestures but cognitive impairments received special education services [67]. For the adolescents with PAE and facial features approximately 11% were eligible for special education services under classification of mild intellectual impairment, 6% were eligible under dual categories, 4% eligible due to identified learning disabilities, 2% eligible for speech or language impairment, and 2% eligible under the classification of moderate intellectual impairment [67]. For the adolescents with PAE without facial features, 5% were eligible for special education services under the classification of mild intellectual impairment, 4% were eligible under emotional or behavioral disorders, 2% were eligible under the classification of learning disabilities, 1% were eligible under the classifications of speech or language impairment or dual category, respectively [67]. A combination of the educational regulations and the variability of needs of school-aged children affected by PAE make it challenging to identify the number of children with FASD who receive special education services and the types of interventions that are effective.

Individuals with Disabilities, Regulations, and Schools

Influenced by civil rights legislation from the 1950s to the mid-1960s, the United States enacted laws to protect the rights of individuals with disabilities. Section 504, Rehabilitation Act, of 1973, as amended in 29 USC § 794 (Section 504), prohibits discrimination against individuals with disabilities by organizations and programs that receive federal assistance [130]. Subsequently, the Americans with Disabilities Act of 1990 and the Amendment Act of 2008 expanded the protection of rights and equal access across public entities of individuals with disabilities and their families regardless of receiving federal funding. These anti-discriminatory laws work alongside the Individuals with Disabilities Education Act (IDEA), which authorizes funding and guides implementation of special education programs and services for infants and school-aged children through secondary school, to protect the rights and ensure services for children and youth with disabilities [130, 131].

Other nations have implemented regulations to protect the rights of individuals with disabilities and provide intervention services. For example, in the United Kingdom, the Special Educational Needs and Disability Act, updated in 2014 outlines the definition of a disability and allocates a continuum of supports for individuals from birth to 25 years of age [132]. However, the implementation of special education services varies within each country of the United Kingdom [132]. Australia passed regulations including the Disability Discrimination Act of 1992 and the Disability Standards for Education in 2005 that provided a definition of a disability, protects the rights of individuals with disabilities, and ensures they receive appropriate instruction and supports to learn in school [133]. Kenya has established policies and frameworks to provide students with disabilities special education services and to remove barriers accessing the services [134]. Due to international efforts of many countries, including Kenya, upholding the United Nations Convention on the Rights of Persons with Disabilities, other nations have established policies to ensure children with disabilities opportunities for equitable and inclusive educational opportunities [135]. For this chapter, the education regulations for the United States in relation to the needs of school-aged children with FASD are discussed.

Definition of Disability

The Americans with Disabilities Act and Section 504 have a similar and broadly defined classification of an individual with a disability [130, 131]. The definition in the Americans with Disabilities Act and Section 504 differs from other legislation granting services and support for individuals with disabilities such as Supplemental Security Income (SSI) or eligibility for special education services. Because Section 504 pertains to entities that receive federal assistance, including the United States Department of Education, schools use their definition when determining whether a student has a disability and is eligible for protections under the law [130].

The disability definition in Section 504 includes physical and mental impairments that significantly impact daily functioning. This would include the effects of PAE. In the law, a physical impairment includes but is not limited to cosmetic disfigurement, or anatomical loss of one or more bodily systems such as neurological, musculoskeletal, cardiovascular, endocrine systems, or impairments with sensory organs [130]. The law provides examples of mental impairments including intellectual disabilities, learning disabilities, mental health disorders, and emotional disorders that substantially interfere with daily activities [131]. The law defines major life activities as actions needed for daily tasks, such as caring for oneself, hearing, seeing, communicating, learning, and working. This includes bodily functions such as breathing and walking [131]. Multiple sources of information are considered to determine if a student has a disability. Medical conditions in remission or improved through treatment or devices does not exclude an individual from meeting the definition of having a disability [130, 131].

Section 504 and Schools

Section 504, 34 CFR Part 104 applies to the education of students with disabilities. The law authorizes students with disabilities equal access to education and opportunities to participate in extracurricular activities with non-disabled peers [130]. To ensure equitable education, Section 504 entitles access to general or special education, support, services, and aides to address the individual needs of students with disabilities [131]. This ensures that students with disabilities have equal opportunities to participate in school-sponsored activities without exclusion, harassment, or bullying because of a disability [131]. Educational entities that receive federal funding are required to comply with Section 504. This includes preschools, public schools, post-secondary schools, adult education programs, and afterschool programs that receive federal assistance from the United States Department of Education [131].

According to Section 504, students with disabilities are to have a free and appropriate education (FAPE) regardless of the severity of the disability [130]. This means that students with disabilities are to be educated with students who are not disabled to the extent possible given their educational needs [130]. The law stipulates periodic evaluations and case reviews to safeguard against misidentification of students with disabilities that might lead to improper educational placement. The law provides students, caregivers, advocates, and monitoring agencies steps to file grievances in cases of noncompliance [131]. The Office of Civil Rights receive the complaints and initiate corrective action [131]. Section 504 does not allocate funding or enforce the implementation of special education programs [130].

In schools, a Section 504 Team is convened to review information when determining if a student's impairment substantially limits functioning in any major life activity regardless of mitigating factors that may offset the impact. A student's high grades or academic performance may not be used to deny 504 accommodations if there are substantial limitations on other life activities [130]. If a student is identified as an individual with a disability under Section 504, then accommodations are provided to ensure equal access to educational opportunities and extracurricular activities. The accommodations, aides, and support must not place undue financial, administrative, or instructional burdens on schools or programs [131]. In some cases, the Section 504 Team may refer the student for consideration for eligibility of special education services as outlined by IDEA [136]. Identification as an individual with a disability does not guarantee that the student is eligible for special education services. If a student is found ineligible for special education services but is identified as having a disability according to Section 504, the student may continue to receive accommodations [130]. Accommodations through Section 504 may be provided throughout an individual's formal educational and into employment [137]. Regarding public education, Section 504 works in coordination with IDEA to meet the educational needs for students until twelfth grade or until their 22nd birthday [137]. A comparison of Section 504 to IDEA is presented in Table 16.1 [138].

Table 16.1 Comparison of Section 504 and IDEA [131, 136–140]

	Section 504 of the Rehabilitation Act of 1973	Individuals with Disabilities Act (2004)
Governmental department	Office of civil rights	United States department of education
Funding provisions	None	Provides federal funding for special education programs for students up to 21 years of age if their 22nd birthday occurs during the summer break, or to their 22nd birthday if it occurs during the school year
Definition of disability	Physical or mental impairment substantially impacting major life activities	Exceptional learners, sometimes including those who are gifted and talented, who exhibit a disability impacting their educational performance
Age-groups	All ages	Infants, children, and youth (0 through to 22nd birthday)
Key elements	Protects the rights of individuals from discrimination based upon their disability Grants access to general education, special education, accommodations, and modifications to ensure equitable educational opportunities of individuals with disabilities Procedures for nonbiased evaluations to determine a disability Safeguards and procedures to ensure appropriate placement and to file grievances	Outlines procedures, including nonbiased evaluations, to identify students in need of specialized instruction, modifications, accommodations, and related services Individualized Education Program (IEP) states the eligible student's instructional goals, objectives, placement for instruction, and related services Provides for instruction in the least restrictive environment Ensures caregiver and when appropriate student participate in decisions Procedural safeguards for caregivers to access to records, participate in school decisions, and provide due process if disagreement or concerns of noncompliance
Free and Appropriate Education (FAPE)	Grants access to general education or special education, accommodations, modifications, services to meet the student with a disability need. Ensures the student with a disability participates with peers without disabilities to the extent possible	Provides special education and related services to eligible students to ensure their educational needs are met to receive a free and appropriate education
Applicable organizations	Educational entities and programs that receive federal assistance. This includes preschools, k-12 public schools, afterschool programs, colleges, and employment	Public schools up to 12th grade, or student's exit from public school if remain until 22nd birthday

The Individuals with Disabilities Education Act (IDEA)

In the United States, special education services for school-aged children are guided by Individuals with Disabilities Education Act (IDEA) Parts B and C and Every Student Succeeds Act of 2015 [141]. Table 16.2 provides a timeline of legislation for school services for children with disabilities.

Table 16.2 Timeline of legislation related to special education services [139, 141–144]

Year	Legislation	Provision summary
1965	Elementary and Secondary Education Act (Pub. L. 89–10)	Funding states to close the achievement gap
1974	The Family Educational Rights and Privacy Act (Pub. L. 93–308)	Commonly referred to as the "Buckley Amendment" established maintain privacy and confidentiality of students and their families. Provided legal guardians the right to examine and challenge school records if they feel they are inaccurate. Protects from release of personally identifiable information to third parties including special education records and Section 504 documentation without consent from legal guardian, parent, or student if reached the age of majority. Transferred rights to the individual with a disability at the age of majority
1975	Education of All Handicapped Children Act (Pub. L. 94–142)	Established free and appropriate education for students with disabilities Mandated Individualized Education Plan (IEP) for students receiving special education services Incorporated caregiver involvement in the education of children with disabilities Established students with disabilities are to be educated in the least restrictive environment. Allocated educational-related services for elementary and secondary school students with disabilities
1986	Amendment to the Education of All Handicapped Children Act (Pub. L. 99–457)	Mandated states to provide services for infants, toddlers, and preschool children with disabilities or at risk for disabilities and not included in the 1975 Education of All Handicapped Children act
1990	Individuals with Disabilities Education Act (Pub. L. 101–336)	Reauthorized the Education of All Handicapped Children Act of 1975. Changed the name to the Individuals with Disabilities Education Act (IDEA). The name used first-person language reflecting changes through advocacy to increase inclusion of individuals with disabilities Expanded the definition of disability and eligibility categories to include autism and traumatic brain injury Mandated transition plans included in IEPs for students with disabilities by age 16
1997	Amendments to the Individuals with Disabilities Education Act (Pub. L. 105–17)	Significant changes regarding disciplining and protecting children with disabilities at school. It is mandated that IEPs must include methods to measure student progress

Table 16.2 (continued)

Year	Legislation	Provision summary
2001	Elementary and Secondary Education Act, no child left behind (Pub. L. 107–110)	Financial resources allocated through Title I for school districts to improve access to quality education for low-income schools. Established schools needed to make Adequately Yearly Progress (AYP) to show student progress with steps provided if AYP was not met. Provided options for parents to move their child to another school if the child attended a school that was considered failing. Allocated supplemental instruction for students who attended schools that were on the "failing list" for 3 years. Linked academic content to standardized testing. Provided criteria for teachers to be considered fully qualified to instruct students Required schools to use scientifically based research to guide programs and instruction. Led to the unsuccessful attempt to establish national academic standards known as Common Core
2004	Individuals with Disabilities Education Improvement Act, (reauthorization of IDEA) (Pub. L. 108–244)	Changed the law to improve the quality of special education and increase academic expectations of students with disabilities to align to the No Child Left Behind Act. Moved to have special education instruction closer to grade level standards. Instruction and interventions must be peer reviewed and scientifically based Data-driven progress monitoring to measure response to the instruction. Allocated steps to prevent overidentification of students in need of special education services because of race or ethnicity. Mandated the IEPs must include measurable annual objectives
2015	Every Student Succeeds Act (Pub. L. 114–95)	Reauthorized the Elementary and Secondary Education Act of 1965, and replaced No Child Left Behind. The law requires every state to measure student performance in reading, mathematics, and science. Each state is required to publish an online report card providing information about each state's educational outcomes, graduation rates, student suspensions, and teacher qualifications. Requires each state to provide the average cost to educate students. Allocates flexibility for states to invest in career and technology education and other student needs. This act is linked to IDEA. It mandates that each state must ensure all children with disabilities are included in state and district assessment programs including those mandated Every Student Succeeds Act. This includes providing appropriate accommodations and alternative assessment

The Individuals with Disabilities Education Act (IDEA) Part B states the provisions of special education services for school-aged children from 3 years of age to 21 years of age. IDEA Part C states the provisions for intervention services for infants and toddlers, from birth to 2-years of age [142]. There are differences between IDEA Part B and IDEA Part C. Some of the differences are described in Table 16.3.

The purpose for IDEA Part B is to ensure that all children with disabilities receive a free and appropriate education with specialized instruction and related services to meet their needs and monitored under public supervision and direction

Table 16.3 Examples of differences between Parts B and C of the Individuals with Disabilities Act [139–143]

IDEA Part B (2006) 34 CFR Part 300 School-aged children 3–21 years of age	IDEA Part C (2011) 34 CFR Part 303 Infants and Toddlers 0–2 years of age
Special education and related services for eligible students	Early intervention services for infants and young children with identified medical, health, and developmental disabilities
Address impact on learning and school through the Individualized Education Program (IEP)	Address impact on development through the Individual Family Service Plan (IFSP)
No mandated coordination of services with community providers	Allocates coordination with community-based agencies and providers
Services provided on a continuum in the least restrictive environment at school	Established minimum of services. Services may be provided in the home, community, or clinic
Both Parts B and C mandate child find, a system to locate and identify children with disabilities in need of services	

[143]. IDEA outlines requirements for use of funding for special education services. It mandates evaluation procedures, eligibility criteria, and exceptions for determining students' eligibility for special education and related services [143]. If a student is found eligible for special education services by the eligibility team, a written plan, the Individualized Education Program (IEP), is developed. The IEP provides an overview of the students' learning strengths and challenges, annual learning goals and coordinated objectives, the types and amount of instructional and related services, settings where the services are provided. Methods to monitor progress, and transition services if the student is at least 16 years of age. The IEP is developed by a team that consists of school personnel, the students' caregivers, and their invitees of other individuals who have knowledge of the students' learning needs. In some cases, the student may be present at the IEP meeting if found appropriate. In addition to program planning, IDEA ensures parental and student rights, procedural safeguards, enforcement to compliance, and steps for due process [141].

The definition of a student with a disability and need for services outlined in IDEA differs from Sect. 504 of the Rehabilitation Act of 1973 and Title II of the Americans with Disabilities Act of 1990. According to IDEA Part B, there are 14 categories used to determined eligibility for special education and related services [141]. A student may be found eligible for services in more than one category. Table 16.4 presents the exceptionalities or eligibility categories, a brief description of each category, and applicable exclusionary factors [138, 141].

To be found eligible for special education services, IDEA mandates that multiple sources of information are considered including students' schoolwork, teacher notes, observation data, performance on school administered assessments, results from psychoeducational evaluations, and medical documentation [141]. Also, evaluations and information from private providers working with a student may be presented for consideration [141].

The law indicates that students would not be considered eligible for special education services if the issues to learning challenges are related to the lack of receiving

Table 16.4 IDEA eligibility exceptionalities [136, 138, 141]

Disability/ exceptionality	Description
Autism	A developmental disability impacting verbal and nonverbal communication and social interaction. Impairments are present before age 3 and impact educational performance. Does not apply if the child has an emotional disturbance that is not related to the disorder
Deaf blindness	Combination of vision and hearing impairments that significantly interfere with communication and other educational needs that cannot be addressed in special education programs for children with only deafness or blindness
Deafness	Impairment in processing linguistic information aurally with or without amplification adversely impacting educational performance
Emotional disturbance	Shows one or more traits of emotional or behavioral disturbance over a long time, harming school functioning. These traits are (1) the inability to learn that cannot be explained by intellectual, sensory, or other health factors; (2) the inability to build or maintain appropriate interpersonal relationships with teachers and classmates; (3) exhibits inappropriate types of behaviors or feeling within every circumstance; (4) shows pervasive depression or unhappiness; and (5) exhibits physical symptoms or fears associated with school problems. Schizophrenia is included within this exceptionality. However, children who are socially maladjusted are excluded unless otherwise identified
Hearing impairment	Fluctuating or permanent loss of hearing impacts educational functioning. This excludes those who meet criteria for deafness
Intellectual disability	Impaired intellectual abilities and adaptive behaviors often noted in early development adversely impacts school functioning
Multiple disabilities (does not include deaf blindness)	Refers to co-occurring impairments (e.g., intellectual disability and blindness) that significantly impact educational performance and cannot be addressed in special education programs that are designed for only one of the impairments
Orthopedic impairment	Severe bone or muscle conditions that often are related to congenital anomalies, disease, or other medical complications adversely impacting educational performance
Other health impairment	Chronic or acute medical conditions that limit strength, vitality, alertness in an educational setting, and impact educational performance
Specific learning disability	A disability in one or more underlying psychological processes that may interfere with listening, thinking, reading, writing, spelling, and mathematics. Students who have learning difficulties related to vision, hearing, motor, intellectual impairment, emotional disturbance, environmental, cultural factors, including limited English language proficiency, or economic disadvantage are excluded
Speech or language impairment	Impairments in aspects of language and communication including articulation, stuttering voice impairment, receptive language, expressive language, that adversely impacts educational performance

(continued)

Table 16.4 (continued)

Disability/ exceptionality	Description
Traumatic brain injury	Brain injury caused by an external physical force resulting in total or partial functional disability, psychosocial impairment or both having a detrimental impact on school functioning. This does not include congenital brain injury, injury from a trauma at birth, or degenerative diseases impacting the brain
Visual impairment including blindness	Impaired vision that adversely impacts educational performance even with correction. Includes partial sight and blindness
Significant developmental delay (only for children ages 3–9)	Young children identified using appropriate diagnostic measures and procedures as having a delay in development in one or more of the following areas: physical development, cognitive development, communication, social-emotional, behavior, and adaptive functioning in need of special education and related services

scientifically based instruction for reading, lack appropriate instruction for math, or if the student has limited English proficiency [141]. In some cases, before determining a student requires special education services, notably for Specific Learning Disability, schools would implement a multi-tiered system of support (MTSS) including response to intervention (RTI) and positive behavioral interventions and supports (PBIS) [141, 145]. This provides multiple tiers of evidenced-based or research-based interventions that increase in intensity according to students' responses to the interventions [145]. Students are referred for consideration for special education services if they show little-to-no progress in response to the interventions [145]. The purpose for MTSS is to prevent misidentification of a student as having a learning disability [143]. There are criticisms about the implementation of MTSS. For example, the implementation of MTSS varies across states and school districts, and often the intervention plans do not clearly define objectives or use appropriate interventions and methods to monitor progress [145].

According to IDEA, special education services are provided on a continuum. Students with disabilities are to be educated within a setting closest to the general education environment to the maximum extent with non-disabled peers [144]. The separation of students with disabilities should only occur when the severity of the disability impedes the student's learning in lesser restrictive settings despite receiving accommodations and other supports [141, 144]. Many students with disabilities are educated in inclusion classes with instruction provided by a general education teacher in coordination with instruction or support through special education [146]. Some critics have suggested that this undermines the purpose for special education by limiting access to specialized interventions and adjustments to materials that some children require [146, 147]. However, many students with disabilities do well in inclusion settings when instruction is on their learning level, and they receive the necessary supports [135].

FASD and IDEA

Given that FASD encompasses the medical and clinical diagnoses of FAS, pFAS, ARND, and ND-PAE, some children with an alcohol-related diagnosis are found eligible under Other Health Impairment (OHI). Other school-aged children with FASD may be found eligible under one or more of the other exceptionalities. Children who have a medical diagnosis but found ineligible for special education services may continue to receive support through a 504 Accommodation Plan or receive supplemental instruction or support that is not funded through IDEA such as Title I early intervening services [141]. The availability of supplemental educational programs vary by school district.

At this time, FASD is not a specific eligibility category listed in the federal IDEA regulation. Advocates are working on the national and state levels to increase awareness, change policy, and improve services for individuals with FASD. In 2021, the FASD Respect Act, to reauthorize and expand funding to increase prevention efforts, research, screening, and identification of FASD was introduced to the 117th United States Congress; however, it was not brought before Congress for a vote by the end of session [148].

In Alaska and California, advocates have had success obtaining recognition of FASD as a medical condition under the exceptionality of OHI for their respective states [149–151]. In addition, Alaska has mandated that all new teacher hires are required to receive training about the impact of FASD [151]. These are steps toward increasing awareness and access to services to improve educational care and outcomes of students affected by PAE.

Educational Care for Individuals with FASD

Educational care for individuals with FASD requires collaboration at the national, state, and local levels to increase awareness, training, research, and access to interventions and supports. For example, systematic efforts to increase public awareness and prevention would help to remove barriers such as social stigma. Regarding research, including FASD within studies examining prevalence or other topics related to developmental disabilities would expand the body of research increasing dissemination of information. Also, providing well designed and inclusive research about FASD would aid in dismantling inaccurate perceptions. Changes in policy, public perception, and approaches to research is only one part of inclusive practices to improve educational care of individuals affected by PAE. Collaborative efforts between educators, caregivers, allied health professionals, and individuals with FASD at local levels are needed as well. A conceptualization of educational care for individuals affected by PAE is presented in Fig. 16.1 [38, 152].

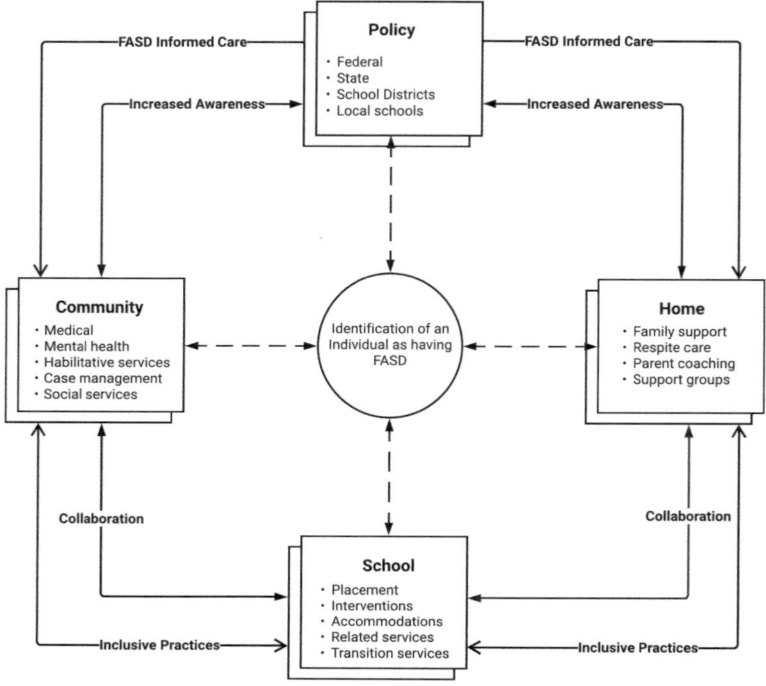

Note: Educational care for school-aged children with FASD requires collaborative efforts among policy makers and stakeholders, medical and community providers, caregivers, and with individuals with FASD (35-36, 38). Policy is needed to increase awareness, disseminate accurate information, and expand access to necessary services (27-28, 38,128). To provide FASD-informed care, policy makers, school administrators, educators, community providers, and caregivers would benefit from training related to their roles in the care of individuals with FASD (35, 36, 122, 128). Educational care requires collaboration between educators, caregivers, allied health professionals, and if developmentally appropriate, the individual with FASD are needed (109-110, 123, 125, 153, 155, 157). This is to provide a collaborative effort to ensure appropriate placement, instructional approaches, related services, accommodations, and transitional plans to improve educational outcomes (153, 155, 162).

Fig. 16.1 Educational care for individuals with FASD

Policy for FASD-Informed Educational Care

The success of advocacy efforts in the states of Alaska and California may be blueprints to expand recognition and training requirements for teachers and others working with children with FASD. The inclusion of FASD in educational regulations and recognized by school systems would provide opportunities to survey and monitor educational trajectories and outcomes. In addition, given the reported prevalence of FASD as 1–5% of school-aged children, with some regions having higher rates, the disorder should be included in research and other policy discussions related to developmental disabilities [5, 30]. This would contribute to disseminating accurate information, open discussions about the disorder, and increase funding to expand opportunities for intervention research to improve educational outcomes.

Currently, training and information about resources for FASD provided in college teacher training programs and professional development within school districts is inconsistent [99]. Incorporating information about FASD into teacher training programs and professional development would be critical to ensure that educators are able to provide the necessary instruction and support to students [29, 35, 36].

Training for Allied Health Professionals, School Personnel, and Caregivers

Studies have shown that providing allied health professionals, educators, and caregivers training about the impact of PAE on development improves managing behavioral and learning needs of children affected by PAE [103, 110]. For professionals and caregivers, training would need to include information about the range of neurodevelopmental deficits attributed to PAE, the complexity of needs, and evidenced-based interventions [37, 153, 154]. As part of the training for allied health professionals and educators, it would be important to discuss how to maintain confidentiality because of sensitive health information. This includes learning how to discuss educational concerns with caregivers who might be sensitive about their children's diagnosis of FASD [124]. Providing quality training would contribute to dispelling misinformation about FASD and facilitate collaboration between caregivers, educators, and allied health providers [34, 124, 153].

For caregivers, training would need to increase their understanding of FASD and how to advocate for their children's needs. Parent training programs such as Families Moving Forward have been found to help caregivers reframe their perceptions of their children's behavior in relation to neurodevelopmental deficits associated with PAE, facilitate positive interactions with their children, and learn to meet the needs of the family [155]. Other intervention programs have incorporated parent training components. For example, researchers provided caregiver training on FASD and how to advocate for their children as part of the Math Interactive Learning Experience (MILE) [110, 111]. For the study, caregivers attended two workshops covering FASD, neurodevelopment, and managing their children's behavior [110]. Incorporated into the training was an overview of IDEA, types of special education services, and other supports children with FASD may require. Caregivers reported they benefitted from the training [110]. To ensure caregivers have tools to advocate for their children with FASD, training would need to include information about educational regulations, limitations of school-based services, and other avenues to obtain services [110, 155]. Also, training would need to include components on how to communicate effectively with schools and educators [34]. Providing caregivers with tools to understand and describe their children's needs might lessen their feelings of frustration and misunderstandings that could lead to potential conflicts with school personnel [156].

Educational Planning for the Individual with FASD

Educational planning begins with a comprehensive evaluation to discern the effects from PAE from other developmental and learning disorders to provide an accurate diagnosis [24, 154]. The evaluation would need to assess cognitive abilities, adaptive functioning, behavior, social-emotional status, and academic achievement [2]. The report from the evaluation would need to be written using terms that caregivers, educators, and other professionals are able to understand [122]. Also, reports would need to discuss the individuals' relative strengths and deficits impacting learning and school functioning [157]. Discussions about individuals' learning strengths and challenges are necessary to guide educational planning [157]. The report recommendations addressing learning and school functioning need to be applicable to the educational setting [29, 122]. This requires the evaluator to understand educational regulations, schools' implementation of special education services, accessibility to supplemental instruction and accommodations that are not part of special education, and the limitations of school service. In some cases, it may be more appropriate for families to seek services from community providers rather than through the school system [156].

Explaining Learning Needs

It is important for caregivers to understand and clearly describe the learning needs of children and adolescents with FASD when advocating for school services. This would include providing caregivers a framework and terms to discuss abilities, or learning strengths, and challenges of their children with FASD when meeting with educators [157]. One framework is the Functional Abilities Classification Tool (FACT) [158].

FACT was developed to be used by allied health professionals, special educators, other clinicians to summarize information gathered from medical records, developmental and psychological evaluations, school records, and student and caregiver input to describe children's functioning and participation in their educational setting [158]. It is based upon the International Classification Functioning, Disability, and Health, Children and Youth (ICF-CY) that considers abilities in terms of participation and engagement in the environment [10, 159]. The ICF-CY refers to disabilities as impairments that restrict engagement and participation. The ICF-CY views the environment as a source of support or barrier to meaningful participation across settings [159]. FACT integrated this perspective into a framework to assist with educational planning [157]. It considers student behaviors as signals indicating that the student may not be receiving the necessary level of interventions or supports or may be mismatched to the classroom expectations or setting for learning [158].

The tool defines abilities as the functions needed to complete or execute a learning task, in areas of verbal communication, literacy, visual cognitive, social skills, executive functioning, and self-regulation [158]. These abilities are rated on a scale of 1–4, with 1 indicating abilities within normal limits or similar to age-matched peers, to 4 indicating that significant modifications are required to ensure learning [158]. FACT defines students' participation as meaningful engagement or participation in structured and unstructured settings that commonly occur in schools. The school settings include individual work, multi-stepped tasks, group work, teacher directed group work, unstructured group work, structured physical activity, such as physical education class, and unstructured physical activities, such as recess. Participation is rated on a scale of 1–4, with 1 indicating the individual engages and participates similar to classmates, and 4 indicating very low quality and frequency of meaningful participation to no engagement [158]. Student perspectives about what they find helpful and challenging at school are incorporated into the summary [158]. The ratings and the student input are summarized to described children's quality of engagement and learning across different school settings and activities. Considering students' learning in terms of the quality and frequency of participation is useful to describe the variability of functioning across settings often noted in school-aged children affected by PAE [1]. This would assist in clarifying the needs of the individual with FASD.

Though FACT may be a useful framework when considering the learning needs of school-aged children with FASD and other disabilities, there are reservations. Studies need to be conducted to examine the tool's validity and reliability. Also, the definitions and constructs need to be reviewed. The tool is subjective and relies on the accuracy of records [158]. Regardless of the tool's limitations, it is a useful framework to consider educational needs by focusing on the individuals' abilities and barriers to learning rather than a diagnostic label. Also, it provides common terminology that may be used by caregivers and others to describe children's learning needs to facilitate negotiations to obtain services.

Educational Placement

As outlined in IDEA, eligibility and special education services including class placement are based upon the needs of the individual [141]. Some children and adolescents with FASD who have significant cognitive impairments or emotional and behavioral needs might benefit from placement in a more restrictive setting such as in a small group, special education class [160]. This is to provide the necessary supervision and highly specialized instruction, such as applied behavioral analysis to improve functional skills, or other interventions that could not be implemented in a larger group setting. Others with FASD do well in inclusion settings or general education settings with accommodations [100]. Educational placement of school-aged children with FASD should be based upon the appropriateness of the classroom and learning expectations to ensure they are maintaining meaningful participation, gaining skills, and interacting with peers in their instructional and school settings [152, 160].

Transition Planning

Given the risks for poor educational outcomes and transition to adulthood experienced by many with FASD, specific plans to move from high school to post-secondary school training are necessary [66, 69, 161]. IDEA mandates that by 16 years of age, the IEP must have a transition plan. However, best practices suggest that it is beneficial to begin when a student is 14 years of age or entering the ninth grade [162, 163]. Also, IDEA indicates that individuals with disabilities may remain in school until their 22nd birthday. For students with FASD and other disabilities, transition planning needs to consider if they should remain in school until the age limit [164].

The purpose for a transition plan is to improve academic and functional skills in preparation to enter post-secondary school activities such as furthering education, participating in vocational training, or entering supported employment or other community programs [163]. A person-centered planning model focusing on the students' strengths and interest is implemented when devising transition plans [164]. This approach not only consider the students' affinities and interests, but also their cognitive, academic, and adaptive functioning to create goals and objectives [164]. Often a vocational assessment is required to evaluate these skills [163]. The assessment would need to examine prevocational and functional skills in addition to surveys to determine the students' interests. Based upon the gathered information, realistic goals and objectives need to be developed to not only improve academic skills but also to build self-determination, or the skills to manage daily life [164]. As part of building self-determining, instructors would need to work with students with FASD to become aware of their strengths, challenges, and interests and set their own goals and objectives [164]. Other objectives to improve adaptive functioning, problem-solving, self-advocacy, and making appropriate social judgments would need to be considered [161, 164]. Transition plan objectives need to be clearly defined, systematically reviewed, and adjusted as the student gains skills [162].

In addition to goals and objectives, a range supports provided at school or in the community may be considered to ensure completion of secondary school and preparation for post-secondary school activities [161, 162]. For example, students might work with mentors, graduation coaches, or school liaisons from vocational rehabilitation programs to complete all prerequisites needed to enter post-secondary school activities. The transition planning team might consider if medical, mental health, social services, and legal advice are needed to make sure the necessary paperwork is correctly completed and submitted so that benefits and other services may be accessed when students reach the age of majority [161]. Also, providing information about peer groups and other social and recreational activities should be included as part of developing their support system [162]. Because of the long-term impact of PAE, many individuals with FASD require support throughout adulthood.

Related Educational Services

Some school-aged children with FASD may require educational-related services to address hearing and vision impairments, weaknesses with speech and language, problems with motor functioning, and other areas [1]. In accordance with IDEA, students who are found eligible may be provided educational-related services at no cost to the caregivers [141]. Examples of school-based services include speech and language therapy, occupational therapy, physical therapy, and assistive technology. Also, students with FASD may benefit from school supports that may not be funded through IDEA. These may include social skills training, afterschool tutoring, or participating in afterschool programs [156]. Availability of these programs vary by school district. In some cases, it may be necessary to seek services from the community or private providers [100].

Individualized Interventions for Children with FASD

There are interventions to improve learning readiness, self-regulation and executive functioning, behavior, as well as early literacy and mathematical skills in children affected by PAE [110, 111, 165]. Many of these interventions are for children 3–12 years of age [165, 166]. There has been little research examining learning challenges and interventions for older school-aged children with FASD [166]. Also, there is little research on the impact of FASD and interventions for academic skills such as expressive writing, reading comprehension, notetaking, or content areas such as history and science [99, 165, 166]. Though studies have shown that children affected by PAE have responded to interventions through serious computer games targeting specific skills, there is little information about the impact of virtual or online learning in comparison to traditional classroom instruction [102, 103]. These are areas for future research to understanding and address the learning needs of school-aged children with FASD.

Research showed that that effective interventions for individuals with FASD share similar traits. The focus for interventions was to build skills by addressing the underlying cognitive deficits mediated by the individuals' relative strengths within the context of a learning or an everyday task [110]. The intervention activities were developmentally appropriate and on the children's learning level [166]. The interventions also focused on changing children's inefficient thinking patterns and improving problem-solving approaches rather than recall of isolated skills [165, 166]. Recognizing common elements of interventions effective for individuals with FASD would be useful to select methods found effective from other learning disorders to address learning challenges associated with PAE [156].

Researchers have examined programs to address challenges with self-regulation and executive functioning associated with the effects of PAE. These interventions may be implemented within a school setting. The Alert Program is used by many occupational therapists to improve children's self-awareness of their arousal level and to use strategies to modify their behavior when they become overwhelmed [167]. Results from studies using this program with children with FASD, between 6 and 12 years of age, have shown improvements with regulating emotions, problem-solving, and with attention [156].

Another program specifically designed for children with FASD, 5–10 years of age is GoFAR [102, 103]. The program used a serious computer game, parent training, and therapeutic sessions with caregivers and their children to improve self-regulation and adaptive behaviors [103]. A key component of GoFAR was to teach children to use the Focus/plan, Act, and Reflect (FAR) framework to approach and systematically work through problems. For each task during the computer game and therapy sessions, children were cued to focus and plan before starting the activity. This directed the children to look at all the information, think about what they are to do, and gather the materials needed to complete the tasks. With this information, the children devised a plan to complete the activity. After making the plan, the children work through the task. They verbalized what they were doing as they completed each step of the task. This was to increase engagement and awareness of their actions. Upon completion of the task, the children reflected upon their actions by recall what they did. The results from the GoFAR studies indicated that children who received the training showed decreases in disruptive behavior, made improvements in their sustained attention, and showed gains in their adaptive skills [102, 103]. The FAR approach is based upon the Plan-Do-Review strategy implemented in the High Scope early childhood programs and is reported to improve children's approaches to solving problems [110]. Similar approaches are used in the Strategies for Enhancing Early Developmental Success (SEEDS) preschool program. Results from a recent case study indicated that program has shown promise to improve parent engagement, self-regulation, and early literacy skills in young children with PAE and involvement with the child welfare system [168].

Academic interventions to improve early reading and mathematics in children affected by PAE have been examined. The Language and Literacy Training program was developed to improve early reading and phonetic skills in young children affected by PAE 9 years of age. The study was conducted in South Africa [169]. Findings from the study indicated that children who received the literacy training made gains in letter knowledge, phonemic awareness, sound-to-symbol association or decoding, spelling, and naming objects and categories. However, there were no group difference between children who received the literacy training and the control group on the overall measure of academic achievement [169].

The Math Interactive Learning Experience (MILE) was developed to improve learning readiness and early mathematical skills in children with FASD 3–10 years of age [110, 111]. Specific instructional approaches were used to address weaknesses with visuospatial processing, encoding, graphomotor skills, working memory, and executive functioning. For example, to improve executive functioning and problem-solving approaches, children were taught to use Focus/Plan, Act, Reflect (FAR) approach used later in the GoFAR study [103, 110]. Through mediated exchanges, children were guided to construct their understanding of the mathematical skills. Carefully selected manipulatives, such as small blocks, were used to provide concrete demonstrations of the skill or concept. As children worked through tasks, they verbalized how they solved the mathematical problems. Once children demonstrated proficiency solving problems using the manipulatives, the instructor directed the children to transform the information into written symbols [110]. Parents were provided direction and activities on how to work with their children at home on the mathematical skills. Results from the study indicated that children made gains on standardized measure of mathematical achievement that were evidence 6 months after participating in the intervention [111]. A study in Canada implemented MILE with children with FASD, 4–10 years of age [170]. The researchers did not incorporate the parent training component. The findings indicated that children who participated in the intervention made gains in their mathematical skills. Specifically, children who were prenatally exposed to alcohol but did not have an FASD diagnosis, who were at the older end of the age range of the study, and had lower intellectual abilities showed greater changes in their mathematic achievement score [170]. The results from MILE indicate that teaching approaches were effective to improve learning readiness and a specific skill deficit that associated with the effects from PAE.

Other studies have examined ways to improve skills related to working memory [171]. Children with FASD, 4–11 years of age, were taught rehearsal strategies to retain information. Children were assigned to either the rehearsal training group or to a control group that did not receive training. A digit span measure requiring the participants to remember strings of numbers that gradually increased in length as the items proceeded were administered to children in each group. Results indicated that both groups performed similar on the digit span measure at the pre-test and at the first post-test. The children who received the rehearsal training performed better than those who did not receive training at the second post-test. The authors concluded that teaching children rehearsal strategies would help to support working memory difficulties in school-aged children with FASD [171].

In addition, many children with FASD are reported to exhibit problems with peer relationships that would interfere with school functioning. The Children's Friendship Training Program was designed for children 6–12 years of age to improve specific skills related to use of prosocial behavior needed to interact with peers [172]. Examples of the skills taught included understanding the rules of social conventions in a group, having conversations, handling teasing, bulling, and unjustified accusations, and negotiating peer conflict. Results from studies conducted in clinical settings and in the community showed children with PAE made improvements in understanding appropriate social skills. Also, parent reports indicated improvement in children's behavior [172, 173]. It is important to note that teacher reports did not indicate improvement in behavior or social skills [172]. The authors suggested that these skills may not be as observable in a structured classroom setting when compared to less structured environments [172, 173]. Overall, these studies show that children with FASD respond to interventions provided in the community or in educational settings to improve academic, behavior, and social interactions that are necessary to function in school.

Classroom Strategies

Because of the variable presentation of the effects from PAE, selecting support strategies would depend upon the individuals' learning strengths and needs [157]. To address the learning and behavioral needs of school-aged children with FASD, it may be necessary to use strategies or approaches found effective for other developmental disabilities or learning disorders. Based upon studies of interventions for children with FASD, classroom instruction would need to be scaffold carefully to help students build upon previous skills [100]. Instructional pacing or presentation of videos when learning online would need to be adjusted to support children's rate of processing [110]. Classroom instruction as well as online learning would need to ensure that there are opportunities for frequent review of the material. Also, tasks would need to be on the individual's learning level. Tasks that are too difficult or too easy may impact behavior and sustained attention [91]. These adjustments may be applied in special education or in general education settings.

Some school-aged children affected by PAE are reported to exhibit behavioral challenges due to the neurodevelopment deficits, experiences of adversity, or other factors that require supports [108, 161]. To assess their behavioral needs, a comprehensive functional behavioral analysis conducted by a behavioral specialist or a trained psychologist to determine the purpose of the behaviors would need to occur. After the functional behavioral analysis is completed, a positive behavioral intervention plan would need to be developed. The behavioral plan would need to be used as a teaching tool to help children with PAE learn specific skills or replacement behaviors to respond and interact effectively at school [101]. Additionally, students may need increased adult supervision and reminders to help them manage the expectations of a school setting [101].

Conclusion

With the necessary support and services, school-aged children with FASD can be successful in their educational setting. The focus of educational interventions is to habilitate skills and support individuals with FASD to meaningfully participate in their learning environment. It requires collaboration between stakeholders, caregivers, school administrators, educators, allied health professionals, and individuals with FASD to make sure funding, policies, recognition of the disorder, and access to services are available. On the individual level, accurate diagnosis and development of a learning profile that incorporates their strengths, talents, and challenges would be necessary to guide educational planning. School-aged children affected by PAE have variable presentations. Therefore, it would be necessary to have educators who are informed about the impact of PAE on learning, behavior, and school functioning and access to resources to provide the necessary interventions. The goals are to provide the necessary educational instruction for all ages to improve outcomes and subsequently the quality of life.

References

1. Mattson SN, Bernes GA, Doyle LR. Fetal alcohol spectrum disorders: a review of the neurobehavioral deficits associated with prenatal alcohol exposure. Alcohol Clin Exp Res. 2019;43(6):1046–62.
2. Kable JA, O'Connor MJ, Olson HC, Paley B, Mattson SN, Anderson SM, et al. Neurobehavioral disorder associated with prenatal alcohol exposure (ND-PAE): proposed DSM-5 diagnosis. Child Psychiatry Hum Dev. 2016;47(2):335–46.
3. Ali S, Kerns KA, Mulligan BP, Olson HC, Astley SJ. An investigation of intra-individual variability in children with fetal alcohol spectrum disorder (FASD). Child Neuropsychol. 2018;24(5):617–37.
4. Coles CD, Kalberg W, Kable JA, Tabachnick B, May PA, Chambers CD. Characterizing alcohol-related neurodevelopmental disorder: prenatal alcohol exposure and the spectrum of outcomes. Alcohol Clin Exp Res. 2020;44(6):1245–60.
5. May PA, Chambers CD, Kalberg WO, Zellner J, Feldman H, Buckley D, et al. Prevalence of fetal alcohol spectrum disorders in 4 US Communities. JAMA. 2018;319(5):474–82.
6. Lange S, Probst C, Gmel G, Rehm J, Burd L, Popova S. Global prevalence of fetal alcohol spectrum disorder among children and youth: a systematic review and meta-analysis. JAMA Pediatr. 2017;171(10):948–56.
7. May PA, Marais AS, De Vries MM, Buckley D, Kalberg WO, Hasken JM, et al. The prevalence, child characteristics, and maternal risk factors for the continuum of fetal alcohol spectrum disorders: a sixth population-based study in the same South African community. Drug Alcohol Depend. 2021;218:108408.
8. Coles CD, Gailey AR, Mulle JG, Kable JA, Lynch ME, Jones KL. A comparison among 5 methods for the clinical diagnosis of fetal alcohol spectrum disorders. Alcohol Clin Exp Res. 2016;40(5):1000–9.
9. Popova S, Lange S, Shield K, Burd L, Rehm J. Prevalence of fetal alcohol spectrum disorder among special subpopulations: a systematic review and meta-analysis. Addiction. 2019;114(7):1150–72.
10. Vale MC, Pereira-da-Silva L, Pimentel MJ, Marques TN, Rodrigues H, Cunha G, et al. Classifying functioning of children and adolescents with intellectual disability: the utility of the international classification of functioning, disability and health for children and youth. J Policy Pract Intellect Disabil. 2017;14(4):285–92.
11. Kable JA, Coles CD. Evidence supporting the internal validity of the proposed ND-PAE disorder. Child Psychiatry Hum Dev. 2018;49(2):163–75.
12. Kundakovic M, Jaric I. The epigenetic link between prenatal adverse environments and neurodevelopmental disorders. Genes (Basel). 2017;8(3):104.
13. Jacobson JL, Akkaya-Hocagil T, Ryan LM, Dodge NC, Richardson GA, Olson HC, et al. Effects of prenatal alcohol exposure on cognitive and behavioral development: findings from a hierarchical meta-analysis of data from six prospective longitudinal U.S. cohorts. Alcohol Clin Exp Res. 2021;45(10):2040–58.
14. Ware AL, Crocker N, O'Brien JW, Deweese BN, Roesch SC, Coles CD, et al. Executive function predicts adaptive behavior in children with histories of heavy prenatal alcohol exposure and attention-deficit/hyperactivity disorder. Alcohol Clin Exp Res. 2012;36(8):1431–41.
15. Kable JA, Mukherjee RA. Neurodevelopmental disorder associated with prenatal exposure to alcohol (ND-PAE): a proposed diagnostic method of capturing the neurocognitive phenotype of FASD. Eur J Med Genet. 2017;60(1):49–54.
16. Doyle LR, Coles CD, Kable JA, May PA, Sowell ER, Jones KL, et al. Relation between adaptive function and IQ among youth with histories of heavy prenatal alcohol exposure. Birth Defects Res. 2018;111(12):812–21.
17. Weyrauch D, Schwartz M, Hart B, Klug M, Burd L. Comorbid mental disorders in fetal alcohol spectrum disorders: a systematic review. J Dev Behav Pediatr. 2017;38(4):283.

18. Mukherjee RAS, Cook PA, Norgate SH, Price AD. Neurodevelopmental outcomes in individuals with fetal alcohol spectrum disorder (FASD) with and without exposure to neglect: clinical cohort data from a national FASD diagnostic clinic. Alcohol. 2019;76:23–8.

19. Flannigan K, Kapasi A, Pei J, Murdoch I, Andrew G, Rasmussen C. Characterizing adverse childhood experiences among children and adolescents with prenatal alcohol exposure and fetal alcohol spectrum disorder. Child Abuse Negl. 2021;112:104888.

20. Streissguth A, Barr HM, Kogan J, Bookstein FL. Understanding the occurrance of secondary disabilities in clients with fetal alcohol syndrome (FAS) and fetal alcohol effects (fAE). Seattle: Washington Univeristy; 1996.

21. Rangmar J, Hjern A, Vinnerljung B, Stromland K, Aronson M, Fahlke C. Psychosocial outcomes of fetal alcohol syndrome in adulthood. Pediatrics. 2015;135(1):e52–8.

22. Karmiloff-Smith A, D'Souza D, Dekker TM, Van Herwegen J, Xu F, Rodic M, et al. Genetic and environmental vulnerabilities in children with neurodevelopmental disorders. Proc Natl Acad Sci U S A. 2012;109(Suppl 2):17261–5.

23. Bakhireva LN, Garrison L, Shrestha S, Sharkis J, Miranda R, Rogers K. Challenges of diagnosing fetal alcohol spectrum disorders in foster and adopted children. Alcohol. 2018;67:37–43.

24. Chasnoff IJ, Wells AM, King L. Misdiagnosis and missed diagnoses in foster and adopted children with prenatal alcohol exposure. Pediatrics. 2015;135(2):264–70.

25. Trent M, Dooley DG, Douge J, Section on Adolescent Health, Council on Community Pediatrics, Committee on Adolescence. The impact of racism on child and adolescent health. Pediatrics. 2019;144(2):e20191765.

26. Malawa Z, Gaarde J, Spellen S. Racism as a root cause approach: a new framework. Pediatrics. 2021;147(1):e2020015602.

27. Roozen S, Stutterheim SE, Bos AER, Kok G, Curfs LMG. Understanding the social stigma of fetal alcohol spectrum disorders: from theory to interventions. Found Sci. 2020;27:753–71.

28. Aspler J, Bogossian A, Racine E. "It's ignorant stereotypes": key stakeholder perspectives on stereotypes associated with fetal alcohol spectrum disorder, alcohol, and pregnancy. J Intellect Dev Disabil. 2021;47(1):53–64.

29. Job JM, Poth CA, Pei J, Caissie B, Brandell D, Macnab J. Toward better collaboration in the education of students with fetal alcohol spectrum disorders: integrating the voices of teachers, administrators, caregivers, and allied professionals. Qual Res Educ. 2013;2(1):38–64.

30. Zablotsky B, Black LI, Maenner MJ, Danielson ML, Bitsko RH, Schieve LA, et al. Prevalence and trends of developmental disabilities among children in the United States: 2009–2017. Pediatrics. 2019;144(4):1–11.

31. Straub L, Bateman BT, Hernandez-Diaz S, York C, Lester B, Wisner KL, et al. Neurodevelopmental disorders among publicly or privately insured children in the United States. JAMA Psychiatry. 2022;79(3):232–42.

32. Popova S, Lange S, Burd L, Nam S, Rehm J. Special education of children with fetal alcohol spectrum disorder. Exceptionality. 2016;24(3):165–75.

33. Duquette C, Stodel E, Fullarton S, Hagglund K. Persistence in high school: experiences of adolescents and young adults with fetal alcohol spectrum disorder. J Intellect Dev Disabil. 2006;31(4):219–31.

34. Cleversey K, Brown J, Kapasi A. Educational services for youth with fetal alcohol spectrum disorder: caregivers' perspectives. Int J Ment Health Addict. 2017;16(5):1156–73.

35. Poth CA, Pei J, Job JM, Wyper K. Toward intentional, reflective, and assimilative classroom practices with students with FASD. Teach Educ. 2014;49:247–64.

36. Cleversey K, Brown J, Kapasi A. Educating adolescents with fetal alcohol spectrum disorder: caregiver support needs. J Child Fam Stud. 2017;26(10):2843–51.

37. Clark E, George MA, Hardy C, Hall WA, MacMillan PD, Wakabayashi S, et al. Exploratory study of the effectiveness of a professional development program on the academic achievement and classroom behavior of students with fetal alcohol spectrum disorder in British Columbia, Canada. Int J Alcohol Drug Res. 2014;3(1):25–34.

38. Boys CJ, Bjorke J, Dole KN, Dalnes C, Terwey S, Chang P-N. Improving educational outcomes in fetal alcohol spectrum disorder through interagency collaboration. J Pediatr Neuropsychol. 2016;2(1–2):50–7.

39. Ylvisaker M, Todis B, Glang A, Urbanczyk B, Franklin C, DePompei R, et al. Educating students with TBI: themes and recommendations. J Head Trauma Rehabil. 2001;16(1):76–93.

40. Kodituwakku PW, Kodituwakku EL. From research to practice: an integrative framework for the development of interventions for children with fetal alcohol spectrum disorders. Neuropsychol Rev. 2011;21(2):204–23.

41. DuPaul GJ, Evans SW, Allan D, Puzino K, Xiang J, Cooper J, et al. High school teacher ratings of academic, social, and behavioral difficulties: factor structure and normative data for the school functioning scale. Sch Psychol. 2019;34(5):479–91.

42. Mayes SD, Calhoun SL, Bixler EO, Zimmerman DN. IQ and neuropsychological predictors of academic achievement. Learn Individ Differ. 2009;19(2):238–41.

43. Ivcevic Z, Brackett M. Predicting school success: comparing conscientiousness, grit, and emotion regulation ability. J Res Pers. 2014;52:29–36.

44. Amso D, Salhi C, Badre D. The relationship between cognitive enrichment and cognitive control: a systematic investigation of environmental influences on development through socioeconomic status. Dev Psychobiol. 2019;61(2):159–78.

45. Vrantsidis DM, Clark CAC, Chevalier N, Espy Andrews K, Wiebe SA. Socioeconomic status and executive function in early childhood: exploring proximal mechanisms. Dev Sci. 2018;23:1–14.

46. Berninger V, Abbott R, Cook CR, Nagy W. Relationships of attention and executive functions to oral language, reading, and writing skills and systems in middle childhood and early adolescence. J Learn Disabil. 2017;50(4):434–49.

47. Pace A, Alper R, Burchinal MR, Golinkoff RM, Hirsh-Pasek K. Measuring success: within and cross-domain predictors of academic and social trajectories in elementary school. Early Child Res Q. 2019;46:112–25.

48. Mayes SD, Frye SS, Breaux RP, Calhoun SL. Diagnostic, demographic, and neurocognitive correlates of dysgraphia in students with ADHD, autism, learning disabilities, and neurotypical development. J Dev Phys Disabil. 2018;30(4):489–507.

49. Decker SL, Roberts AM, Roberts KL, Stafford AL, Eckert MA. Cognitive components of developmental writing skill. Psychol Sch. 2016;53(6):617–25.

50. Duckworth AL, Quinn PD, Tsukayama E. What no child left behind leaves behind: the roles of IQ and self-control in predicting standardized achievement test scores and report card grades. J Educ Psychol. 2012;104(2):439–51.

51. Duckworth AL, Seligman MEP. The science and practice of self-control. Perspect Psychol Sci. 2017;12(5):715–8.

52. Finch JE, Obradović J. Independent and compensatory contributions of executive functions and challenge preference for students' adaptive classroom behaviors. Learn Individ Differ. 2017;55:183–92.

53. Hofmann W, Schmeichel BJ, Baddeley AD. Executive functions and self-regulation. Trends Cogn Sci. 2012;16(3):174–80.

54. Willoughby MT, Wylie AC, Little MH. Testing longitudinal associations between executive function and academic achievement. Dev Psychol. 2019;55(4):767–79.

55. Miyake A, Friedman NP. The nature and organization of individual differences in executive functions: four general conclusions. Curr Dir Psychol Sci. 2012;21(1):8–14.

56. Hartung J, Engelhardt LE, Thibodeaux ML, Harden KP, Tucker-Drob EM. Developmental transformations in the structure of executive functions. J Exp Child Psychol. 2020;189:104681.

57. Montroy JJ, Bowles RP, Skibbe LE, McClelland MM, Morrison FJ. The development of self-regulation across early childhood. Dev Psychol. 2016;52(11):1744–62.

58. Reid N, Petrenko CLM. Applying a developmental framework to the self-regulatory difficulties of young children with prenatal alcohol exposure: a review. Alcohol Clin Exp Res. 2018;42(6):987–1005.

59. Mischel W, Ayduk O, Berman MG, Casey BJ, Gotlib IH, Jonides J, et al. 'Willpower' over the life span: decomposing self-regulation. Soc Cogn Affect Neurosci. 2011;6(2):252–6.
60. Park D, Yu A, Baelen RN, Tsukayama E, Duckworth AL. Fostering grit: perceived school goal-structure predicts growth in grit and grades. Contemp Educ Psychol. 2018;55:120–8.
61. Bandura A. Perceived self-efficacy in cognitive development and functioning. Educ Psychol. 1993;28(2):117–48.
62. Cattelino E, Morelli M, Baiocco R, Chirumbolo A. From external regulation to school achievement: the mediation of self-efficacy at school. J Appl Dev Psychol. 2019;60:127–33.
63. Meltzer L, Reddy R, Pollica LS, Roditi B, Sayer J, Theokas C. Positive and negative self-percetions: is there a cylical relationship between teachers' and students' perceptions of effort, strategy use, and academic performance? Learn Disabil Res Pract. 2004;19(1):33–44.
64. Hwang S, White SF, Nolan ZT, Sinclair S, Blair RJ. Neurodevelopmental changes in the responsiveness of systems involved in top down attention and emotional responding. Neuropsychologia. 2014;62:277–85.
65. Flannigan K, Wrath A, Ritter C, McLachlan K, Harding KD, Campbell A, et al. Balancing the story of fetal alcohol spectrum disorder: a narrative review of the literature on strengths. Alcohol Clin Exp Res. 2021;45(12):2448–64.
66. McLachlan K, Flannigan K, Temple V, Unsworth K, Cook JL. Difficulties in daily living experienced by adolescents, transition-aged youth, and adults with fetal alcohol spectrum disorder. Alcohol Clin Exp Res. 2020;44(8):1609–24.
67. Howell KK, Lynch ME, Platzman KA, Smith GH, Coles CD. Prenatal alcohol exposure and ability, academic achievement, and school functioning in adolescence: a longitudinal follow-up. J Pediatr Psychol. 2006;31(1):116–26.
68. Expulsion rates by school board. Government of Ontario. 2007–2020. https://data.ontario.ca/dataset/2d2c39a7-9318-4db1-8555-a5d105e48619/resource/50549b35-0e39-4853-8842-d55b3cbbecba/download/enbrd_expulsions_0708_1920.xlsx. Accessed 14 Sept 2022.
69. Lynch ME, Kable JA, Coles CD. Prenatal alcohol exposure, adaptive function, and entry into adult roles in a prospective study of young adults. Neurotoxicol Teratol. 2015;51:52–60.
70. Snyder TD, de Brey C, Dillow SA. Digest of education statistics 2015. In: Institute of Educational Sciences USDoE, editor. National Center for Education Statistics. 51st ed. Washington, DC: Institute of Educational Sciences; 2016.
71. Nissinen NM, Gissler M, Sarkola T, Kahila H, Autti-Ramo I, Koponen AM. Completed secondary education among youth with prenatal substance exposure: a longitudinal register-based matched cohort study. J Adolesc. 2021;86:15–27.
72. Kable JA, Coles CD, Cifasd. Prefrontal cortical responses in children with prenatal alcohol-related neurodevelopmental impairment: a functional near-infrared spectroscopy study. Clin Neurophysiol. 2017;128(11):2099–109.
73. Biffen SC, Warton CMR, Lindinger NM, Randall SR, Lewis CE, Molteno CD, et al. Reductions in corpus callosum volume partially mediate effects of prenatal alcohol exposure on IQ. Front Neuroanat. 2018;11:132.
74. Wozniak JR, Mueller BA, Mattson SN, Coles CD, Kable JA, Jones KL, et al. Functional connectivity abnormalities and associated cognitive deficits in fetal alcohol spectrum disorders (FASD). Brain Imaging Behav. 2017;11(5):1432–45.
75. Kodali VN, Jacobson JL, Lindinger NM, Dodge NC, Molteno CD, Meintjes EM, et al. Differential recruitment of brain regions during response inhibition in children prenatally exposed to alcohol. Alcohol Clin Exp Res. 2017;41(2):334–44.
76. Biffen SC, Dodge NC, Warton CMR, Molteno CD, Jacobson JL, Meintjes EM, et al. Compromised interhemispheric transfer of information partially mediates cognitive function deficits in adolescents with fetal alcohol syndrome. Alcohol Clin Exp Res. 2022;46(4):517–29.
77. Burden MJ, Westerlund A, Muckle G, Dodge N, Dewailly E, Nelson CA, et al. The effects of maternal binge drinking during pregnancy on neural correlates of response inhibition and memory in childhood. Alcohol Clin Exp Res. 2011;35(1):69–82.

78. Coles CD, Li Z. Functional neuroimaging in the examination of effects of prenatal alcohol exposure. Neuropsychol Rev. 2011;21(2):119–32.
79. Coles CD, Platzman KA, Lynch ME, Freides D. Auditory and visual sustained attention in adolescents prenatally exposed to alcohol. Alcohol Clin Exp Res. 2002;26(2):263–70.
80. Lewis CE, Thomas KG, Dodge NC, Molteno CD, Meintjes EM, Jacobson JL, et al. Verbal learning and memory impairment in children with fetal alcohol spectrum disorders. Alcohol Clin Exp Res. 2015;39(4):724–32.
81. Dodge NC, Thomas KGF, Meintjes EM, Molteno CD, Jacobson JL, Jacobson SW. Spatial navigation in children and young adults with fetal alcohol spectrum disorders. Alcohol Clin Exp Res. 2019;43(12):2536–46.
82. Infante MA, Moore EM, Bischoff-Grethe A, Tapert SF, Mattson SN, Riley EP. Altered functional connectivity during spatial working memory in children with heavy prenatal alcohol exposure. Alcohol. 2017;64:11–21.
83. Newcombe NS, Huttenlocher J. Making space. The development of spatial representation and resoning. Cambridge: MIT Press; 2000.
84. Doyle LR, Moore EM, Coles CD, Kable JA, Sowell ER, Wozniak JR, et al. Executive functioning correlates with communication ability in youth with histories of heavy prenatal alcohol exposure. J Int Neuropsychol Soc. 2018;24(10):1026–37.
85. Kippin NR, Leitao S, Watkins R, Finlay-Jones A. Oral and written communication skills of adolescents with prenatal alcohol exposure (PAE) compared with those with no/low PAE: a systematic review. Int J Lang Commun Disord. 2021;56(4):694–718.
86. Jacobson JL, Dodge NC, Burden MJ, Klorman R, Jacobson SW. Number processing in adolescents with prenatal alcohol exposure and ADHD: differences in the neurobehavioral phenotype. Alcohol Clin Exp Res. 2011;35(3):431–42.
87. Meintjes EM, Jacobson JL, Molteno CD, Gatenby JC, Warton C, Cannistraci CJ, et al. An FMRI study of number processing in children with fetal alcohol syndrome. Alcohol Clin Exp Res. 2010;34(8):1450–64.
88. Woods KJ, Meintjes EM, Molteno CD, Jacobson SW, Jacobson JL. Parietal dysfunction during number processing in children with fetal alcohol spectrum disorders. Neuroimage Clin. 2015;8:594–605.
89. Crocker N, Riley EP, Mattson SN. Visual-spatial abilities relate to mathematics achievement in children with heavy prenatal alcohol exposure. Neuropsychology. 2015;29(1):108–16.
90. Glass L, Moore EM, Akshoomoff N, Jones KL, Riley EP, Mattson SN. Academic difficulties in children with prenatal alcohol exposure: presence, profile, and neural correlates. Alcohol Clin Exp Res. 2017;41(5):1024–34.
91. Zentall SS. Theory- and evidence-based strategies for children with attentional problems. Psychol Sch. 2005;42(8):821–36.
92. Ritfeld GJ, Kable JA, Holton JE, Coles CD. Psychopharmacological treatments in children with fetal alcohol spectrum disorders: a review. Child Psychiatry Hum Dev. 2021;53(2):268–77.
93. Mattson SN, Crocker N, Nguyen TT. Fetal alcohol spectrum disorders: neuropsychological and behavioral features. Neuropsychol Rev. 2011;21(2):81–101.
94. Glass L, Graham DM, Deweese BN, Jones KL, Riley EP, Mattson SN. Correspondence of parent report and laboratory measures of inattention and hyperactivity in children with heavy prenatal alcohol exposure. Neurotoxicol Teratol. 2014;42:43–50.
95. Kully-Martens K, Denys K, Treit S, Tamana S, Rasmussen C. A review of social skills deficits in individuals with fetal alcohol spectrum disorders and prenatal alcohol exposure: profiles, mechanisms, and interventions. Alcohol Clin Exp Res. 2012;36(4):568–76.
96. Kautz-Turnbull C, Petrenko CLM. A meta-analytic review of adaptive functioning in fetal alcohol spectrum disorders, and the effect of IQ, executive functioning, and age. Alcohol Clin Exp Res. 2021;45(12):2430–47.
97. Jirikowic TL, Thorne JC, McLaughlin SA, Waddington T, Lee AKC, Astley Hemingway SJ. Prevalence and patterns of sensory processing behaviors in a large clinical sample of children with prenatal alcohol exposure. Res Dev Disabil. 2020;100:103617.

98. Hofer M. Goal conflicts and self-regulation: a new look at pupils' off-task behaviour in the classroom. Educ Res Rev. 2007;2(1):28–38.

99. Lees B, Riches J, Mewton L, Elliott EJ, Allsop S, Newton N, et al. Fetal alcohol spectrum disorder resources for educators: a scoping review. Health Promot J Austr. 2021;33(3):797–809.

100. Green J. Fetal alcohol spectrum disorders: understanding the effects of prenatal alcohol exposure and supporting students. J Sch Health. 2007;77(3):103–8.

101. Hutton L. Improving the behavior of children with fetal alcohol spectrum disorders. Teach Except Child. 2021;54(2):97–105.

102. Kable JA, Taddeo E, Strickland D, Coles CD. Improving FASD children's self-regulation: piloting phase 1 of the GoFAR intervention. Child Fam Behav Ther. 2016;38(2):124–41.

103. Coles CD, Kable JA, Taddeo E, Strickland DC. A metacognitive strategy for reducing disruptive behavior in children with fetal alcohol spectrum disorders: GoFAR pilot. Alcohol Clin Exp Res. 2015;39(11):2224–33.

104. Fuglestad AJ, Whitley ML, Carlson SM, Boys CJ, Eckerle JK, Fink BA, et al. Executive functioning deficits in preschool children with fetal alcohol spectrum disorders. Child Neuropsychol. 2015;21(6):716–31.

105. Thorne JC, Coggins TE. Cohesive referencing errors during narrative production as clinical evidence of central nervous system abnormality in school-aged children with fetal alcohol spectrum disorders. Am J Speech Lang Pathol. 2016;25(4):532–46.

106. Kjellmer L, Olswang LB. Variability in classroom social communication: performance of children with fetal alcohol spectrum disorders and typically developing peers. J Speech Lang Hear Res. 2013;56(3):982–93.

107. Olswang L, Svensson L, Astley S. Observation of classroom social communication: do children with fetal alcohol spectrum disorders spend their time differently than their typically developing peers? J Speech Lang Hear Res. 2010;53:1687–703.

108. Flannigan K, Pei J, McLachlan K, Harding K, Mela M, Cook J, et al. Responding to the unique complexities of fetal alcohol spectrum disorder. Front Psychol. 2022;12:778471.

109. Kautz-Turnbull C, Adams TR, Petrenko CLM. The strengths and positive influences of children with fetal alcohol spectrum disorders. Am J Intellect Dev Disabil. 2022;127(5):355–68.

110. Kable JA, Coles CD, Taddeo E. Socio-cognitive habilitation using the math interactive learning experience program for alcohol-affected children. Alcohol Clin Exp Res. 2007;31(8):1425–34.

111. Coles CD, Kable JA, Taddeo E. Math performance and behavior problems in children affected by prenatal alcohol exposure: intervention and follow-up. J Dev Behav Pediatr. 2009;30:7–15.

112. Goldschmidt L, Richardson GA, Stoffer DS, Geva D, Day NL. Prenatal alcohol exposure and academic achievement at age six: a nonlinear fit. Alcohol Clin Exp Res. 1996;20(4):763–70.

113. Goldschmidt L, Richardson GA, Cornelius MD, Day NL. Prenatal marijuana and alcohol exposure and academic achievement at age 10. Neurotoxicol Teratol. 2004;26(4):521–32.

114. O'Leary CM, Taylor C, Zubrick SR, Kurinczuk JJ, Bower C. Prenatal alcohol exposure and educational achievement in children aged 8–9 years. Pediatrics. 2013;132(2):e468–75.

115. Jacobson SW, Jacobson JL. The risk of low-to-moderate prenatal alcohol exposure on child academic underachievement and behavior may be difficult to measure and should not be underestimated. Evid Based Med. 2014;19(2):1–2.

116. Zuccolo L, Lewis SJ, Smith GD, Sayal K, Draper ES, Fraser R, et al. Prenatal alcohol exposure and offspring cognition and school performance. A 'Mendelian randomization' natural experiment. Int J Epidemiol. 2013;42(5):1358–70.

117. von Hinke Kessler SS, Wehby GL, Lewis S, Zuccolo L. Alcohol exposure in utero and child academic achievement. Econ J. 2014;124:634–67.

118. Glass L, Graham DM, Akshoomoff N, Mattson SN. Cognitive factors contributing to spelling performance in children with prenatal alcohol exposure. Neuropsychology. 2015;29(6):817–28.

119. Yu X, Dunstan J, Jacobson SW, Molteno CD, Lindinger NM, Turesky TK, et al. Distinctive neural correlates of phonological and reading impairment in fetal alcohol-exposed adolescents with and without facial dysmorphology. Neuropsychologia. 2022;169:108188.

120. Rasmussen C, Bisanz J. The relation between mathematics and working memory in young children with fetal alcohol spectrum disorders. J Spec Educ. 2011;45(3):184–91.

121. Swart S, Hall WA, McKee WT, Ford L. Caregivers' management of schooling for their children with fetal alcohol spectrum disorder. Qual Health Res. 2014;24(11):1540–52.

122. Pei J, Job JM, Poth C, Atkinson E. Assessment for intervention of children with fetal alcohol spectrum disorders: perspectives of classroom teachers, administrators, caregivers, and allied professionals. Psychology. 2013;04(03):325–34.

123. Duquette C, Stodel E, Fullarton S, Hagglund K. Secondary school experiences of individuals with foetal alcohol spectrum disorder: perspectives of parents and their children. Int J Incl Educ. 2007;11(5–6):571–91.

124. Skorka K, McBryde C, Copley J, Meredith PJ, Reid N. Experiences of children with fetal alcohol spectrum disorder and their families: a critical review. Alcohol Clin Exp Res. 2020;44(6):1175–88.

125. Ryan S, Ferguson D. On, yet under the radar: students with fetal alcohol spectrum disorders. Except Child. 2006;72(3):363–79.

126. Dybdahl C, Ryan S. Inclusion for students with fetal alcohol syndrome: classroom teachers talk about practice. Prev Sch Fail. 2009;53(3):185–95.

127. Duquette CA, Stodel EJ, Fullarton S, Hagglund K. Educational advocacy among adoptive parents of adolescents with fetal alcohol spectrum disorder. Int J Incl Educ. 2012;16(11):1203–21.

128. Van Schalkwyk I, Marais S. Educators' relational experiences with learners identified with fetal alcohol spectrum disorder. S Afr J Educ. 2017;37(3):1–9.

129. Greenmyer JR, Klug MG, Kambeitz C, Popova S, Burd L. A multicountry updated assessment of the economic impact of fetal alcohol spectrum disorder: costs for children and adults. J Addict Med. 2018;12(6):466–73.

130. U.S. Department of Education. Parent and educator resource guide to Section 504 in public elementary and secondary schools. Washington, DC: U.S. Department of Education; 2016.

131. U.S. Department of Education. Protecting students with disabilities. Frequently asked questions about Section 504 and the Education of Children with Disabilities. 2020. https://www2.ed.gov/about/offices/list/ocr/504faq.html#:~:text=Section%20504%20is%20a%20federal%20law%20designed%20to,assistance%20from%20the%20U.S.%20Department%20of%20Education%20%28ED%29.

132. Education Df. Special Educational Needs and Disability Code of Practice: 0–25 years In: Education Df, Health Df, editors. United Kingdon Open Government Licence v3.0; 2015. p. 1–292.

133. Australian Government Department of Education S, and Employment Final Reprot of the 2020 Review of the Disability Standards for Education 2005. Australia Australian Government Department of Education, Skills, and Employment; 2021.

134. Kiru EW. Special education in Kenya. Interv Sch Clin. 2018;54(3):181–8.

135. Buchner T, Shevlin M, Donovan MA, Gercke M, Goll H, Šiška J, et al. Same progress for all? Inclusive education, the United Nations convention on the rights of persons with disabilities and students with intellectual disability in European countries. J Policy Pract Intellect Disabil. 2020;18(1):7–22.

136. U.S. Department of Education. IDEA individuals with Disabilities Education Act. Washington, DC: U.S. Department of Education; 2022. https://sites.ed.gov/idea/about-idea/

137. U.S. Department of Education. Supporting students with disabilities and avoiding the discriminatory use of student discipline under Section 504 of the rehabilitation Act in: rights. Washington, DC: U.S. Department of Education; 2022. p. 1–32.

138. Hallahan DP, Pullen PC, Kauffman JM, Badar J. Exceptional learners: an introduction to special education. Upper Saddle River: Pearson; 2020. p. 1–29.

139. Zirkel PA. A comprehensive comparison of the IDEA and Section 504/ADA. Wests Educ Law Report. 2012;282:767–84.
140. deBettencourt LU. Understanding the difference between IDEA and Section 504. Teach Except Child. 2002;34(3):16–23.
141. Yell ML, Katsiyannis A, Bradley MR. The individuals with disabilities education act. In: Kauffman JM, Hallahan DP, Pullen Cullen P, editors. Handbook of special education. 2nd ed. New York: Routledge; 2017.
142. Individuals with Disabilities Education Act Pub. L. No. 108–446 (2006, 2004).
143. Yell ML, Katsiyannis A, Bradley RM. The individuals with disabilities education act: the evaluation of special education law. In: Kauffman JM, Hallahan DP, editors. Handbook of special education. New York: Taylor & Francis; 2011. p. 61–76.
144. Education USDo. IDEA. Individuals with disabilities education act. Topic areas. Least restrictive environment. 2022. https://sites.ed.gov/idea/topic-areas/#LRE.
145. Kauffman JM. The promises and limitations of educational tiers for special and inclusive education. Educ Sci. 2021;11(7):323.
146. Kauffman JM, Hornby G. Inclusive vision versus special education reality. Educ Sci. 2020;10(9):258.
147. Kauffman JM, Anastasiou D, Maag JW. Special education at the crossroad: an identity crisis and the need for a scientific reconstruction. Exceptionality. 2016;25(2):139–55.
148. FASD Respect Act Senate, 117 Sess. 2021.
149. Health UoAACo. Alaska fetal alcohol spectrum disorders data systems development: gaps, opportunities, and recommendations Authority AMHT; 2021.
150. Senate Bill California State Legislature (2021).
151. Group AFSPW. Alaska Fetal Alcohol Spectrum Disorders (FASD) Strategic Plan 2017–2022. In: Education GsCoDaS, editor. 2018. p. 2–13.
152. Millar JA, Thompson J, Schwab D, Hanlon-Dearman A, Goodman D, Koren G, et al. Educating students with FASD: linking policy, research and practice. J Res Spec Educ Needs. 2017;17(1):3–17.
153. Reid N, White C, Hawkins E, Crawford A, Liu W, Shanley D. Outcomes and needs of health and education professionals following fetal alcohol spectrum disorder-specific training. J Paediatr Child Health. 2020;56(2):317–23.
154. Pei J, Baugh L, Andrew G, Rasmussen C. Intervention recommendations and subsequent access to services following clinical assessment for fetal alcohol spectrum disorders. Res Dev Disabil. 2017;60:176–86.
155. Petrenko CL. Positive behavioral interventions and family support for fetal alcohol spectrum disorders. Curr Dev Disord Rep. 2015;2(3):199–209.
156. Millians MN. Educational needs and care of children with FASD. Curr Dev Disord Rep. 2015;2(3):210–8.
157. Kully-Martens K, McNeil A, Pei J, et al. Toward a strengths-based cognitive profile of children with fetal alcohol spectrum disorders: implications for intervention. Curr Dev Disord Rep. 2022;9:53–62.
158. Klein B, Kraus de Camargo O. A proposed functional abilities classification tool for developmental disorders affecting learning and behaviour. Front Educ. 2018;3:2018.
159. de Schipper E, Lundequist A, Wilteus AL, Coghill D, de Vries PJ, Granlund M, et al. A comprehensive scoping review of ability and disability in ADHD using the international classification of functioning, disability and health-children and youth version (ICF-CY). Eur Child Adolesc Psychiatry. 2015;24(8):859–72.
160. Zigmond NP, Kloo A. General and special education are (and should be) different. In: Kauffman JM, Hallahan DP, Pullen PC, editors. Handbook of special education. 2nd ed. New York: Routledge; 2017. p. 249–61.
161. Flannigan K, Rebus M, Gear A, Basisty B, Couling K, Whitford C, et al. Understanding adverse experiences and providing school-based supports for youth who are at high risk with and without FASD. Int J Spec Educ. 2017;21(4):842–56.

162. Cavendish W, Connor D. Toward authentic IEPs and transition plans: student, parent, and teacher perspectives. Learn Disabil Q. 2017;41(1):32–43.
163. Prince AMT, Katsiyannis A, Farmer J. Postsecondary transition under IDEA 2004. Interv Sch Clin. 2013;48(5):286–93.
164. Avellone LE, Taylor T. Transitioning students with low-incidence disabilities to community living. In: Kauffman JM, Hallahan DP, Pullen Cullen P, editors. Handbook of special education. New York: Routledge; 2017. p. 758–70.
165. Petrenko CL, Alto ME. Interventions in fetal alcohol spectrum disorders: an international perspective. Eur J Med Genet. 2017;60(1):79–91.
166. Reid N, Dawe S, Shelton D, Harnett P, Warner J, Armstrong E, et al. Systematic review of fetal alcohol spectrum disorder interventions across the life span. Alcohol Clin Exp Res. 2015;39(12):2283–95.
167. Wells AM, Chasnoff IJ, Schmidt CA, Telford E, Schwartz LD. Neurocognitive habilitation therapy for children with fetal alcohol spectrum disorders: an adaptation of the alert program. Am J Occup Ther. 2012;66(1):24–34.
168. Hajal NJ, Paley B, Delja JR, Gorospe CM, Mogil C. Promoting family school-readiness for child-welfare involved preschoolers and their caregivers: case examples. Child Youth Serv Rev. 2019;96:181–93.
169. Adnams CM, Sorour P, Kalberg WO, Kodituwakku P, Perold MD, Kotze A, et al. Language and literacy outcomes from a pilot intervention study for children with fetal alcohol spectrum disorders in South Africa. Alcohol. 2007;41(6):403–14.
170. Kully-Martens K, Pei J, Kable J, Coles CD, Andrew G, Rasmussen C. Mathematics intervention for children with fetal alcohol spectrum disorder: a replication and extension of the math interactive learning experience (MILE) program. Res Dev Disabil. 2018;78:55–65.
171. Loomes C, Rasmussen C, Pei J, Manji S, Andrew G. The effect of rehearsal training on working memory span of children with fetal alcohol spectrum disorder. Res Dev Disabil. 2008;29(2):113–24.
172. O'Connor MJ, Frankel F, Paley B, Schonfeld AM, Carpenter E, Laugeson EA, et al. A controlled social skills training for children with fetal alcohol spectrum disorders. J Consult Clin Psychol. 2006;74(4):639–48.
173. O'Connor MJ, Laugeson EA, Mogil C, Lowe E, Welch-Torres K, Keil V, et al. Translation of an evidence-based social skills intervention for children with prenatal alcohol exposure in a community mental health setting. Alcohol Clin Exp Res. 2012;36(1):141–52.

Chapter 17
The Justice System and FASD

Jacqueline Pei, Jessica J. Joseph, Kaitlyn McLachlan, and Mansfield Mela

Individuals with FASD are viewed as a particularly vulnerable group within the criminal justice system [1–4]. Overrepresented and often misunderstood, adverse outcomes such as justice system involvement have been a dominant storyline in the FASD literature, yet increasingly families and professionals assert that this is neither a necessary nor inevitable outcome. Instead, increased understandings of the mechanisms that influence development and behavior, including both criminal and noncriminal behavior, should inform our recognition and response to this population, which may in turn help reduce these intersections with the justice system. Equally importantly, this will also foster an FASD-informed response within the system to avoid cumulative impacts often reported once individuals are engaged within the system.

J. Pei (✉)
Department of Educational Psychology, University of Alberta, Edmonton, AB, Canada

Department of Pediatrics, University of Alberta, Edmonton, AB, Canada

Canada FASD Research Network, Vancouver, BC, Canada

6-131 Education North, University of Alberta, Edmonton, AB, Canada
e-mail: jpei@ualberta.ca

J. J. Joseph
6-131 Education North, University of Alberta, Edmonton, AB, Canada
e-mail: jjjoseph@ualberta.ca

K. McLachlan
Department of Psychology, University of Guelph, Guelph, ON, Canada
e-mail: kkmclac02@uoguelph.ca

M. Mela
Department of Psychiatry, College of Medicine, University of Saskatchewan, Saskatoon, Canada
e-mail: Mam865@mail.usask.ca

For years, biopsychosocial models have aided in furthering our understanding of the complex and intersecting nature of the biological and environmental underpinnings that shape human development and behavior [5, 6]. These frameworks illustrate that human behavior is a product of complex transactions between our biological functioning and the environmental influences around us, including family, peers, systems, and policies [5–7]. Understanding the unique nature of these transactions is foundational to supporting individuals with FASD toward healthy outcomes.

The present chapter will provide a synthesizing review of the vulnerabilities that exist for individuals with fetal alcohol spectrum disorder (FASD) and their involvement with the criminal justice system. Then, we discuss strategies for mitigating criminal justice system involvement and the commission of crimes and explore a reasoned, compassionate, and evidence-informed approach for effectively responding to criminal behavior among those with FASD. "Vulnerabilities for Intersecting with the Criminal Justice System" provides a brief overview of the risk factors that exist for intersecting with the criminal justice system in the general population, followed by an overview of why those with FASD are particularly vulnerable. Next, "Intersections with the Justice System" provides a synthesizing review of the literature regarding the heightened vulnerability for those with FASD at every level of the criminal justice system. This will include discussions on the vulnerability many people with FASD experience during interactions with the police, the formal adjudication, incarceration, and reintegration into the community. Finally, "Responding to the Call for Improved Practices" unifies the key themes discussed in the chapter and provides recommendations that inform how forensic mental health and criminal justice professionals should respond to and support individuals with FASD in justice contexts. Overall, the intent of this chapter is to increase public awareness and facilitate action from policy developers, clinicians, correctional personnel, and forensic professionals. The onus is on us.

Vulnerabilities for Intersecting with the Criminal Justice System

Jason is spending his day with Frank and the guys. He is thrilled to finally be 'one of the guys.' He's used to being made fun of, or worse, ignored, and feels he does not fit in anyway. His frequent foster home moves growing up had been confusing to him, and he has simply learned he is a 'bad kid.' So, when Frank invited him to come alone, Jason thought maybe he would finally fit in. He happily mirrored the look and attitude of his new peers and was pleased to see the reactions of others to his group—he was now a person to be taken seriously! Jason has had trouble securing a job, since leaving high school early, so the added promise of money to help make ends meet sealed the deal. On this particular day when his friends asked him to help break into a car, Jason did not think to ask who it may belong to or what might happen; it was not unusual for Jason to act first and consider the consequences later. Particularly now that he was one of the guys. When Jason started to drive, he savoured the thrill that came with the risk he was taking. Then he heard the sirens. Jason's adrenaline jumped in—his ability to reason or consider his actions, disappeared. He was in flight mode. He drove fast, he did not, and could not, see the risks. Even as he saw the roadblock ahead, he simply pressed the gas, hitting the police cars, and injuring an adjacent officer, before hitting a tree and coming to a stop.

Vulnerabilities for Engaging in Criminal Behavior

Multiple factors have been associated with an increased likelihood for criminal behavior, that, as noted above, tend to operate in a transactional manner. This applies for all populations, and in fact consideration of the associations generally described in the literature provides a first step in later considering ways in which those with FASD may uniquely present within the justice system.

Both individual-level and environmental factors have been associated with criminal justice system involvement. Individual factors are diverse and often nested within environmental or contextual vulnerabilities and include both brain-based and mental health risk. Brain-based contributions to offending behavior [8, 9], such as cognitive vulnerabilities [10–12], are important for adaptive responses to ambiguous situations and/or stimuli [13]. For example, a highly sensitized threat response system may be useful for rapid response to risk within a dangerous context, but then may contribute to inappropriate and excessive responses within low-risk contexts. Moreover, exceptionally high rates of mental health disorders are identified for incarcerated individuals in large systematic and meta-analytic reviews for both youth and adults [14–16]. Bridging both mental health associations, and environmental vulnerabilities, is exposure to trauma. In fact, researchers have suggested that one of the most salient predictors of contact with the criminal justice system is trauma [17], particularly exposure to cumulative adverse (or traumatic) childhood experiences (i.e., ACEs) [18, 19]. The link between cumulative ACEs and crime is apparent for both justice-involved youth [18] and adults [20]. In addition, other family variables also predict offending behaviors in the general population such as disruptions to family structure and caregiver changes, which might include divorce/separation, single parenthood, early child rearing (e.g., teenage parents), foster parenting, parental absence, and family death [21].

Feeling socially isolated or not connected to peer networks [22] is related to offending behavior. Conversely, having peer networks who hold pro-criminal attitudes or having peers who have committed crimes in the past [23] are frequently related to offending behavior. Other environmental influences, outside of relationships, also introduce vulnerabilities for criminal behavior, including school and/or employment difficulties such as academic failure, unemployment, or truancy [24]; a lack of prosocial recreation, leisure, or extracurricular activities [25]; and poverty or low socioeconomic status are all prominent predictors of offending behavior in the general population.

Considering the transactional nature of offending, criminal behavior recursively impacts an individual's cognitive and environmental vulnerabilities. For example, challenges in the family might lead to poor academic achievement [26], with its attendant social disadvantage, which could then lead to criminal behavior [27], which then introduces and exacerbates problems within the family [28].

FASD and the Justice System

FASD is often described as a hidden disability due to individuals frequently going undetected or misdiagnosed; although an individual may have many complex areas of need, they may not "look" different, and in many cases the extent of their difficulties may be masked. Nonetheless, emerging research suggests that individuals with FASD are identified as overrepresented in the justice systems internationally [29–33]. Moreover, although the research is limited, one study of justice-involved youth with FASD found they encountered the justice system earlier, and engaged in a higher number of offending behaviors compared to justice-involved youth without FASD [34]. Rates of legal difficulties and contact with the criminal justice system have also been shown to be elevated among individuals accessing FASD diagnostic clinics and services. In a recent Canadian study, 30% of adolescents and adults with FASD indicated having legal problems with offending at the time of their diagnostic assessment, and 3% indicated experiencing difficulties with incarceration [35]. Similarly, in a 25-year follow-up of those diagnosed with FASD in the United States, 60% had been in contact with the law and 35% had been incarcerated [4, 36]. High rates of FASD in incarcerated youth have also been observed internationally [30, 37].

Although these numbers provide information on current estimates of prevalence, experts believe that these statistics underestimate the prevalence of FASD in the justice system, such that there is an even greater number of undiagnosed and/or misdiagnosed people in both youth and adult correctional facilities. Conversely, others identify additional factors that may lead to over-incarceration of individuals with FASD, such as elevated risk of false confessions, potentially resulting in wrongful conviction [38]. Either way it is clear that improved identification is needed in order to pave the way for improved understanding and responses.

Limited access to informed psychological assessment and screening practices also puts individuals with FASD at further risk, particularly through a specialized forensic mental health lens whereby both legal and clinical factors can be evaluated and understood in synthesis [39]. Assessment and screening practices meet complementary but distinct needs. Screening practices provide a necessary step in identification of individuals with FASD, while assessment provides the in-depth functional information needed to support informed case management and intervention planning [40–42]. Without identification and a comprehensive understanding of the individual with FASD, our ability to understand and respond is limited. The needs of the individual may remain hidden, which further perpetuates their vulnerability [42], and can lead to deleterious consequences such as an increased likelihood of long-term involvement with the justice system [41, 43].

Seeing FASD—Individual Characteristics That Impact Functioning

Individuals with FASD experience a broad range of difficulties (e.g., cognitive, behavioral, emotional, social) [44, 45] that interact to perpetuate their vulnerabilities to engaging in offending behaviors. Among those who have engaged in offending behaviors, individuals with FASD often exhibit more neurocognitive deficits compared to justice-involved individuals without FASD [46]. Prenatal alcohol exposure results in central nervous system (CNS) dysfunction [47, 48], including smaller brain volumes, disorganized brain connectivity, and impairments in several neurotransmitter systems [49]. Specifically, brain regions that regulate executive function and emotional regulation are also altered by prenatal alcohol exposure such as frontal-temporal structures [44], the hippocampus [50], the thalamus [51], and the amygdala [52]. The many teratogenic effects of alcohol on the developing brain lead to a diverse and heterogeneous array of cognitive and behavioral consequences for these individuals [44] that can impact their ability to experience success within school and work environments, while also increasing their social vulnerability. For instance, individuals with FASD often have difficulties with social communication and displaying appropriate social skills [53], as well as difficulties correctly interpreting social situations (i.e., hostile attribution bias) [54]. Therefore, those with FASD are less likely to accurately evaluate their social actions elevating their risk of susceptibility to peer influence [53], as well as manipulation and alignment with antisocial peer groups, including engaging in criminal activities to "fit-in" [55]. Moreover, deficits in working memory [56], source memory (i.e., remembering where a message comes from) [57], and long-term memory and memory integration [58], may impact compliance with rules and expectations.

Certainly the deficits in problem-solving, set shifting, emotion regulation, and cognitive flexibility typically reported for this population [44, 56, 59] may impact problem-solving and adaptability, which are critical skills for daily functioning, particularly through older adolescence and the transition to adulthood at which point consideration of consequences for ones actions is paramount within social structures of behavioral control. The many, complex, and inter-related neurocognitive needs of this population not only impact their ability to function as expected but may also influence their self-perceptions and increase vulnerability to mental health difficulties.

High rates of mental illness are often present among individuals with FASD more broadly, including those who engage in criminal behaviors [2, 60], including internalizing disorders such as depression and anxiety [61], externalizing disorders such as ADHD [62], and substance abuse disorders [63]. In fact, with rates as high as 94% of those with FASD having comorbid mental disorders [63], concurrent difficulties is the proverbial "rule and not the exception" for those with FASD. In addition, elevated rates of physical health problems and comorbidity highlight the complexity and depth of need concerning whole-person care for individuals with FASD [64], including those who become justice-involved [31, 65, 66].

The environmental vulnerabilities for those with FASD spans family, peer, and societal disadvantages [41, 67, 68]. Social-contextual factors exist for those with FASD including [69] low socioeconomic status, un(der)employment, and difficulties in independent living [35, 69]. Prenatal alcohol exposure in an individual is also often associated with an increased vulnerability to environmental stress and adversity [63, 67]. Individuals with FASD are reported to experience higher rates of trauma, particularly higher rates of adverse childhood experiences (ACEs), and cumulative ACEs, relative to peers without FASD [70–72]. Youth with FASD who intersect with government systems and services, such as children's services or the justice system, are also more vulnerable to ACEs than those without similar involvement [72].

The complex intersection of cognitive and environmental vulnerabilities, occurring at elevated levels and without the right supports in place, creates a "perfect storm" for a propensity or vulnerability toward becoming engaged in the criminal justice system [4]. Applying a transactional framework [6] to these vulnerabilities allows us to consider two key themes (1) in what way is an individual's unique profile of needs contributing to their behavior? And (2) how might their functioning interact with environmental vulnerabilities? [67].

Current evidence-based intervention practices utilized within the justice system are limited in their effectiveness for those with FASD. For instance, not only are specific, relevant symptoms not necessarily being targeted, but a combination of cognitive and behavior therapy is often employed for those with FASD, especially in the criminal justice context [73]. This raises two concerns: first, the use of traditional cognitive therapies, without applying an FASD-informed lens or recognizing that an individual may experience substantial neurocognitive dysfunction as a result of PAE, may (incorrectly) operate from the assumption that an individual understands and is able to readily identify and reflect on their own thoughts, beliefs, emotions, and actions [73]. This is problematic because those with FASD often struggle with executive functioning, adaptive functioning, and attention [44]. Consequently, they may have difficulty benefitting as expected from intervention strategies that place heavy emphasis on cognition in therapy without modification or accommodation [74].

Second, the behavioral components of many therapeutic techniques often heavily depend on creating rigid routines, structure, and consistency that are externally enforced. In doing so there is a heavy reliance on changes and support from people in the individual's environment. This can again be problematic without applying an FASD-informed lens and explicitly identifying the specific vulnerabilities and needs for an individual client with FASD within their environment outside of the justice system. This may be of particular concern for those who may not have access to safe and supportive structured environments and care providers [75] or may place a high burden on stable caregivers in the community. Ultimately, "failed" treatment experiences increase the risk of labeling an individual with FASD as being "difficult" or "unreceptive" to intervention, as well as impacting an individual's motivation and likelihood of wanting to engage in future programs and supports. More broadly, limited access to FASD treatment resources both within and beyond the justice context, including therapists and appropriate programming, has also been shown in multiple international settings, such as Australia [76], New Zealand [77], and South Africa [78],—ultimately, this culminates in an increased vulnerability for offending behavior.

Individuals with FASD may experience stigma and discrimination from various sectors, including the public, the education system, mental health and social service systems, and the media [79]; the justice system is no exception. Stigma for this group can be further perpetuated by public and media perceptions that reinforce that FASD is a result of an individual's behavior or that individuals with FASD are unable to care for themselves or lead positive, healthy, and successful lives [70]. Even well-intentioned efforts to support individuals with FASD "so they don't end up in the justice system" can fuel mis-perceptions that justice system involvement is somehow inevitable for individuals with FASD. The public and media's representation of individuals with FASD can sensationalize individual behaviors and often suggests that all individuals with FASD are the same, detracting from the efficacy of intervention and support, and the reality that many individuals with FASD experience healthy outcomes and contribute positively to society [80]. Social media can further contribute to stigma, as inaccurate and often misleading information about FASD and individuals with FASD can be shared on a public and viral scale [79].

There is a call for *all* legal and forensic professionals to better understand the vulnerabilities associated with FASD [66, 81]. Recognizing and acknowledging the needs of this underserved population may equip us to more effectively enact systematic approaches to support healthy outcomes, including reduced recidivism. More details and recommendations for doing so will be discussed in the last section of this chapter.

Intersections with the Justice System

Jason's car was surrounded. His panic intensified. Flinging open his door he searched for a gap in the perimeter. He was unable to understand the words being yelled at him. All he knew was that he was trapped and needed to escape. And that he was probably in a lot of trouble. He ran towards a gap. As the volume of voices shouting around him grew, he simply ran faster—his brain was not allowing him to process the information. As the police officers neared, his panic escalated. He flailed as he was tackled and restrained.

Later Jason found himself in the police station. He could not remember how he got there. It was a blur. Police were talking to him. Yelling at him. He had trouble making it all out and understanding what they were saying. He knew he was in big trouble. He wondered where his friends were. Thinking of his friends reminded him he is tough. Swearing is a good way to get people to leave you alone. He didn't want to speak to anyone, not his Uncle, not a lawyer. Lawyers don't help anyhow, and plus, he didn't have one. They made him speak to someone on the phone who said she was a lawyer. She told him not to talk to the police and to be quiet. But, it was Friday and he was going to have to sit in a holding cell through the weekend. He was probably going to jail anyhow. He dozed in the interview room for an hour, and when the detectives came back, they promised that it would be better for him if he just came clean and said what he did. They promised they would put in a good word with the judge, that everyone makes mistakes. Jason wasn't going to get his friends in trouble. That would mean trouble for him. But he wanted the judge to take it easy. He decided to tell the police what happened, and thought, who knows, maybe it would look good for his case and he would get released over the weekend on bail. He bet his Uncle would be able to come up with the money and post it for him. He would pay him back.

The Impact of FASD When in Contact with the Police

FASD is often associated with a variety of interacting cognitive and environmental challenges [44, 67] with relevance for interactions with police. This may be most evident in initial police interactions and police investigations.

Initial Police Interactions

Police interactions can be highly charged for all parties. Elevated emotionality, combined with cognitive vulnerabilities for individuals with FASD, can set the stage for rapid escalation of interactions. When these vulnerabilities are not identified or engaged effectively, they may inflame interactions and lead to worsening outcomes [82]. In the context of interactions with law enforcement agents, this might include resisting arrest charges, and assault or violence toward the police [83]. Moreover, lower IQ as well as reading and language comprehension difficulties has been known to impede one's ability to navigate interactions with legal professions, particularly among those with FASD, and is linked with poor understanding legal rights on arrest [1, 83], as well as understanding the actions, procedures, and consequences levied by the police [83]. For example, fines, conversations, and written warnings are often articulated using specialized and complex language that is typically presented at a grade 6–12 level [84] which may be incomprehensible for many youth and those with cognitive deficits, including those with FASD [1].

Environmental contributors often associated with FASD may also lead to vulnerabilities during police encounters. For example, some but not all individuals with FASD may be exposed to criminal behavior, violence, and victimization by family, caregivers, and peers. Additionally, they may demonstrate immature interpersonal skills such as being easily intimidated or having a desire to please those in authority [4, 85], which may significantly increase their vulnerability when interacting with police. In turn, they may then be more likely to acquiesce and endorse what they have been told without fact checking. Adverse life problems are experienced at elevated rates among people with FASD, including low SES and difficulties related to employment [35, 86], which often make tickets, fines, and other fiscal consequences near impossible for them to resolve and again result in further legal consequences [41].

Police Investigation Considerations

Perhaps the most informative illustration of the ways in which the cognitive and environmental contributors associated with FASD intersect to produce vulnerability during police encounters is during police questioning/interrogation. In particular, coercive techniques may pose a greater risk for individuals with FASD, necessitating a different kind of support and protection.

Risk factors that increase a suspect's vulnerability to coercive interrogation methods include younger age, impaired cognitive abilities, and mental health difficulties [87, 88]. These are applicable to the deficits found in many individuals with FASD. In general, coercive police techniques are an important risk factor associated with the potential for false confessions [89, 90], particularly, as articulated by Drake and colleagues [91], as false confessions typically arise when a suspect struggles with internal factors such as lower IQ, hyperactivity, and/or inattention, and/or external factors such as wanting questioning to stop and to go home, protecting the identity of the true perpetrator, and succumbing to police pressure and manipulation, are present [92]. Youth in general, and those with cognitive impairments in particular, are often less strategic in their decision-making due to immature development of higher order thinking [93], impulsivity, and reduced foresight for consequences of their actions [94]. For youth with FASD, these risk factors converge [53]. Contributing to this, they have been identified as having immature social skills [95], as being easily manipulated by others [96], and as having a desire to please authority [4]. As such it is proposed that those with FASD may be at a particular disadvantage during police interrogation. Indeed, one study of 50 youth and young adults with FASD found that 40% admitted that they had made at least one false confession to the police [1]. These numbers are consistent among youth without FASD [1], further suggesting a call for improved police investigation methods among vulnerable populations.

The Impact of FASD During the Formal Adjudication Process

During the formal adjudication process, the interacting cognitive and environmental factors present for those with FASD [67] impact how these individuals behave and are perceived, in varying ways. This includes considerations related to courtroom proceedings, administrative and compliance issues, and competencies/fitness to stand trial.

Courtroom and Proceeding Considerations

The courtroom can be an unfamiliar, strange, and overwhelming environment that places the defendant at the center of attention [83]. In general, younger people and individuals with impairments in cognitive functioning often demonstrate high rates of deficits in their psycholegal capacities [1, 97], as do those diagnosed with learning disabilities, attention problems, and externalizing behaviors [97, 98]. These difficulties are particularly problematic during formal adjudication proceedings [99, 100] and may be pronounced for those with FASD [83]. For instance, specialized language in the courtroom often includes extensive legal jargon and advanced level grammar and diction [83], which can be difficult for many individuals with FASD to comprehend. Given that FASD is often associated with difficulties in language comprehension and working memory [101], those with FASD may also have deficits in their ability to meaningfully engage and participate during legal proceedings [1, 83] or even comprehend the purpose and process of the legal proceedings in the first place [102]. In addition, the pace of courtroom proceedings can be dynamic, such that it transitions from a slow to fast pace unpredictably, without a warning or an opportunity to ask questions [83]. The changes of pace can be confusing and difficult to follow at the best of times as it requires processing information ridden with jargon without the opportunity to confer with supporters, such as a lawyer and ensure adequate comprehension [83].

The courtroom is also a busy place that is filled with an assortment of noise and distractions, including bright lights, people coming and going, multiple conversations going on at once, and a lot of background noise [83]. The additional stimulation that exists in the courtroom then paves the way for further challenges with attention, impulsivity, and a potential sensory overload. Considering that sensory processing difficulties are often associated with FASD [103], those with FASD may become overwhelmed by the language, pace, and overstimulating environment of the courtroom. Overall, the difficulties of those with FASD could then translate to inappropriate impulsive or aggressive behaviors being exhibited during legal proceedings, which may then be misconstrued as intentionally hostile toward legal professionals—and thereby potentially add additional consequences for them [83].

Even outside of the courtroom, executive function deficits, common in accused with FASD, present unique challenges in limiting the decision-making abilities relating to pleas. Either impulsively or without fully estimating and grasping the implications, individuals may offer a plea in the mistaken assumption that their case will be settled quickly and favorably [104]. Negotiations necessary for plea bargains are dependent on cognitive abilities that, when impaired, leave the accused in a precariously disadvantaged situation. Lawyers, unaware of the disparity between receptive and expressive language of affected persons may mistake apparent competent verbal communication with discernment of communicated words. This is especially relevant if the accused also manifests desire and eagerness to please and may consequently agree to the lawyer's inquiry "do you understand."

Competencies and Fitness to Stand Trial

Mental health assessments may be administered to identify whether an individual has the capacity to comprehend the legal process [82, 83]. In Canada, the United Kingdom, and many commonwealth nations, the assessment is referred to as Fitness to Stand Trial (i.e., Competence to Stand Trial in the United States) [105]. Fitness (or Competence) to stand trial assessments are put in place to protect the rights of the accused by ensuring that they are competent to appear in front of the courtroom; in effect, whether the suspect understands the nature of the proceedings, the possible consequences of the proceedings, and is able to communicate with counsel [106]. However, despite these intentions, there are limitations with the utility of these assessments, such that (1) these assessments are not aimed at identifying/

understanding the unique vulnerabilities that exist for those with FASD [95] and (2) the criteria to be deemed "unfit" or unable to comprehend legal proceedings is extremely conservative and tends to focus most heavily on overt and extreme mental health symptoms (e.g., psychosis, intellectual disability) and thus is much less often applied in the context of FASD [82, 107]. When an "unfit" label is applied to those who are assessed, these individuals then begin interventions that are aimed at increasing their ability to stand trial [106, 108]. These methods are problematic because the congenital brain injury that occurs after prenatal alcohol exposure requires a dedicated, tailored, and purposeful combination of psychopharmacology and psychoeducation to elicit cognitive growth [109]. For those placed in more restrictive settings after a finding of unfit to stand trial, delays, or challenges in remediation may be particularly problematic given the serious deprivation of liberty.

Administrative and Compliance Considerations

Environmental factors such as low SES, unemployment, and homelessness also further impact those with FASD during adjudication [2, 68]. Fines, bail, or other socio-economic factors, such as being able to demonstrate and maintain a fixed address, coupled with potentially diminished or lacking support systems, may also further impact compliance with the adjudication process [68, 83]. Difficulties with executive functioning, working memory, and planning for those with FASD may be associated with missing court dates and not paying fines on time [83]. Furthermore, difficulties with language and communication may impact interactions with probation/parole/police officers that they might be working with [83]. All these factors therefore result in further consequences for these vulnerable individuals.

The Impacts of the Vulnerabilities in the Forensic Mental Health Sector

To establish whether a crime was committed and if the perpetrator was wholly, partially, or not responsible, most western adversarial systems recognize the role of mental disorder in impacting criminal responsibility. Terms such as not guilty by reason of insanity, guilty but insane, and not criminally responsible due to mental disorder are used for those designated as having acted under the provisions that interfere with the mental aspect of crime (mens rea). The criteria outlined in legislation across most common law legal systems align with the criteria that the accused "was labouring under such a defect of reason, from disease of the mind, as not to know the nature and quality of the act he was doing; or if he did know it, that he did not know he was doing what was wrong" [110]. However, this approach has been criticized as a net "too narrow" to identify those with a vast array of mental conditions that may impact degrees of responsibility, including those with FASD. Traditionally, disorders related to delusions, hallucinations, and severe cognitive symptoms easily constitute the deficits needed to designate someone as not criminally responsible. Alternatively, disorders such as PTSD, antisocial personality disorder, and autism spectrum disorder rarely result in an accused being found not criminally responsible under the law [111].

Similarly, FASD in many accused rarely constitutes grounds for referral, assessment, determination, and a verdict to exempt from criminal responsibility. The threshold is high because the individual declared not criminally responsible is supposed to have acted without awareness of the consequences and without knowledge that their actions or omissions were either legal or morally wrong or both. While the reasons for this may seem obvious, much debate has begun to challenge this traditional legal conceptualization of criminal responsibility. For instance, it has been recommended that the deficits of FASD should be sufficient to declare the accused, at most, to have partial responsibility in some cases. In a case report, the court in Australia reversed a conviction to grant a verdict of diminished responsibility which ultimately mitigated against the sentence the accused received [112]. After reviewing the criteria and aligning those with the common FASD cognitive deficits, diminished responsibility was conceptualized with a two-prong advantage; first for the accused with FASD and second for reducing the repeated incarceration of individuals with a hidden disability like FASD [113]. Individuals so declared will benefit from the comprehensive community care similar to those with other mental health diagnoses.

Current therapeutic jurisprudence (TJ) principles seek to apply the law in assisting individuals. Recognizing that multiple factors come together to place certain accused at a disadvantage, TJ approaches serve as a solution to the revolving door phenomenon also related to offending patterns in those with FASD [114, 115]. FASD and its manifestations challenge the traditional assumptions of the criminal justice system. The adjudication process should accommodate manifestations such as unawareness of consequences, cognitively induced impulse control and inattention, which contribute to certain criminal behavior. With the proliferation of mental health courts, diversion is now possible for those with FASD so that they are better supported in the community. In turn, FASD-informed mental health and addiction teams in collaboration with experienced FASD community networks are better placed to best manage individuals with FASD who offend in the community. Housing, rehabilitative employment opportunities, and resources that adjust their offerings to the unique needs of individuals with FASD are also more likely to result in successful outcomes, reaching beyond the important, but narrow and insufficient goal of reducing recidivism, so commonly seen as solely paramount in offending contexts [116]. It is also possible that, by the nature of comorbidity and misdiagnosis, individuals with FASD form part of the population of those already found not criminally responsible. This invites research to identify what features qualify for the verdict, alone or in combination with other symptoms of mental disorder.

The Impacts of FASD During Incarceration

Being incarcerated is considered the most serious sanction and is usually reserved for cases where it is absolutely needed to reach goals of justice and protect the public. Yet, incarceration is often the default system for many individuals with FASD [117]. This is problematic because individuals with FASD do not do well during incarceration [117], and many have advocated that incarceration and punishment without consideration for the unique needs of those with FASD may not be functional or effective [68], especially among youth [118]. Not only are individual vulnerabilities for individuals with FASD potentially problematic as they may increase risk of victimization, but the goals of sentencing may also not be appropriately achieved without specialized consideration by the courts [3, 102]. Accordingly, consideration for impacts within correctional settings, rehabilitation and intervention, and risk assessment is particularly important.

Managing Within a Correctional Setting

Although some have suggested that the rigid and consistent schedules imposed on those who are incarcerated may have a beneficial impact for individuals with FASD, evidence suggests that not only is incarceration harmful to health and well-being, it constitutes the most serious deprivation of liberty [119]. Individuals with FASD may have increased vulnerability in the correctional context due to difficulties with comprehension, working memory, and processing speed that are often inflamed in high pressure situations like incarceration [120], as well as challenges adjusting, complying, and remembering the expectations and routines around them during incarceration [119]. Furthermore, these difficulties may be misinterpreted as intentional hostility, non-compliance, and rule-breaking by correctional staff [119]. As a result, those with FASD may experience a greater number of disciplinary sanctions during incarceration, coupled with an increased likelihood of becoming incarcerated again and sooner (i.e., 6 months sooner) than those without FASD [120].

Interacting with cognitive vulnerabilities are a unique set of social, and environmental, challenges for those with FASD while incarcerated. Given that individuals with FASD are often vulnerable to antisocial peer influence, and often seek to "fit-in" and be well liked by others [55], they become vulnerable to influence and victimization during incarceration with antisocial peers [68]. This may translate to being used and manipulated by peers, as well as taking the blame for more sophisticated inmates—which in turn, may result in more punitive consequences for the individual with FASD [119]. Furthermore, susceptibility to antisocial influence may also result in those with FASD spending more time with disruptive inmates and an increased involvement with antisocial peer groups [119]. Those with FASD are also vulnerable to victimization while incarcerated, including becoming the victim of physical, sexual, and emotional abuse [119, 121].

Rehabilitation and Intervention Considerations

The most influential model informing effective justice-context programs and interventions is the Risk-Needs-Responsivity framework (RNR) [122]. The RNR framework generally asserts that understanding, prevention, and intervention within the justice system is grounded in abiding by key principles, including: (1) identifying an individual's overall level of risk, as well as the specific risk factors that contribute to and/or drive criminal behavior; and (2) using tailored intervention strategies that specifically target the *relevant* underlying mechanism(s) that drove the criminal behavior to rehabilitate the offender [41, 123]; and that providing care or interventions for irrelevant factors, may actually be more deleterious [43]; and (3) ensuring that interventions are provided in a manner so as to be appropriately responsive to the capacities of the person receiving the intervention. However, there are limitations in applying this framework to individuals with FASD that include limited awareness of FASD among professionals, challenges with assessment practices, and poorly matched intervention efforts and approaches to individual needs and capacities [41].

In conjunction with practices that occur before sentencing, incarceration also presents a valuable opportunity for forensic professionals to apply a comprehensive case management framework. From this perspective, assessment may be viewed as a form of intervention [82], such that our ability to provide meaningful interventions for those with FASD who are incarcerated is contingent on understanding the unique underlying mechanisms and factors that drove the offending behavior [68, 82]. With regard to the RNR framework, this means that our ability to implement programs with appropriate attention and planning for *responsivity*, or strategies that specifically target the relevant vulnerabilities present for the individual in a manner likely to result in effective impact, are significantly impaired [82]. This is particularly important because many professionals in the justice system mistakenly attribute offending behaviors to factors, or vulnerabilities, that are not actually present for the individual they are responding to [124]. Providing interventions that target typical, but irrelevant risk factors may inadvertently lead to unintended deleterious consequences such as increased offending behavior during incarceration and when reintegrating into the community [124].

Due to limited knowledge of functioning across neurodevelopmental and social domains, interventions that are selected may prove to be a poor fit for individuals with FASD. For instance, current correctional interventions may employ cognitive behavior therapeutic techniques that place too heavy of an emphasis on the cognitive components, making interventions less effective for those with FASD [74]. In addition, present justice-based intervention approaches for individuals with FASD often aim to be "quick-fix" solutions to modify behavior [108]. Given that FASD may be conceptualized as a brain injury resulting from the prenatal exposure to alcohol [44], it has been argued that these "quick-fix" intervention strategies are frequently ineffective for those with FASD, particularly in the absence of additional system level supports and resources [83, 125]. Consequently, our current approaches to help support those with FASD who have offended may often not be serving their intended purpose [41].

The Impacts of FASD for Community Reintegration

The limited research available at this time reveals that many individuals with FASD, without appropriate supports, are potentially at increased risk to reoffend, and reoffend sooner than individuals reintegrating into the community who do not have FASD [34, 120, 126]. In fact, the frequency of recidivism among those with FASD and the ensuing re-involvement with the justice system have left many to argue that there is a "revolving door" phenomenon for those with FASD and the justice system [114, 115]. More specifically, without appropriate supports and skills in place, individuals with FASD are at risk of continuing to engage in offending behaviors and become reacquainted with the justice system, with an inability to break the cycle of offending [127].

Current research provides insight into cognitive factors that may impact the ability of individuals with FASD to meet post-release expectations [83, 121]. First, deficits in working memory and comprehension may make it difficult to meet the demands of their release conditions (e.g., court dates, appointments, meetings with probation, and/or parole officers) [41]. Furthermore, it has been noted that difficulties with self-regulation and impulsivity also make it difficult for those with FASD to comply with community reintegration steps, such as working in an unstructured and unmonitored way with parole and/or probation officers [41]. In addition, difficulties with language comprehension and memory also impede their ability to interact and communicate with the probation/parole officers that they might be working with, paralleling their vulnerabilities at the police level [82, 83]. This is important because these difficulties often lead to misunderstandings, breached conditions, and strained relationships with law enforcement, as well as potential further negative consequences as a result of these infractions [82].

Intersecting with cognitive vulnerabilities are environmental risk factors. This is a population who often struggle with poverty and marginalization that proves to be a substantial barrier to success upon their release. Without safe and secure housing, income supports, and employment training opportunities, individuals with FASD will remain vulnerable. Lack of connections to community resources, treatment programs, and supports to assist in access to these programs aggravates this vulnerability. These basic needs, when unmet in individuals with FASD, require specific consideration and planning to facilitate community reintegration. Without such support these individuals may remain more vulnerable to affiliation with secure threat groups (gangs) and other deviant social groups during their time in incarceration [128] and consequently have a wider social circle of criminally involved peers when released back into the community [74]. Similarly, they may utilize the lessons that they have learned from peers during incarceration and adopt more "street-wise" behaviors and versatile offending skills while incarcerated that they then employ in the community on release [74]. Unsurprisingly, these behaviors then lead to future interactions with the police and the justice system [82, 121].

System Wide Gaps

Broadly speaking, the justice system affords us many opportunities to support improved outcomes for individuals with FASD by addressing gaps in the system. In particular, the need for consistent identification, comprehensive assessment, and access to training for criminal justice professionals is reported as common barriers to best practice [45, 104, 129].

Identification At present, there are limited procedures in place to identify FASD within the justice system [42, 82, 83], despite high prevalence rates and concerns regarding high rates of unidentified individuals within the system. Moreover, assessment is seldomly included as part of the adjudication process [82, 95], and when it is, typically involves a combination of informal screening and assessments aimed at identifying whether the individual has the capacity to generally comprehend the legal process [82, 83].

Assessment for Intervention Limited assessment services also mean that those with FASD often make their way through incarceration without any form of functional, nor comprehensive assessment to identify needs that may be addressed to mitigate risk [82]. Furthermore, once released from incarceration, those with FASD have limited access to assessment, intervention, or community support [82, 130], but are still expected to follow-through with their court orders. Researchers have noted that this practice gap exists despite requests for the court to implement appropriate and life-long community support for those with FASD who have engaged in offending behavior [82]. Assessment of cognitive and mental health functioning would facilitate access to a dedicated, tailored, and purposeful intervention plans to elicit meaningful growth and address areas of risk and need [39, 109]. Without proper assessment of the vulnerabilities that exist [39, 82], coupled with tailored intervention plans that result from the assessments that do take place [108], those with FASD are again left at increased risk of being misunderstood and vulnerable.

Access to Training A lack of training for forensic professionals is reported for every level of the criminal justice system, which also impacts our ability to recognize and respond to the needs of these vulnerable individuals [35, 104, 129]. For example, many police officers do not receive training regarding the unique vulnerabilities that exist for those with FASD and how these vulnerabilities may play-out during police encounters and questioning [83, 131]. Furthermore, lawyers, judges, and court officials may be under trained on the presentation of FASD and the vulnerabilities that exist for these individuals, inside the courtroom. A lack of understanding of FASD by lawyers, judges, and other members of the court may lead to an increased likelihood of criminal convictions and the ensuing jail/prison sentences [132]. Training is improving among judges [102]. There is also a need to educate correctional staff, and forensic mental health professionals, on the vulnerabilities and behaviors of individuals with FASD who are incarcerated [133]. The call for training also extends to probation officers, parole officers, and community support workers, particularly life-long supports [130, 134], to help them navigate their reintegration into the community on release.

Responding to the Call for Improved Practices

Jason's case highlights a number of key issues and difficulties relevant for individuals with FASD, and a range of legal and justice professionals, across adjudicative stages in the legal system. Importantly, effective responses and scaffolding must be put in place long before risk for engaging in crime and becoming involved in the criminal justice system occurs. Although Jason experienced many difficulties shared by individuals with FASD, it does not appear that he was identified, nor did he ultimately have the opportunity to undergo a fulsome and multifaceted evaluation of his functioning, strengths and needs. Understanding these factors for Jason, through a strengths-based lens, particularly at an early age, coupled with the provision of appropriate proactive supports and resources within his family prior to child welfare involvement, may have made a critical impact for Jason in shifting his early trajectory. In particular, his experience of disruptive and destabilizing and frequent moves may have proved much more harmful and difficult for Jason compared to a child without similar neurodevelopmental difficulties and needs. Without the right supports in place, Jason then also experienced school disruption, and other common difficulties experienced by individuals with unrecognized complex needs, including difficulties related to employment, housing, and income.

Ultimately, these challenges and unmet needs in respect to positive and meaningful opportunities for socialization and relationships with prosocial peers may have contributed to Jason becoming enmeshed with criminally-involved peers, and ultimately, the current legal trouble. Training for police officers to recognize when they are engaging with a person who has complex neurodevelopmental needs may have resulted in more effective de-escalation following the car crash. Enhanced legal safeguards and procedural protections, including FASD-informed legal counsel present with Jason during police interview, and the use of non-coercive interview techniques by police during interrogation may have reduced the chances of Jason acquiescing and admitting guilt, without fulsome understanding and appreciation of his legal rights as a suspect. Moving forward, a comprehensive evaluation of Jason's functional cognitive and mental health needs should inform next legal steps and decisions, including a tailored evaluation of the risks and needs he experiences not only in relation to his offending risk, but also to inform the provision of appropriate services and interventions to support not only desistance from crime, but also healthy outcomes including stable housing, meaningful employment, and healthy peer relationships. In the section that follows, we outline a number of key themes and recommendations that may prove helpful for facilitating action to improve outcomes for individuals with FASD involved in the criminal justice system, and across all recommendations, emphasize the importance of a strengths-based and preventative lens.

Intersections with the criminal justice system, particularly for those with FASD, are complex and multidimensional with a variety of underlying cognitive [44], environmental [67], and system level [2] vulnerabilities that interact in unique ways to increase the likelihood of offending (or perceived offending) behavior in this population. Importantly, while a variety of vulnerabilities exist for those with FASD, these individuals often have strengths such as friendliness, kindness, affection, work ethic, and generosity, just to name a few [135] that need to be fostered, considered, and leveraged when interpreting and responding to offending behavior for those with FASD. To help facilitate an integrated understanding and improve our ability to respond, a synthesis of the key themes and calls to action discussed in this chapter, and recommendations for better responding, follows.

Synthesizing the Key Themes and Recommendations to Facilitate Action

Theme 1: Primary Intervention and Prevention Throughout the chapter, we have discussed various frameworks that are important to consider in the context of FASD in the criminal justice system. A transactional/dynamic paradigm [5–7] should be employed when considering the cognitive, environmental, and system level vulnerabilities, and the unique ways that these vulnerabilities interact to increase the propensity toward offending behavior among those with FASD. Recognizing this dynamic process not only poises us to respond in meaningful ways—but to also engage in primary intervention and prevention that may reduce the likelihood for intersection with the justice system. Healthy outcomes may be facilitated through shared understanding and support for the unique needs of individuals balanced by appreciation for their strengths and capacities, applied proactively and collaboratively throughout the lifespan across all developmental domains [136]. Strong familial cohesion and attachment, adapted school environments, well suited mental health supports, and safe and stable housing and employment are a few areas in which support may be provided, and healthy outcomes nurtured. Justice system involvement is not an inevitable outcome for individuals with FASD, nor a final endpoint for those who do experience legal difficulties.

Theme 2: A Call for Adopting an FASD Lens Accordingly, the aim of this chapter was to outline not only the vulnerabilities that exist for those with FASD across various levels of the justice system, but to convey that each of these vulnerabilities do not operate in isolation. In fact, many individuals with FASD are at a particular disadvantage in having a unique and complex interplay of neurocognitive functioning and environmental conditions that they are faced with [67, 109], that many have referred to as a "double jeopardy" [2, 137]. Ergo, intentionally understanding and reflecting on how the vulnerabilities at play for each individual with FASD interact with one another in such complex, and involuntary ways, will help those in the justice system adopt a needed FASD lens when working with this vulnerable group. Appreciation of the reciprocal, or transactional, interaction of factors may be best situated with a biopsychosocial model, thus highlighting not only the many transactions that may occur between factors but also the many domains from which these factors may arise. Similar to applying a transactional lens, understanding individuals with FASD who are justice-involved or at risk of becoming involved, through a biopsychosocial model, will also allow professionals in the criminal justice sector to appreciate the complex interplay of vulnerabilities that exist for those with

FASD. In particular, the use of a biopsychosocial model has been recommended for enhancing our ability to respond and provide effective intervention strategies for those with FASD [82], which will be discussed in more detail below.

Theme 3: Moving Toward an Informed Understanding of FASD in the Justice System As discussed throughout this chapter, those with FASD are up against a variety of cognitive [44, 46], developmental [68], social [54], and system [125] challenges that increase the likelihood that they will intersect with the justice system [41, 82]. Consequently, these vulnerabilities significantly compromise the ability of those with FASD to function effectively and be understood properly, within all levels of the traditional justice system. Accordingly, a common theme that arose is the call to *educate and train* professionals, at every level of the justice system, to allow for an informed understanding and appreciation for FASD in the justice system [66]. In general, this might include the implementation of FASD education within university and other professional curriculums, as suggested by several researchers [42, 133, 138].

At the *police level*, education/training on FASD may be disseminated through guidebooks for police officers, such as those offered through No FASD in Australia [139], that include an informed understanding of how interacting with those with FASD, through an FASD lens, might be utilized. Alternatively, professional development courses, such as those offered through CanFASD [140] that provide research and informative video content to help inform officers may also be considered. These recommendations could also be applied at the *adjudication level*, such that guides could be created, by future researchers and policy makers, that specifically target judges and lawyers with an informed understanding of the interplay of factors involved in working with those with FASD. The use of training programs, such as those through CanFASD [140], aimed at educating judges and lawyers may also be considered. Researchers have also advocated for training judges to understand and intentionally consider FASD in the courtroom [141]. Borrowing from a pilot project in Manitoba, Canada, interested legal aid lawyers could also elect to dedicate themselves to FASD clients, where they are able to gain additional education and take on less clients to help support those with FASD [142].

Similarly, these resources could be shared with corrections officers and other staff who interact with FASD offenders while they are *incarcerated*, as well as extended to social, community, and family support workers to help them support those with FASD *reintegrate into the community* after incarceration [45, 133]. These tools, strategies, and resources, that help facilitate an informed understanding of FASD could be accessed/shared through FASD dedicated and accredited resources such as CANFASD in Canada [140], NoFASD in Australia [139], or FASD United— an international organization and resource center that specializes in an informed understanding of FASD [143].

Theme 4: Identification and Assessment Another common theme that arose throughout this chapter was the need for approaches to identification and assessment to help facilitate recognition of needs and informed responses [66, 82]. This necessarily includes consideration of the relevant and appropriate level of risk factors involved for each individual case in order to inform mitigation strategies [34, 40]. Currently, there is no systematic approach used within the justice system, although modifications and specifiers exist in the DSM that clinicians (i.e., forensic psychologists and psychiatrists) can utilize [82, 112], including applying the *other specified* and/or *unspecified* classification to a Neurodevelopmental Disorder (NDD) diagnosis; or, for those with low IQ and adaptive functioning, applying the Intellectual Developmental Disorder using the specification of severity and etiology of prenatal exposure; or, for those who demonstrate significant externalizing behavior concerns, applying a neurobehavioral disorder diagnosis, associated with prenatal alcohol exposure (e.g., ND-PAE) [117, 144].

In conjunction with these limitations to assessment and diagnosis, there is also a call for comprehensive, functional assessment (as opposed to the current surface level screenings that take place, if at all) to become a mandatory part of the criminal justice system [66, 82], specifically beginning with screening before adjudication [41]. A recommendation for doing so might include encouraging judges to intentionally be asking about whether FASD is present in the courtroom [141], and order mandatory comprehensive, functional assessments to those who enter the courtroom and may be vulnerable [82]. For example, organizations like the Centerpoint program in Edmonton, Canada could be employed to help facilitate education and the administration of the assessments for the courts [82, 145]. Implementing these recommendations will also then allow our present system to consider assessment as a form of intervention, particularly when strengths and protective factors that may be leverage are identified, in order to support community reintegration [4].

Theme 5: Rethinking the System It has been suggested that coercive police tactics [89], overwhelming courtrooms [83], punishment [118], and incarceration [82] approaches are not effective means of interacting with, nor modifying the behavior of, those with FASD. Accordingly, there is a call for change and a call for the use of therapeutic jurisprudence or using the law to support those with FASD by providing alternative, supportive, and rehabilitative focused strategies to better respond and reduce offending behavior(s) of these individuals [82]. Recommendations to help improve our response in this regard include four key levels. First, to address the potentially problematic traditional interrogation techniques associated with increased risk of false confessions and vulnerability for those with FASD, it is recommended that our police officers are not only trained (as above), but that interrogation methods be carefully considered. For instance, the use of the PEACE model in the United Kingdom [146], which is aimed at eliciting information to gain a better understanding of the situation as opposed to applying pressure or using manipulation, could be considered in more jurisdictions. This may help alleviate the consequences for the coercive techniques presently being used in jurisdictions such as North America [83]. It should also be recommended that those with FASD, or even suspected FASD, have access to support during interrogation [82]. Here, the use of forensic mental health professionals [82], mentors [130], or lawyers dedicated to FASD [141] may help facilitate support in this regard.

Secondly, to begin addressing the adjudication level difficulties for those with FASD, the consideration of a problem-solving courts with either a mental health focus, or FASD specific focus, may be recommended [130]. The essence of a separate or problem-solving court approach would be to incorporate an informed understanding of FASD and the underlying factors that may have contributed to the offending behavior, the use of verdicts that place less responsibility on the defendant with FASD, and verdicts that reduce punitive consequences and instead focus on aligning the individual with services and people that support them and promote prosocial behavior [130]. Furthermore, modifications to our current adult court proceedings that borrow from the practices currently employed in the youth court systems may also be considered [83]. For example, reducing the pace and level of language used inside the courtroom, making courtrooms private to limit the amount of people/distractions that are present; employing the use of dedicated FASD lawyers who specialize in working with the vulnerabilities associated with FASD; allowing time for intentionally investigating whether the suspect with FASD comprehends the proceedings; and employing verdicts that prioritize rehabilitation and long-term support over punishment and incarceration [83]. Additionally, programs such as the Alexis FASD Justice Program (AFJP) in rural Canada, which utilizes information from neurocognitive assessments to inform court decisions for adults with FASD, may also be employed at the adjudication level [147].

Efforts to enact these recommendations are beginning to emerge. For instance, a special FASD-designated problem-solving court in Manitoba, Canada, recently opened. All members of the court, including the lawyers and judge, are FASD-informed, and opportunities for a range of accommodations to support meaningful participation during the adjudicative process are being provided. Additionally, as a solution-focused court, defendants can be connected with the FASD Justice Program, through which they can receive support and navigational assistance with clinical and community services necessary for effective sentences and rehabilitation. Evaluation of program outcomes is planned, in order to continue the process of developing evidence-informed problem-solving courts, including mental health courts and even competency-related subprograms, as they are being applied with increasing frequency and may provide more optimal adjudicative environments for many individuals with FASD [148].

Third, inclusion of a rehabilitative approach is needed for individuals with FASD [117]. Although the idea of rehabilitation of individuals with FASD has at times been met with confusion and dismissal [149], this is increasingly identified as a necessary response to those with FASD who have engaged in offending behavior [150]. This may include using assessment as a form of intervention [4], to allow professionals to specifically map and target the cognitive, environmental, and system level barriers that contributed to the offending behavior that align with the bio-psychosocial model [82], and are beneficial, supportive, and helpful for the individual [41]. In addition, restorative justice approaches have increasingly been considered for more effectively addressing the needs of individuals with FASD [104, 151]. In general, although the research remains limited, researchers advise against "quick-fix" approaches [108]. Consideration for approaches that merge both environmental supports with efforts to support behavioral change that are FASD-informed have been suggested. For instance, use of behaviorist techniques, such as structure, consistency, and predictability that are individualized and involve behavioral reinforcement, and promote adaptive, prosocial functioning [152] could be utilized. Strategies used can leverage the individual's strengths and focus on physical learning and building skills to replace problematic patterns should also be considered [152]. Skill-based programs that allow for social skills training, education, upgrading, and future employment opportunities should be considered when responding to those with FASD who have intersected with the justice system [82]. In conjunction with these psychosocial interventions, many psychopharmacological interventions may be efficacious for those with FASD (e.g., stimulants, dexamphetamine) [109] and may be considered in the criminal justice context [82].

Finally, it is imperative to note that support, responding, and rehabilitation should not end with incarceration, but should extend into the community to help support those with FASD long-term. At present, once the individual is released back into the community, not all individuals have the same access to support or intervention [130], some will return to difficult social, economic, and personal circumstances, and without the right support may return to risky activities and may associate with the deviant peer groups they met during incarceration [55]. To help alleviate these struggles, researchers have recommended that reintegration into the community needs to begin with intensive supports such as intensive case management and continued psychosocial and psychopharmacological interventions, which can then be followed by continued support and management that progressively (if/when possible) becomes more hands-off over time [82]. To do so, community forensic mental health support centers such as Centerpoint in Edmonton, Canada [145], or the use of an informed and relatable mentor [112] could be employed to support the individual with FASD as they navigate reintegrating into society after incarceration. In addition, peer monitoring may be used to help support those with FASD reintegrate in the community [60].

Theme 6: Adopting an International Response to FASD in the Justice System This is an evolving field. We are at our best when we work and learn together. Throughout this chapter, there were many instances which demonstrated that some regions are experiencing different levels of success in supporting FASD within their respective criminal justice systems than others. In other words, there are a variety of opportunities for us to learn from one another, and continued research initiatives, to identify better practices moving forward. For example, the difficulties with awareness and training that exist in Australia [76] and South Africa [78] could be supported by having initiatives such as the Commonwealth FASD Strategy that is currently in place in Australia [125], or adopting some of the training strategies, such as those offered through CanFASD [140], that promote awareness and prevention in Canada. It should also be noted that, across regions, there are also practices that are being offered in youth justice systems (e.g., focus on rehabilitation, supports during interrogation, incarceration, and reintegration) [83] that could be adopted and utilized in the adult justice system. Taken together, it is recommended that we work together and learn from one another, on an international level, to adopt and modify our current practices to help support and accommodate those with FASD, who are most vulnerable in our present justice systems.

Concluding Remarks

When we alter our understanding and response, through education, appreciate the transactional complexity of FASD, operate from a shared understanding, and work together we position ourselves to transform the justice system to support individuals with FASD. As discussed throughout this chapter, living with FASD is often accompanied by a complex and dynamic set of biological, environmental, and system level factors that interact in unique ways to produce a particularly salient vulnerability for engaging in offending behavior among those with FASD. By adopting an FASD lens and implementing some of the recommendations discussed in this chapter, the hope is to provide an opportunity for police officers, lawyers, judges, doctors, and other forensic mental health professionals to learn about FASD and utilize an informed perspective to promote support, growth, and change among those with FASD who intersect with the justice system. Although the justice system is often viewed as a "destination" or the "end of the line," particularly among those with FASD, it does not have to be. Therefore, we leave readers with the reminder that the onus should **not** be on the individual struggling to navigate their vulnerabilities and behaviors in the justice system. The onus is on us as professionals to adopt an informed FASD lens and to focus on justice as an opportunity for rehabilitation and growth.

References

1. McLachlan K, Roesch R, Viljoen JL, Douglas KS. Evaluating the psycholegal abilities of young offenders with fetal alcohol spectrum disorder. Law Hum Behav. 2014;38(1):10–22. https://doi.org/10.1037/lhb0000037.
2. Pei J, Leung WS, Jampolsky F, Alsbury B. Experiences in the Canadian criminal justice system for individuals with fetal alcohol spectrum disorders: double jeopardy? Can J Criminol Crim Justice. 2016;58(1):56–86. https://doi.org/10.3138/cjccj.2014.E25.
3. Roach K, Bailey A. The relevance of fetal alcohol spectrum disorder in Canadian criminal law from investigation to sentencing. UBCL Rev. 2009;42(1):1–68.
4. Streissguth A, Barr H, Kogan J, Bookstein F. Primary and secondary disabilities in fetal alcohol syndrome. The challenge of fetal alcohol syndrome: overcoming secondary disabilities. In: Streissguth AP, Kanter J, editors. The challenge of fetal alcohol syndrome: overcoming secondary disabilities. Seattle: University of Washington Press; 1997. p. 25–39.
5. Bronfenbrenner U. Toward an experimental ecological framework. Am Psychol. 1977;32(7):513–31. https://doi.org/10.1037/0003-066X.32.7.513.
6. Sameroff AJ. The transactional model. In: Sameroff A, editor. The transactional model of development: how children and contexts shape each other. Washington, DC: American Psychological Association; 2009. p. 3–21.

7. Sameroff AJ. Ecological perspectives on developmental risk. In: Osofsky JD, editor. WAIMH handbook of infant mental health, vol. 4. New York: Wiley; 2000. p. 1–33.

8. Beaver KM, Boutwell BB, Barnes JC, Cooper JA. The biosocial underpinnings to adolescent victimization: results from a longitudinal sample of twins. Youth Violence Juvenile Justice. 2009;7(3):223–38.

9. Beaver KM, DeLisi M, Wright JP, Vaughn MG. Gene—environment interplay and delinquent involvement: evidence of direct, indirect, and interactive effects. J Adolesc Res. 2009;24(2):147–68.

10. Bergvall ÅH, Wessely H, Forsman A, Hansen S. A deficit in attentional set-shifting of violent offenders. Psychol Med. 2001;31(6):1095–105. https://doi.org/10.1017/S0033291701004317.

11. Brower MC, Price BH. Neuropsychiatry of frontal lobe dysfunction in violent and criminal behaviour: a critical review. J Neurol Neurosurg Psychiatry. 2001;71(6):720–6. https://doi.org/10.1136/jnnp.71.6.720.

12. Giancola PR, Zeichner A. Neuropsychological performance on tests of frontal-lobe functioning and aggressive behavior in men. J Abnorm Psychol. 1994;103(4):832–5.

13. Séguin JR, Arseneault L, Tremblay RE. The development of self-regulation: toward the integration of cognition and emotion. Cogn Dev. 2007;22:401–5.

14. Beaudry G, Yu R, Långström N, Fazel S. An updated systematic review and meta-regression analysis: mental disorders among adolescents in juvenile detention and correctional facilities. J Am Acad Child Adolesc Psychiatry. 2021;60(1):46–60. https://doi.org/10.1016/j.jaac.2020.01.015.

15. Fazel S, Seewald K. Severe mental illness in 33,588 prisoners worldwide: systematic review and meta-regression analysis. Br J Psychiatry. 2012;200(5):364–73. https://doi.org/10.1192/bjp.bp.111.096370.

16. Fazel S, Hayes AJ, Bartellas K, Clerici M, Trestman R. Mental health of prisoners: prevalence, adverse outcomes, and interventions. Lancet Psychiatry. 2016;3(9):871–81. https://doi.org/10.1016/S2215-0366(16)30142-0.

17. Hammersley R. Pathways through drugs and crime: desistance, trauma and resilience. J Crim Just. 2011;39(3):268–72. https://doi.org/10.1016/j.jcrimjus.2011.02.006.

18. Baglivio MT, Wolff KT, DeLisi M, Jackowski K. The role of adverse childhood experiences (ACEs) and psychopathic features on juvenile offending criminal careers to age 18. Youth Violence Juvenile Justice. 2020;18(4):337–64. https://doi.org/10.1177/1541204020927075.

19. Garbarino J. ACEs in the criminal justice system. Acad Pediatr. 2017;17(7):32–3. https://doi.org/10.1016/j.acap.2016.09.003.

20. Taillieu TL, Davila IG, Struck S. ACEs and violence in adulthood. Adverse Childhood Exp. 2020;1:119–42. https://doi.org/10.1016/B978-0-12-816065-7.00007-0.

21. Wong SK. Reciprocal effects of family disruption and crime: a panel study of Canadian municipalities. West Criminol Rev. 2011;12(1):43–63.

22. Leo C, Goff C. Inner city decay, poverty, social isolation and crime: a research design. In: Proceedings of the annual meeting of the American Sociological Association. San Francisco: American Sociological Association; 1998. p. 1–19. https://files.eric.ed.gov/fulltext/ED425259.pdf.

23. Andrews DA, Dowden C. The risk–need–responsivity model of assessment and human service in prevention and corrections: crime-prevention jurisprudence. Can J Criminol Crim Justice. 2007;49(4):439–64. https://doi.org/10.3138/cjccj.49.4.439.

24. Andrews DA, Bonta J, Wormith JS. The recent past and near future of risk and/or need assessment. Crime Delinq. 2006;52(1):7–27. https://doi.org/10.1177/0011128705281756.

25. Mahoney JL. School extracurricular activity participation as a moderator in the development of antisocial patterns. Child Dev. 2000;71(2):502–16. https://doi.org/10.1111/1467-8624.00160.

26. Duke NN. Adolescent adversity, school attendance and academic achievement: school connection and the potential for mitigating risk. J Sch Health. 2020;90(8):618–29. https://doi.org/10.1111/josh.12910.

27. Savage J, Ferguson CJ, Flores L. The effect of academic achievement on aggression and violent behavior: a meta-analysis. Aggress Violent Behav. 2017;37:91–101. https://doi.org/10.1016/j.avb.2017.08.002.
28. Farmer M. The importance of strengthening female offenders' family and other relationships to prevent reoffending and reduce intergenerational crime. London: Ministry of Justice; 2019. https://assets.publishing.service.gov.uk/government/uploads/system/uploads/attachment_data/file/642244/farmer-review-report.pdf
29. Burns L, Breen C, Bower C, O'Leary C, Elliott EJ. Counting fetal alcohol spectrum disorder in Australia: the evidence and the challenges. Drug Alcohol Rev. 2013;32(5):461–7. https://doi.org/10.1111/dar.12047.
30. Bower C, Watkins RE, Mutch RC, Marriott R, Freeman J, Kippin NR, et al. Fetal alcohol spectrum disorder and youth justice: a prevalence study among young people sentenced to detention in Western Australia. BMJ Open. 2018;8(2):e019605.
31. McLachlan K, McNeil A, Pei J, Brain U, Andrew G, Oberlander TF. Prevalence and characteristics of adults with fetal alcohol spectrum disorder in corrections: a Canadian case ascertainment study. BMC Public Health. 2019;19(43):1–10. https://doi.org/10.1186/s12889-018-6292-x.
32. Bagley K. Responding to FASD: what social and community service professionals do in the absence of diagnostic services and practice standards. Adv Dual Diagn. 2019;12(1/2):14–6. https://doi.org/10.1177/1541204020927075.
33. Popova S, Lange S, Shield K, Burd L, Rehm J. Prevalence of fetal alcohol spectrum disorder among special subpopulations: a systematic review and meta-analysis. Addiction. 2019;114(7):1150–72. https://doi.org/10.1111/add.14598.
34. McLachlan K, Gray AL, Roesch R, Douglas KS, Viljoen JL. Lutheation of the predictive validity of the SAVRY and YLS/CMI in justice-involved youth with fetal alcohol spectrum disorder. Psychol Assess. 2018;30(12):1640–51.
35. McLachlan K, Flannigan K, Temple V, Unsworth K, Cook JL. Difficulties in daily living experienced by adolescents, transition-aged youth, and adults with fetal alcohol spectrum disorder. Alcohol Clin Exp Res. 2020;44(8):1609–24. https://doi.org/10.1037/pas0000612.
36. Streissguth AP, Barr HM, Kogan J, Bookstein FL. Final report: understanding the occurrence of secondary disabilities in clients with fetal alcohol syndrome (FAS) and fetal alcohol effects (FAE). Washington, DC: University of Washington Publication Services; 1996.
37. May PA, Blankenship J, Marais AS, Gossage JP, Kalberg WO, Barnard R, De Vries M, Robinson LK, Adnams CM, Buckley D, Manning M. Approaching the prevalence of the full spectrum of fetal alcohol spectrum disorders in a South African population-based study. Alcohol Clin Exp Res. 2013;37(5):818–30. https://doi.org/10.1111/acer.12033.
38. Santtila P, Alkiora P, Ekholm M, Niemi P. False confession to robbery: the roles of suggestibility, anxiety, memory disturbance and withdrawal symptoms. J Forensic Psychiatry. 1999;10(2):399–415. https://doi.org/10.1080/09585189908403692.
39. Holland L, Reid N, Smirnov A. Neurodevelopmental disorders in youth justice: a systematic review of screening, assessment and interventions. J Exp Criminol. 2021;21:1–40. https://doi.org/10.1007/s11292-021-09475-w.
40. Bonta J, Andrews DA. Risk-need-responsivity model for offender assessment and rehabilitation. Rehabilitation. 2007;6(1):1–22.
41. Pei J, Burke A. Risk, needs, responsivity: rethinking FASD in the criminal justice system. In: Jonsson E, Clarren S, Binnie I, editors. Ethical and legal perspectives in fetal alcohol spectrum disorders (FASD). New York: Springer; 2018. p. 269–85. https://doi.org/10.1007/978-3-319-71755-5_16.
42. McLachlan K, Amlung M, Vedelago L, Chaimowitz G. Screening for fetal alcohol spectrum disorder in forensic mental health settings. J Forensic Psychiatry Psychol. 2020;31(5):643–66. https://doi.org/10.1080/14789949.2020.1781919.
43. Fast DK, Conry J. Fetal alcohol spectrum disorders and the criminal justice system. Dev Disabil Res Rev. 2009;15(3):250–7. https://doi.org/10.1002/ddrr.66.

44. Mattson SN, Bernes GA, Doyle LR. Fetal alcohol spectrum disorders: a review of the neurobehavioral deficits associated with prenatal alcohol exposure. Alcohol Clin Exp Res. 2019;43(6):1046–62. https://doi.org/10.1111/acer.14040.

45. Pedruzzi RA, Hamilton O, Hodgson HH, Connor E, Johnson E, Fitzpatrick J. Navigating complexity to support justice-involved youth with FASD and other neurodevelopmental disabilities: needs and challenges of a regional workforce. Health Justice. 2021;9(1):1–2. https://doi.org/10.1186/s40352-021-00132-y.

46. Mela M, Flannigan K, Anderson T, Nelson M, Krishnan S, Chizea C, et al. Neurocognitive function and fetal alcohol spectrum disorder in offenders with mental disorders. J Am Acad Psychiatry Law. 2020;48(2):195–208. https://doi.org/10.29158/JAAPL.003886-20.

47. Gupta KK, Gupta VK, Shirasaka T. An update on fetal alcohol syndrome—pathogenesis, risks, and treatment. Alcohol Clin Exp Res. 2016;40(8):1594–602. https://doi.org/10.1111/acer.13135.

48. Lange S, Rehm J, Anagnostou E, Popova S. Prevalence of externalizing disorders and autism spectrum disorders among children with fetal alcohol spectrum disorder: systematic review and meta-analysis. Biochem Cell Biol. 2018;96(2):241–51. https://doi.org/10.1139/bcb-2017-0014.

49. Hagerman RJ. Psychopharmacological interventions in fragile X syndrome, fetal alcohol syndrome, Prader–Willi syndrome, Angelman syndrome, Smith–Magenis syndrome, and Velocardiofacial syndrome. Ment Retard Dev Disabil Res Rev. 1999;5(4):305–13. https://doi.org/10.1002/(SICI)1098-2779(1999)5:4<305::AID-MRDD8>3.0.CO;2-L.

50. Donald KA, Fouche JP, Roos A, Koen N, Howells FM, Riley EP, et al. Alcohol exposure in utero is associated with decreased gray matter volume in neonates. Metab Brain Dis. 2016;31(1):81–91. https://doi.org/10.1007/s11011-015-9771-0.

51. Roussotte FF, Sulik KK, Mattson SN, Riley EP, Jones KL, Adnams CM, et al. Regional brain volume reductions relate to facial dysmorphology and neurocognitive function in fetal alcohol spectrum disorders. Hum Brain Mapp. 2012;33(4):920–37.

52. Nardelli A, Lebel C, Rasmussen C, Andrew G, Beaulieu C. Extensive deep gray matter volume reductions in children and adolescents with fetal alcohol spectrum disorders. Alcohol Clin Exp Res. 2011;35(8):1404–17. https://doi.org/10.1111/j.1530-0277.2011.01476.x.

53. Kully-Martens K, Denys K, Treit S, Tamana S, Rasmussen C. A review of social skills deficits in individuals with fetal alcohol spectrum disorders and prenatal alcohol exposure: profiles, mechanisms, and interventions. Alcohol Clin Exp Res. 2012;36(4):568–76. https://doi.org/10.1111/j.1530-0277.2011.01661.x.

54. Runions KC, Keating DP. Anger and inhibitory control as moderators of children's hostile attributions and aggression. J Appl Dev Psychol. 2010;31(5):370–8. https://doi.org/10.1016/j.appdev.2010.05.006.

55. Schonfeld AM, Paley B, Frankel F, O'Connor MJ. Executive functioning predicts social skills following prenatal alcohol exposure. Child Neuropsychol. 2006;12(6):439–52. https://doi.org/10.1080/09297040600611338.

56. Rasmussen C, Bisanz J. Executive functioning in children with fetal alcohol spectrum disorders: profiles and age-related differences. Child Neuropsychol. 2009;15(3):201–15. https://doi.org/10.1080/09297040802385400.

57. Kully-Martens K, Pei J, Job J, Rasmussen C. Source monitoring in children with and without fetal alcohol spectrum disorders. J Pediatr Psychol. 2012;37(7):725–35. https://doi.org/10.1093/jpepsy/jsr123.

58. Pei J, Job J, Kully-Martens K, Rasmussen C. Executive function and memory in children with fetal alcohol spectrum disorder. Child Neuropsychol. 2011;17(3):290–309. https://doi.org/10.1080/09297049.2010.544650.

59. Mattson SN, Crocker N, Nguyen TT. Fetal alcohol spectrum disorders: neuropsychological and behavioral features. Neuropsychol Rev. 2011;21(2):81–101. https://doi.org/10.1007/s11065-011-9167-9.

60. Tait CL, Mela M, Boothman G, Stoops MA. The lived experience of paroled offenders with fetal alcohol spectrum disorder and comorbid psychiatric disorder. Transcult Psychiatry. 2017;54(1):107–24. https://doi.org/10.1177/1363461516689216.
61. Woltering S, Lishak V, Hodgson N, Granic I, Zelazo PD. Executive function in children with externalizing and comorbid internalizing behavior problems. J Child Psychol Psychiatry. 2016;57(1):30–8. https://doi.org/10.1111/jcpp.12428.
62. Saylor KE, Amann BH. Impulsive aggression as a comorbidity of attention-deficit/hyperactivity disorder in children and adolescents. J Child Adolesc Psychopharmacol. 2016;26(1):19–25. https://doi.org/10.1089/cap.2015.0126.
63. Pei J, Denys K, Hughes J, Rasmussen C. Mental health issues in fetal alcohol spectrum disorder. J Ment Health. 2011;20(5):473–83. https://doi.org/10.3109/09638237.2011.577113.
64. Weyrauch D, Schwartz M, Hart B, Klug MG, Burd L. Comorbid mental disorders in fetal alcohol spectrum disorders: a systematic review. J Dev Behav Pediatr. 2017;38(4):283–91. https://doi.org/10.1097/DBP.0000000000000440.
65. Himmelreich M, Lutke CJ, Hargrove ET. The lay of the land: fetal alcohol spectrum disorder (FASD) as a whole-body diagnosis. In: Begun AL, Murray MM, editors. The Routledge handbook of social work and addictive behaviors. 1st ed. London: Routledge; 2020. p. 191–215.
66. Reid N, Kippin N, Passmore H, Finlay-Jones A. Fetal alcohol spectrum disorder: the importance of assessment, diagnosis and support in the Australian justice context. Psychiatry Psychol Law. 2020;27(2):265–74. https://doi.org/10.1080/13218719.2020.1719375.
67. Dixon DR, Kurtz PF, Chin MD. A systematic review of challenging behaviors in children exposed prenatally to substances of abuse. Res Dev Disabil. 2008;29(6):483–502. https://doi.org/10.1016/j.ridd.2007.05.006.
68. Wyper K, Pei J. Neurocognitive difficulties underlying high risk and criminal behaviour in FASD: clinical implications. In: Nelson M, Trussler M, editors. Fetal alcohol spectrum disorders in adults: ethical and legal perspectives. Cham: Springer; 2016. p. 101–20.
69. Olson HC, Oti R, Gelo J, Beck S. "Family matters": fetal alcohol spectrum disorders and the family. Dev Disabil Res Rev. 2009;15(3):235–49. https://doi.org/10.1002/ddrr.65.
70. Flannigan K, Kapasi A, Pei J, Murdoch I, Andrew G, Rasmussen C. Characterizing adverse childhood experiences among children and adolescents with prenatal alcohol exposure and fetal alcohol spectrum disorder. Child Abuse Negl. 2021;112:104888. https://doi.org/10.1016/j.chiabu.2020.104888.
71. Kambeitz C, Klug MG, Greenmyer J, Popova S, Burd L. Association of adverse childhood experiences and neurodevelopmental disorders in people with fetal alcohol spectrum disorders (FASD) and non-FASD controls. BMC Pediatr. 2019;19(1):1–9. https://doi.org/10.1186/s12887-019-1878-8.
72. Tan GK, Symons M, Fitzpatrick J, Connor SG, Cross D, Pestell C. Adverse childhood experiences, associated stressors and comorbidities in children and youth with fetal alcohol spectrum disorder across the child protection. Res Square. 2021;2021:738216. https://doi.org/10.21203/rs.3.rs-738216/v1.
73. Day A, Ward T, Shirley L. Reintegration services for long-term dangerous offenders: a case study and discussion. J Offender Rehabil. 2011;50(2):66–80. https://doi.org/10.1080/10509674.2011.546225.
74. Boland FJ. Fetal alcohol syndrome: implications for correctional service. Washington, DC: U.S. Department of Justice; 1998. p. 96.
75. Baumbach J. Some implications of prenatal alcohol exposure for the treatment of adolescents with sexual offending behaviors. Sex Abuse J Res Treat. 2002;14(4):313–27. https://doi.org/10.1023/A:1019969503528.
76. Fitzpatrick JP, Pestell CF. Neuropsychological aspects of prevention and intervention for fetal alcohol spectrum disorders in Australia. J Pediatr Neuropsychol. 2017;3(1):38–52. https://doi.org/10.1007/s40817-016-0018-8.

77. Bagley K. Responding to FASD: what social and community service professionals do in the absence of diagnostic services and practice standards. Adv Dual Diagn. 2018;12(1/2):14–26. https://doi.org/10.1177/1541204020927075.

78. Olivier L, Curfs LM, Viljoen DL. Fetal alcohol spectrum disorders: prevalence rates in South Africa. S Afr Med J. 2016;106(6):103–6.

79. Choate P, Badry D. Stigma as a dominant discourse in fetal alcohol spectrum disorder. Adv Dual Diagn. 2019;12(1/2):36–52. https://doi.org/10.1108/ADD-05-2018-0005.

80. Aspler J, Zizzo N, Bell E, Di Pietro N, Racine E. Stigmatisation, exaggeration, and contradiction: an analysis of scientific and clinical content in Canadian print media discourse about fetal alcohol spectrum disorder. Can J Bioethics/Revue canadienne de bioéthique. 2019;2(2):23–35. https://doi.org/10.7202/1058140ar.

81. McLachlan K, Mullally K, Ritter C, Mela M, Pei J. Fetal alcohol spectrum disorder and neurodevelopmental disorders: an international practice survey of forensic mental health clinicians. Int J Forensic Ment Health. 2021;20(2):177–97. https://doi.org/10.1080/14999013.2020.1852342.

82. Mela M. Medico-legal interventions in management of offenders with fetal alcohol spectrum disorders (FASD). In: Nelson M, Trussler M, editors. Fetal alcohol spectrum disorders in adults: ethical and legal perspectives. Cham: Springer; 2016. p. 121–38.

83. McLachlan K, Rasmussen C. Understanding the neurobehavioral deficits and psycholegal capacities of individuals with FASD in the criminal justice system. In: Nelson M, Trussler M, editors. Fetal alcohol spectrum disorders in adults: ethical and legal perspectives, vol. 2016. Cham: Springer; 2018. p. 145–61.

84. Eastwood J, Snook B, Luther K. Measuring the reading complexity and oral comprehension of Canadian youth waiver forms. Crime Delinq. 2015;61(6):798–828. https://doi.org/10.1177/0011128712453689.

85. Brown NN, Gudjonsson G, Connor P. Suggestibility and fetal alcohol spectrum disorders: I'll tell you anything you want to hear. J Psychiatry Law. 2011;39(1):39–71. https://doi.org/10.1177/009318531103900103.

86. Streissguth A, Bookstein F, Barr H, Sampson P, OMalley K, Young J. Risk factors for adverse life outcomes in fetal alcohol syndrome and fetal alcohol effects. J Dev Behav Pediatr. 2004;25(4):228–38.

87. Appelbaum KL, Appelbaum PS. Criminal-justice-related competencies in defendants with mental retardation. J Psychiatry Law. 1994;22(4):483–503. https://doi.org/10.1177/009318539402200402.

88. Drizin SA, Leo RA. The problem of false confessions in the post-DNA world. N C Law Rev. 2003;82:891–1007.

89. Inbau FE, Reid JE, Buckley JP, Jayne BC. Essentials of the Reid technique: criminal interrogation and confessions. 2nd ed. Massachusetts: Jones & Bartlett Publishers; 2013. p. 216.

90. Leo RA. Police interrogation and American justice. Cambridge: Harvard University Press; 2009. p. 384.

91. Drake KE, Gonzalez RA, Sigurdsson JF, Sigfusdottir ID, Gudjonsson GH. A national study into temperament as a critical susceptibility factor for reported false confessions amongst adolescents. Pers Individ Differ. 2017;111(1):220–6. https://doi.org/10.1016/j.paid.2017.02.022.

92. Redlich AD, Summers A, Hoover S. Self-reported false confessions and false guilty pleas among offenders with mental illness. Law Hum Behav. 2010;34(1):79–90. https://doi.org/10.1007/s10979-009-9194-8.

93. Peterson-Badali M, Abramovitch R. Children's knowledge of the legal system: are they competent to instruct legal counsel? Can J Criminol. 1992;34(2):139–60. https://doi.org/10.3138/cjcrim.34.2.139.

94. Cauffman E, Sternberg L. Immaturity of judgment in adolescence: why adolescents may be less culpable than adults. In: Grisso T, Schwartz RG, editors. Youth on trial: a developmental perspective on juvenile justice. Illinois: University of Chicago Press; 2000. p. 325–43. https://doi.org/10.1002/bsl.416.

95. Brown JM, Haun J, Zapf PA, Brown NN. Fetal alcohol spectrum disorders (FASD) and competency to stand trial (CST): suggestions for a 'best practices' approach to forensic evaluation. Int J Law Psychiatry. 2017;52:19–27. https://doi.org/10.1016/j.ijlp.2017.04.002.

96. Greenspan S, Driscoll JH. Why people with FASD fall for manipulative ploys: ethical limits of interrogators' use of lies. In: Nelson M, Tressler M, editors. Fetal alcohol spectrum disorders in adults: ethical and legal perspectives, vol. 2016. Cham: Springer; 2016. p. 23–38.

97. Cunningham KA. Advances in juvenile adjudicative competence: a 10-year update. Behav Sci Law. 2020;38(4):406–20. https://doi.org/10.1002/bsl.2478.

98. Ryba NL, Zapf PA. The influence of psychiatric symptoms and cognitive abilities on competence-related abilities. Int J Forensic Ment Health. 2011;10(1):29–40. https://doi.org/10.1080/14999013.2010.550982.

99. Pirelli G, Gottdiener WH, Zapf PA. A meta-analytic review of competency to stand trial research. Psychol Public Policy Law. 2011;17(1):1–53. https://doi.org/10.1037/a0021713.

100. Viljoen JL, Roesch R. Competence to waive interrogation rights and adjudicative competence in adolescent defendants: cognitive development, attorney contact, and psychological symptoms. Law Hum Behav. 2005;29(6):723–42. https://doi.org/10.1007/s10979-005-7978-y.

101. Wyper KR, Rasmussen CR. Language impairments in children with fetal alcohol spectrum disorder. J Popul Ther Clin Pharmacol. 2011;18(2):364–76.

102. Gagnier KR, Moore TE, Green JM. A need for closer examination of FASD by the criminal justice system: has the call been answered? J Popul Ther Clin Pharmacol. 2011;18(3):426–39.

103. Jirikowic T, Olson HC, Kartin D. Sensory processing, school performance, and adaptive behavior of young school-age children with fetal alcohol spectrum disorders. Phys Occup Ther Pediatr. 2008;28(2):117–36. https://doi.org/10.1080/01942630802031800.

104. Evans J, Bourgon N. Exploring the use of restorative justice practices with adult offenders with fetal alcohol spectrum disorder. Ottawa: Department of Justice Canada, Research and Statistics Division; 2020. p. 22.

105. Stafford KP, Sellbom MO. Assessment of competence to stand trial. In: Otto RK, editor. Forensic psychology. 2nd ed. New Jersey: Wiley; 2012. p. 412–39.

106. Mackay R, Brookbanks W. Fitness to plead: international and comparative perspectives. Oxford: Oxford University Press; 2018. p. 319.

107. Roesch R, Ogloff JR, Hart SD, Dempster RJ, Zapf PA, Whittemore KE. The impact of Canadian criminal code changes on remands and assessments of fitness to stand trial and criminal responsibility in British Columbia. Can J Psychiatry. 1997;42(5):509–14. https://doi.org/10.1177/070674379704200508.

108. Zapf PA, Roesch R. Future directions in the restoration of competency to stand trial. Curr Dir Psychol Sci. 2011;20(1):43–7. https://doi.org/10.1177/0963721410396798.

109. Mela M, Okpalauwaekwe U, Anderson T, Eng J, Nomani S, Ahmed A, et al. The utility of psychotropic drugs on patients with fetal alcohol spectrum disorder (FASD): a systematic review. Psychiatry Clin Psychopharmacol. 2018;28(4):436–45. https://doi.org/10.1080/24750573.2018.1458429.

110. Wettstein RM, Mulvey EP, Rogers R. A prospective comparison of four insanity defense standards. Am J Psychiatry. 1991;148(1):21–7. https://doi.org/10.1176/ajp.148.1.21.

111. Berger O, McNiel DE, Binder RL. PTSD as a criminal defense: a review of case law. J Am Acad Psychiatry Law Online. 2012;40(4):509–21.

112. Scott R. Fetal alcohol syndrome disorder: diminished responsibility and mitigation of sentence. Australas Psychiatry. 2018;26(1):20–3. https://doi.org/10.1177/1039856217716289.

113. Mela M, Luther G. Fetal alcohol spectrum disorder: can diminished responsibility diminish criminal behaviour? Int J Law Psychiatry. 2013;36(1):46–54. https://doi.org/10.1016/j.ijlp.2012.11.007.

114. Jampolsky F. Introduction; FASD and the revolving door of criminal justice. In: Jonsson E, Clarren S, Binnie I, editors. Ethical and legal perspectives in fetal alcohol spectrum disorders (FASD). Springer: Cham; 2018. p. 187–200.

115. Public Health Agency of Canada. Fetal alcohol spectrum disorder: a framework for action. Ottawa: Public Health Agency of Canada; 2005. p. 25.
116. Mela M. Prenatal alcohol exposure: a clinician's guide. Washington, DC: American Psychiatric Association Publishing; 2021. p. 472.
117. Luther G, Mela M. The top ten issues in law and psychiatry. Saskatchewan Law Rev. 2006;69(2):401–26.
118. Gatti U, Tremblay RE, Vitaro F. Iatrogenic effect of juvenile justice. J Child Psychol Psychiatry. 2009;50(8):991–8. https://doi.org/10.1111/j.1469-7610.2008.02057.x.
119. Fast D, Conry J. The challenge of fetal alcohol syndrome in the criminal legal system. Addict Biol. 2004;9(2):161–6. https://doi.org/10.1080/13556210410001717042.
120. MacPherson PH, Chudley AE, Grant BA. Fetal alcohol spectrum disorder (FASD) in a correctional population: prevalence, screening and diagnosis. Ottawa: Correctional Service Canada; 2011.
121. Brown J, Long-McGie J, Wartnik A, Oberoi P, Wresh J, Weinkauf E, Falconer G, Kerr A. Fetal alcohol spectrum disorders in the criminal justice system: a review. J Law Enforcement. 2014;3(6):1–10.
122. Ward T, Melser J, Yates PM. Reconstructing the risk–need–responsivity model: a theoretical elaboration and evaluation. Aggress Violent Behav. 2007;12(2):208–28. https://doi.org/10.1016/j.avb.2006.07.001.
123. Russell NK, Yee Tan K, Pestell CF, Connor S, Fitzpatrick JP. Therapeutic recommendations in the youth justice system cohort diagnosed with foetal alcohol spectrum disorder. Youth Justice. 2021;23:e14732254211036195.
124. Lowenkamp CT, Latessa EJ. Evaluation of Ohio's community based correctional facilities and halfway house programs. Ohio: University of Cincinnati; 2002. p. 315.
125. Reid N. Fetal alcohol spectrum disorder in Australia: what is the current state of affairs? Drug Alcohol Rev. 2018;37(7):827–30. https://doi.org/10.1111/dar.12855.
126. Ogilvie JM, Stewart AL, Chan RC, Shum DH. Neuropsychological measures of executive function and antisocial behavior: a meta-analysis. Criminology. 2011;49(4):1063–107. https://doi.org/10.1111/j.1745-9125.2011.00252.x.
127. Passmore HM, Giglia R, Watkins RE, Mutch RC, Marriott R, Pestell C, et al. Study protocol for screening and diagnosis of fetal alcohol spectrum disorders (FASD) among young people sentenced to detention in Western Australia. BMJ Open. 2016;6(6):e012184. https://doi.org/10.1136/bmjopen-2016-012184.
128. Mitten R. Fetal alcohol spectrum disorders and the justice system. Saskatchewan: Commission on First Nations and Metis Peoples and Justice Reform; 2004. p. 38. http://www.justicereformcomm.sk.calvolume2/12section9.pdf
129. Bibr C. Knowledge of Northern Ontario School of Medicine students on the subject of fetal alcohol spectrum disorder. Sudbury: Laurentian University; 2019. p. 136. https://zone.biblio.laurentian.ca/handle/10219/3173
130. Luther G, Mela M, Bae V. Literature review on therapeutic justice and problem solving courts. Saskatoon: University of Saskatchewan Faculty of Law; 2013. p. 24. https://cfbsjs.usask.ca/documents/Lit%20Review%20MHC%20Saskatoon%20Academic%20Dec%202013.pdf
131. Stewart M, Glowatski K. Front-line police perceptions of fetal alcohol spectrum disorder in a Canadian province. Police J. 2014;87(1):17–27. https://doi.org/10.1350/pojo.2014.87.1.648.
132. Brown NN, Wartnik AP, Connor PD, Adler RS. A proposed model standard for forensic assessment of fetal alcohol spectrum disorders. J Psychiatry Law. 2010;38(4):383–418. https://doi.org/10.1177/009318531003800403.
133. Passmore HM, Mutch RC, Watkins R, Burns S, Hall G, Urquhart J, et al. Reframe the behaviour: evaluation of a training intervention to increase capacity in managing detained youth with fetal alcohol spectrum disorder and neurodevelopmental impairments. Psychiatry Psychol Law. 2020;28(3):382–407. https://doi.org/10.1080/13218719.2020.1780643.
134. Passmore HM, Mutch RC, Burns S, Watkins R, Carapetis J, Hall G, Bower C. Fetal alcohol spectrum disorder (FASD): knowledge, attitudes, experiences and practices of the Western

Australian youth custodial workforce. Int J Law Psychiatry. 2018;59:44–52. https://doi.org/10.1016/j.ijlp.2018.05.008.
135. Flannigan K, Hardy K, Reid D. Strengths among individuals with FASD. Family Advisory Committee; 2018. https://canfasd.ca/wp-content/uploads/2018/10/Strengths-Among-Individuals-with-FASD.pdf. Accessed 4 Feb 2022.
136. Pei J, Kapasi A, Kennedy KE, Joly V. Towards healthy outcomes for individuals with fetal alcohol spectrum disorder. The Canada FASD research network in collaboration with the University of Alberta. Vancouver: University of Alberta; 2019. https://canfasd.ca/wp-content/uploads/2019/11/Final-Towards-Healthy-Outcomes-Document-with-links.pdf
137. Coggins TE, Timler GR, Olswang LB. A state of double jeopardy: impact of prenatal alcohol exposure and adverse environments on the social communicative abilities of school-age children with fetal alcohol spectrum disorder. Lang Speech Hear Serv Sch. 2007;38(2):117–27. https://doi.org/10.1044/0161-1461(2007/012.
138. Mutch RC, Jones HM, Bower C, Watkins RE. Fetal alcohol spectrum disorders: using knowledge, attitudes and practice of justice professionals to support their educational needs. J Popul Ther Clin Pharmacol. 2016;23(1):77–89.
139. NoFASD. Fetal alcohol spectrum disorder: FASD guidebook for police officers. Ottawa (ON): Royal Canadian Mounted Police; 2018. 36 p. https://www.nofasd.org.au/wp-content/uploads/2018/05/Foetal_alcohol_syndrome_guide_for_police_Canada_2005.pdf. Accessed 19 Sept 2021.
140. Canada FASD Research Network. Vancouver (BC):CanFASD; 2021. https://canfasd.ca/online-learners/. Accessed 19 Sept 2021.
141. Malbin DV. Fetal alcohol spectrum disorder (FASD) and the role of family court judges in improving outcomes for children and families. Juv Fam Court J. 2004;55(2):53–63. https://doi.org/10.1111/j.1755-6988.2004.tb00161.x.
142. Department of Justice. The FASD youth justice pilot project. Ottawa: Government of Canada; 2021. https://www.justice.gc.ca/eng/fund-fina/cj-jp/yj-jj/sum-som/r4.html
143. FASD United. FASD united policy and training center: changing the landscape on prenatal substance exposure. Washington, DC: FASD United; 2021. https://nofaspolicycenter.org
144. Kable JA, Mukherjee RA. Neurodevelopmental disorder associated with prenatal exposure to alcohol (ND-PAE): a proposed diagnostic method of capturing the neurocognitive phenotype of FASD. Eur J Med Genet. 2017;60(1):49–54. https://doi.org/10.1016/j.ejmg.2016.09.013.
145. Centerpoint. Alberta: Justice Resource Institute; 2021. https://jri.org/services/acute-care-and-juvenile-justice/irtp/centerpoint. Accessed 19 Sept 2021.
146. Milne B, Bull R. Investigative interviewing: psychology and practice. Chichester: Wiley; 1999. p. 223.
147. Flannigan K, Pei J, Rasmussen C, Potts S, O'Riordan T. A unique response to offenders with fetal alcohol spectrum disorder: perceptions of the Alexis FASD Justice Program. Can J Criminol Crim Justice. 2018;60(1):1–33. https://doi.org/10.3138/cjccj.2016-0021.r2.
148. Heilbrun K, Giallella C, Wright HJ, DeMatteo D, Griffin PA, Locklair B, et al. Treatment for restoration of competence to stand trial: critical analysis and policy recommendations. Psychol Public Policy Law. 2019;25(4):266–83. https://doi.org/10.1037/law0000210.
149. Chartrand LN, Forbes-Chilibeck EM. The sentencing of offenders with fetal alcohol syndrome. Health Law J. 2003;11:35–70.
150. Stewart LA, Wilton G, Sapers J. Offenders with cognitive deficits in a Canadian prison population: prevalence, profile, and outcomes. Int J Law Psychiatry. 2016;44:7–14. https://doi.org/10.1016/j.ijlp.2015.08.026.
151. Blagg H, Tulich T, May S. Aboriginal youth with foetal alcohol spectrum disorder and enmeshment in the Australian justice system: can an intercultural form of restorative justice make a difference? Contemp Justice Rev. 2019;22(2):105–21. https://doi.org/10.1080/10282580.2019.1612246.
152. Brown N, Connor PD, Adler RS. Conduct-disordered adolescents with fetal alcohol spectrum disorder: intervention in secure treatment settings. Crim Justice Behav. 2012;39(6):770–93. https://doi.org/10.1177/0093854812437919.

Index

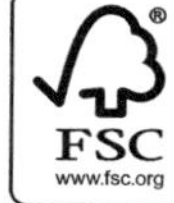